Principles of Healthcare Reimbursement

Fifth Edition

Anne B. Casto, RHIA, CCS

and

Elizabeth Forrestal, PhD, RHIA, CCS, FAHIMA

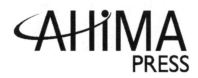

ISBN: 978-1-58426-434-7
AHIMA Product No.: AB202014

AHIMA Staff:
Caitlin Wilson, Assistant Editor
Jason O. Malley, Vice President, Business and Innovation
Ashley R. Latta, Production Development Editor
Pamela Woolf, Director of Publications

For more information, including updates, about AHIMA Press publications, visit http://www.ahima.org/publications/updates.aspx

American Health Information Management Association
233 North Michigan Avenue, 21st Floor
Chicago, Illinois 60601-5809
ahima.org

Contents

Detailed Contents

About the Authors

The Foundation of Research and Education (FORE) Triumph Awards are national awards designed to recognize special individuals who have made a difference in the health information management (HIM) field. Specifically, the Legacy Award honors significant contribution to the knowledge base of the HIM field through an insightful recent publication, building on the enduring tradition of the Edna K. Huffman Literary Award.

The 2007 recipients of the Legacy Award were Anne B. Casto, RHIA, CCS, and Elizabeth Forrestal, PhD, RHIA, CCS, FAHIMA, who authored this publication, *Principles of Healthcare Reimbursement*, Fifth Edition. This publication makes a complex topic understandable for students and practitioners and helps clarify the US healthcare reimbursement maze.

Anne B. Casto, RHIA, CCS, is president of Casto Consulting, LLC. Before founding the firm, Casto was program manager of the HIMS division at the Ohio State University School of Allied Medical Professions. Casto taught healthcare reimbursement, ICD-9-CM coding, and CPT coding courses for several years. Additionally, Casto was responsible for curriculum revisions in the areas of chargemaster management, clinical data management, and healthcare reimbursement.

Additionally, Casto was the vice president of Clinical Information for Cleverley & Associates, where she worked very closely with APC regulations and guidelines, preparing hospitals for the implementation of the new Medicare PPS. Casto was also the clinical information product manager for CHIPS/Ingenix. She joined CHIPS/Ingenix in 1998 and spent the majority of her time developing coding compliance products for the inpatient and outpatient settings.

Casto has been responsible for inpatient and outpatient coding activities in several large hospitals, including Mt. Sinai Medical Center (NYC), Beth Israel Medical Center (NYC), and The Ohio State University. She has worked extensively with CMI, quality measures, physician documentation, and coding accuracy efforts at these facilities.

Casto received her degree in health information management at The Ohio State University in 1995. She received her Certified Coding Specialist credential in 1998 from the American Health Information Management Association. Additionally, Casto received the ICD-10-CM/PCS trainer certificate in 2009 from the American Health Information Management Association. Casto received the 2008 OHIMA Distinguished Member Award and the 2011 Professional Achievement Award honoring her commitment, creativity, and leadership to the HIM profession.

Elizabeth Forrestal, PhD, RHIA, CCS, FAHIMA, is a professor in the Department of Health Services and Information Management at East Carolina University, Greenville, North Carolina.

She had previously worked at Hennepin County Medical Center and the University of Minnesota Hospitals, both in Minneapolis, Minnesota, from 1974 through 1990. Dr. Forrestal worked in several departments, such as third-party reimbursement, credit and collections, account auditing, outpatient registration, inpatient admissions, research studies, and quality management.

In 1990, Dr. Forrestal joined the faculty of the Georgia Regents University (formerly Medical College of Georgia) in Augusta, Georgia. While on the faculty, she also consulted for the Physicians' Practice Group. Dr. Forrestal successfully sat for the first CCS examination in 1992. In 2001, she was awarded the designation of Fellow of the American Health Information Management Association, one of the first two individuals in the country to receive this award. She was the first editor of *Perspectives in Health Information Management* and has delivered presentations at numerous AHIMA events.

Dr. Forrestal earned her baccalaureate degree from the University of Minnesota. While working, she returned to school to earn her associate's degree in medical record technology. She completed St. Scholastica's progression program to earn her post-baccalaureate certificate in health information administration. She earned her master's degree in organizational leadership from the College of St. Catherine's and her doctorate in higher education from Georgia State University.

Acknowledgments

AHIMA Press would like to thank Mary Juenemann, MS, RHIA, CCS for her review and feedback on this textbook.

Foreword

William O. Cleverley, PhD
Professor Emeritus, The Ohio State University

I have taught healthcare financial management to graduate students for 30 years and have always believed that the critical area of understanding was reimbursement. When I first started teaching, the primary—perhaps exclusive—focus was on hospitals, but that has changed. Financing and organizational patterns have shifted to create large healthcare firms in other sectors, such as medical groups, nursing facilities, imaging centers, surgery centers, home health firms, and many others. The primary focal point of difference between healthcare firms and businesses in other industries, however, is still payment. Healthcare firms are very unique in how they receive compensation for the services that they provide. When I started teaching, 30 years ago, I could not find any other industry that had as complex a revenue function as healthcare firms—nor can I today. In fact, the level of complexity for healthcare firms has increased exponentially over the last 30 years.

Noting that the revenue function, or reimbursement, is complex for a healthcare firm does not explain why this is critical. Let's examine the very basis of management in any business. Simply stated, management must control the difference between revenue and cost, which we call profit. It makes little difference whether the firm is taxable or tax-exempt. Viable businesses must manage the profit function. Although there are clearly differences in cost functions between healthcare firms and firms in other industrial sectors, the differences are not all that significant. Generic principles for cost management might apply equally in a software firm or a hospital. The revenue function is, however, a completely different manner.

Why is the revenue function so different for healthcare firms compared to other industries? I believe there are at least four reasons. First, the vast majority of payment is paid not by the client (patient), but rather by a third party on behalf of the patient. Second, the level of payment for a set of identical services may vary dramatically depending on the specific third-party payer. Third, the actual determination of payment for a specific third-party payer is often complex, based on preestablished or negotiated rules of payment frequently related to the codes entered upon a patient's bill or claim. Fourth, the government is often the largest single payer and does not negotiate payment, but simply defines the rules for payment pursuant to which it will render compensation for services provided to its beneficiaries.

To get a partial view of the complexity of reimbursement in the healthcare industry, let's describe a typical managed care contract with a hospital. Let's assume this payer pays for inpatient services on a per diem basis, with separate rates for medical and surgical cases. In addition, carve-outs are present for cardiology diagnosis-related groups (DRGs). Finally, obstetrics and nursery care services are paid on case rates. To provide some additional risk protection to the hospital, a stop-loss provision is also inserted after total charges exceed a certain limit. Outpatient services are paid on a mix of fee schedules and discounted billed charges. Outpatient surgical cases are paid on a fee schedule based on designated ambulatory surgical groups. Emergency visits are also on a fee schedule, based on level of service. Other fee schedules exist for specific imaging procedures, and everything else is paid on a discounted, billed-charge basis. Multiply this one payer by 100 to recognize other payers and throw in Medicare and Medicaid payment rules, and you have a nightmare in administration. It may be a nightmare, but it is very real to most healthcare firms; yet their very financial viability is contingent upon successful management of this complex revenue function.

Coding and billing issues are central to most of the present reimbursement plans. In fact, many healthcare firms can lose substantial sums of money because they are not coding their patients' claims in an accurate and complete manner. For example, failing to code an additional diagnosis can result in assignment of a lower DRG and thus lost revenue. Though some healthcare executives may fail to understand the importance of the coding function, it would behoove them to acquire an appreciation of coding, because much of their revenue function is related to what is done by coders. Conversely, many people in health information management may understand the technical side of what they do, but they don't appreciate their role in the overall financial success of the health firm in which they work.

This background explains why I am so excited about the publication of this book. Anne Casto and Elizabeth Forrestal have put together a much-needed text on reimbursement that fills a void. I believe that this text is a first. It provides a comprehensive review of the reimbursement world for healthcare firms of multiple types. It also provides very specific material on the actual completion of claims and the rules for final payment determination. Medicare payment provisions are covered in great detail, but the text also includes other payers. It covers payment provisions for hospitals, but it also covers payment for other payers, including managed care plans.

I believe this book is a must-read reference for healthcare executives who need a comprehensive reference on payment in the healthcare industry. It will be a fine supplement for healthcare management students who need to know how the firms they will manage will be paid and how coding and billing functions can affect results. It is also a critical text for health information managers and students. It is often easy to lose sight of the forest when you are engaged in tree cutting. This text provides a clear, concise description of the payment landscape for healthcare firms, which will enable health information managers to better integrate their functions into the overall organizational strategic position of the healthcare firms where they work. A large number of specific examples are also provided to help cement conceptual frameworks with operational reality. Another great feature of this text is its explanation of the myriad acronyms and jargon used in the healthcare industry. Short, concise definitions are given for everything from APCs to RBRVS.

This text met and exceeded the three Rs that I use in evaluation. First, the text is very readable and easy to understand. Second, the text is especially relevant to all healthcare managers as they seek to improve financial performance. Third, the text is rich in detail and practical illustrations. This book will occupy a prominent position on my bookshelf and will be a great reference.

William O. Cleverley, PhD
Professor Emeritus
The Ohio State University

Preface

Health information management (HIM) professionals play a critical role in the delivery of healthcare services in the United States. To be fully effective in their roles, however, HIM professionals need an in-depth understanding of healthcare reimbursement systems, reimbursement methodologies, and payment processes throughout the healthcare industry.

Principles of Healthcare Reimbursement integrates information about all US healthcare payment systems into one authoritative source. It examines the complex financial systems within today's healthcare environment and provides an understanding of the basics of health insurance and public funding programs, managed care contracting, and how services are paid. Not only does the text provide step-by-step detail about how each payment system functions, but the history behind each is provided. This gives the reader an appreciation for the complexity of reimbursement systems and an understanding of the profound effect they have had on providers and payers, consumers, public-sector policymakers, and the development of classification and information technology systems over the years.

Healthcare leaders and administrators often have to learn about healthcare payment systems on-the-job and on-the-fly. Other texts feature healthcare finance and healthcare economics, but not the bottom line and nitty-gritty of the healthcare payment systems themselves. This book fills that gap.

Chapter 1, Healthcare Reimbursement Methodologies, introduces and explains the basic concepts and principles of healthcare reimbursement in step-by-step, simple terms. This introduction provides the reader with the solid foundation needed to understand the more detailed and complex discussions that follow in later sections of the book.

Chapter 2, Clinical Coding and Coding Compliance, presents baseline information about today's approved code sets and their functionality and explains the complex interrelationships between reimbursement, coded data, and compliance with the rules and regulations of public and private third-party payers.

Chapter 3, Voluntary Healthcare Insurance Plans, explains private or commercial healthcare insurance plans and Blue Cross/Blue Shield plans and provides the reader with a detailed understanding of the sections of a healthcare insurance policy.

Chapter 4, Government-Sponsored Healthcare Programs, differentiates among the various government-sponsored healthcare programs in effect today, explains their effect on the American healthcare system, and presents the history of Medicare and Medicaid programs in America.

Chapter 5, Managed Care Plans, describes the origins, evolution, and principles of managed care and discusses the numerous types of plans that have emerged through the integration of administrative, financial, and clinical systems to both deliver and finance healthcare services.

Chapter 6, Medicare-Medicaid Prospective Payment Systems for Inpatients, explains common models and policies of payment for inpatient Medicare and Medicaid prospective payment systems and defines basic language associated with reimbursement under PPSs in acute care hospitals and inpatient psychiatric facilities.

Chapter 7, Ambulatory and Other Medicare-Medicaid Reimbursement Systems, explains common models and policies of payment for Medicare and Medicaid healthcare payment systems for physicians and outpatient settings, including physician offices, ambulance services, hospital outpatient services, ambulatory surgery centers, end-stage renal disease services, services of safety-net providers, and hospice care.

Chapter 8, Medicare-Medicaid Prospective Payment Systems for Postacute Care, describes the federal payment systems for the settings that provide care for patients recovering from inpatient acute care. These settings include skilled nursing facilities, long-term care hospitals, inpatient rehabilitation facilities, and home health agencies. The basic language of postacute is defined. Grouping models and payment formulae are explained in detail.

Chapter 9, Revenue Cycle Management, explains the components of the revenue cycle, defines revenue cycle management, and describes the connection between effective revenue cycle management and providers' fiscal stability.

Chapter 10, Value-Based Purchasing, provides a history of systems for pay for performance and value-based purchasing in the American healthcare system. Additionally, CMS quality initiatives for the hospital inpatient and outpatient settings that have been recently implemented are discussed in detail.

A complete glossary of reimbursement terminology is included at the end of the book. Throughout the text chapters, boldfaced type is used to indicate the first substantial reference to key terms included in the glossary. A detailed content index is also included at the conclusion of the text.

About the Online Resources

For Students

The online resources that accompany this book include an electronic student workbook. Go to http://ahimapress .org/Casto4347/, and register your unique student code on the interior cover of this text to download the files.

For Instructors

AHIMA provides supplementary materials for educators who use this book in their classes. Materials include the student materials listed above, as well as an instructor manual with lesson plans and test banks for each chapter, PowerPoint notes for lectures, and complete answer keys. Each chapter contains "Check Your Understanding" questions for discussion and to help the reader focus on important points within the text. The answers to these questions are included at the end of the book.

Review quizzes also follow each chapter, and the answer key for the review quizzes is included in the Instructor Guide, which contains other materials, including PowerPoint slides for classroom lectures and an exercise test bank. Visit http://www.ahima.org/publications/educators.aspx for instruction on requesting instructor materials. If you have any questions regarding the instructor materials, please contact AHIMA Customer Relations at (800) 335-5535 or submit a customer support request at https://secure.ahima.org/contact/contact.aspx.

Chapter 1
Healthcare Reimbursement Methodologies

Objectives

- To differentiate common national models of healthcare delivery
- To appreciate the size and complexity of the US healthcare delivery sector
- To appreciate the influence of the federal government in the US healthcare sector
- To define health insurance
- To differentiate payment methods on unit of payment, time frame, and risk

- To identify types of healthcare reimbursement methodologies
- To differentiate fee-for-service reimbursement from episode-of-care reimbursement
- To describe trends in the healthcare sector
- To define terms associated with healthcare reimbursement methodologies

Key Terms

Accountable care organization (ACO)
Affordable Care Act (ACA)
Allowable charge
Bad debt
Block grant
Bundling
Capitated payment method
Capitation
Case
Case-based payment
Charge
Charity care
Claim
Copayment
Customary, prevailing, and reasonable (CPR)
Deductible
Dependent (family) coverage
Discounted fee-for-service
Episode-of-care reimbursement
Fee
Fee schedule
Fee-for-service reimbursement

First mover
Global payment method
Guarantor
Health disparity
Health Care and Education Reconciliation Act of 2010
    (P.L. 111–152): see Affordable Care Act (ACA)
Individual (single) coverage
Insurance
Manager's amendment
Meaningful use
Medical tourism
Medicare-severity diagnosis-related group (MS-DRG)
National health service (Beveridge) model
Patient Protection and Affordable Care Act of 2010
    (P.L. 111–148): see Affordable Care Act (ACA)
Payer
Per diem payment
Policy
Premium
Private health insurance model
Prospective payment method
Provider

Reimbursement
Resource-based relative value scale (RBRVS)
Retrospective payment method
Risk pool
Self-insured plan
Self-pay
Single-payer health system
Social insurance (Bismarck) model

Third-party payer
Third-party payment
Transparency
Uncompensated care
Underserved area
Universal healthcare coverage
Usual, customary, and reasonable (UCR)

Introduction to Healthcare Reimbursement

Health personnel who understand the US healthcare reimbursement systems can assist their patients and clients, their organizations, and their own families. This book is a guide to healthcare reimbursement. The book divides healthcare reimbursement into its essential systems, such as inpatient payment systems, ambulatory systems, and postacute care systems. In this chapter and the following chapters, readers will learn about healthcare reimbursement methodologies; clinical coding and compliance; voluntary healthcare insurance plans; government-sponsored healthcare programs; managed care plans; Medicare–Medicaid prospective payment systems for inpatients, ambulatory, and other Medicare–Medicaid reimbursement systems; revenue cycle management; and models of quality, performance, and payment. It is essential that health personnel understand the reimbursement systems in the US healthcare sector because of their potential effects on people's lives.

A systematic approach makes the complexity of the healthcare reimbursement systems manageable. To put the systems in context, the background and key historical events in the development of each system and its payment methods are briefly described. Then, in straightforward language, the payment methods for each system are explained clearly and in detail. Step by step, the reader is walked through the procedures of each payment method. Terms, abbreviations, and acronyms are clearly defined. Accuracy, however, is not sacrificed for simplicity. Readers can feel confident as members of the healthcare team.

National Models of Healthcare Delivery

Three national models for delivering healthcare services exist: social insurance, national health service, and private health insurance (Kulesher and Forrestal 2014, 127). These models can be seen in various permutations in countries around the world. The models vary by sources of funding, number and type of payers involved, and levels of healthcare services. Here are descriptions of the three national models:

- **Social insurance model**, or the Bismarck model. Introduced in 1883 by German Chancellor Otto von Bismarck, this model is the oldest in the world (Frogner et al. 2011, 72). The foundation of this model is **universal healthcare coverage** for a set of benefits defined by the national government. In this model, every worker and employer must contribute to sickness funds, agencies that collect and redistribute money per government regulations; they are a form of social security. The amounts of the contributions are proportionate to workers' and employers' incomes. Workers can choose among competing sickness funds (Frogner et al. 2011, 72). With varying modifications, France, Japan, the Netherlands, and many other countries have adopted this German model.

- **National health service model**, or the Beveridge model. In 1946, Sir William Beveridge created the national health service model for the United Kingdom (UK) (Frogner et al. 2011, 72). In the UK, the government owns the clinics and hospitals and pays the doctors and health personnel who work in these public facilities. This government-run model is a **single-payer health system**—the UK government is the only payer. The healthcare system is financed by the country's general revenues. The general revenues come from taxes that increase in proportion to income (progressive tax) (Frogner et al. 2011, 72). With varying modifications, Spain and the Scandinavian countries have adopted this model.

- **Private health insurance model**. In this model, many private health insurance companies exist. The private health insurance companies collect premiums to create a pool of money. This pool of money is used to pay health claims. Much as with the Bismarck model, workers and employers contribute to the pool. Unlike the Bismarck system, the insurance company determines the contribution, and this contribution is not based on the employees' incomes (Frogner et al. 2011, 73). The United States and Switzerland use the private health insurance model. In Switzerland, governmental regulation of health insurance is more extensive than in the United States (Frogner et al. 2011, 73).

No country's system is a pure version of these models (Kulesher and Forrestal 2014, 127). For example, a hybrid combining aspects of the Bismarck and Beveridge models exists. This hybrid is used in Canada, South Korea, and other countries. Generally, however, one model can be determined as dominating each country's system.

These national delivery models are often discussed in the healthcare sector. Healthcare policy makers compare the US model to these models and, depending on the policy maker's view, the comparison reflects negatively or positively on the US model. For example, the Canadian system is "considerably" simpler than the US system (Sessions and Detsky 2010, 2078). On the other hand, "one-fourth or more of Canadian … adults reported having to wait six days or more to see a doctor or nurse when sick," compared with US adults, who reported "quick access" (Schoen et al. 2010, 2328). Therefore, healthcare personnel should be aware of these models because they are often referenced during discussions of healthcare delivery.

US Healthcare Sector

Four characteristics are key to understanding the US healthcare sector. These characteristics are the size of this economic sector, its complexity, intricate payment methods and rules, and broad program scopes.

First, the US healthcare sector is large. In 2012, the US healthcare sector accounted for $2.8 trillion, or 17.2 percent of the nation's gross domestic product (GDP). To put these amounts in understandable terms, $8,915 was spent for each person in the United States (Martin et al. 2014, 67).

Second, in addition to being large, the US healthcare system is complex. Factors in the system's complexity are its fragmentation (France 2008, 676) and the sets of intricate interactions among these "fragments" (parts). These fragments are actually subsystems. For example, the system includes subsystems representing sources of health services, such as physicians, large and small hospitals, rehabilitation specialists, chiropractors, and medical equipment companies, to name a few. Just as numerous as the sources of health services are the subsystems that pay for services. These **payers** include Medicare, private health insurance, Blue Cross and Blue Shield, workers' compensation, Indian Health Services, and private individuals—just to begin the list. Thus, the US healthcare system is inherently complex

because it is actually multiple subsystems rather than a single system.

Third, the subsystems interact using many varied and complicated payment methods and rules. For example, a physician's office might have "at least a dozen separate contracts for providing healthcare services" (Washburn 1999, 35). Typical midsize and large payers, such as Blue Cross or health insurance companies, may have thousands of contracts with physicians, hospitals, and other **providers** of services (Kongstvedt 2013, 59). Moreover, the payment rates and clauses of these contracts can be revised, updated, or renewed on different timetables, such as mid-year, annually, or after multiple years (Jones and Mills 2006, 52, 54) Managing these contracts often requires specialized computer software (Kongstvedt 2013, 60). Thus, payment methods and rules change unpredictably—and often.

Example: Noted Healthcare Economist's Description of the US Healthcare System

Henry J. Aaron describes the US healthcare system as an administrative monstrosity, a truly bizarre mélange of thousands of payers with payment systems that differ for no socially beneficial reason, as well as staggeringly complex public systems with mind-boggling administered prices and other rules expressing distinctions that can only be regarded as weird (Aaron 2003, 802).

Fourth, some of the organizations within the sector have programs with broad scopes and responsibilities (Medicare Payment Advisory Committee 2001, 3). For example, some health plans, widening their scope beyond providing hospital care, take responsibility for the health of entire populations and communities (Lynn and Kamp 2014, 6). Moreover, the Centers for Medicare and Medicaid Services (CMS) is an operating division within the Department of Health and Human Services (HHS). The CMS is responsible for the two largest federal healthcare programs, Medicare and Medicaid, as well as for the Children's Health Insurance Program (CHIP). The CMS estimates that 123 million individuals are covered by Medicare, Medicaid, or CHIP—more than one in three Americans (Mitchell 2014, 1).

Illustrating the size of the healthcare sector, its complexity, intricate payment methods and rules, and programs' broad scopes are table 1.1 and table 1.2.

Although the content of table 1.1 dates to 2001, the volumes and complexity of federal payment systems have not lessened. In fact, since 2001, as table 1.2 shows, the federal payment systems have become more complex, with several new federal payment systems having been implemented.

Table 1.1.   2001—Examples of complexity in federal payment methods

Example	Complexity as Represented by Volume
Recognized entities for payment	30
U.S. Federal Law Code	More than 600 pages
Code of Federal Regulations (CFR)	Two volumes
Three pages of new regulations for providers	100 pages of explanation
Medicare claims processing	900 million claims from more than 700,000 providers per year
Contractors for the Centers for Medicare and Medicaid Services (CMS)	116 private contractors to administer, regulate, and monitor Medicare program

Source: Medicare Payment Advisory Committee. 2001. A Report to the Congress: Reducing Medicare Complexity and Regulatory Burden. www .medpac.gov/publications/congressional_reports/dec2001RegBurden.pdf, pp. 4, 5, 7, 15.

Dominance of Federal Healthcare Payment Methods

The US federal government is the dominant player in the healthcare sector. The federal Medicare program is the largest single payer for health services (Calcagno 2014, 5). Medicare is a health insurance program for senior citizens, people who have disabilities, and people who have end-stage kidney disease (see chapter 4 for a full description). Medicare also "provides significant funds for medical education, research, and the care of disadvantaged and vulnerable people" (Mayes and Berenson 2006, 2). In addition, Medicaid, a joint state–federal program, is the largest source of federal revenue for states (Kaiser Family Foundation 2013a, 31). Medicaid provides reimbursement for health services received by low-income persons and families (see chapter 4 for a full description). In 2011, federal and state Medicaid spending, excluding administrative costs, totaled $414 billion (Kaiser Family Foundation

2013a, 25). Moreover, the federal government also pays for health services for other populations, including active-duty and retired military personnel and their families, veterans, Native Americans, and injured and disabled workers (Knickman 2011, 55). Thus, much of the healthcare sector relies on the federal government for reimbursement.

Because of the size of the federal role in healthcare reimbursement, any changes that the federal government makes in its reimbursement methods profoundly affect providers, other health insurers, and the healthcare system. The federal government is the **first mover** in the US healthcare system (Mayes and Berenson 2006, 2). For instance, other payers follow Medicare's lead in changes to payment methods (Calcagno 2014, 5).

Health Insurance

Generally, **reimbursement** for healthcare services depends on patients having health **insurance**. Insurance is a system of reducing a person's exposure to risk of loss by having another party (insurance company or insurer) assume the risk. In healthcare, the risk that the healthcare insurance company assumes is the unknown cost of healthcare for a person or group of persons.

However, the insurance company that assumes the risk reduces its own risk by distributing the risk among a larger group of persons (insureds). This group of persons has similar risks of loss and is known as a **risk pool**. In healthcare, the variability of health statuses across many people allows the healthcare insurance company to make a better estimate of the average costs of healthcare.

The insurance company, however, receives a **premium** payment in return for assuming the insureds' exposure to risk of loss. The premium payments for all the insureds in the group are combined in a pool of money. Insurers use actuarial data to calculate the premiums so that the pool of money is sufficiently large to pay losses of the entire group. Thus, specific to healthcare, the risk is the potential that a person will get sick or require health services and will incur bills (costs) associated with his or her treatment or services. The premium payments for health insurance are calculated to pay for all the potential covered healthcare costs for an entire group of patients.

Table 1.2.   Selected federal payment systems

Site	System	Rate Method		Abbreviation	Effective Date
		Relative Weighted Group	Per Diem or Treatment		
Hospital Inpatient Settings					
Inpatient Acute Care Hospital	Inpatient prospective payment system (IPPS)	Diagnosis-related group		DRG	October 1, 1983
		Medicare-severity diagnosis related group (enhancement)		MS-DRG	October 1, 2007
Inpatient Psychiatric Facility	Inpatient psychiatric facility prospective payment system (IPF PPS)		Per diem with facility-level and patient-level adjustments		April 1, 2005
Postacute Settings					
Skilled Nursing Facility	Skilled nursing facility prospective payment system (SNF PPS)	Resource utilization group		RUG	July 1, 1998
Home Health Agency	Home health prospective payment system (HHPPS)	Home health resource group		HHRG	October 1, 2000
Inpatient Rehabilitation Facility	Inpatient rehabilitation facility prospective payment system (IRF PPS)	Case mix group		CMG	January 1, 2002
Long-Term Care Hospital	Long-term care hospital prospective payment system (LTCH PPS)	Diagnosis related group		LTC-DRG	October 1, 2002
		Medicare-severity diagnosis related group (enhancement)		MS-LTC-DRG	October 1, 2007
Ambulatory Settings					
Outpatient Hospital Service	Outpatient prospective payment system (OPPS)	Ambulatory payment classification group		APC	August 1, 2000
Ambulatory Surgery Center	Ambulatory surgery center (ASC) payment method	Ambulatory surgery center group		ASC	1982
		Ambulatory payment classification group (integrated into outpatient prospective payment system)		APC	January 1, 2008
Physicians and Health Professional Non-physician Providers	Resource-based relative value scale (RBRVS)	Relative value unit		RVU	January 1, 1992
Medicare End-Stage Renal Disease Facilities	End-stage renal disease prospective payment system (ESRD PPS)		Per treatment base rate with facility-level and patient-level adjustments		January 1, 2011
Federally Qualified Health Centers	Federally qualified health center prospective payment system (FQHC PPS)		Per diem		October 1, 2014
Hospice	Hospice services payment system		Four categories of per diems matched to intensity of care		October 1, 1983
Ambulance Services	Ambulance services payment system	Relative value unit		RVU	April 1, 2002

1. True or False? The national health service (Beveridge) model is different from the social insurance (Bismarck) model because the Beveridge model is financed by general revenue funds from fiscal taxes, whereas the Bismarck model is financed by workers' and employers' compulsory payroll contributions into sickness funds.

2. What are the four characteristics of the US healthcare sector?

3. True or False? The federal role in the healthcare sector is limited to paying providers for the healthcare costs of senior citizens.

4. What do insurers receive in return for assuming the insureds' exposure to risk or loss?

5. Insurers pool premium payments for all the insureds in a group, then use actuarial data to calculate the group's premiums so that
   a. Premium payments are lowered for insurance plan payers
   b. The pool is large enough to pay losses of the entire group
   c. Accounting for the group's plan is simplified
   d. All of the above

Historical Perspectives

Health insurance in the United States has been made available to help offset the expenses of the treatment of illness and injury. One health systems expert characterizes the development of health insurance in the United States as "accidental" (Gabel 1999, 63). The first "sickness" clause was inserted in an insurance document in 1847. However, health insurance did not become established until 1929, when Blue Cross first covered schoolteachers in Texas. In 1932, a citywide plan was begun in Sacramento, California. In the 1940s, during World War II, the executive and judicial branches of government issued a series of acts to address a labor shortage (Gabel 1999, 63). These acts became the basic structure of health insurance in the United States. Moreover, these acts resulted in today's linkage of health insurance and employment. Thus, as an industry, health insurance became widespread in the United States after World War II (Longest and Darr 2014, 42). Such accidental evolution did not occur in other countries, such as Great Britain, Canada, and Germany, where specific legislative acts created health insurance systems (Gabel 1999, 63).

Health Insurance and Employment

In the United States, health insurance is usually tied to employment. Many larger employers, as part of a package of employment benefits, pay a portion of the health insurance premium. Health insurance that covers only the employee is known as **individual (single) coverage**. Employees may be required to pay extra for health insurance for a spouse or children. Health insurance for a spouse or children or both is known as **dependent (family) coverage**. Medicare is also considered insurance because payroll taxes, through both employers' and employees' contributions, finance one portion of Medicare coverage. Premiums paid by eligible individuals and matched by the federal government also finance Medicare's supplemental medical insurance program.

When people lose their jobs, they often lose their health insurance. Although people can continue their health insurance by paying for the insurance entirely by themselves, the payments are expensive. In certain circumstances, under the Consolidated Omnibus Budget Reconciliation Act (COBRA) of 1985, people can extend their health insurance for a limited period or, under the Affordable Care Act (ACA) of 2010, they may enroll in federal marketplace healthcare insurance.

Example: Effect of Loss of Health Insurance on Public Healthcare Spending

People's loss of health insurance affects us all, not just people who are unemployed. For example, Medicaid is a joint federal and state program that provides medical and health services to the poor. During an economic downturn between 2000 and 2003, more people were eligible for Medicaid. Their enrollment in Medicaid resulted in a 34 percent increase in Medicaid spending, from $205.7 billion to $275.5 billion. In the economic crisis of 2008, every 1 percent increase in the number of Americans unemployed equaled the loss of employer-sponsored health insurance for approximately 2.5 million workers and their dependents, according to the American Hospital Association. Comparing the periods of July through September, the amount of unreimbursed (uncompensated) care that hospitals provided increased by 8 percent, from $853.5 million in 2007 to $923.6 million in 2008. Thus people's loss of health insurance results in greater public spending on healthcare (Holahan, J., and A. Ghosh, 2005, W5-61).

For some employed people, the adequacy of the health insurance is an issue. Some health insurance plans require patients or their families to pay 20 percent or more of the costs of their healthcare. Healthcare costs can easily be in the thousands of dollars; 20 percent of

$10,000 is $2,000, which is a sizable sum for many people. Other employees work for employers that do not offer health benefits. These persons must purchase their own insurance at an extremely high rate. Obtaining and retaining adequate health insurance are problems for many US workers.

Compensation for Healthcare

Reimbursement is the healthcare term referring to compensation or repayment for healthcare services. Reimbursement is being repaid or compensated for expenses already incurred or, as in the case of healthcare, for services that have already been provided. In healthcare, services are often provided before payment is made. Unlike the car dealership, in which customers pay for a car or arrange a loan before driving the car off the lot, patients walk out of the hospital treated, without making payment arrangements. Therefore, the physicians and clinics must seek to be paid back for services that they have already provided and for incurred expenses, such as the cost for supplies used. These physicians, clinics, hospitals, and other healthcare organizations and practitioners are requesting reimbursement for health services.

Third-Party Payment

Experts in healthcare finance refer to **third-party payment** or **third-party payers**. Who or what are these parties? Discussions of third-party payers can be confusing because no mention is made of first parties and second parties. A party is an entity that receives, renders, or pays for health services. The first party is the patient himself or herself or the person, such as a parent, responsible for the patient's health bill. The second party is the physician, clinic, hospital, nursing home, or other healthcare entity rendering the care. These second parties are often called **providers** because they provide healthcare. The third party is the payer, an uninvolved insurance company or health agency that pays the physician, clinic, or other second-party provider for the care or services rendered to the first party (patient). Examples of third-party payers are health insurance companies, workers' compensation, and Medicare.

Characteristics of Reimbursement Methodologies

Three characteristics describe various methods of healthcare reimbursement. These characteristics are the unit of payment, the time orientation, and the degree

of financial risk for the parties (Wouters et al. 1998, 3) (table 1.3). The unit of payment can range from a payment for each service, such as a payment for each laboratory test, to a block payment for an entire population for a period of time, such as a governmental budget transfer to the state health department. The time orientation is retrospective versus prospective. In **retrospective payment methods**, the payer learns of the costs of the health services after the patient has already received the services. The provider also receives payment after the services have been provided. In a **prospective payment method**, the payments are preset before care is delivered. Financial risk refers back to the definition of health insurance. When the costs of health services are learned after the care is provided, the third-party payer (health insurance entity) is at risk. When providers must project the costs of treating patients into the future and contract to provide all care for those estimated costs, the provider is at risk. Patients assume risk because they must pay higher and higher percentages of the costs as their share.

Table 1.3.   Characteristics of reimbursement methodologies

Characteristic	Description
Unit of payment	Element that is the basis of payment; ranges in aggregation from single service, such as a laboratory test, to an entire clinic visit to an episode of care to hospitalization to, finally, an entire population
Time orientation	Retrospective (learned after care or services provided) or Prospective (determined in advance of care or services)
Degree of financial risk	Level of uncertainty related to the cost of healthcare or to a potential financial loss or harm

Types of Healthcare Reimbursement Methodologies

This section discusses the fundamental concepts in healthcare reimbursement methodologies. The section is organized by the two major types of unit of payment: **fee-for-service reimbursement** and **episode-of-care reimbursement** (table 1.4). Also briefly addressed are the other characteristics of healthcare payment methods: time frame and risk. The chapter concludes with a peek into the future of healthcare reimbursement.

Table 1.4. Major types of reimbursement methodologies

Fee-for-Service	Episode-of-Care
Self-pay	Capitated payment
Traditional retrospective payment	Global payment
Managed care*	Prospective payment

*Some forms.

Fee-for-Service Reimbursement

Fee-for-service reimbursement is a healthcare payment method in which providers receive payment for each service rendered. Fee-for-service is a common method of calculating healthcare reimbursement.

A **fee** is a set amount or a set price. Fee-for-service means a specific payment is made for each specific service provided or rendered. In the fee-for-service method, the provider of the healthcare service (the second party) charges a fee for each type of service, and the health insurance company pays each fee for a covered service. These fees or prices are known as **charges** in healthcare. Sometimes, there is little relationship between the actual costs to provide a service and its charge.

Typically, the physician, healthcare organization, or other practitioner bills for each service provided on a **claim** that lists the fees or charges for each service. The claim is sent to the third-party payer (health insurance company or health agency). In healthcare, sending the claim to the third-party payer is known as submitting a claim. Within the stipulations of the health insurance **policy** (contract) or the governmental regulations, the third party pays the claim. The majority of US physicians, healthcare organizations, and other practitioners use this method of billing.

People who have health insurance that reimburses on the basis of fee-for-service have the advantage of great independence. Their health insurance plans allow them to make almost all health decisions about which physician to see and about which conditions to have treated. The patient or the provider submits a claim to the health insurance company, and, if the service is covered in the health insurance policy, the patient or provider receives reimbursement. For the patient, the disadvantage of fee-for-service is that fee-for-service plans often have higher **deductibles** or **copayments** than other types of health insurance, such as managed care plans.

For health insurance plans, fee-for-service has the disadvantage of uncertainty. The costs of reimbursing the providers are unknown because the services that patients will receive are unknown. Moreover, costs will increase if the providers increase the fees for each service, if patients receive more services than expected, or if more expensive services are substituted for less expensive services. Examples of fee-for-service reimbursement are self-pay, traditional retrospective payment, and managed care.

Self-Pay

Self-pay is a type of fee-for-service because the patients or their **guarantors** (responsible persons, such as parents for children) pay a specific amount for each service received. The patients or guarantors make such payments themselves to the providers, such as physicians, clinics, or hospitals that rendered each service. There are two situations in which self-pay occurs.

In the first situation, the patients or guarantors have health insurance. However, the patients or guarantors choose to pay the healthcare provider themselves and to subsequently seek reimbursement directly from their private health insurance or from the governmental agency that covers their health benefits.

In the second situation, the patients or guarantors choose not to use their health insurance. For example, they may want to have cosmetic surgery or some other health service not covered under health insurance. For these individuals, self-pay results because no third party payer is paying for their health services.

The outcome, though, in both situations is self-pay. Some patients and guarantors may seek recompense from a third-party payer, and others may bear the burden of the costs of their healthcare themselves. Thus, in self-pay, the patients or guarantors directly pay their healthcare providers for the costs of their healthcare.

A related concept is the **self-insured plan**. A self-insured plan is one in which the employer eliminates the middleman. The employer administers its own health insurance benefits. Rather than shift the risk to a health insurance entity, the employer (or other entity, such as a professional association) assumes the costs of healthcare for its employees or members and their dependents.

Traditional Retrospective Payment

The traditional retrospective payment method of reimbursement pays providers after the services have been rendered. Retrospective reimbursement is a type of fee-for-service because the providers are reimbursed for each service rendered. Third-party payers reimburse providers for charges previously incurred. The reimbursement payments are based on the charges for the services provided. This method has historically been the traditional method of reimbursement.

Fee Schedule

In a fee-for-service environment, third-party payers establish a **fee schedule**. A fee schedule is a predetermined list of fees that the third-party payer allows for payment for all healthcare services. The **allowable charge** represents the average or maximum amount the third-party payer will reimburse providers for the service.

Discounted Fee-for-Service Payment

To begin to control costs, the third-party payers negotiated reduced fees for their members or insureds. The payment method using these reduced fees is known as **discounted fee-for-service**. Versions of the discounted fee-for-service payment method are the **usual, customary, and reasonable (UCR)**, **the customary, prevailing, and reasonable (CPR)**, and the **resource-based relative value scale (RBRVS)** (Blount and Waters 2001, 6).

UCR is defined as usual in the provider's practice, customary in the community, and reasonable for the situation. CPR is defined as customary in the providers' practice, prevailing in the community, and reasonable as the provider's lowest actual charge. The UCR and the CPR are methods of payment within the type of traditional retrospective payment. Both methods are based on data from past claims. Private insurance companies use the UCR method. Prior to the implementation of its current payment methods, Medicare employed CPR. Both UCR and CPR are becoming rare.

Established in 1992, the RBRVS is a discounted fee schedule that Medicare uses to reimburse physicians. The RBRVS is a payment method that classifies health services based on the cost of providing physician services in terms of effort, practice expenses (overhead), and malpractice insurance.

Uncertainty for Third-Party Payers

For third-party payers, the retrospective fee-for-service payment method has the disadvantage of great uncertainty. The payers have no way of knowing the total charges that will be incurred and for which they must reimburse the providers.

Criticism of Fee-for-Service Reimbursement

Critics of fee-for-service reimbursement assert that the method provides few incentives to control costs. In a fee-for-service environment, providers are reimbursed for each service they provide. The more services a provider renders, the more reimbursement the provider receives. Moreover, critics argue that there is little incentive to order less expensive services rather than more expensive services. Therefore, some experts contend that fee-for-service reimbursement inappropriately inflates the costs of healthcare because the payment method rewards providers for more services regardless of whether such services are warranted.

Managed Care

In managed care reimbursement methods (discussed fully in chapter 5), third-party payers "manage" both the costs of healthcare and the outcomes of care. By managing care, these methods begin to address the criticism of fee-for-service reimbursement. In managed care plans, the third-party payer has implemented some provisions to control the costs of healthcare while maintaining quality care.

Features of Managed Care

Common features of managed care include

- Comprehensiveness
- Coordination and planning
- Education of patients and providers
- Assessment of quality
- Control of costs

Purposes of Managed Care

The two purposes of the management or control are to reduce the costs of healthcare for which the third-party payer must reimburse the providers and to ensure continuing quality of care.

Managed care payers have instituted many means to control the costs and quality of healthcare. One example of a provision is the requirement that patients obtain prior approvals for surgeries. Another example is a hybrid of the discounted fee-based system in which the payer reimburses the provider up to a percentage of the allowable fee and the insured must pay the remaining percentage (Koch 2002, 109). Finally, having one primary care provider to coordinate all aspects of healthcare supports the quality of healthcare by reducing fragmentation and enhancing integration.

Forms of Managed Care

There are numerous forms of managed care. These forms include health maintenance organizations (HMOs), exclusive provider organizations (EPOs), point-of-service plans (POSs), and preferred provider organizations (PPOs). One can imagine these forms as a continuum of control, with the HMOs representing the most controlled and the PPOs representing the least controlled.

Criticisms of Managed Care

Some critics of managed care argue that managed care too severely limits the following capabilities:

- Patients' access to care and their freedom to choose healthcare providers

- Providers' ability to order diagnostic tests and therapeutic procedures

These critics contend that administrators, rather than medical and health personnel, are making decisions about patients' health futures.

Episode-of-Care Reimbursement

Episode-of-care reimbursement is a healthcare payment method in which providers receive one lump sum for all the services they provide related to a condition or disease. In the episode-of-care payment method, the unit of payment is the episode, not each individual health service. Thus the episode-of-care payment method eliminates individual fees or charges. The episode-of-care payment method is an attempt to correct perceived faults in the fee-for-service reimbursement method. Thus, the episode-of-care reimbursement method controls costs on a grand or systematic scale.

An episode of care is the health services that a patient receives

- For a particular health condition or illness

- During a period of relatively continuous care from a provider

In the episode of care, one amount is set for all the care associated with the condition or illness. Forms of episode-of-care reimbursement are the capitated

payment method, the global payment method, and the prospective payment method.

Occasionally, an episode of care is defined as a specific number of days. The federal government's payment method for home care services is an example. The per-episode home health payment covers all home care services and nonroutine medical supplies delivered to the patient during a 60-day period.

Capitated Payment Method

The **capitated payment method**, or **capitation**, is a method of payment for health services in which the third-party payer reimburses providers a fixed, per capita amount for a period. "Per capita" means "per head" or "per person." A common phrase in capitated contracts is "per member per month" (PMPM). The PMPM is the amount of money paid each month for each individual enrolled in the health insurance plan. Capitation is characteristic of HMOs.

In capitation, the actual volume or intensity of services provided to each patient has no effect on the payment. More services do not increase the payment, nor do fewer services decrease the payment. If the provider contracts with a third-party payer to provide services to a group of workers for a capitated rate, the provider receives the payments for each member of the group regardless of whether all the members receive the provider's services. There are no adjustments for the complexity or extent of the health services.

Example:

Z Company has a health insurance plan for its workers and their families through Wellness HMO. Wellness HMO has contracted with Dr. T to provide health services (care) to members of the Z Company group for the capitated rate of $15 per month ($15 PMPM).

Dr. T is under contract to receive $15 per month for every member of the Z group. The members of the Z group total 100. Each month Dr. T receives $1,500 ($15 × 100 members) from Wellness HMO for the Z group. Dr. T receives $1,500 regardless of whether no members of the group see him in the clinic or all the members of the group see him in the clinic. Dr. T receives $1,500 whether all the members receive complex care for cancer or all the members receive simple care for preventive flu shots.

The advantages of capitated payment are that the third-party payer has no uncertainty and that the provider has a guaranteed customer base. The third-party payer knows exactly what the costs of healthcare for the group will be, and the providers know that they will have a certain group of customers. However, for the provider, there is also great uncertainty because the patients' usage of provider services is unknown and the complexities and costs of services are unknown.

Global Payment Method

In the **global payment method**, the third-party payer makes one combined payment to cover the services of multiple providers who are treating a single episode of care. Thus, this payment method consolidates payments. A **block grant** is a fixed amount of money given or allocated for a specific purpose. For example, in a block grant, there is a transfer of governmental funds to cover health services. In the global payment method, there is no additional payment for higher volumes of services or more expensive or complex services.

Medicare's payment system for home health services is an example of a global payment method. Various types of home health services are consolidated into the single payment. These services include all speech therapy, physical therapy, and occupational therapy; skilled nursing visits; home health aide visits; medical social services, and nonroutine medical supplies.

The most comprehensive version of the global payment system is the total-episode-of-care. For an episode of care, the total-episode-of-care payment rate is a single price that covers costs across the continuum of care, which could include all of the following:

- Facility costs across the continuum of care, such as hospital, nursing home, clinic, and outpatient rehabilitation

- Technical and professional components of procedures in radiology, pathology, and the laboratory

- Physician professional fees for anesthesia, surgery, and consultation

- Home care costs

Less comprehensive versions of the global payment method exist. For example, some global payment methods include only ambulatory costs or only inpatient costs, termed the ambulatory-episode-of-care and inpatient-episode-of-care methods, respectively.

Another less comprehensive version is a global surgical package. The global surgical package encompasses an operation, local or topical anesthesia, a preoperative clinic visit, immediate postoperative care, and usual postoperative follow-up. In outpatient dialysis facilities, **bundling** combines into a single prospective payment the costs of dialysis services, injectable drugs, laboratory tests, and medical equipment and supplies (Medicare Payment Advisory Commission 2013, 1). In the special-procedure package, all the costs associated with a diagnostic or therapeutic procedure are included in the payment. Examples include extracorporeal shock wave lithotripsy and vasectomy. Another common package is for obstetrical services. An ambulatory-visit package includes all ambulatory services, including physicians' charges, laboratory tests, x-rays, and other ambulatory services associated with one clinic visit. The per-episode home health payment is also a less comprehensive global payment rate. The single payment covers all home care services and nonroutine medical supplies that a patient receives during a 60-day period.

As can be seen, third-party payers and providers have created multiple variations of the global payment method. The multiple variations, however, have added to the complexity of healthcare reimbursement.

Prospective Payment Method

In the prospective payment method, payment rates for healthcare services are established in advance for a specific time period. The predetermined rates are based on average levels of resource use for certain types of healthcare. It is important to note that prospective payment methods are based on averages. On individual patients, providers can lose money or make money, but over time, providers should come out even. Payment is determined by the resource needs of the average patient for a set period of time or given set of conditions or diseases. Prospective payment methods representing these two situations are per diem payment and case-based payment, respectively.

Providers are paid the preestablished rates regardless of the costs they actually incur. Thus, prospective payment is another method in which the actual number or intensity of the services does not affect a preestablished compensation. The intent of prospective payment methods is to reduce the likelihood that charges will increase because limits on payments are preset for the future period.

Per Diem Payment

Per diem payment, or per day (daily rate), is a limited type of prospective payment method. The third-party payer reimburses the provider a fixed rate for each day during which a covered member is hospitalized. Traditionally, the per diem payment method has been used to reimburse providers for inpatient hospital services. Examples of per diem payments are Medicare's payment method for inpatient psychiatric facilities, as well as some supplemental health insurance plans.

Third-party payers set the per diem rates using historical data. For example, to establish an inpatient per diem, the total costs for all inpatient services for a population during a period are divided by the sum of the lengths of stay in the period. To determine the payment, the per diem rate is multiplied by the number of days of hospitalization. In the absence of historical data, third-party payers and providers must consider several factors to establish per diem rates. These factors include costs, lengths of stay, volumes of service, and patients' severity of illness.

Critics of the per diem payment method contend that the method encourages providers to increase the number of inpatient admissions, to extend the lengths of stay, or both. These strategies would result in increased reimbursements. Another prospective payment method, case-based reimbursement, corrects the flaws perceived in the per diem payment method.

Case-Based Payment

In the **case-based payment** method, providers receive a fixed, preestablished payment for each case. **Cases** are patients, residents, or clients who receive health services for a condition or disease. Third-party payers reimburse providers for each case rather than for each service (fee-for-service) or per diem.

Example:

Two patients were hospitalized with pneumonia. One patient was hospitalized for three days, the other for 30 days. Each patient is a case. The third-party payer has established a payment rate for cases with pneumonia. The hospital would receive two payments, exactly the same, for the two cases.

The payment is determined by the historical resource needs of the average patient for a given set of conditions or diseases. Case-based payment can be one flat rate per case or can be multiple rates that represent categories of cases (sets of conditions or diseases).

An example of the case-based payment system built on categories of cases is Medicare's method of payment for inpatient hospital services (prospective payment system, or PPS). This method of payment is based on categories of payment called **Medicare-severity diagnosis-related groups (MS-DRGs)**. Each MS-DRG categorizes patients who are homogeneous in terms of clinical profiles and requisite resources. Thus, patients classified to the same group have similar diagnoses and treatments, consumption of resources, and lengths of stay. Each MS-DRG has a payment rate called a weight. Weights are relative to one another. Higher weights are associated with groups in which patients require more resources for care and treatment. Higher resource consumption is related to higher intensity of services due to the severity of illness or the types of services needed for care and treatment, such as expensive equipment or medications. Higher weights translate into higher payments.

MS-DRGs are sensitive to resource complexity and severity of illness (Bowman 2007, 16). To make MS-DRGs sensitive to resource complexity and severity of illness, diagnosis codes were classified into three hierarchical levels in terms of their severity. The extent to which these diagnoses increased consumption of hospital resources was then evaluated. Next, the MS-DRGs' weights were aligned to their consumption of resources due to their resource complexity or severity of illness. Higher weights were assigned to MS-DRGs that required higher resource consumption, with lower weights being assigned to MS-DRGs that required fewer resources. The relatively weighted group is the basic unit of payment. Higher relative weights link to higher payment rates.

Several US federal payment methods are case-based prospective payment methods. For example, in table 1.2, the following payment systems are some of the case-based prospective methods: inpatient acute-care hospital, skilled nursing facility, home health agency, outpatient hospital services, inpatient rehabilitation facility, and long-term care hospital.

The case-based payment method rewards effective and efficient delivery of health services and penalizes ineffective and inefficient delivery. The case-based payment rates are based on averages of costs for patients within the group. Generally, costs for providers that treat patients efficiently and effectively are beneath the average costs. The providers make money in this situation. On the other hand, providers that typically exceed average costs lose money. Inefficiencies include duplicate laboratory work, scheduling delays, and lost reports. Many healthcare organizations have implemented procedures to streamline the delivery of health services to offset inefficiencies. Poor clinical diagnostic skills are an example of ineffectiveness. Thus, the more efficiently and effectively a provider delivers care, the greater its operating margin will be.

Criticisms of Episode-of-Care Reimbursement

Some consumer advocates have voiced concerns about episode-of-care reimbursement, noting that the payment method creates incentives to substitute less expensive diagnostic and therapeutic procedures and laboratory and radiological tests and to delay or deny procedures and treatments. Healthcare analysts, on the other hand, point out the savings associated with eliminating wasteful or unnecessary procedures and tests, noting that volume and expense do not necessarily define quality.

Check Your Understanding 1.2

1. Where and when did health insurance become established in the United States?

2. What is the term for health insurance that only covers the employee?

3. What term in healthcare means compensation or repayment for rendering healthcare services?

4. Who is the third party in healthcare situations?
   a. Patient
   b. Provider
   c. Payer
   d. Cannot be determined

5. All of the following are types of episode-of-care reimbursement except
   a. Global payment
   b. Prospective payment
   c. Capitation
   d. Self-insured plan

6. What discounted fee schedule does Medicare use to reimburse physicians?

7. Name and describe some versions of the global payment method.

Trends in Healthcare Reimbursement

Five trends affect the entire healthcare sector:

- Constantly increasing healthcare spending
- Efforts to reform the healthcare system
- Initiatives to expand the sector's adoption and use of health information and communication technologies
- Medical tourism
- Transparency

The first trend underlies the second and third trends. This section describes these trends.

Constantly Increasing Healthcare Spending

Each year, national spending on healthcare increases. This increased spending is a concern because money is a limited resource. As spending on healthcare increases, the money available for other sectors of the economy, such as education or roads, decreases. Experts at the Health Care Cost Institute (HCCI), a nonprofit, nonpartisan research institute, state that "rising health care costs are stifling economic growth, consuming increasing portions of the nation's gross domestic product, and putting added burdens on businesses, the public sector, individuals, and families" (HCCI 2015). Thus, this constantly increasing healthcare spending negatively affects the country's economy and thereby its people.

The trend of increased spending on healthcare has been consistent for more than a decade. Table 1.5 shows the percentage increases for selected years. Although the percentages appear small, they represent billions of dollars. For example, in 2012, $2.8 trillion was spent on healthcare, or $8,915 per person in the United States (Martin et al. 2014, 67). At this rate of increase, healthcare spending is projected to reach 19.6 percent of the gross domestic product (GDP) by 2019, up from 13.7 percent in 1993 (Sisko et al. 2010, 1937).

Over the past decade, the rate of increase has gradually decelerated. This slightly slowed rate of increase is shown by the decreasing percentage of increase per year (table 1.5). Primary factors in this slowing rate of increase are the effect of the economic recession and its modest recovery (Martin et al. 2014, 67). It should be

Table 1.5. Percentage increase in total national healthcare spending over time (selected years)

2002	2004	2006	2008	2010	2012
9.3%[a]	7.9%[b]	6.7%[c]	4.7%[d]	3.9%[e]	3.7%[f]

[a]Smith, C., et al. 2005. (January–February). Health spending slows in 2003. *Health Affairs* 24(1):185–194.

[b]Smith, C., Cowan, C., Heffler, S., and Catlin, A. 2006. (January–February). National health spending in 2004: Recent slowdown led by prescription drug spending. *Health Affairs* 25(1):186–196.

[c]Catlin, A., et al. 2008. (January–February). National health spending in 2006: A year of change for prescription drugs. *Health Affairs* 27(1):14–29.

[d]Martin, A., et al. 2011. (January–February). Recession contributes to slowest annual rate of increase in health spending in five decades. *Health Affairs* 30(1):11–22.

[e]Martin, A.B., et al. 2012. (January). Growth in US health spending remained slow in 2010; health share of gross domestic product was unchanged from 2009. *Health Affairs* 31(1):208–219.

[f]Martin, A.B., et al. 2014. (January). National health spending in 2012: Rate of health spending growth remained low for the fourth consecutive year. *Health Affairs* 33(1):67–77.

emphasized, however, that despite this deceleration, the trend of increasing healthcare expenditures continues.

Healthcare Reform

The belief that continued increases in healthcare spending are unsustainable keeps policy makers focused on the issue of healthcare reform. In addition, the economic crisis beginning in 2008 stimulated discussion of healthcare reform as a means to save money at multiple levels: federal and state governments, employers, and individuals. The exact parameters and framework of healthcare reform are an ongoing debate.

Background

The US health system has three core problems: excessive cost; unsafe, inequitable, and poor-quality care; and lack of access (Ricketts and Nielsen 2010, 214). The first problem is easily understood considering the discussion, earlier in this chapter, of ever-increasing healthcare spending. The second problem has been documented in reports of the Institute of Medicine (IOM). The third problem has also been reported by HHS and independent experts. Selected examples of the latter two problems are provided in the next few paragraphs.

Two reports from the IOM particularly highlighted unsafe and poor-quality care in the US health system. In its 2000 report *To Err Is Human*, the IOM reported that research studies had shown that between 44,000 and 98,000 people die per year as a result of medical errors (Institute of Medicine 2000, 1). More people died from medical errors than from motor vehicle accidents (43,458) or from breast cancer (42,297) (Institute of Medicine 2000, 1). The IOM's second landmark report, *Crossing the Quality Chasm*, showed that thousands of Americans frequently do *not* receive medical care to meet their needs or care based on the best scientific knowledge (Institute of Medicine 2001, 1). Per the report, "quality problems are everywhere and affecting many patients" (Institute of Medicine 2001, 1). More than a gap, a chasm exists between the care that Americans should receive and what they actually receive (Institute of Medicine 2001, 1). The two reports did affect the US healthcare delivery system. In the decade since the publication of *To Err Is Human*, healthcare organizations have slightly progressed in reducing harm and increasing patient safety (Wachter 2010, 172). Similarly, slight progress has been made in bridging the quality chasm. There are "pockets of excellence ... in particular services at individual health care facilities" (Chassin and Loeb 2011, 562). However, "maintaining consistently high levels of ... quality over time and across all health care services and settings" has eluded the health system (Chassin and Loeb 2011, 562).

International comparisons support the IOM's assessment of the US healthcare system's quality. Generally, Americans have shorter lives and poorer health than residents of many other high-income countries (Woolf and Aron 2013, 1). For example, experts reviewed reports and analyzed health-related data from several countries, including Australia, Canada, several European countries, New Zealand, and the United States (Avendano and Kawachi 2014, 308). The information was compiled from multiple international surveys on the health of countries' populations. The reports and analyses presented information on various dimensions of healthcare, such as quality, access, efficiency, equity, and healthy lives (Avendano and Kawachi 2014, 308; Davis et al. 2014, 7–9). In terms of overall quality, the performance of the US healthcare system is in the middle. For example, the US system ranks third in effective care and seventh in safe care. As indicated by these analyses, the US healthcare system, despite being the most expensive among these 11 countries, does not result in superior outcomes (Davis et al. 2014, 7–8, 13–15).

Health disparities represent an inequity in the US healthcare system. Health disparities are defined as "population-specific differences in the presence of disease, health outcomes, quality of healthcare and access to healthcare services—that exist across racial and ethnic groups" (National Conference of State Legislatures 2014, n.p.). Recently, the term "health inequities" has come into use as an alternative to the term "health disparities" (Adler and Stewart 2010, 6).

A significant body of research prompted Congress to request that the IOM assess the extent of racial and ethnic differences in healthcare and evaluate potential sources of these differences. The result was the IOM's 2003 report, *Unequal Treatment: Confronting Racial and Ethnic Disparities in Health Care* (Smedley et al. 2003, 3–4). Factors associated with health disparities are inadequate access to care, poor quality of care, genetics, residence in an **underserved area** or community, and personal behaviors (National Conference of State Legislatures 2014, n.p.). More recently, the IOM sponsored a workshop to assess progress in reducing disparities. The findings of the workshop were published in the IOM report, *How Far Have We Come in Reducing Health Disparities? Progress Since 2000: Workshop Summary* (Anderson 2012). A key theme of the workshop's participants was that health disparities are persistent and exist across people's entire lives. Moreover, "members of racial and ethnic minorities have access to a lower quality of healthcare services than majority group members" (Anderson 2012, 7).

Health disparities represent inefficiencies in the healthcare delivery system and result in unnecessary costs to all patients, providers, and payers (National Conference of State Legislatures 2014, n.p.). For example, using data from the Medical Expenditure Panel Survey and the National Vital Statistics Reports, health policy analysts calculated the unnecessary costs of men's health disparities. Specifically, they estimated the potential cost savings of eliminating health disparities for male racial and ethnic minorities. The total direct medical care expenditures "for African American men were $447.6 billion of which $24.2 billion was excess medical care expenditures" (Thorpe et al. 2013, 195). Additionally, estimated excess indirect costs to the U.S. economy due to health disparities for African American, Asian, and Hispanic men totaled $436.3 billion (Thorpe et al. 2013, 203). In summary, "disparities are unjust, unethical, costly, and unacceptable" (Betancourt et al.

2014, 144). Experts, conducting the previously described analysis of international data, found that Americans lack access to their healthcare system more than any other country in the report (Davis et al. 2014, 20). Per the report, "a higher percentage of people in the U.S. go without needed care because of cost than in any other surveyed nation. Americans were the most likely to say they had access problems because of cost" (Davis et al. 2014, 20). Lack of access to care can result from many factors (Adler and Stewart 2010, 11–12). One factor is a lack of healthcare insurance. People who lack healthcare insurance may be either uninsured (no insurance) or underinsured (inadequate insurance with limited benefits or very high premiums or other fees). Other factors include lack of transportation and language barriers.

Uncompensated care is healthcare organizations' total costs for unreimbursed services to medically indigent or underinsured patients and clients (American Hospital Association 2014, 2). No payments are received for these services from the patient, client, or third-party payer. Uncompensated care is the sum of the healthcare organization's **bad debts** and **charity care** (American Hospital Association 2014, 1). Bad debts are services for which healthcare organizations expected, but did not receive, payment (American Hospital Association 2014, 2). Charity care consists of services for which healthcare organizations did not expect payment because they had previously determined the patients' or clients' inability to pay (American Hospital Association 2014, 2). Uncompensated care represents a significantly *increasing* cost to healthcare organizations. For example, between 2011 and 2012, uncompensated care increased 11.7 percent, from $41.1 billion to $45.9 billion (American Hospital Association 2014, 3; ACA International n.d., n.p). Across all providers, health policy analysts estimated that uncompensated care in 2013 totaled between $74.9 billion and $84.9 billion (Coughlin et al. 2014, 807). Thus, providers across the continuum of care are bearing the significant costs of uncompensated care.

Affordable Care Act

In 2010, healthcare reform legislation passed the US Congress and was signed by President Barack Obama. This legislation was the **Patient Protection and Affordable Care Act of 2010 (P.L. 111–148)**, as amended by the **Health Care and Education Reconciliation Act of 2010 (P.L. 111–152)**. Collectively, these two acts are known as the **Affordable Care Act** (**ACA** or PPACA; sometimes they are erroneously referred to as the Accountable Care Act). Commonly the Affordable Care Act is known as "Obamacare."

Purposes

The ACA builds on existing systems to address the US health system's problems of excessive cost, poor quality, and lack of access (Silberman et al. 2011, 155). Therefore, the purposes of the ACA are to

- Decelerate the rate of increase in healthcare costs

- Improve population health, healthcare access, and healthcare quality (Silberman et al. 2011, 155)

Provisions

The Patient Protection and Affordable Care Act as amended by the Health Care and Education Reconciliation Act has 10 titles (chapters) (US Government Printing Office 2010a, 2010b). These 10 titles are subdivided into subtitles, parts (only occasionally), and sections. The number of subdivisions among the titles varies depending on the extent and complexity of the title's content. The requirements in the titles and their subdivisions are being phased in between 2010 and 2020 (National Rural Health Association, n.d.). Brief overviews of key points in the titles follow:

- Title I: Quality, Affordable Health Care for All Americans
  - Makes purchasing health insurance easier and more affordable for many people and small businesses.
  - Defines an essential benefits package (Kaiser Family Foundation 2011, 5). *Update: Specific coverage requirements were delayed by actions of federal agencies until 2016 (Redhead and Kinzer 2014b, 2).*
  - Requires most US citizens and legal residents to have health insurance (tax penalties for noncoverage begin in 2014). *Update: Penalties for noncoverage were delayed by actions of federal agencies until 2016 (Redhead and Kinzer 2014b, CRS-5).*
  - Extends health insurance benefits to dependent children up to age 26 (Kaiser Family Foundation 2011, 1, 4).

  - Includes premium and cost-sharing credits (subsidies) for eligible poor individuals and families.
  - Creates state-based health insurance exchanges (American Health Benefit Exchanges and Small Business Health Options Program—SHOP—Exchanges).
  - Strengthens the system of employer-based health insurance (assesses penalty against employers with 50 or more full-time employees who do not offer health insurance benefit beginning 2014). *Update: Penalties were delayed until 2015 by actions of federal agencies (Redhead and Kinzer 2014b, 2).*
  - Provides a tax credit to employers with less than 25 employees and average annual wages of less than $50,000 that purchase health insurance for employees (Kaiser Family Foundation 2011, 3).

- Title II: Role of Public Programs
  - Extends Medicaid coverage to uninsured people, such as low-income adults (up to 133 percent of federal poverty level) who had previously been excluded from Medicaid coverage (see chapter 4 for full discussion of Medicaid) (Kaiser Family Foundation 2011, 1; Silberman et al. 2011, 155). *Update: In June 2012, the Supreme Court ruled that the states' expansion of their Medicaid programs was optional, effectively minimizing the effect of this provision (Jacobs and Callaghan 2013, 1024).*
  - Requires states to maintain current income eligibility levels for children in Medicaid and Children's Health Insurance Program (CHIP) until 2019 and to extend funding for CHIP through 2015 (Kaiser Family Foundation 2011, 2).
  - Provides states new options for offering home and community health services through Medicaid (Kaiser Family Foundation 2011, 11).
  - Includes protections for American Indians and Alaska Natives.

- Title III: Improving the Quality and Efficiency of Health Care
  - Focuses on enhancing Medicare by improving quality and controlling costs.

- ° Links quality outcomes and payment across the continuum of care.
- ° Gradually closes gap (donut hole) for coverage of prescription drugs (closed in 2020) (Jackson 2010, 244).
- ° Expands Medicare coverage for screenings and preventive services (Jackson 2010, 244).
- ° Incrementally reduces higher payments of Medicare managed care until they equal fee-for-service payments (Jackson 2010, 243).
- ° Establishes, as an investigation into controlling costs, a national pilot program on payment bundling that includes inpatient physician services, outpatient hospital services, and postacute care services (Silberman et al. 2010, 228).
- ° Establishes a national strategy to improve the delivery of healthcare services, patient health, and population health, which includes redesignating the National Center on Minority Health and Health Disparities as the National Institute on Minority Health and Health Disparities (NIMHD) (National Institute on Minority Health and Health Disparities n.d.).
- ° Establishes a shared savings program through **accountable care organizations (ACOs)**. (ACOs are primary care–led physician and hospital organizations that voluntarily form networks.)
- ° ACOs provide coordinated care for at least 5,000 Medicare fee-for-service beneficiaries (Meyer 2011, 1227).
- ° ACOs "receive a share of the savings they produce for Medicare if they meet quality and cost targets" (Meyer 2011, 1227).

- Title IV: Prevention of Chronic Disease and Improving Public Health
  - ° Creates Prevention and Public Health Fund to expand prevention, wellness, and public health activities (funds increase from $500 million in 2010 to $2 billion in 2015) (Silberman et al. 2010, 226).
  - ° Includes initiatives related to improving population health, particularly as recommended by the US Preventive Services Task Force (Silberman et al. 2010, 226).
  - ° Supports innovation in prevention and public health, including data collection and analysis to understand health disparities.

- Title V: Health Care Workforce
  - ° Expands existing sections of the Public Health Service Act to further increase supply of health workforce (Ricketts and Walker 2010, 251).
  - ° Provides, through the Departments of Labor, Education, and Treasury, a combination of grants, loans, work-study, tax credits, and student loan forgiveness (Kaiser Family Foundation 2013b).
  - ° Establishes commission to coordinate supply and demand of health workforce (Ricketts and Walker 2010, 251).

- Title VI: Transparency and Program Integrity
  - ° Requires disclosure of ownership or investment interests.
  - ° Enhances federal integrity programs to eliminate fraud, waste, and abuse in Medicare, Medicaid, and the Children's Health Insurance Program.
  - ° Creates new research institute that evaluates and funds research that compares outcomes, effectiveness, and risks of medical treatments, services, drugs, and biological and medical devices (Silberman et al. 2010, 227).

- Title VII: Improving Access to Innovative Medical Therapies
  - ° Includes provision for approval of biosimilars (generic biological agents) and expands the affordable medicines program.

- Title VIII: CLASS (Community Living Assistance Services and Support) Act
  - ° Establishes a national, voluntary health insurance program for purchasing community living assistance and supports (Kaiser Family Foundation 2011, 11). *Update: the American Taxpayer Relief Act of 2013 repealed the CLASS Act prior to its implementation because of concerns about the program's long-term financial viability (Reaves and Musumeci 2014, 9).*

- Title IX: Revenue Provisions
  - Includes provisions that affect the Internal Revenue Code, such as excise taxes on high-cost, employer-based health insurance plans; inclusion on W-2 forms; use of health savings and flexible spending accounts; fees on health insurance providers; and hospital insurance tax on high-income taxpayers.

- Title X: Strengthening Quality, Affordable Care for All Americans
  - Is known as the **manager's amendment** (Slifkin 2010, 5).
  - Is a legislative mechanism in which a package of numerous, individual, previously agreed-upon amendments is added to a bill (Mandal 2007, 278).
  - With the Health Care and Education Reconciliation Act amends and supersedes the previous titles (Slifkin 2010, 5).

Implementation

The ACA is a comprehensive framework addressing the core problems of the healthcare sector. As some experts state, the ACA is "the most sweeping piece of healthcare legislation since the enactment of Medicare and Medicaid in 1965" (Silberman et al. 2010, 215). Yet the ACA is still a work in progress (Gorin 2011, 83; Silberman et al. 2011, 215). Federal agencies have been developing regulations to implement the ACA. Moreover, the details of these regulations will be worked out over several years. The ACA is not "perfect"; it "does not address all of our current health system woes" (Silberman et al. 2010, 230). Revisions should be expected as providers, analysts, and policy makers learn what works and what needs to be changed.

Full implementation of the healthcare reforms in the ACA is not ensured. The United States has a 90-year history of failure in healthcare reform (Fuchs 2009, W183). As early as 1912, President Theodore Roosevelt's Bull Moose Party had universal health insurance as a plank in its campaign platform (Cansler 2011, 152). Prior to President Obama, Presidents Franklin Roosevelt, Truman, Eisenhower, Kennedy, Johnson, Nixon, Carter, and Clinton have all participated in the national healthcare debate (Cansler 2011, 152).

A leading obstacle to healthcare reform is that Americans lack an understanding of their healthcare system. "Most Americans do not have a good understanding of how the health care system works, how the new legislation will affect them, which provisions will be implemented when, and how the expanding system will be financed" (Sparer 2011, 43). A second important obstacle is the sheer size and complexity of the US healthcare system. These characteristics make single, across-the-board changes difficult to implement without unintended consequences. Other experts also list "partisan bickering," obstructionism by special interest groups, and the public's fear of "big government" as potential obstacles (Cooper and Castle 2009, W170–W171). Other significant obstacles include the lingering economic recession, constitutional challenges—more than 80 in 2013 alone regarding contraceptive coverage, and lack of appropriations (funding) (Sobel and Salganicoff, 2013). Finally, since the enactment of the ACA, Republican members of the House of Representatives have passed multiple acts to defund, delay, and repeal it in its entirety, or some of its individual provisions (Redhead and Kinzer 2014a, 11–15).

Use of Health Information and Communication Technologies

Effective use of health information and communication technologies allows clinical data to follow patients throughout the continuum of care. This electronic flow of health information fosters coordination and efficiency in the delivery of health services. For example, the availability of key clinical data at the point-of-service may increase quality and reduce costs by preventing readmissions, improving diagnoses, reducing duplicate testing, and preventing medication errors (Walker et al. 2005, W5-13–W5-14; Frisse et al. 2012, 331). Thus the **meaningful use** of health information and communication technologies is thought to be key to coordinating health services.

In meaningful use, providers use health information and communication technologies to enter basic patient data, apply software programs to improve safety and quality, exchange health information, and submit quality and other measures. Experts therefore propose meaningful use as a way to improve the quality of care and to reduce its cost. However, in 2008 and 2009, a national survey of physicians revealed that only 4 percent had fully functional EHR systems and that only 13 percent had basic EHR systems (DesRoches et al. 2008, 50). Similarly, a national survey of hospitals revealed that only 1.5 percent of hospitals had comprehensive EHR systems and that a mere 7.6 percent had basic EHR systems (Jha et al. 2009, 1628). Little diffusion of health information and communication technologies existed.

To address this lack of significant diffusion, full implementation of health information and communication technologies became a national priority (Fleming et al. 2011, 481). Therefore, in 2009, as part of the American Reinvestment and Recovery Act (ARRA), Congress passed the Health Information Technology for Economic and Clinical Health (HITECH) Act. The HITECH Act promoted the adoption and use of EHRs and other health information and communication technologies. The ACA built upon the HITECH Act. The HITECH Act included $19.2 billion for health IT (Blumenthal 2009, 1477). Of the $19.2 billion, $17.2 billion was for financial incentives to physicians and hospitals. These incentives were processed through the federal reimbursement systems for physicians and hospitals. An additional $2 billion in grants and loans was administered through the Office of the National Coordinator (ONC) for Health Information Technology (Steinbrook 2009, 1058).

A core goal of the HITECH Act was to improve the quality and efficiency of healthcare by fostering the electronic flow of patients' data to the patients' sites of care (Williams et al. 2012, 527). An infrastructure to support the electronic flow and exchange of health information across healthcare organizations, such as hospitals and physician offices, is a health information exchange. To facilitate the establishment of health information exchanges, the HITECH Act provided grants to states to design health information exchanges (Adler-Milstein and Jha 2014, 26). Progress has been made in the diffusion of health information and communication technologies. In 2012, 44 percent of hospitals reported having and using at least a basic EHR system (DesRoches et al. 2013, 1478). In terms of the health information exchanges, a recent survey found that across all 50 states, 30 percent of medical–surgical, nonfederal hospitals shared data with providers not affiliated (not associated) with the hospital (Adler-Milstein and Jha 2014, 26). Participation in the exchanges was not evenly distributed across the states. Delaware, Indiana, New York, and Rhode Island had widespread participation, whereas Alaska, Minnesota, New Hampshire, North Dakota, and Wyoming had minimal participation. Thus, although progress has been made in implementing widespread use of

health information and communication technologies, the potential gains in quality, efficiency, and cost-effectiveness have yet to be fully realized.

Medical Tourism

Medical tourism dates to the ancient Greeks, who traveled to seek care from their god of medicine, Aesculapius (McGuire 2013, 496). More recently, outbound medical tourism has occurred in the United States for many years. However, the globalization of medical tourism is recent and its development rapid (Hopkins et al. 2010, 187).

Medical tourism is traveling across borders to receive healthcare. Other terms for medical tourism include health tourism and medical travel. Motivations for medical tourism include lower cost, avoidance of long wait times, or receipt of specialized services not locally available (Hopkins et al. 2010, 185). "The age of global comparison shopping for health services has arrived" (Turner 2010, 465).

From a US perspective, types of medical tourism include the following:

- Inbound: Patients coming from other countries to the United States to receive services at US healthcare organizations. Inbound tourists are primarily from the Middle East, South America, and Canada (Keckley and Underwood 2008, 19).

- Outbound: Patients leaving the United States to receive services in other countries' healthcare organizations. Four of the most common destinations are India, Costa Rica, Thailand, and Mexico (Alleman et al. 2011, 495; Larocco and Pinchera 2011, 27).

- Domestic: Patients leaving their local areas to receive healthcare services in other states. For many years, healthcare organizations, such as the Mayo Clinic, Johns Hopkins Health System, and the Cleveland Clinic, have been domestic medical tourist destinations (Fottler et al. 2014, 50, 52).

Inbound tourists typically come to US healthcare organizations for specialized medical or surgical care that is unavailable in their own countries and that requires inpatient hospitalization. Other primary reasons that medical tourists come to US healthcare organizations are to avoid long waiting periods and to access the organizations' high-quality health services (Keckley and Underwood 2008, 20). The most common types of care that US outbound tourists seek are orthopedic procedures, cardiac procedures, infertility services, and cosmetic surgery (Alleman et al. 2011, 495). Additionally, for dental procedures, US medical tourists visit Mexico (Larocco and Pinchera 2011, 27).

Few hard data exist on the size of the medical tourism market (Hopkins et al. 2010, 194). Based on estimations from the Deloitte Center for Health Solutions, outbound medical tourists are projected to increase from 6 million in 2010 to 15.75 million in 2017 (Keckley and Underwood 2008, 3, 14). Considering the increasing out-of-pocket costs for US consumers, outbound medical tourism may grow, as suggested by the Deloitte Center's estimates. US healthcare organizations, to offset the potential revenues lost to outbound tourism, have partnered with international healthcare organizations (Keckley and Underwood 2008, 16, 17). Inbound medical tourists represent 2 percent of users of US hospital services (Keckley and Underwood 2008, 19). Thus, inbound and domestic medical tourism is a burgeoning niche in the healthcare industry. Accordingly, this niche could be a new source of revenues for US healthcare organizations. Health personnel should monitor this trend because their organizational leaders may develop marketing initiatives to mine the potential revenue streams from inbound, outbound, or domestic tourists.

Transparency

Experts propose that the healthcare industry adopt a "transparency imperative" (Kocher and Emanual 2013, 296). A transparency imperative is needed for stakeholders to receive full value from the US healthcare system. These healthcare stakeholders include oversight entities, payers, purchasers, consumers, providers, and health-related organizations. The transparency imperative requires that "all data on price, utilization, and quality of healthcare should be made available to the public unless there is a compelling reason not to do so" (Kocher and Emanuel 2013, 296). Moreover, healthcare leaders agree with these experts. Per a Commonwealth Fund Survey, "transparency in health care—including collecting and reporting public information on the quality and price of healthcare services—is essential for moving toward a higher-performing healthcare system in the US" (Shea et al. 2007, 2).

The IOM describes healthcare **transparency** as

making available to the public, in a reliable and understandable manner, information on the healthcare system's quality, efficiency, and consumer experience with care, which includes price and quality data, so as to influence the behavior of patients, providers, payers, and others to achieve better outcomes, such as quality and cost of care (Kirschner 2010, 3; Institute of Medicine 2001, 8).

Healthcare transparency is sharing information about the cost and quality of healthcare with stakeholders, such as patients, consumers, and payers, so that they can make informed choices when selecting physicians, hospitals, insurance companies, and other health decisions (Arnold 2014, 79; Leavitt 2008, 12).

Healthcare transparency is not new, but its extent and importance are a current development. As early as 1863, Florence Nightingale published mortality rates for principal hospitals in England (Nightingale 1863, 3; Dehmer et al. 2014, 1239). More recently, each year, from 1987 through 1994, the CMS (then known as Health Care Financing Administration, HCFA) published a report on observed hospital-specific mortality rates for Medicare acute care hospitals and compared the rate to predicted rates obtained from modeling nationwide data (Cleves and Golden 1996, 40). Currently, CMS posts quality data on its Compare website for many types of healthcare organizations, such as acute care hospitals, nursing homes, home health agencies, and physicians (Centers for Medicare and Medicaid Services n.d.). In terms of cost and use data, in 2014, the CMS released detailed information on use and cost for more than 880,000 physicians and other health care providers (such as audiologists, physician assistants, and other health professionals) (Brennan et al. 2014, 99). This release "was unprecedented in its size and scope: it included nearly 10 million records accounting for more than $77 billion in Medicare payments" (Brennan et al. 2014, 99). In the three months after its release, the information, available at a CMS website, had been downloaded or accessed more than 300,000 times (Brennan et al. 2014, 99).

Quality, cost, and use are not the only issues affected by healthcare transparency. A policy paper from the American College of Physicians lists multiple other aspects, such as safety, efficiency, patients' experiences, professionalism (such as licensure, special certifications, and adverse legal actions), and potential financial conflicts of interest (Kirschner 2010, 4).

Many stakeholders believe that healthcare transparency has the potential to ultimately improve the delivery of healthcare (Dehmer et al. 2014, 1239). Accordingly, this trend merits the attention of health personnel.

Chapter 1 Review Quiz

1. Which one of the three models of healthcare delivery is used in the United States?

2. Why is the US federal government a dominant player in the healthcare sector?

3. Who are the first, second, and third parties in healthcare situations?

4. Compare the UCR and CPR payment systems.

5. Describe the two purposes of managed care.

6. Why have many insurers replaced retrospective health insurance plans with group plans such as HMOs and PPOs?

7. What are advantages of capitated payments for providers and payers?

8. How do third-party payers set per diem payment rates?

9. Describe the major benefits of episode-of-care reimbursement according to its advocates, as well as the major concerns about episode-of-care reimbursement expressed by its critics.

10. Why is the constant trend of increased national spending on healthcare a concern?

References

Aaron, H.J. 2003. The costs of health care administration in the United States and Canada—Questionable answers to a questionable question. *New England Journal of Medicine* 349(8):801–803.

ACA International, the Association of Credit and Collections Professionals. n.d. Hospitals' uncompensated care costs increased to $45.9 billion. http://www.acainternational.org/healthcaremarket-hospitals-uncompensated-care-costs-increased-to-459-billion-30841.aspx.

Adler, N.E., and J. Stewart. 2010. Health disparities across the lifespan: Meaning, methods, and mechanisms. *Annals of the New York Academy of Sciences* 1186(1):5–23.

Adler-Milstein, J., and A.K. Jha. 2014. Health information exchange among U.S. hospitals: Who's in, who's out, and why? *Healthcare* 2(1):26–32.

Alleman, B.W., T. Luger, H.S. Reisinger, R. Martin, M.D. Horowitz, and P. Cram. 2011. Medical tourism services available to residents of the United States. *Journal of General Internal Medicine* 26(5):492–497.

American Hospital Association. 2014. Uncompensated Hospital Care Cost Fact Sheet. http://www.aha.org/content/14/14uncompensatedcare.pdf.

Anderson, K.M. 2012. *How Far Have We Come in Reducing Health Disparities?: Progress Since 2000: Workshop Summary*. Washington, DC: National Academies Press.

Arnold, P. 2014. Quality and safety in high-reliability organizations. Chapter 3 in *Introduction to Quality and Safety Education for Nurses: Core Competencies*. Edited by Kelly, P., and B.A. Vottero, and C. Christie-McAuliffe. New York: Springer Publishing Company.

Avendano, M., and I. Kawachi. 2014. Why do Americans have shorter life expectancy and worse health than do people in other high-income countries? *Annual Review of Public Health* 35:307–325.

Betancourt, J.R., J. Corbett, and M.R. Bondaryk. 2014. Addressing disparities and achieving equity: cultural competence, ethics, and health-care transformation. *Chest* 145(1):143–148.

Blount, L.L., and J.M. Waters. 2001. *Managing the Reimbursement Process*, 3rd ed. Chicago: AMA Press.

Blumenthal, D. 2009. Stimulating the adoption of health information technology. *New England Journal of Medicine* 360(15):1477–1479.

Bowman, S. 2007. Severity-adjusted DRGs for FY08? CMS proposes DRG refinements based on severity of illness. *Journal of AHIMA* 78(7):16–20.

Brennan, N., P.H. Conway, and M. Tavenner. 2014 (July 10). The Medicare physician-data release—context and rationale. *New England Journal of Medicine* 371(2):99–101.

Calcagno, A. 2014. Medicare—the federal financial gorilla. *Vital Signs* 19(3):5. http://www.massmed.org/news-and-publications/vital-signs/vital-signs-march-2014-(pdf).

Cansler, L.M. 2011. North Carolina's preparation for gaining the benefits and meeting the requirements of national health care reform. *North Carolina Medical Journal* 72(2):152–154.

Catlin, A., C. Cowan, M. Hartman, and S. Heffler. 2008. National health spending in 2006: A year of change for prescription drugs. *Health Affairs* 27(1):14–29.

Centers for Medicare and Medicaid Services. n.d. Find Doctors, Providers, Hospitals, Plans & Suppliers. http://www.medicare.gov.

Chassin, M.R., and J.M. Loeb. 2011. The ongoing quality improvement journey: Next stop, high reliability. *Health Affairs* 30(4):559–568.

Cleves, M.A., and W.E. Golden. 1996 (April). Assessment of HCFA's 1992 Medicare hospital information report of mortality following admission for hip arthroplasty. *Health Services Research* 31(1):39–48.

Cooper, J., and M. Castle. 2009. Health reform: A bipartisan view. *Health Affairs* 28(2):W169–W172.

Coughlin, T.A., J. Holahan, K. Caswell, and M. McGrath. 2014. An estimated $84.9 billion in uncompensated care was provided in 2013; ACA payment cuts could challenge providers. *Health Affairs* 33(5):807–814.

Davis, K., K. Stremikis, D. Squires, and C. Schoen. 2014 (June). Mirror, mirror on the wall: How the performance of the U.S. health care system compares internationally. http://www.commonwealthfund.org/~/media/files/publications/fund-report/2014/jun/1755_davis_mirror_mirror_2014.pdf.

Dehmer, G.J., J.P. Drozda, R.G. Brindis, F.A. Masoudi, J.S. Rumsfeld, L.E. Slattery, and W.J. Oetgen. 2014 (April 8). Public Reporting of Clinical Quality Data. *Journal of the American College of Cardiology* 63(13):1239–1245.

DesRoches, C.M., E.G. Campbell, S.R. Rao, K. Donelan, T.G. Ferris, A. Jha, R. Kaushal, D.E. Ley, S. Rosenbaum, A.E. Shields, and D. Blumenthal. 2008. Electronic health records in ambulatory care—A national survey of physicians. *New England Journal of Medicine* 359(1):50–60.

DesRoches, C.M., D. Charles, M.F. Furukawa, M.S. Joshi, P. Kralovec, F. Mostashari, C. Worzala, A.K. Jha. 2013. Adoption of electronic health records grows rapidly, but fewer than half of US hospitals had at least a basic system in 2012. *Health Affairs* 32(8):1478–1485.

Fleming, N.S., S.D. Culler, R. McCorkle, E.R. Becker, and D.J. Ballard. 2011. The financial and nonfinancial costs of implementing electronic health records in primary care practices. *Health Affairs* 30(3):481–489.

Fottler, M.D., D. Malvey, Y. Asi, S. Kirchner, and N.A. Warren. 2014 (January–February). Can inbound and domestic medical tourism improve your bottom line? Identifying the potential of a U.S. tourism market. *Journal of Healthcare Management* 59(1):49–63.

France, G. 2008. The form and context of federalism: Meanings for health care financing. *Journal of Health Politics, Policy and Law* 33(4):649–705.

Frisse, M.E., K.B. Johnson, H. Nian, C.L. Davison, C.S. Gadd, K.M. Unertl, P.A. Turri, and Q. Chen. 2012. The financial impact of health information exchange on emergency department care. *Journal of the American Medical Informatics Association* 19(3):328–333.

Frogner, B.K., H.R. Waters, and G.F. Anderson. 2011. Comparative health systems. Chapter 4 in *Jonas & Kovner's Health Care Delivery in the United States*, 10th ed. Edited by Kovner, A.R., and J.R. Knickman. New York: Springer Publishing Company.

Fuchs, V.R. 2009. Health reform: Getting the essentials right. *Health Affairs* 28(2):W180–W183.

Gabel, J.R. 1999. Job-based health insurance, 1977–1998: The accidental system under scrutiny. *Health Affairs* 18(6):62–74.

Gorin, S.H. 2011. The Affordable Care Act: Background and analysis. *Health and Social Work* 36(2):83–86.

Health Care Cost Institute [HCCI]. 2015. *Introducing HCCI.* http://www.healthcostinstitute.org.

Holahan, J., and A. Ghosh. 2005. Understanding the recent growth in Medicaid spending, 2000–2003. *Health Affairs Suppl Web Exclusives*, W5-52–W5-62.

Hopkins, L., R. Labonte, V. Runnels, and C. Packer. 2010. Medical tourism today: What is the state of existing knowledge? *Journal of Public Health Policy* 31(2):185–198.

Institute of Medicine, Committee on Quality of Health Care in America. 2000. *To Err Is Human: Building a Safer Health System.* Washington, DC: National Academy Press.

Institute of Medicine, Committee on Quality of Health Care in America. 2001. *Crossing the Quality Chasm: A New Health System for the 21st Century.* Washington, DC: National Academy Press.

Jackson, B. 2010. Health reform impacts and improvements affecting Medicare beneficiaries. *North Carolina Medical Journal* 71(3):243–245.

Jacobs, L.R., and T. Callaghan. 2013. Why states expand Medicaid: party, resources, and history. *Journal of Health Politics, Policy & Law* 38(5):1023–1050.

Jha, A.K., C.M. DesRoches, E.G. Campbell, K. Donelan, S.R. Rao, T.G. Ferris, A. Shields, S. Rosenbaum, and D. Blumenthal. 2009. Use of electronic health records in U.S. hospitals. *New England Journal of Medicine* 360(16):1628–1638.

Jones, C.L., and T.L. Mills. 2006. Negotiating a contract with a health plan. *Family Practice Management* 13(10):49–55.

Kaiser Family Foundation. 2011. Summary of new health reform law. http://www.kff.org/healthreform/upload/8061.pdf.

Kaiser Family Foundation. 2013a. *Medicaid a Primer: Key Information on the Nation's Health Coverage Program for Low-Income People.* http://kff.org/medicaid/issue-brief/medicaid-a-primer/.

Kaiser Family Foundation. 2013b. Summary of the Affordable Care Act. http://kff.org/health-reform/fact-sheet/summary-of-the-affordable-care-act/.

Keckley, P.H., and H.R. Underwood. 2008. *Medical Tourism: Consumers in Search of Value.* http://www.deloitte.com/assets/Dcom-Croatia/Local%20Assets/Documents/hr_Medical_tourism.pdf

Kirschner, N. 2010. *Healthcare transparency-focus on price and clinical performance information.* Policy paper of the American College of Physicians. Philadelphia, PA: American College of Physicians. http://www.acponline.org/advocacy/current_policy_papers/assets/transparency.pdf.

Knickman, J.R. 2011. Health care financing. Chapter 3 in *Jonas & Kovner's Health Care Delivery in the United States*, 10th ed. Edited by Kovner, A.R., and J.R. Knickman. New York: Springer Publishing Company.

Koch, A. L. 2002. Financing health services. In *Introduction to Health Services*, 6th ed. Edited by S.J. Williams and P.R. Torrens. Albany, NY: Delmar.

Kocher, R.P., and E.J. Emanuel. 2013. The transparency imperative. *Annals of Internal Medicine* 159(4):296–297.

Kongstvedt, P.R. 2013. The provider network. Chapter 4 in *Essentials of Managed Health Care*, 6th ed. Edited by P.R. Kongstvedt. Burlington, MA: Jones and Bartlett Learning Company.

Kulesher, R., and E. Forrestal. 2014. International models of health systems financing. *Journal of Hospital Administration* 3(4):127–139.

Larocco, S.A., and B.J. Pinchera. 2011 (June). The emerging trend of medical tourism. *Nursing Management* 42(6):24–29.

Leavitt, M.O. 2008. Building a value-based health care system: Prologue series. http://archive.hhs.gov/secretary/prologueseries/buildingvaluehc.pdf.

Longest, B.B., and K. Darr. 2014. *Managing Health Services Organizations and Systems*, 6th ed. Baltimore, MD: Health Professions Press.

Lynn, G., and P.H. Kamp. 2014. Joining the payer world. *Trustee* 67(2):6–7.

Mandal, U.C. 2007. *Dictionary of Public Administration*. New Delhi, India: Sarup and Sons.

Martin, A., D. Lassman, L. Whittle, and A. Catlin. 2011. Recession contributes to slowest annual rate of increase in health spending in five decades. *Health Affairs* 30(1):11–22.

Martin, A.B., D. Lassman, B. Washington, and A. Catlin. 2012. Growth in US Health Spending Remained Slow in 2010; Health Share of Gross Domestic Product Was Unchanged from 2009. *Health Affairs* 31(1):208–219.

Martin, A.B., M. Hartman, L. Whittle, and A. Catlin. 2014. National health spending in 2012: Rate of health spending growth remained low for the fourth consecutive year. *Health Affairs* 33(1):67–77.

Mayes, R., and R.A. Berenson. 2006. *Medicare Prospective Payment and the Shaping of U.S. Health Care*. Baltimore, MD: Johns Hopkins University Press.

McGuire, M.F. International accreditation of ambulatory surgical centers and medical tourism. 2013. *Clinics in Plastic Surgery* 40(3):493–498.

Medicare Payment Advisory Committee. 2001. A report to the Congress: Reducing Medicare complexity and regulatory burden. http://www.medpac.gov/documents/contractor-reports/report-to-the-congress-reducing-medicare-complexity-and-regulatory-burden-(december-2001).pdf.

Medicare Payment Advisory Commission. 2013. Outpatient dialysis services payment system. http://www.medpac.gov/documents/payment-basics/outpatient-dialysis-services-payment-system.pdf?sfvrsn=0

Meyer, H. 2011. Accountable care organization prototypes: Winners and losers? *Health Affairs* 30(7):1227–1231.

Mitchell, A. 2014 (May 15). Congressional Research Service. Centers for Medicare and Medicaid Services: President's FY2015 Budget. Report R43446. http://fas.org/sgp/crs/misc/R43446.pdf

National Conference of State Legislatures. 2014. Health disparities overview. http://www.ncsl.org/default.aspx?tabid=14494.

National Institute on Minority Health and Health Disparities [NIMHD]. n.d. About NIMHD. http://www.nimhd.nih.gov/about/nimhdHistory.html

National Rural Health Association. n.d. Government Affairs, Health Reform and You. Health Care Reform Timeline. http://www.ruralhealthweb.org/go/left/government-affairs/health-reform-and-you/health-care-reform-timeline.

Nightingale, F. 1863. *Notes on Hospitals*. London, UK: Longman, Green, Longman, Roberts, and Green. https://archive.org/details/notesonhospital01nighgoog.

Reaves, E.L., and M. Musumeci. 2014. *Medicaid and Long-Term Services and Supports: A Primer*. http://kff.org/medicaid/report/medicaid-and-long-term-services-and-supports-a-primer/.

Redhead, C.S., and J. Kinzer. 2014a. Legislative Actions to Repeal, Defund, or Delay the Affordable Care Act. http://fas.org/sgp/crs/misc/R43289.pdf

Redhead, C.S., and J. Kinzer. 2014b. Implementing the Affordable Care Act: Delays, Extensions, and Other Actions Taken by the Administration. http://fas.org/sgp/crs/misc/R43474.pdf.

Ricketts, T.C., and C. Nielsen. 2010. What does health reform mean for North Carolina? *North Carolina Medical Journal* 71(3):214.

Ricketts, T.C., and E. Walker. 2010. Health reform and workforce. *North Carolina Medical Journal* 71(3):250–253.

Schoen, C., R. Osborn, D. Squires, M.M. Doty, R. Pierson, and S. Applebaum. 2010. How health insurance design affects access to care and costs, by income, in eleven countries. *Health Affairs* 29(12):2323–2334.

Sessions, S.Y., and A.S. Detsky. 2010. Washington, Ottawa, and health care reform: A tale of two capitals. *Journal of the American Medical Association* 303(2):2078–2079.

Shea, K.K., A. Shih, and K. Davis. 2007. Health care opinion leaders' views on the transparency of health care quality and price information in the United States. Commonwealth Fund Data Brief. http://www.commonwealthfund.org/~/media/files/publications/data-brief/2007/nov/health-care-opinion-leaders-views-on-the-transparency-of-health-care-quality-and-price-information-i/shea_hcoltransparencysurveydatabrief_1078-pdf.pdf.

Silberman, P., C.E. Liao, and T.C. Ricketts. 2010. Understanding health reform: A work in progress. *North Carolina Medical Journal* 71(3):215–231.

Silberman, P., L.M. Cansler, W. Goodwin, B. Yorkery, K. Alexander-Bratcher, and S. Schiro. 2011. Implementation of the Affordable Care Act in North Carolina. *North Carolina Medical Journal* 72(2):155–159.

Sisko, A.M., C.J. Truffer, S.P. Keehan, J.A. Poisal, M.K. Clemens, and A.J. Madison. 2010. National health spending projections: The estimated impact of reform through 2019. *Health Affairs* 29(1):1933–1941.

Slifkin, R. 2010. Healthcare reform update. Chapel Hill, NC. Council for Allied Health in North Carolina. http://www.med.unc.edu/ahs/cahnc/files/presentations/HealthCare%20Reform%20Update%2005-05-2010.pdf.

Smedley, B.D., A.Y. Stith, and A.R. Nelson, eds. 2003. Institute of Medicine Committee on Understanding and Eliminating Racial and Ethnic Disparities in Health Care. *Unequal Treatment: Confronting Racial and Ethnic Disparities in Health Care.* Washington, DC: National Academy Press.

Smith, C., C. Cowan, A. Sensenig, and A. Catlin. 2005. Health spending slows in 2003. *Health Affairs* 24(1):185–194.

Smith, C., C. Cowan, S. Heffler, and A. Catlin. 2006. National health spending in 2004: Recent slowdown led by prescription drug spending. *Health Affairs* 25(1):186–196.

Sobel, L., and A. Salganicoff. 2013 (December). Issue Brief. *A Guide to the Supreme Court's Review of the Contraceptive Coverage Requirement.* http://kaiserfamilyfoundation.files.wordpress.com/2013/12/8523-guide-to-the-supreme-courts-review-of-the-contraceptive-coverage-requirement1.pdf.

Sparer, M.S. 2011. Health policy and health reform. Chapter 2 in *Jonas & Kovner's Health Care Delivery in the United States*, 10th ed. Edited by Kovner, A.R., and J.R. Knickman. New York: Springer Publishing Company.

Steinbrook, R. 2009. Health care and the American Recovery and Reinvestment Act. *New England Journal of Medicine* 360(11):1057–1060.

Thorpe, R.L., P. Richard, J.V. Bowie, T.A. LaVeist, and D.J. Gaskin. 2013. Economic burden of men's health disparities. *International Journal of Men's Health* 12(3):195–212.

Turner, L. 2010. Medical tourism and the global marketplace in health services: U.S. patients, international hospitals, and the search for affordable health care. *International Journal of Health Services* 40(3):443–467.

U.S. Government Printing Office. 2010a. Public Law 111-152—Health Care and Education Reconciliation Act of 2010. http://www.gpo.gov/fdsys/pkg/PLAW-111publ152/content-detail.html.

U.S. Government Printing Office. 2010b. Public Law 111-148—Patient Protection and Affordable Care Act of 2010. http://www.gpo.gov/fdsys/pkg/PLAW-111publ148/html/PLAW-111publ148.htm.

Wachter, R.M. 2010. Patient safety at ten: Unmistakable progress, troubling gaps. *Health Affairs* 29(1):165–173.

Walker, J., E. Pan, D. Johnston, J. Adler-Milstein, D.W. Bates, and B. Middleton. 2005. The value of health care information exchange and interoperability. *Health Affairs* 24 (Suppl Web Exclusives):W5-10–W5-18.

Washburn, E.R. 1999. The coming medical apocalypse. *Physician Executive* 25(1):34–39.

Williams, C., F. Mostashari, K. Mertz, E. Hogin, and P. Atwal. 2012. From the Office of the National Coordinator: The strategy for advancing the exchange of health information. *Health Affairs* 31(3):527–536.

Woolf, S.H., and L. Aron, eds. 2013. *U.S. Health in International Perspective: Shorter Lives, Poorer Health.* Washington, DC: National Academies Press.

Wouters, A., S. Bennett, and C. Leighton. 1998. Alternative payment methods: Incentives for improving health care delivery. *PHR Primer for Policymakers.* http://www.phrplus.org/Pubs/pps1.pdf.

Other resources

Agency for Healthcare Quality and Research. 2015. National Healthcare Quality & Disparities Reports. http://www.ahrq.gov/research/findings/nhqrdr/index.html.

Chapter 2
Clinical Coding and Coding Compliance

Objectives

- To differentiate the different code sets approved by the Health Insurance Portability and Accountability Act of 1996

- To describe the structure of approved code sets

- To examine coding compliance issues that influence reimbursement

- To explain the roles of various Medicare improper payment review entities

Key Terms

Abuse
AHA Coding Clinic for ICD-9-CM
AHA Coding Clinic for ICD-10-CM and ICD-10-PCS
AHA Coding Clinic for HCPCS
AHIMA Standards of Ethical Coding
Balanced Budget Act (BBA) of 1997
Benchmarking
Category I code (CPT)
Category II code (CPT)
Category III code (CPT)
Centers for Medicare and Medicaid Services (CMS)
Classification system
Coding compliance plan
Compliance
Compliance officer
Compliance Program Guidance
Comprehensive Error Rate Testing (CERT) program
CPT Assistant
Current Procedural Terminology (CPT)
False Claims Act
Fraud
Healthcare Common Procedure Coding System (HCPCS)

Health Insurance Portability and Accountability Act (HIPAA) of 1996
ICD-10-CM Coordination and Maintenance Committee
Improper payment reviews
International Classification of Diseases, Ninth Revision, Clinical Modification (ICD-9-CM)
International Classification of Diseases, Tenth Revision, Clinical Modification (ICD-10-CM)
International Classification of Diseases, Tenth Revision, Procedure Coding System (ICD-10-PCS)
Medicare administrative contractor (MAC)
Medicare integrity program
Modifier
Mortality
National Center for Health Statistics (NCHS)
Office of Inspector General (OIG)
Office of Inspector General Workplan
Operation Restore Trust
Recovery Audit Contractor (RAC)
World Health Organization (WHO)

The Clinical Coding–Reimbursement Connection

Simply put, reimbursement is payment to healthcare providers and facilities for services rendered to patients. Communication of the services provided is transmitted from the provider to the third-party payer, public or private, via coded information. Using standardized coding systems allows for a stable and efficient payment process. Payment methodologies and systems used to determine coverage of services and supplies vary, but the code sets used remain constant across all the different healthcare settings.

One need not be a coding expert per se to be able to understand healthcare reimbursement. However, just using the designated code set is not enough. Physicians and healthcare facilities will receive accurate reimbursement for the services they render to patients only if claims submitted comply with the guidelines and conventions published for the various clinical coding sets. To fully understand the intricate workings of the various Medicare prospective payment systems (PPSs) and private payer systems, baseline knowledge of the approved code sets and their functionality is essential. The **Health Insurance Portability and Accountability Act (HIPAA) of 1996** designated the code sets for healthcare services reporting to public and private insurers. The HIPAA-compliant code sets are listed in table 2.1.

The *International Classification of Diseases*

HIPAA designates the ***International Classification of Diseases, Clinical Modification* (ICD)** to report diagnoses in all healthcare settings and procedures for inpatient encounters (table 2.1). The ICD coding and **classification system** is used throughout the world

Table 2.1. HIPAA-designated code sets

Provider	Inpatient		Outpatient	
	Diagnosis	Procedure	Diagnosis	Procedure
Physician	ICD*	CPT	ICD	CPT
Facility	ICD	ICD	ICD	HCPCS (CPT and HCPCS Level II)

*The clinical modification version in current use is ICD-9-CM; ICD-10-CM/PCS is expected to be implemented on October 1, 2015, barring any legislative action from Congress amending the implementation date.

for **mortality** reporting. ICD is maintained by the **World Health Organization (WHO)** and is updated approximately every 10 years.

ICD-10-CM/PCS

The current international version of ICD is in the 10th revision and is referred to as ICD-10. The United States, however, adopted the ninth revision of ICD (ICD-9), modified it clinically, and continues to use it as the method for communicating diagnoses and inpatient procedures for public and private reimbursement systems. However, on Friday, January 16, 2009, the US Department of Health and Human Services (DHHS) published a final rule for the adoption of ICD-10-CM and ICD-10-PCS code sets to replace the ICD-9-CM code sets under rules 45 CFR Parts 160 and 162 of HIPAA. The effective date for the use of ICD-10-CM and ICD-10 procedure coding system (ICD-10-PCS) is no sooner than October 1, 2015. The new structure of ICD-10-CM will provide greater detail and granularity that will allow more accurate code submission. This not only benefits healthcare facilities, but also will allow payers to better measure quality outcomes and expand pay-for-reporting and pay-for-performance programs. The new format for ICD-10-PCS is very different from the ICD-9-CM Volume 3 format and will allow the United States to realize benefits of interoperability standards specified by the Healthcare Information Technology Standards Panel (HITSP). In addition, the new procedure classification system allows for all procedures to be coded and reported with limited use of "not elsewhere classified" options. The final rule, HIPAA Administrative Simplification: Modifications to Medical Data Code Set Standards to Adopt ICD-10-CM and ICD-10-PCS, can be downloaded for review from http://edocket.access.gpo.gov/2009/pdf/E9-743.pdf.

The clinical modification (CM) of ICD-10 was developed by the **National Center for Health Statistics (NCHS)** and is slated for implementation in 2015. Although the international version of ICD focuses on acute illnesses and mortality, ICD-10-CM was expanded to include morbidity or chronic conditions and procedure reporting. ICD-10-PCS was developed by CMS to provide a new methodology and code structure for reporting procedures in the United States. There are several new features in ICD-10-CM that will allow for a greater level of specificity and clinical detail than ICD-9-CM, such as laterality, additional combination codes, and expanded code categories

(Casto 2015). There are many benefits to transitioning to ICD-10-CM and ICD-10-PCS, which will allow for more precise capture of healthcare data:

- Improved ability to measure heath care service, including quality and safety data

- Augmented sensitivity when refining grouping and reimbursement methodologies

- Expanded ability to conduct public health surveillance

- Decreased need to include supporting documentation with claims

- Strengthened ability to distinguish advances in medicine and medical technology

- Enhanced detail on socioeconomic, family relationships, ambulatory care conditions, problems related to lifestyle, and the results of screening tests

- Increased use of administrative data to evaluate medical processes and outcomes, to conduct biosurveillance, and to support value-based purchasing initiatives (AHA 2015)

The clinical modification of ICD has several uses:

- Classifying morbidity and mortality information for statistical purposes

- Classifying diagnosis and procedure information for epidemiological and clinical research

- Indexing hospital records by disease and surgical procedure

- Reporting information to various healthcare reimbursement systems

- Analyzing resource consumption patterns

- Analyzing adequacy of reimbursement for health services (AHA 2004)

Providers use the clinical modification of ICD coding to determine payment categories for various PPSs, including the following:

- Hospital inpatient: Medicare-severity diagnosis-related groups (MS-DRGs)

- Hospital rehabilitation: case-mix groups (CMGs)

- Long-term care: long-term care Medicare-severity diagnosis-related groups (LTC-MS-DRGs)

- Home health: home health resource groups (HHRGs)

Structure of ICD-10-CM

ICD-10-CM contains two volumes:

- The Tabular List of Diseases and Injuries

- The Alphabetic Index to Diseases

Table 2.2 lists the contents of each volume.

Table 2.2.   ICD-10-CM codebook structure

Volume 1—Tabular List of Diseases and Injuries	Volume 2—Alphabetic Index to Diseases
Classification of Diseases and Injuries	Index to Diseases and Injuries
	Table of Neoplasms
	Table of Drugs and Chemicals
	External Cause of Injuries Index

ICD-10-CM diagnosis codes vary in length from three to seven characters, with a decimal point placed after the third character. The first three characters are a category code. The fourth and fifth characters are subcategory codes that provide the specificity necessary to accurately describe a patient's clinical condition. Some codes have a seventh character to further describe the circumstances of the condition. If a code requires a seventh character and is not six characters in length, a placeholder X must be used to fill in the empty character slot (figure 2.1).

Figure 2.1.   ICD-10-CM diagnosis code structure

S10.11XA	
S10	Superficial injury of neck
S10.1	Other and unspecified superficial injuries of throat
S10.11	Abrasion of throat
S10.11XA	Abrasion of throat, initial encounter

Structure of ICD-10-PCS

ICD-10-PCS contains four sections: Index, Tables, Code Listings, and Appendices. ICD-10-PCS has a logical, consistent code structure. Coders use the index to locate the appropriate table for code selection, using

Figure 2.2.   02BG0ZX Excision of mitral valve, open approach, diagnostic

Character 1	Character 2	Character 3	Character 4	Character 5	Character 6	Character 7
Section	Body System	Operation	Body Part	Approach	Device	Qualifier
0	2	B	G	0	Z	X
Medical and Surgical	Heart and Great Vessels	Excision	Mitral Valve	Open	No Device	Diagnostic

the procedure's root operation as the main term. The first three characters of the code identify the table to be used for code assignment. After the table is identified, codes must be constructed by choosing accurate values to complete the seven-character code. The spaces of the code are called characters and are filled with individual letters and numbers called values (figure 2.2).

Using the example in figure 2.2, the procedure is an excision (partial removal) of the mitral valve. Using the index, the coder would locate the main term "Excision" and subterm "Valve" to see that the table to be used to construct the code is Table 02B. The coder would review the value choices for the remaining four characters in Table 02B and make the final determination based on the medical record documentation in the health record.

Maintenance of ICD-10-CM/PCS

The **ICD-10-CM/PCS Coordination and Maintenance Committee**, composed of NCHS and the **Centers for Medicare and Medicaid Services (CMS)**, is responsible for maintaining the US clinical modification version of the code set. NCHS makes determinations regarding diagnosis issues, whereas CMS maintains the procedures. Advisory in nature, the committee was created in 1985 to discuss possible updates and revisions to ICD-9-CM. It has transitioned to the maintenance of ICD-10-CM/PCS. Final determinations are made by the director of the NCHS and the administrator of the CMS.

The committee holds public meetings every year in March and September, and suggestions for new codes, modifications, and deletions are submitted by members of both public and private sectors. Proposals for code changes are submitted before the semiannual meetings and include a description of the diagnosis or procedure and rationale for the requested modification. Supporting references, literature, statistics, and cost information may also be submitted. Requests must follow industry-accepted ICD-10-CM/PCS coding conventions. Each year after the December meeting, the committee determines code modifications to become

effective October 1 of the following year. In addition, CMS has the option to add new codes in April every year. This additional opportunity was added to address healthcare community concerns about limitations of code maintenance. Meeting materials and proposals for diagnosis issues are located on the NCHS portion of the Centers for Disease Control and Prevention website (http://www.cdc.gov). Meeting materials and proposals for procedure issues are located on the CMS website (http://www.cms.hhs.gov).

ICD-10-CM and ICD-10-PCS Coding Guidelines

Because ICD-10-CM/PCS codes serve as the communication vehicle between providers and insurers, it is vital to follow ICD-10-CM/PCS guidelines at all times. Accurate reimbursement depends on timely, accurate, and complete coding of the services and procedures provided to beneficiaries. The Official Coding Guidelines for ICD-10-CM are available for download from the NCHS website. The Official Coding Guidelines for ICD-10-PCS are available for download from the CMS website. Additionally, the Cooperating Parties—NCHS, CMS, American Hospital Association (AHA), and American Health Information Management Association (AHIMA)—and the Editorial Advisory Board are responsible for publishing additional coding guidelines for ICD-10-CM/PCS. These additional coding guidelines are published by the AHA in *Coding Clinic for ICD-10-CM and ICD-10-PCS*, the only official publication for ICD-10-CM/PCS coding guidelines and advice. *Coding Clinic* is published quarterly and includes the following information (AHA 2015):

- Official coding advice and official coding guidelines

- Correct code assignments for new technologies and newly identified diseases

- Articles and topics that offer practical information and improve data quality

- Conduit for disseminating coding changes and corrections to hospitals and other parties

- "Ask the Editor" questions addressed using practical examples

Coding Clinic should be a component of all coding education and **compliance** programs for healthcare provider and facility coding units.

Healthcare Common Procedure Coding System

The **Healthcare Common Procedure Coding System (HCPCS)** is a two-tiered system of procedural codes used primarily for ambulatory care and physician services. A third tier, pertaining to codes developed by local payers, was eliminated as of December 31, 2003, in compliance with HIPAA standard procedure code requirements. HCPCS codes are frequently attached to inpatient and outpatient charge description masters (CDMs) for convenience and to facilitate communication between providers and payers about services and supplies included in the CPT or HCPCS Level II system.

CPT (HCPCS Level I)

Current Procedural Terminology (CPT) is used throughout the United States to report diagnostic and surgical services and procedures. Created and first published by the American Medical Association (AMA) in 1966, CPT was designed to be a means of effective and dependable communication among physicians, patients, and third-party payers (LaTour and Eichenwald 2013, 393). The terminology provides a uniform coding scheme that accurately describes medical, surgical, and diagnostic services. The CPT coding system is used by physicians to report services and procedures performed in the hospital inpatient and outpatient setting and by facilities for outpatient services and procedures (table 2.1). CPT has several uses:

- Communication vehicle for public and private reimbursement systems

- Development of guidelines for medical care review

- Basis for local, regional, and national use comparisons

- Medical education and research

The code set was adopted into HCPCS in 1985 and became the HCPCS Level I code set for Medicare

reporting, so CPT is referred to as HCPCS Level I as well as CPT in the coding and reimbursement communities.

Structure of CPT

The terminology is divided into six main sections, known as **Category I codes**, plus two types of supplementary codes (**Category II** and **Category III codes**), and **modifiers**.

Category I CPT codes consist of the following six sections:

- Evaluation and Management

- Anesthesia

- Surgery

- Radiology

- Pathology and Laboratory

- Medicine

The Surgery section is further divided as follows:

Integumentary System	10021 to 19499
Musculoskeletal System	20005 to 29999
Respiratory System	30000 to 32999
Cardiovascular System	33010 to 39599
Digestive System	40490 to 49999
Urinary System	50010 to 53899
Male Genital System	54000 to 55980
Female Genital System	56405 to 58999
Maternity Care and Delivery	59000 to 59899
Endocrine System	60000 to 60699
Nervous System	61000 to 64999
Eye and Ocular Adnexa	65091 to 68899
Auditory System	69000 to 69979
Operating Microscope	69990

Table 2.3 contains a listing of the top 10 CPT codes reported to Medicare in 2010.

Each of the three code categories in the CPT coding system serves a different and unique purpose.

Category I codes describe a procedure or service that is consistent with contemporary medical practice and that is performed by many physicians in clinical practice in multiple locations (Beebe 2003, 84). The specific use of devices and drugs for all services in this category must be approved by the US Food and Drug Administration (FDA). Category I codes are represented by a five-character numeric code.

Within Category I codes there are unlisted codes. Unlisted codes are used to report services and

Table 2.3. CPT codes

Medicare Top 10 Procedures by Unit of Service—CY 2013	
36415	Routine venipuncture
85025	Complete CBC
80053	Comprehensive metabolic panel
85610	Prothrombin time
80048	Metabolic panel, total calcium
80061	Lipid panel
93005	Electrocardiogram, tracing
84484	Assay of troponin, quantitative
99213	Established outpatient visit level 3
85027	Blood count; complete (CBC), automated

Adapted from Hospital Outpatient Prospective Payment System (OPPS) 2013 data set provided by Health Policy Analytics, LLC.

procedures that are not represented by an existing code. Typically, unlisted codes are used for new or innovative procedures that have not been added to the CPT coding system. When an unlisted code is reported, supporting documentation should be submitted to the third-party payer to establish correct coding and medical necessity for that service.

Category II codes were created to facilitate data collection for certain services and to test results that contribute to positive health outcomes and high-quality patient care (Beebe 2003, 84). This category of codes is a set of optional tracking codes for performance measurement. The services included in this category are often part of the Evaluation and Management service or other component part of a service. Category II codes have been implemented to help medical practices and facilities reduce operational costs by replacing time-consuming medical record documentation reviews and surveys with this streamlined code tracking system (Beebe 2003, 84). Use of Category II codes is optional, and they may not be used as substitutes for Category I codes. Category II codes are represented by a five-character alphanumeric code with the alpha character F in the last position—for example, (1234F).

Category III codes represent emerging technologies. This category of codes was created to help facilitate data collection and assessment of new services and procedures (Beebe 2003, 85). To qualify for inclusion in this category, a service or procedure must have relevance for research, either ongoing or planned. Like

Category II codes, Category III codes are represented by an alphanumeric five-character code with the alpha character T in the last field—for example, (1234T).

In addition to the three categories of codes, CPT contains modifiers for use by physicians and other healthcare providers. A modifier is a two-character numeric or alphanumeric character designed to give Medicare and other third-party payers additional information needed to process a claim. A physician or facility uses a modifier to flag a service provided to a patient that has been altered by some special circumstance(s) but for which the basic code description itself has not changed. Following are common reasons to use a modifier (AMA 2005, xiv):

- A service or procedure has been increased or reduced.
- Only part of a service was performed.
- A bilateral procedure was performed.
- A service or procedure was performed more than once.
- Unusual events occurred during a procedure or service.

Medical record documentation must support the use of a modifier because the modifier may change the reimbursement for the service or procedure. For example, modifier 91 is used to indicate that a clinical laboratory test was repeated. Rules governing the usage of this modifier specify that it may not be used when an equipment or testing failure has occurred, but rather only when the test has been reordered to determine whether a change in the result has occurred. Accordingly, using modifier 91 relays to the third-party payer that the duplicate code reported was not accidental or fraudulent but instead was correct, and that the physician ordered the test twice based on medically necessary foundations. However, failure to have supporting documentation in the medical record that establishes medical necessity can result in claim denials and fraud or abuse penalties.

Maintenance of CPT

The CPT Editorial Research and Development Department supports the modification process for the code set. A 16-member CPT Editorial Panel meets four times yearly to consider proposals for changes to CPT. The Editorial Panel is supported by the CPT Advisory Committee, which comprises representatives of more than 90 medical specialty societies and other healthcare professional organizations. To stay current with new technologies and pioneering procedures, CPT is revised each year, with changes going into effect the following January 1.

Requesting a Code Modification for CPT

CPT coding modifications are submitted to the CPT Editorial Research and Development Department at the AMA. The Coding Change Request Form found on the AMA website (http://www.ama-assn.org) must be used and submitted along with supporting documentation and clinical vignettes. A coding modification may be requested for all three categories of codes. After the Coding Change Request Form is received, it is reviewed for completeness by the AMA staff. If the form is complete, Coding Change Request Forms for Category I and Category III codes are forwarded to the CPT Advisory Committee for a detailed review.

Coding Change Request Forms for Category II CPT Codes are sent to the Performance Measurement Advisory Group for review. These requests must receive a two-thirds majority opinion from the advisory group before they are passed on to the CPT Advisory Committee. The AMA established the Performance Measurement Advisory Group to help create and maintain the performance measurement codes (Beebe 2003, 84). The group consists of representatives from various organizations, AMA's CPT and clinical quality improvement staffs, the CPT Editorial Panel, health services researchers, and other knowledgeable experts.

After review by the CPT Advisory Committee, those requests that warrant final review are submitted to the CPT Editorial Panel responsible for final decisions on all coding modifications (AMA 2004). A calendar for code submission deadlines and regular meetings for the CPT Advisory Committee and the CPT Editorial Panel is posted on the AMA website.

CPT Coding Guidelines

The AMA provides several resources regarding the appropriate use of CPT. The official publication for CPT coding issues and guidance is *CPT Assistant* (AMA 1989–2014). *CPT Assistant* contains the following helpful features:

- Coding communication that provides up-to-date information on codes and trends

- Clinical vignettes that offer insight into confusing coding and modifier usage scenarios

- Coding consultation that covers the most frequently asked questions

All coding education and compliance programs should include the use of *CPT Assistant*.

HCPCS Level II

HCPCS was developed by CMS in the 1980s to report services, supplies, and procedures not represented in the CPT (HCPCS Level I) code set but submitted for reimbursement (CMS 2004a). The descriptions identify items or services rather than specific brand names and do not endorse any manufacturer. This alphanumeric code set is a standardized coding system that provides an established environment for claims submission and processing. The system is managed by both private and public health insurers. The existence of a particular code does not guarantee or indicate coverage/reimbursement by Medicare, Medicaid, or other third-party payers. There are two types of codes within the HCPCS Level II system: permanent and temporary.

HCPCS Level II Permanent Codes

HCPCS Level II permanent codes may be used by all public and private health insurers. Permanent codes are alphanumeric, with five characters with an alpha character in the first position—for example, A2345. The alpha character designates the category to which the code is classified. Table 2.4 lists the categories of permanent HCPCS codes.

Within the permanent codes are "miscellaneous/not otherwise classified" codes. These codes enable suppliers and healthcare providers to report items/services that have not been incorporated into the coding system but that nonetheless have been approved for marketing by the FDA (CMS 2004a). Miscellaneous codes are manually reviewed and must be submitted with accompanying pricing and documentation of medical necessity.

Current Dental Terminology (CDT4), commonly known as dental codes, constitutes a separate category of national permanent codes. The codes are copyrighted and maintained by the American Dental Association (ADA). Dental codes are easily identified: because they begin with the letter D.

HCPCS Level II Temporary Codes

HCPCS Level II temporary codes are used to meet the immediate and short-term operational needs of individual insurers, public and private (CMS 2004a).

Table 2.4.   Permanent HCPCS codes

Permanent Code Categories	Covers	Insurers
A codes	Ambulance and transportation services, medical and surgical supplies, administrative, and miscellaneous and investigational services and supplies	All payers
B codes	Enteral and parenteral therapy	All payers
D codes	Dental	All payers
E codes	Durable medical equipment	All payers
J codes	Drugs that cannot ordinarily be self-administered, chemotherapy, immunosuppressive drugs, inhalation solutions	All payers
L codes	Orthotic and prosthetic procedures and devices	All payers
M codes	Office services and cardiovascular and other medical services	All payers
P codes	Pathology and laboratory services	All payers
R codes	Diagnostic radiology	All payers
V codes	Vision, hearing, and speech-language pathology services	All payers

Table 2.5.   Temporary HCPCS codes

Temporary Code Categories	Covers	Insurers
C codes	Items that may qualify for pass-through payment under HOPPS	Medicare hospital outpatient claims
G codes	Professional healthcare procedures and services	Medicare hospital outpatient claims
Q codes	Drugs, biological agents, medical equipment	Medicare hospital outpatient claims
K codes	Durable medical equipment	DMERCs—durable medical equipment regional carriers
S codes	Drugs, services, and supplies	BCBSA and AHIP and Medicaid
H codes	Mental health services	State Medicaid agencies
T codes	Items for which there are no permanent national codes	State Medicaid agencies and private insurers

Table 2.6.   HCPCS Level II codes

Medicare Top 10 Services, Procedures, or Supplies by Unit of Service—CY 2013	
Code	Description
J2405	Injection ondansetron hydrochloride
J3010	Injection fentanyl citrate
J2250	Injection, midazolam HCl
Q9967	LOCM 300–399 mg/mL iodine
G0378	Hospital observation per hour
J7030	Normal saline solution infusion
J1644	Injection, heparin sodium
J0690	Injection cefazolin sodium
J1170	Injection hydromorphone
J2270	Injection, morphine sulfate

Adapted from Hospital Outpatient Prospective Payment System (OPPS) 2013 data set provided by Health Policy Analytics, LLC.

Temporary codes are also alphanumeric, with five characters and an alpha character in the first position. As in permanent codes, the alpha character designates the category to which the code is classified. Table 2.5 lists the categories of temporary HCPCS codes. Temporary codes may remain so indefinitely. However, if deemed necessary, a permanent code will be created to replace the temporary code, and the temporary code will then be deleted. The top 10 HCPCS codes reported to Medicare in 2010 are found in table 2.6.

HCPCS Level II Modifiers

Like CPT, HCPCS Level II allows for modifiers. HCPCS Level II modifiers are two-character alpha or alphanumeric codes. A modifier is designed to give Medicare and other third-party payers additional information needed to process a claim. Many HCPCS Level II modifiers indicate body areas that allow for specific information to be provided to third-party payers. Table 2.7 provides examples of HCPCS Level II modifiers.

Maintenance of HCPCS Level II Coding System

Permanent codes are maintained jointly by America's Health Insurance Plans (AHIP), the Blue Cross and Blue Shield Association (BCBSA), and CMS. Together these organizations comprise the National Panel (CMS 2004a). Permanent National Codes are updated annually every January 1. Temporary codes, which make up 35 percent of HCPCS Level II codes, are

Table 2.7.   HCPCS Level II modifier examples

HCPCS Level II Modifiers	
LT	Left side
RT	Right side
E1	Upper left, eyelid
F1	Left hand, second digit

maintained by the individual members of the National Panel rather than by the group (CMS 2004a). For example, the HCPCS Workgroup, a part of the CMS workgroup, makes the decisions about temporary codes for Medicare. Temporary codes can be added, changed, or deleted on a quarterly basis.

Requesting a Code Modification for HCPCS Level II

There are three types of coding modifications to HCPCS Level II codes that users can request: a code may be added to the code set, the language used to describe an existing code may be changed, and an existing code may be deleted. The HCPCS Level II coding review process is a continual process. The review cycle runs from April 2 through the following April 1.

Requests for code changes may be submitted any time during the year. The proper request format can be found on the CMS website (http://www.cms.hhs.gov). Requests for coding modifications are submitted to the Alpha-Numeric HCPCS Coordinator at the CMS. After a request is submitted, it is reviewed by the CMS HCPCS Workgroup at one of its regular monthly meetings. After considering the request, the HCPCS Workgroup will make a recommendation to the HCPCS National Panel. The HCPCS Workgroup may also create a temporary Medicare national code pending the National Panel action. The HCPCS Workgroup's recommendations usually fall into one of the following categories:

- Add a code
- Use an existing code that describes the item or service
- Use an existing code for miscellaneous items or services
- Revise an existing code
- Delete an existing code

The National Panel is responsible for approving all coding modifications. All three members of the National Panel must agree on all requests before a change may be made. After the decision is made regarding a request, the panel will send a decision letter to the requester. If the requester is unsatisfied with the decision, a new request with new supporting information may be submitted for reconsideration and evaluation (CMS 2004a).

HCPCS Level II Coding Guidelines

AHA Coding Clinic for HCPCS is a resource newsletter that provides coding advice for the users of HCPCS Level II. This quarterly newsletter was first introduced in March 2001 and is published by the Central Office of ICD-9-CM. The newsletter includes an "Ask the Editor" section providing actual examples, correct code assignment for new technologies, articles, and a bulletin of coding changes and corrections (AHA 2004). Although this is not official coding guidance, it is expert. There is no official coding resource for HCPCS Level II other than coverage determinations issued by CMS and its **Medicare administrative contractors (MACs)**. MACs contract with Medicare to process claims for a specific area or region. The MAC determines costs and reimbursement amounts, conducts reviews and audits, and makes payments to providers for covered services on behalf of Medicare. It is important to keep in mind that coding does not dictate coverage of medical services or reimbursement policies.

Coding Systems as Communication Facilitators

Clinical coding systems serve as the communication vehicle between healthcare providers and public and private third-party payers. This solid and reliable communication enables providers and facilities to be accurately reimbursed in a timely manner. Understanding the basics of clinical coding systems enables coding, billing, and reimbursement professionals to fully grasp reimbursement principles and concepts.

Check Your Understanding 2.1

1. The code sets to be used for healthcare services reporting by both public and private insurers were designated by what legislation?

2. The first three characters in an ICD-9-CM diagnosis code represent its
    a. Subclassification
    b. Subcategory
    c. Category
    d. Modifier

3. What organizations maintain the ICD-10-CM/PCS code set?

4. Where are the ICD-10-CM/PCS coding guidelines published?

5. What code set was incorporated into the Healthcare Common Procedure Coding System as HCPCS Level I?

Coding Compliance and Reimbursement

For coding, billing, and reimbursement professionals, being compliant means performing job functions according to the laws, regulations, and guidelines set forth by Medicare and other third-party payers. Today, being compliant with the rules and regulations is just one component of being proficient at a healthcare professional's job, but it is an indication that, as a professional, the person is able to perform at an acceptable skill level and ethical standard. It is the responsibility of coding, billing, and reimbursement professionals to perform their jobs with integrity at all times. The appendix to this chapter, *AHIMA Standards of Ethical Coding*, sets forth guidelines that all coding, billing, and reimbursement professionals should understand and ponder during ethical decision making.

Fraud and Abuse

Medicare defines **fraud** as "an intentional representation that an individual knows to be false or does not believe to be true and makes, knowing that the representation could result in some unauthorized benefit to himself/herself or some other person" (CMS 2004b). An example of fraud is billing for a service that was not rendered.

Abuse occurs when a healthcare provider unknowingly or unintentionally submits an inaccurate claim to for payment. Abuse generally results from unsound medical, business, or fiscal practices that directly or indirectly result in unnecessary costs to the Medicare program. An example of abuse involves inadvertently reporting a procedure code that describes a service that was more extensive than the procedure performed. In Medicare, the most common forms of fraud and abuse include the following (CMS 2004b):

- Billing for services not furnished

- Misrepresenting the diagnosis to justify payment

- Soliciting, offering, or receiving a kickback

- Unbundling or "exploding" charges

- Falsifying certificates of medical necessity, plans of treatment, and medical records to justify payment

- Billing for a service not furnished as billed (known as upcoding)

The mid-1980s through late 1990s brought about a wave of legislation targeted at fighting Medicare and Medicaid fraud and abuse.

Legislative Background

It is important to explore and understand the legislative history of fraud and abuse. In an effort to eliminate erroneous healthcare spending for the Medicare and Medicaid programs, Congress passed several acts targeting fraud and abuse. Not only did the revamped and newly created legislation show a commitment to protecting the Medicare Trust Fund by Congress, but it gave CMS the resources and penalties necessary to battle fraud and abuse.

False Claims Act

The **False Claims Act** was passed during the Civil War to penalize contractors of all kinds who knowingly filed a false or fraudulent claim, used a false record or statement, or conspired to defraud the US government (Schraffenberger and Kuehn 2007, 254). Today, the False Claims Act provides the support for the federal government to rebuke abusers of the Medicare and Medicaid systems. The Medicare and Medicaid Patient and Program Protection Act of 1987 supports the use of civil monetary penalties for acts of fraud and abuse against the Medicare and Medicaid programs. This act allows for fines up to $10,000 per violation and exclusions from Medicare participation.

Office of Inspector General Compliance Program Guidance

In 1991, the **Office of Inspector General (OIG)** released seven elements that the office believed should serve as the foundation of an effective corporate compliance plan (OIG 1991). These elements are

- Written policies and procedures

- Designation of a **compliance officer**

- Education and training
- Communication
- Auditing and monitoring
- Disciplinary action
- Corrective action

In response to numerous laboratory investigations for improper coding and billing, *Compliance Program Guidance for Clinical Laboratories* was released in February 1997 and then revised in February of the following year. The guidance provides principles for compliant documentation and coding practices in laboratories. For example, laboratories were instructed that they must not use diagnostic information from earlier dates of service on current laboratory testing orders. At the time, this was common practice, but it is a compliance risk because a patient's condition warranting a procedure may change from visit to visit.

In February 1998, the OIG released *Compliance Program Guidance for Hospitals*. This document highlighted several coding and billing areas that were at risk for noncompliance. Some examples are upcoding services, unbundling services, and reporting incorrect discharge destination.

Since 1998, numerous other **Compliance Program Guidance** documents have been released for various healthcare settings, including hospice, home health, physician practices, and skilled nursing facilities.

Several years have passed since the *Compliance Program Guidance for Hospitals* was released. In January 2005, CMS released the *Supplemental Compliance Program Guidance for Hospitals* in the *Federal Register*. Because hospitals' operations and reimbursement systems have changed since 1998, the OIG decided to revise the *Program Guidance*. Although expanded, the original seven elements continue to be the basis for an effective hospital compliance plan (DHHS 2005, 4874–4876):

- Designation of a compliance officer and compliance committee
- Development of compliance policies and procedures, including standard of conduct
- Development of open lines of communication
- Appropriate training and education
- Internal monitoring and auditing

- Response to detected deficiencies
- Enforcement of disciplinary standards

The *Supplemental Compliance Program Guidance for Hospitals* provides further detail about compliance risk areas for outpatient procedure coding, admissions and discharge criteria, supplemental payment considerations, and use of information technology (DHHS 2005, 4860–4862). A copy of the *Supplemental Compliance Program Guidance for Hospitals* can be found on the OIG website (http://www.oig.hhs.gov).

Operation Restore Trust

A joint effort of the DHHS, OIG, CMS, and Administration on Aging (AOA), **Operation Restore Trust** was released in 1995 to target fraud and abuse among healthcare providers. The program originally focused on five states (California, Illinois, Florida, New York, and Texas), where a third of the Medicare and Medicaid population resided. Within the first two years, Operation Restore Trust spent $7.9 million and recovered $188 million—a 24:1 return on investment. This major push for accurate coding and billing eventually spread to become a nationwide effort. In addition to fraud and abuse investigations, Operation Restore Trust paved the way for implementation of a national toll-free fraud and abuse hotline, the Voluntary Disclosure Program, and Special Fraud Alert documents.

Health Insurance Portability and Accountability Act of 1996

Although HIPAA is widely known for its security and privacy provisions, a large portion of the act focused on fraud and abuse prevention. HIPAA created the **Medicare Integrity Program**. Not only did Medicare continue to review provider claims for fraud and abuse, but the focus expanded to cost reports, payment determinations, and the need for ongoing compliance education (Schraffenberger and Kuehn, 2007).

Balanced Budget Act of 1997

One objective of the **Balanced Budget Act (BBA) of 1997** was to improve program integrity for Medicare. The provisions within the BBA attempted to educate Medicare beneficiaries about their role in preventing and reporting fraudulent acts. Beneficiaries were advised to review Medicare Summary Notices (MSNs; formerly Explanations of Medicare Benefits, or EOMBs) for errors and to report errors to the secretary of DHHS.

In addition, they were notified of their right to request copies of detailed bills for healthcare services and informed of the implementation of a toll-free fraud and abuse hotline. The BBA also initiated a data collection program to collect fraud and abuse information in the healthcare sector as mandated by HIPAA.

As legislation regarding healthcare fraud and abuse became more prevalent, the need for a stronger workforce behind the laws was inevitable. Personnel were added to the Department of Justice (DOJ) and Federal Bureau of Investigation (FBI) to keep up with the warranted reviews.

Improper Payments Legislation

The Improper Payments Information Act (IPIA; P.L. 107–300), enacted on November 26, 2002, requires that all federal agencies provide an estimate of improper payments and what actions are being taken to reduce improper payments. The Improper Payments Elimination and Recovery Act (IPERA; P.L. 111–204), enacted on July 22, 2010, amended IPIA. CMS has developed or modified existing programs to comply with both of these acts. For example, the Office of Management and Budget (OMB) identified Medicaid's Children's Health Insurance Program (CHIP; program discussed further in chapter 4) as a program that has a significant potential for improper payments. Therefore, CMS created the Payment Error Rate Measurement (PERM) program for Medicaid to comply with IPIA. Educational materials, statistics, and reports regarding the PERM program can be found at https://www.cms.gov/perm/. In addition, the Medicare Comprehensive Error Rate Testing (CERT) program complies with IPERA for the Medicare fee-for-service programs. CERT is discussed further in this chapter, as it is part of the Medicare Review and Education program. Additionally, the Improper Payments Elimination and Recovery Improvement Act (IPERIA: P.L.112-248), enacted on January 10, 2013 further strengthened and intensify efforts to identify, prevent and recover payment errors, waste, fraud, and abuse. These acts have greatly affected the Medicare Integrity Program. To learn more about the program, view the Medicare Program Integrity Manual, available for download at http://www.cms.gov.

Oversight of Medicare Claims Payments

Not only is CMS is required by the act to protect the Medicare Trust Fund, but legislative acts such as IPERA and IPERIA also provide specific requirements for reporting and correcting improper payments. To complete the numerous requirements, CMS has established the Medicare Review and Education program. Under this program, CMS uses a variety of entities, such as MACs, to complete medical reviews, which are also known as **improper payment reviews**. All entities completing medical reviews and providing education are referred to as Medicare contractors. Figure 2.3 provides a snapshot of the roles of the various entities included in medical reviews/improper payment reviews. The Medical Review and Education Program is based on Progressive Corrective Action (PCA), an operational principle that includes the following steps:

- Data analysis
- Error detection
- Validation of errors
- Provider education
- Determination of review type
- Sampling of claims
- Payment recovery

The goal of the program is to reduce Medicare payment errors by identifying and eliminating billing errors made by providers. Medicare contractors focus reviews on preidentified areas that have been determined by contractor data analysis, CERT findings, OIG/Government Accountability Office (GAO) reports, and **Recovery Audit Contractor (RAC)** vulnerabilities work. Medical reviews consist of the Medicare contractors collecting information and performing a clinical review to determine whether Medicare's coverage, coding, and medical necessity requirements are met.

The major causes of improper payments include physician orders missing, signatures being illegible or missing, **National Coverage Determinations (NCDs)/Local Coverage Determinations (LCDs)** requirements not being met, and medical records documentation not supporting medical necessity. NCDs and LCDs communicate coverage and medical necessity requirements. NCDs, LCDs, and other compliance guidance documents are discussed in greater detail under "Compliance" in chapter 9 of this text. Additionally, review entities look for unbundling and upcoding of services. **Unbundling** is the process in which individual component codes are submitted for reimbursement rather than a single comprehensive code.

Figure 2.3.   Roles of Various Medicare Improper Payment Review Entities

	Types of Claims	How selected	Volume of Claims	Type of Review	Purpose of Review	Other Functions
QIO	Inpatient Hospital claims only	All claims where hospital submits an adjusted claim for a higher-weighted DRG Expedited Coverage Reviews requested by beneficiaries	**Very small**	• Prepay & Concurrent (Patient still in hospital) • Complex only	To prevent improper payments through DRG upcoding To resolve discharge disputes between beneficiary and hospital	Quality Reviews
CERT*	All Medical Claims	**Randomly**	**Small**	• Postpay only • Complex only	To **measure** improper payments	None
PERM*	All Medical Claims Randomly	**Randomly**	**Small**	• Postpay only • Complex only	To **measure** improper payments	None
Medical Review Units* at MACs	All Medicare FFS Claims	Targeted	Depends on number of claims with possible improper payments for this provider	• Prepay & Postpay • Automated, & Complex	To **prevent future** improper payments	• Education • Appeals
Medicare Recovery Auditors*	All Medicare FFS Claims	Targeted	Depends on number of claims with possible improper payments for this provider	• Postpay • Automated and Complex	To detect and correct past improper payments	None
PSC/ZPICS	All Medicare FFS Claims	Targeted	Depends on number of potentially fraudulent claims submitted by provider	• Prepay and Postpay • Automated and Complex	To identify potential fraud	----
OIG	All Claims	Targeted	Depends on number of potentially fraudulent claims submitted by provider	• Postpay • Complex	To identify fraud	----

*Overseen by OFM/PCG

Reference: Centers for Medicare and Medicaid Services. 2011c. Overview of Improper Payment Reviews Conducted by Medicare and Medicaid Review Contractors. Slide 5. http://www.cms.gov/CERT/downloads/Overview_Review.pdf.

Unbundling is discussed in more detail in conjunction with the National Correct Coding Initiative in chapter 9 of this text. **Upcoding** is the fraudulent process of submitting codes for reimbursement that indicates more complex or higher-paying services than those that the patient actually received. Upcoding is discussed in more detail under "Revenue Cycle Analysis" in chapter 9 of this text.

Provider education is a key component of this program. After areas of concern or vulnerabilities are identified, Medicare contractors are expected to publish LCDs to provide guidance to the medical community regarding coverage, coding, and medical necessity requirements. In addition, Medicare Learning Network (MLN) articles should be created in an effort to improve transparency of the medical review process.

Comprehensive Error Rate Testing Program

CERT was first a responsibility of the OIG, and national error rates were calculated by the OIG from 1996 to 2002. The program was transitioned to Medicare beginning in 2001. The IPIA of 2002 solidified the program, and Medicare released its first report in 2003. Recently, the program was enhanced to meet requirements under the IPERA of 2010 (P.L. 111–204). The purpose of CERT is to measure improper payments, not to measure fraud. During each reporting period, claims are randomly selected for review from each of the types of Medicare contractors, as illustrated in figure 2.4. CERT identifies improper payments as

• Payment that should not have been made

• Payment made in an incorrect amount

- Payment to an ineligible recipient
- Payment for an ineligible service
- Duplicate payment
- Payment for service that was not received

National error rates are calculated each year and are published with the associated financial effect of improper payments. Figure 2.5 provides a listing of the past national error rates. The error rate has varied from year to year, and the error rate for 2013 was 10.5 percent ($36.0 billion). The primary error identified by the CERT was lack of documentation to support reported services. Such figures indicate that there continues to be a need for this program as well as for continued Medicare claims reviews.

Office of Inspector General Reports

Although the OIG no longer executes CERT, the agency does provide relevant reports to the Medical Review and Education Program for continued review. Significant OIG reports are communicated via Medicare transmittals to Medicare contractors for use in their medical review activities. Each year, the OIG provides its Work Plan, which outlines the areas of focus for the upcoming year. Providers and facilities can use the Work Plan to construct their own compliance reviews on these topics of interest. The OIG Work Plan is published each year at http://www.oig.hhs.gov.

National Recovery Audit Program

What started out as a demonstration project is now a fully implemented CMS program that encompasses all areas of Medicare fee-for-service and Medicaid. The National Recovery Audit Program is executed under the Medicare Integrity Program and is designed as another CMS avenue to prevent improper payments and ultimately to protect the Medicare Trust Fund.

RAC Program

With the overwhelming success of the RAC demonstration program and the modifications to the program, Section 302 of the Tax Relief and Healthcare Act (TRHCA) of 2006 made the RAC

Figure 2.4.   The CERT process

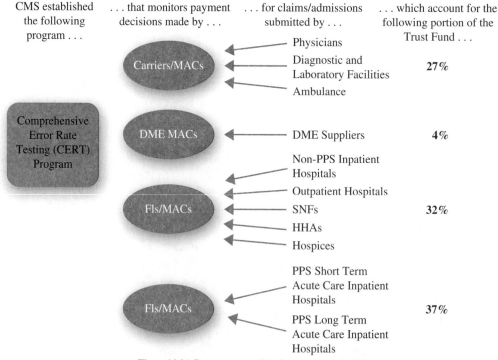

Fls and MACs are responsible for payment decisions on inpatient hospital claims beginning with the November 2009 report

Reference: Centers for Medicare and Medicaid Services. 2011a. CERT 101. Slide 7. http://www.cms.gov/CERT/Downloads/CERT_101.pdf.

Figure 2.5.   CERT error rates by year, 1996–2010

Year	Error Rate	Total Dollars Paid	Total Improper Payments
1996	14.2%	$168.1 B	$23.8 B
1997	11.8%	$177.9 B	$20.9 B
1998	8.4%	$177.0 B	$14.9 B
1999	8.6%	$168.9 B	$14.5 B
2000	9.4%	$174.6 B	$16.4 B
2001	8.8%	$191.3 B	$16.8 B
2002	8.0%	$212.8 B	$17.1 B
2003	6.4%*	$199.1 B	$12.7 B*
2004	10.1%	$213.5 B	$21.7 B
2005	5.2%	$234.1 B	$12.1 B
2006	4.4%	$246.8 B	$10.8 B
2007	3.9%	$276.2 B	$10.8 B
2008	3.6%	$288.2 B	$10.4 B
2009	12.4%	$308.4 B	$35.4 B
2010	10.5%	$326.4 B	$34.3 B

*These entries have been adjusted to account for the high provider non-response rate in 2003. Had the adjustment not been made, the improper payments would have been $21.5 billion, and the national paid claims error rate would have been 10.8 percent.

Reference: Centers for Medicare and Medicaid Services. 2011a. CERT 101. Slide 9. http://www.cms.gov/CERT/Downloads/CERT_101.pdf.

Table 2.8.   Recovery audit contractors

Region	Recovery Audit Contractor	Contingency Fee
Region A	Performant Recovery	12.45%
Region B	CGI Technologies and Solutions, Inc.	12.50%
Region C	Connolly Consulting Associates, Inc.	9.00%
Region D	HealthDataInsights, Inc.	9.49%

program permanent. Unlike other improper payment review entities, recovery auditors are reimbursed via a contingency fee based on the amount of improper payments identified and successfully collected. Table 2.8 provides the RAC contractors and subcontractors by region, along with the settled contingency fee. Figure 2.6 provides the RAC jurisdictions.

Figure 2.6.   RAC jurisdictions

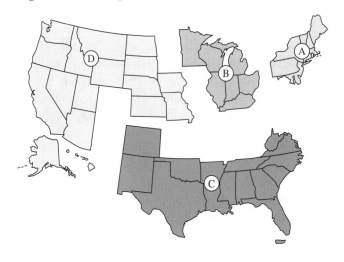

The RAC program has five key program components. The first component is to ensure accuracy. It is imperative that the RACs accurately identify improper payments. RACs must have a physician medical director as well as certified coders on staff. For medical necessity reviews, many RACs use registered nurses or other clinical staff. Additionally, a RAC must have review issues, also known as vulnerabilities, approved by the recovery audit validation contractor before performing audits. The RACs must publish all vulnerabilities on their websites before the vulnerabilities can be used in audits. The RAC must ensure that the program operates efficiently and effectively. This key component is in place to ensure constant and high-quality communication between all stakeholders. Additionally the program works to improve the RAC Data Warehouse and the use of Electronic Submission of Medical Documents (esMD) for medical records requests. The next key component is to maximize transparency. The RACs prepare and post quarterly newsletters online. The quarterly newsletters provide the amount of overpayments and underpayments for each RAC for each quarter. Additionally, the top issue for each RAC is provided. Another key component is to minimize provide burden. Any given medical record or encounter may be reviewed by only one improper payment review entity for a given issue. Therefore, if a MAC has reviewed an encounter for medical necessity the encounter cannot be reviewed by the RAC. However, the encounter may be reviewed by the RAC for another issue, such as improper coding. Additionally, RACs must establish a customer service center to answer queries from facilities and practices. The last key component is to develop robust provide education. The RACs and MACs collaborate to ensure that policies are correctly interpreted. There are scheduled conference calls between RACs, MACs, CMS policy staff, and CMS clinical staff to ensure uniformity in policy application across improper payment review entities.

The RAC process begins with a review. There are three types of reviews.

- Automated—RACs use claims data analysis to identify improper payments.

- Semi-automated—RACs initiate the review through claims data analysis but then require the submission of the medical record documents to substantiate the improper payment.

- Complex—Require the review of clinical medical record documents to confirm the improper payment.

For a semi-automated review or complex review, the RAC will request medical records from the facility or provider. The provider must follow a strict timetable when submitting records to the RAC. Documents can be submitted through esMD, or hard copies can be mailed to the RAC. After the RAC review is complete and an improper payment has been identified the MACs issues a demand letter to the facility or provider. The demand letter requests a specific amount to be repaid,

provides a detailed rationale for the improper payment, and includes instructions for adjudication or appeal. Facilities or providers that disagree with the improper payment can appeal the RAC decision. The appeal process can be a five-level process:

- Redetermination—performed by the MAC

- Reconsideration—performed by a qualified independent contractor (QIC)

- Administrative law judge (ALJ) review

- Appeals council review

- Final judicial review—performed by federal district court

Appeals can be time-consuming and costly to the facility or provider. However, successful appeals provide valuable information that can be used to improve medical record document and to support future appeals.

For fiscal year 2013, the RACs collected $3.75 billion in improper payments (up from $92.3 million in 2010). Of this total, $3.65 billion resulted from overpayments to providers. A total of $102.4 million of improper payments resulted from underpayments to providers (CMS 2013). These figures appear to be very high, but when put into perspective, the RAC program collected less than 1 percent of the total expenditures ($481 billion) for Part A and Part B in 2013 (CMS 2013). Figure 2.7 shows the collections by

Figure 2.7. RAC collections by Recovery Auditor for 2013

Corrections by Recovery Auditor					
	Overpayments Collected		Underpayments Restored		Total Corrected	
Recovery Auditor	No. of Claims	Amount Collected	No. of Claims	Amount Restored	No. of Claims	Amount Corrected
Performant	365,435	$762,312,114	3,823	$14,708,223	369,258	$777,020,336
CGI	132,787	$528,731,497	2,416	$7,781,593	135,203	$536,513,091
Connolly	537,690	$1,219,049,512	23,203	$43,358,754	560,893	$1,267,408,266
HDI	453,622	$1,140,665,285	13,167	$31,521,627	456,789	$1,172,187,913
Unknown*	104	$155,217	2	$38,307	106	$193,524
Total	1,489,638	$3,650,914,625	42,611	$102,408,504	1,532,249	$3,753,323,129

Reference: Centers for Medicare and Medicaid Services. 2013. Recovery Auditing in Medicare for Fiscal Year 2013; FY2013 Report to Congress. Page 11. http://www.cms.gov/Research-Statistics-Data-and-Systems/Monitoring-Programs/Medicare-FFS-Compliance-Programs/Recovery-Audit-Program/Downloads/FY-2013-Report-To-Congress.pdf.

Figure 2.8.   RAC corrections by provider type for 2013

Corrections by Provider Type			
Claim Type	Overpayments Collected	Underpayments Restored	Total Amount Corrected
Inpatient	$3,437,554,670	$86,149,338	$3,523,704,008
SMF	$1,840,735	$19,567	$1,860,302
Hospice	$34,858	-	$34,858
Outpatient	$46,637,617	$5,071,482	$51,709,099
Home Health	$6,386,724	$4,037,775	$10,424,498
Physician	$56,836,203	$1,241,449	$58,077,652
DME	$73,849,883	$225,754	$74,075,638
Unknown	$27,773,935	$5,663,139	$33,437,075
Total	$3,650,914,625	$102,408,504	$3,753,323,129

Reference: Centers for Medicare and Medicaid Services. 2013. Recovery Auditing in Medicare for Fiscal Year 2013; FY2013 Report to Congress. Page 35. http://www.cms.gov/Research-Statistics-Data-and-Systems/Monitoring-Programs/Medicare-FFS-Compliance-Programs/Recovery-Audit-Program/Downloads/FY-2013-Report-To-Congress.pdf.

Figure 2.9.   Top issue per region, Q4 2014

Region A:	**Cardiovascular Procedures:** (Medical Necessity) Medicare pays for inpatient hospital services that are medically necessary for the setting billed. Medical documentation for patients undergoing cardiovascular procedures needs to be complete and support all services provided in the setting billed.
Region B:	**Cardiovascular Procedures:** (Medical Necessity) Medicare pays for inpatient hospital services that are medically necessary for the setting billed. Medical documentation for patients undergoing cardiovascular procedures needs to be complete and support all services provided in the setting billed.
Region C:	**Cardiovascular Procedures:** (Medical Necessity) Medicare pays for inpatient hospital services that are medically necessary for the setting billed. Medical documentation for patients undergoing cardiovascular procedures needs to be complete and support all services provided in the setting billed.
Region D:	**Minor Surgery and other treatment billed as Inpatient:** (Medical Necessity) When beneficiaries with known diagnoses enter a hospital for a specific minor surgical procedure or other treatment that is expected to keep them in the hospital for less than 24 hours, they are considered outpatient for coverage purposes regardless of the hour they presented to the hospital, whether a bed was used, and whether they remained in the hospital after midnight.

Reference: Centers for Medicare and Medicaid Services. 2014. National Recovery Audit Program Quarterly Newsletter July 1, 2014 through September 30, 2014. http://www.cms.gov/Research-Statistics-Data-and-Systems/Monitoring-Programs/Medicare-FFS-Compliance-Programs/Recovery-Audit-Program/Downloads/Medicare-FFS-Recovery-Audit-Program-4th-qtr-2014.pdf.

recovery auditor as reported to Congress. Figure 2.8 provides the corrections by type of provider for 2013 as reported to Congress. Figure 2.9 provides the top issue per region reported in the fourth-quarter 2014 RAC newsletter.

Providers challenged 30.7 percent of all claims with an overpayment determination in review year 2013. Furthermore, 18.1 percent of claims were overturned in the provider's favor (CMS 2013). With such statistics, it is clear that facilities must continue to closely monitor RAC determinations at their facilities. Facilities must incorporate issues identified by RACs and other Medicare contractors into their coding compliance plans.

In September 2012, the Recovery Auditor Prepayment Review Demonstration began. During this three-year demonstration project, recovery auditors review claims before payment. The program includes eleven states: Florida, California, Michigan, Texas, New York, Louisiana, Illinois, Pennsylvania, Ohio, North Carolina, and Missouri. The recovery auditors started the program by reviewing short-stay inpatient hospital claims for specified MS-DRGs. A short stay admission is one in which the length of stay is two days or fewer. Initial results reported in the RAC 2013 Report to Congress revealed that more than 58 percent of the reviewed claims were improperly billed. The improper billing resulted in $22.3 million in saving to the Medicare Trust Fund (CMS 2013). CMS continues to evaluate the results and savings from this demonstration project until its completion in 2015.

Other Third-Party Payer Reviews

As with CMS, other payers have developed medical review programs to ensure that payments are warranted and accurate. However, unlike with Medicare, for which the review programs, issues under review, and review results for the regions and nation are available for the healthcare community to review online, commercial payers typically do not publish such information for all to see. Review criteria are developed by the individual payers based on their own historical data and audits. Commercial payers may incorporate issues that have previously been identified by Medicare but that are applicable to their beneficiary profile into their own review portfolio. For example, excisional debridement vulnerabilities identified by RACs may be used by a commercial payer, but criteria for newborn or pregnancy reviews would need to be developed by the commercial payers, the volume for these cases being so low for the Medicare population. When commercial payer reviews are executed at a healthcare facility, the review topics, as well as the findings, should be incorporated into the coding compliance plans.

Coding Compliance Plan

Every coding unit should have a **coding compliance plan**, a component of the health information management (HIM) department compliance plan and the overall corporate compliance plan at its facility. The plan should focus on the unique regulations and guidelines with which coding professionals must comply. As discussed previously, the DHHS has released several versions of *Compliance Program Guidance* for various healthcare settings. The model provided by the OIG guidance is also applicable to individual coding units. Building a complete compliance plan is essential for establishing a solid coding team. The core areas of the coding compliance plan are policies and procedures, education and training, and auditing and monitoring.

Policies and Procedures

Well-designed and complete policies and procedures provide employees with consistent guidance to perform their assigned tasks. Without such guidance, employees may complete their tasks in different ways, causing major confusion, inefficiencies, and possibly noncompliance. Managers should perform a job analysis to ensure that every task has an established policy or procedure to govern it. Because coding has so many rules and official guidelines, it is critical that this section of the coding compliance plan be methodically compiled. Following is a far from exhaustive list of issues that should be included in a coding compliance plan:

- Physician query process
- Coding diagnoses not supported by medical documentation
- Upcoding
- Unbundling
- Coding medical records without complete documentation
- Assignment of discharge destination codes
- Correct use of encoding software
- Complete process for using scrubber software

Education and Training

A good education plan is essential to succeeding as a coding team. To be compliant, coding, billing, and reimbursement professionals must continually participate in their education. Rules and regulations for public and private payers are released almost daily. Recognized means of communication of this vital information must be established in the coding compliance plan. A sample of issues that should be placed on the continuous education schedule includes

- Public and private payer guidelines
- LCDs
- NCDs
- Official Coding Guidelines for ICD-10-CM, CPT, and HCPCS Level II codes
- Quarterly and yearly code changes
- Quarterly and yearly prospective payment system changes
- OIG work plan issues
- National Correct Coding Initiative (NCCI)

Special attention should be paid to the work of new coders. Every coding manager must assess a new employee's compliance level and degree of understanding. Education must be provided to bring deficient coders up to speed with expected guidelines. Completion of required educational sessions should be built into annual evaluations/reviews for all coding, billing, and reimbursement employees.

Auditing and Monitoring

Managers must be diligent at auditing and monitoring compliance in the coding unit. During the auditing phase, the coding manager gathers information about the department's compliance with policies and procedures. Incorporating internal and external auditing into the coding compliance plan has proven the best strategy. Internal auditing enables managers to see firsthand where their units' strengths and weaknesses lie. External auditing provides an unbiased view of a department's performance. Together, internal and external audits help coding managers build effective education plans for their units.

Two forms of **benchmarking** can help a manager determine the staff's level of compliance: internal and external benchmarking. Internal benchmarking or trending allows the manager to examine reporting rates over time. This exercise helps the manager pinpoint the specific period when a compliance issue arose. External benchmarking or peer comparison helps a manager to know how his or her team has performed compared with peers. Issues can reveal, for example, whether **coding practices** put the facility at risk. Benchmarking will help establish reasonable parameters. Target areas for internal and external benchmarking should correlate with those highlighted in the policies and procedures and education and training sections of the coding compliance plan, along with problem areas identified during routine internal and external audits.

Check Your Understanding 2.2

1. The new coding assistant at the Glen Ellyn Medical Group office coded and submitted a claim to Blue Cross for an initial evaluation and management office visit when, in fact, the patient was established with the practice and was seen strictly for a follow-up medical check. The resulting error was an example of _____.

2. All of the following are efforts to fight healthcare fraud and abuse *except*
   a. Operation Restore Trust
   b. Medicare Integrity Program
   c. Tax Equity and Fiscal Responsibility Act (TEFRA) of 1982
   d. Medicare and Medicaid Patient and Program Protection Act of 1987

3. What legislation supports the CERT program?

4. What differentiates recovery auditors from other entities performing improper payment reviews?

5. What are the core areas of the coding compliance plan?

Chapter 2 Review Quiz

For questions 1, 2, and 3, match each coding system on the left with its description of uses on the right.

1. ICD   ____   a. Medical and surgical supplies

2. HCPCS Level II   ____   b. Physician inpatient or outpatient procedures

3. CPT   ____   c. Diagnoses and inpatient procedures

4. Common forms of fraud and abuse include all of the following *except*
   a. Upcoding
   b. Unbundling
   c. Refiling claims after denials
   d. Billing for services not furnished to patients

5. Name and describe three of the seven OIG elements of an effective compliance plan.

6. The CERT program was established to correct improper payments. True or false?

7. Describe the importance of the RAC prepayment review demonstration project.

8. What resource can managers use to discover current target areas of compliance?

9. What two forms of benchmarking can be using to determine a staff's level of compliance?

10. The ICD is maintained by the American Medical Association. True or false?

References

American Hospital Association. 2004. AHA Central Office. http://www.hospitalconnect.com.

American Hospital Association. 2015. AHA Central Office. http://www.ahacentraloffice.org/codes/ICD10.shtml.

American Medical Association. 2004. http://www.ama-assn.org.

American Medical Association. 2005. *Current Procedural Terminology*. Chicago: AMA.

American Medical Association. 1989 to 2014. *CPT Assistant*. Chicago: AMA.

Beebe, M. 2003. CPT Category III codes cover new, emerging technologies: New codes developed to address issues in light of HIPAA. *Journal of AHIMA* 74(9):84–85.

Casto, A. 2015. *ICD-10-CM Code Book*: Chicago: AHIMA Press.

Centers for Medicare and Medicaid Services. 2004a. Healthcare Common Procedure Coding System (HCPCS). http://www.cms.hhs.gov/medicare/hcpcs.

Centers for Medicare and Medicaid Services. 2004b. Fighting fraud and abuse. http://www.cms.hhs.gov/providers/fraud.

Centers for Medicare and Medicaid Services. 2011a. CERT 101. http://www.cms.gov/CERT/Downloads/CERT_101.pdf.

Centers for Medicare and Medicaid Services. 2011b. Implementation of recovery auditing at the Centers for Medicare and Medicaid Services: FY2010 report to Congress. https://www.cms.gov/Recovery-Audit-Program/Downloads/FY2010ReportCongress.pdf.

Centers for Medicare and Medicaid Services. 2011c. Overview of improper payment reviews conducted by Medicare and Medicaid review contractors. http://www.cms.gov/CERT/downloads/Overview_Review.pdf.

Centers for Medicare and Medicaid Services. 2013. Recovery Auditing in Medicare for Fiscal Year 2013; FY2013 Report to Congress.

Centers for Medicare and Medicaid Services. 2014. National Recovery Audit Program Quarterly Newsletter July 1, 2014 through September 30, 2014.

Department of Health and Human Services. 2005. OIG supplemental compliance program guidance for hospitals. *Federal Register* 70(19):4858–4876.

LaTour, K., and S. Eichenwald, eds. 2013. *Health Information Management: Concepts, Principles, and Practice*. Chicago: AHIMA.

Office of the Inspector General (OIG). 1991. *Compliance Program Guidance*.

Schraffenberger, L.A., and L. Kuehn. 2007. *Effective Management of Coding Services*, 3rd ed. Chicago: AHIMA.

Additional Resources

AHIMA ICD-10-CM/PCS Academic Transition Workgroup. 2009. Transitioning to ICD-10-CM/PCS—An academic timeline. *Journal of AHIMA* 80(4):59–64.

Centers for Medicare and Medicaid Service. 2006. Status on the use of Recovery Audit Contractors (RACs) in the Medicare program. http://www.cms.hhs.gov/RAC/Downloads/RACStatusDocumentFY2006.pdf.

Centers for Medicare and Medicaid Services. 2007. Crosswalk from CMS DRGs to MS-DRGs. http://www.cms.hhs.gov/AcuteInpatientPPS/FFD/.

Centers for Medicare and Medicaid Services. 2011. Comprehensive error rate testing. http://www.cms.gov/cert.

Centers for Medicare and Medicaid Services. 2011. Medical review and education. http://www.cms.gov/Medical-Review/.

Centers for Medicare and Medicaid Services. 2011. Recovery audit program. http://www.cms.gov/Recovery-Audit-Program/.

Centers for Medicare and Medicaid Services. 2015. ICD-10-PCS Official Guidelines for Coding and Reporting. http://www.cms.gov/Medicare/coding/ICD10/Downloads/2015-PCS-guidelines.pdf.

First Coast Service Options. 1999. *Medicare Fraud and Abuse: A Practical Guide of Proactive Measures to Avoid Becoming a Victim*. Washington, DC: Health Care Financing Administration.

United States Congress. 2002. Public Law 107-300. Improper Payments Information Act of 2002. http://www.dol.gov/ocfo/media/regs/IPIA.pdf.

United States Congress. 2010. Public Law 111-204. Improper Payments Elimination and Recovery Act of 2010. http://frwebgate.access.gpo.gov/cgi-bin/getdoc.cgi?dbname=111_cong_bills&docid=f:s1508enr.txt.pdf.

United States Congress. 2013. Public Law 112-248. Improper Payments Elimination and Recovery Act of 2013. http://www.ssa.gov/improperpayments/documents/IPERIA--PLAW-112publ248.pdf.

Appendix 2A
American Health Information Management Association Standards of Ethical Coding

Introduction

The Standards of Ethical Coding are based on the American Health Information Management Association's (AHIMA's) Code of Ethics. Both sets of principles reflect expectations of professional conduct for coding professionals involved in diagnostic or procedural coding or other health record data abstraction.

A Code of Ethics sets forth professional values and ethical principles and offers ethical guidelines to which professionals aspire and by which their actions can be judged. Health information management (HIM) professionals are expected to demonstrate professional values by their actions to patients, employers, members of the healthcare team, the public, and the many stakeholders they serve. A Code of Ethics is important in helping guide the decision-making process and can be referred to by individuals, agencies, organizations, and bodies (such as licensing and regulatory boards, insurance providers, courts of law, government agencies, and other professional groups).

The AHIMA Code of Ethics (available on AHIMA's website) is relevant to all AHIMA members and credentialed HIM professionals and students regardless of their professional functions, the settings in which they work, and the populations they serve. Coding is a core HIM function, and due to the complex regulatory requirements affecting the health information coding process, coding professionals are frequently faced with ethical challenges. The AHIMA Standards of Ethical Coding are intended to assist coding professionals and managers in decision-making processes and actions, outline expectations for making ethical decisions in the workplace, and demonstrate coding professionals' commitment to integrity during the coding process regardless of the purpose for which the codes are being reported. They are relevant to all coding professionals and to those who manage the coding function, regardless of the healthcare setting in which they work or whether they are AHIMA members or nonmembers.

These Standards of Ethical Coding have been revised to reflect the current healthcare environment and modern coding practices. The previous revision was published in 1999.

Standards of Ethical Coding

Coding professionals should:

1. Apply accurate, complete, and consistent coding practices for the production of high-quality healthcare data.

2. Report all healthcare data elements (for example, diagnosis and procedure codes, present on admission indicator, discharge status) required for external reporting purposes (for example, reimbursement and other administrative uses, population health, quality and patient safety measurement, and research) completely and accurately, in accordance with regulatory and documentation standards and requirements and applicable official coding conventions, rules, and guidelines.

3. Assign and report only the codes and data that are clearly and consistently supported by health record documentation in accordance with applicable code set and abstraction conventions, rules, and guidelines.

4. Query provider (physician or other qualified healthcare practitioner) for clarification and additional documentation prior to code assignment when there is conflicting, incomplete, or ambiguous information in the health record regarding a significant reportable condition or procedure or other reportable data element dependent on health record documentation (for example, present on admission indicator).

5. Refuse to change reported codes or the narratives of codes so that meanings are misrepresented.

6. Refuse to participate in or support coding or documentation practices intended to inappropriately increase payment, qualify for insurance policy coverage, or skew data by means that do not comply with federal and state statutes, regulations, and official rules and guidelines.

7. Facilitate interdisciplinary collaboration in situations supporting proper coding practices.

8. Advance coding knowledge and practice through continuing education.

9. Refuse to participate in or conceal unethical coding or abstraction practices or procedures.

10. Protect the confidentiality of the health record at all times and refuse to access protected health information not required for coding-related activities (examples of coding-related activities include completion of code assignment, other health record data abstraction, coding audits, and educational purposes).

11. Demonstrate behavior that reflects integrity, shows a commitment to ethical and legal coding practices, and fosters trust in professional activities.

Revised and approved by the House of Delegates 09/08.

All rights reserved. Reprint and quote only with proper reference to AHIMA's authorship.

Resources
AHIMA Code of Ethics. Available at http://www.ahima.org/about/ethics.asp

ICD-9-CM Official Guidelines for Coding and Reporting. http://www.cdc.gov/nchs/datawh/ftpserv/ftpicd9/icdguide07.pdf

AHIMA's position statement on Quality Health Data and Information. Available at http://www.ahima.org/dc/positions

AHIMA's position statement on Uniformity and Consistency of Healthcare Data (DRAFT)

AHIMA Practice Brief titled "Managing an Effective Query Process." Available at http://www.ahima.org/infocenter/briefs.asp

How to Interpret the Standards of Ethical Coding
The following ethical principles are based on the core values of the American Health Information Management Association and the AHIMA Code of Ethics and apply to all coding professionals. Guidelines for each ethical principle include examples of behaviors and situations that can help to clarify the principle. They are not meant as a comprehensive list of all situations that can occur.

1. ***Apply accurate, complete, and consistent coding practices for the production of high-quality healthcare data.***

    Coding professionals and those who manage coded data shall:

    1.1. Support selection of appropriate diagnostic, procedure and other types of health service related codes (for example, present on admission indicator, discharge status).

    Example:
    Policies and procedures are developed and used as a framework for the work process, and education and training is provided on their use.

    1.2. Develop and comply with comprehensive internal coding policies and procedures that are consistent with official coding rules and guidelines, as well as reimbursement regulations and policies, and prohibit coding practices that misrepresent the patient's medical conditions and treatment provided or are not supported by the health record documentation.

    Example:
    Code assignment resulting in misrepresentation of facts carries significant consequences.

    1.3. Participate in the development of institutional coding policies and ensure that coding policies complement, and do not conflict with, official coding rules and guidelines.

    1.4. Foster an environment that supports honest and ethical coding practices, resulting in accurate and reliable data.

    Coding professionals **shall not**:

    1.5. Participate in improper preparation, alteration, or suppression of coded information.

2. ***Report all healthcare data elements (for example, diagnosis and procedure codes, present on admission indicator, discharge status) required for external reporting***

purposes (for example, reimbursement and other administrative uses, population health, public data reporting, quality and patient safety measurement, research) completely and accurately, in accordance with regulatory and documentation standards and requirements and applicable official coding conventions, rules, and guidelines.

Coding professionals **shall**:

2.1. Adhere to the ICD coding conventions, official coding guidelines approved by the Cooperating Parties,[1] the CPT rules established by the American Medical Association, and any other official coding rules and guidelines established for use with mandated standard code sets.

Example:
Appropriate resource tools that assist coding professionals with proper sequencing and reporting to stay in compliance with existing reporting requirements are available and used.

2.2. Select and sequence diagnosis and procedure codes in accordance with the definitions of required data sets for applicable healthcare settings.

2.3. Comply with AHIMA's standards governing data reporting practices, including health record documentation and clinician query standards.

3. *Assign and report only the codes that are clearly and consistently supported by health record documentation in accordance with applicable code set conventions, rules, and guidelines.*

Coding professionals **shall**:

3.1. Apply skills, knowledge of currently mandated coding and classification systems, and official resources to select the appropriate diagnostic and procedural codes (including applicable modifiers), and other codes representing healthcare services (including substances, equipment, supplies, or other items used in the provision of healthcare services).

Example:
Failure to research or confirm the appropriate code for a clinical condition not indexed in the classification, or reporting a code for the sake of

convenience or to affect reporting for a desired effect on the results, is considered unethical.

4. *Query provider (physician or other qualified healthcare practitioner) for clarification and additional documentation prior to code assignment when there is conflicting, incomplete, or ambiguous information in the health record regarding a significant reportable condition or procedure or other reportable data element dependent on health record documentation (for example, present on admission indicator).*

Coding professionals **shall**:

4.1. Participate in the development of query policies that support documentation improvement and meet regulatory, legal, and ethical standards for coding and reporting.

4.2. Query the provider for clarification when documentation in the health record that impacts an externally reportable data element is illegible, incomplete, unclear, inconsistent, or imprecise.

4.3. Use queries as a communication tool to improve the accuracy of code assignment and the quality of health record documentation, not to inappropriately increase reimbursement or misrepresent quality of care.

Example:
Policies regarding the circumstances when clinicians should be queried are designed to promote complete and accurate coding and complete documentation, regardless of whether reimbursement will be affected.

Coding professionals **shall not**:

4.4. Query the provider when there is no clinical information in the health record prompting the need for a query.

Example:
Query the provider regarding the presence of gram-negative pneumonia on every pneumonia case, regardless of whether there are any clinical indications of gram-negative pneumonia documented in the record.

5. *Refuse to change reported codes or the narratives of codes so that meanings are misrepresented.*

Coding professionals **shall not**:

5.1. Change the description for a diagnosis or procedure code or other reported data element so that it does not accurately reflect the official definition of that code.

Example:
The description of a code is altered in the encoding software, resulting in incorrect reporting of this code.

6. *Refuse to participate in or support coding or documentation practices intended to inappropriately increase payment, qualify for insurance policy coverage, or skew data by means that do not comply with federal and state statutes, regulations, and official rules and guidelines.*

Coding professionals **shall**:

6.1. Select and sequence the codes such that the organization receives the optimal payment to which the facility is legally entitled, remembering that it is unethical and illegal to increase payment by means that contradict regulatory guidelines.

Coding professionals **shall not**:

6.2. Misrepresent the patient's clinical picture through intentional incorrect coding or omission of diagnosis or procedure codes, or the addition of diagnosis or procedure codes unsupported by health record documentation, to inappropriately increase reimbursement, justify medical necessity, improve publicly reported data, or qualify for insurance policy coverage benefits.

Examples:
A patient has a health plan that excludes reimbursement for reproductive management or contraception; so rather than report the correct code for admission for tubal ligation, it is reported as a medically necessary condition with performance of a salpingectomy. The narrative descriptions of both the diagnosis and procedures reflect an admission for tubal ligation and the procedure (tubal ligation) is displayed on the record.

A code is changed at the patient's request so that the service will be covered by the patient's insurance.

Coding professionals **shall not**:

6.3. Inappropriately exclude diagnosis or procedure codes in order to misrepresent the quality of care provided.

Examples:
Following a surgical procedure, a patient acquired an infection due to a break in sterile procedure; the appropriate code for the surgical complication is omitted from the claims submission to avoid any adverse outcome to the institution.

Quality outcomes are reported inaccurately in order to improve a healthcare organization's quality profile or pay-for-performance results.

7. *Facilitate interdisciplinary collaboration in situations supporting proper coding practices.*

Coding professionals **shall**:

7.1. Assist and educate physicians and other clinicians by advocating proper documentation practices, further specificity, and resequence or include diagnoses or procedures when needed to more accurately reflect the acuity, severity, and the occurrence of events.

Example:
Failure to advocate for ethical practices that seek to represent the truth in events as expressed by the associated code sets when needed is considered an intentional disregard of these standards.

8. *Advance coding knowledge and practice through continuing education.*

Coding professionals **shall**:

8.1. Maintain and continually enhance coding competency (for example, through participation in educational programs, reading official coding publications such as the Coding Clinic for ICD-9-CM, and maintaining professional certifications) in order to stay abreast of changes in codes, coding guidelines, and regulatory and other requirements.

9. *Refuse to participate in or conceal unethical coding practices or procedures.*

Coding professionals **shall**:

9.1. Act in a professional and ethical manner at all times.

9.2. Take adequate measures to discourage, prevent, expose, and correct the unethical conduct of colleagues.

9.3. Be knowledgeable about established policies and procedures for handling concerns about colleagues' unethical behavior. These include policies and procedures created by AHIMA, licensing and regulatory bodies, employers, supervisors, agencies, and other professional organizations.

9.4. Seek resolution if there is a belief that a colleague has acted unethically or if there is a belief of incompetence or impairment by discussing their concerns with the colleague when feasible and when such discussion is likely to be productive. Take action through appropriate formal channels, such as contacting an accreditation or regulatory body and/or the AHIMA Professional Ethics Committee.

9.5. Consult with a colleague when feasible and assist the colleague in taking remedial action when there is direct knowledge of a health information management colleague's incompetence or impairment.

Coding professionals **shall not**:

9.6. Participate in, condone, or be associated with dishonesty, fraud and abuse, or deception. A non-exhaustive list of examples includes:

- ° Allowing inappropriate patterns of retrospective documentation to avoid suspension or increase reimbursement
- ° Assigning codes without supporting provider (physician or other qualified healthcare practitioner) documentation
- ° Coding when documentation does not justify the diagnoses and/or procedures that have been billed
- ° Coding an inappropriate level of service
- ° Miscoding to avoid conflict with others
- ° Adding, deleting, and altering health record documentation
- ° Copying and pasting another clinician's documentation without identification of the original author and date

- ° Knowingly reporting incorrect present on admission indicator
- ° Knowingly reporting incorrect patient discharge status code
- ° Engaging in negligent coding practices

10. ***Protect the confidentiality of the health record at all times and refuse to access protected health information not required for coding-related activities (examples of coding-related activities include completion of code assignment, other health record data abstraction, coding audits, and educational purposes).***

Coding professionals **shall**:

10.1. Protect all confidential information obtained in the course of professional service, including personal, health, financial, genetic, and outcome information.

10.2. Access only that information necessary to perform their duties.

11. ***Demonstrate behavior that reflects integrity, shows a commitment to ethical and legal coding practices, and fosters trust in professional activities.***

Coding professionals **shall**:

11.1. Act in an honest manner and bring honor to self, peers, and the profession.

11.2. Truthfully and accurately represent their credentials, professional education, and experience.

11.3. Demonstrate ethical principles and professional values in their actions to patients, employers, other members of the healthcare team, consumers, and other stakeholders served by the healthcare data they collect and report.

[1] The Cooperating Parties are the American Health Information Management Association, American Hospital Association, Centers for Medicare & Medicaid Services, and National Center for Health Statistics.

Source:
AHIMA House of Delegates. "AHIMA Standards of Ethical Coding." September 2008.

Chapter 3
Voluntary Healthcare
Insurance Plans

Objectives

- To discuss major types of voluntary healthcare insurance plans

- To differentiate individual healthcare plans from employer-based healthcare plans

- To describe types of Blue Cross and Blue Shield plans

- To describe state healthcare plans for the medically uninsurable

- To explain the provisions of healthcare insurance policies and the elements of a healthcare insurance identification card

- To describe the filing of a healthcare insurance claim

- To discuss remittance advices and explanations of benefits

- To define basic language associated with reimbursement by commercial healthcare insurance plans and by Blue Cross and Blue Shield plans

Key Terms

Actual charge
Adjudication
Adjustment
Adverse selection
Allowable charge
Appeal
Assignment of benefits
Benefit
Benefit cap
Benefit period
Catastrophic expense limit
Center of excellence
Certificate holder
Certificate number
Certificate of insurance
Claim
Claim attachment
Claim submission
Clean claim
Clearinghouse
Coinsurance

Consumer-directed (consumer-driven) healthcare plan (CDHP)
Contracted discount rate
Coordination of benefits (COB)
Copayment
Cost sharing
Covered condition
Covered service
Deductible
Dependent
Dirty claim
Edit
Editor
Electronic claim submission
Electronic funds transfer (EFT)
Electronic remittance advice (ERA)
Eligibility
Endorsement
Enrollment
Exclusion
Explanation of benefits (EOB)

Family coverage
Flexible spending (saving) account (FSA)
Formulary
Guaranteed issue
Group number
Guarantor
Health reimbursement arrangement (HRA)
Health savings account (HSA)
High-deductible health plan (HDHP)
High-risk pool
Indemnity health insurance
In-network
Insured
Late enrollee
Limitation
Maximum out-of-pocket cost
Medical emergency
Medical necessity
Medically uninsurable
Medigap
Member
Moral hazard
Nonsingle coverage
Open enrollment (election) period
Other party liability (OPL)
Out-of-network
Out-of-pocket
Point-of-service healthcare insurance

Policy
Policyholder
Pre-certification
Pre-existing condition
Pre-existing condition exclusion
Preferred drug list
Premium
Primary insurer (payer)
Prior approval
Prudent layperson standard
Qualifying life event (QLE)
Remittance advice
Rider
Risk
Risk pool
Secondary insurer (payer)
Single coverage
Special enrollment (election) period
State healthcare insurance plan
Stop–loss benefit
Subscriber
Summary of Benefits and Coverage (SBC)
Supplemental insurance
Tier
Waiting period
Wellness program
Wraparound
Write-off

Introduction to Voluntary Healthcare Insurance

Voluntary health insurance (VHI) is the umbrella term that includes private or commercial healthcare insurance plans and Blue Cross and Blue Shield plans. Voluntary health insurance is private and denotes employment (Koch 2002, 96). VHI is differentiated from social health insurance and public welfare. Social health insurance comprises government programs based on current or past employment. Public welfare is assistance to categories of low-income people or other defined subpopulations.

Payments from voluntary health insurance plans account for approximately 33 percent of healthcare expenditures in the United States (Martin et al. 2014, 74). Accordingly, understanding this form of healthcare insurance is integral to understanding healthcare reimbursement.

Before the 1970s, almost all voluntary health insurance was **indemnity health insurance**. Indemnity healthcare insurance plans are also called retrospective fee-for-service, as described in chapter 1. Indemnity health plans offer individuals the freedom to choose their healthcare professionals.

Types of Voluntary Healthcare Insurance

Healthcare insurance companies sell healthcare plans to both individuals and groups of people. Also, healthcare insurance companies allow people to purchase healthcare coverage for

- Themselves only, which is known as **single coverage** or, alternatively, as self-only coverage, individual coverage, or an individual plan

- Themselves and their dependents, which is known as **nonsingle coverage** or **dependent coverage** and can be the purchaser-plus-one coverage or **family coverage**

Dependents are spouses and other family members. Nonsingle coverage costs more than single coverage.

This chapter investigates two major categories of voluntary health insurance—private or commercial healthcare insurance plans and Blue Cross and Blue Shield plans—organized in three classifications as illustrated in figure 3.1. A third minor category, state-sponsored plans for medically uninsurable persons, is also described.

Figure 3.1.   Three classifications of voluntary healthcare insurance

Commercial (private*) individual (private*) healthcare insurance plan
Commercial (private*) employer-based healthcare insurance plan
Blue Cross and Blue Shield Plans

*Private is used two ways in the healthcare insurance industry: (1) as a synonym for commercial healthcare insurance and (2) to mean purchased by an individual rather than by an employer for a group.

The first major category is private or commercial healthcare insurance, which contains two classifications: individual (private) healthcare insurance plans and employer-based healthcare insurance plans. Employer-based healthcare insurance plans are also termed group plans.

Differentiating the two classifications of private or commercial healthcare insurance is the size of the **risk pool**. A risk pool is a group of individual entities, such as individual persons, employers, or associations, whose healthcare costs are combined for evaluating financial history and estimating future costs (American Academy of Actuaries 2006, 2). There are three types of pools:

- Individual pools—These are pools of individuals, such as self-employed people or people who work for companies that do not offer healthcare insurance. The people in these pools are similar because they are all seeking health insurance, so these pools tend to be the least diverse or most homogeneous of the three types (American Academy of Actuaries 2006, 2–4).

- Large-employer pools—Employees of one employer, typically 1,000 members or more. These pools are large and diverse (heterogeneous).

- Multiple-employer pools—Employees from several midsize employers or small employers or groups of associations. These pools are smaller and less diverse than the large-employer pools are.

Smaller pools do not provide a sufficiently wide range of diversity in terms of age, sex, and health status, so they are at risk for **adverse selection**. Adverse selection is having disproportionate numbers of sick people. On the other hand, the diversity of the large-employer pools provides stable trends in utilization and financial impact. A key point is that the larger the pool, the more able it is to balance a wide variety of **risks** (from healthy persons to persons with chronic conditions or catastrophic illnesses). The risk is distributed across more entities.

Thus, individual (private) healthcare insurance plans are known as individual insurance because the pool is at the individual level. Conversely, employer-based healthcare insurance plans are called group plans because the risk pools are large-employer pools or multiple-employer pools.

Confusing Terminology

Classifications of voluntary healthcare insurance and terminology can be confusing in the healthcare industry. First, classifications overlap because commercial healthcare insurance plans and Blue Cross and Blue Shield plans often have multiple divisions that offer options both to private individuals and to employers. For example, both Aetna and Blue Cross and Blue Shield of Florida have healthcare insurance plans for individuals and families and for groups of employees. These diversified offerings make clear distinctions between the types of healthcare insurance plans difficult. Second, members of the healthcare industry give the same words different meanings in different situations:

- The word *individual* is used two ways: to mean "nongroup" and also to mean "single coverage" or "no dependent coverage."

- The word *private* is also used two ways: to mean commercial healthcare insurance and to mean healthcare insurance purchased by an individual versus healthcare insurance purchased by an employer for a group of employees.

Most important, classification of a healthcare insurance plan depends on the provisions of the healthcare insurance plan and how the plan functions, rather than on its name.

Individual Healthcare Plans

Individuals and self-employed businesspersons purchase healthcare insurance for themselves and their families. Thus, individual healthcare plans are termed *individual plans* because individuals purchase them. For some

people, the individual healthcare plan is their only plan for self and family. Other people purchase individual healthcare plans to supplement their employer-based group insurance or their Medicare.

In general, individual healthcare insurance plans provide fewer **covered services** at a higher cost than employer-based group healthcare insurance plans (see the next section). Thus, **policyholders** of individual healthcare insurance pay higher **premiums** to obtain and maintain healthcare insurance. Premiums are the periodic payments that a policyholder or certificate holder must make to an insurer in return for healthcare coverage. Also higher are the **deductibles** that the policyholder must pay before the healthcare insurance will assume its share of liability for the remaining costs.

Employer-Based (Group) Healthcare Plans

Employer-based (or employer-sponsored) healthcare plans are group plans for groups of employees or members. Employer-based healthcare insurance is the most common means of coverage for the nonelderly in the United States (Claxton et al. 2013, 1667). Of the population younger than 65 years old, 58.3 percent have employer-based healthcare insurance (Gould 2013, 603). As the name implies, an employer-based healthcare plan is based on people's employment. However, occasionally *employer-based healthcare plan* is a misnomer because the type includes all plans that cover groups. Individuals may form groups through professional associations and other entities. Generally, though, employer-based healthcare insurance is an employment benefit (like vacation time or a retirement plan).

Employer-based healthcare plans have lower premiums and deductibles and greater **benefits** than individual healthcare plans. Moreover, the employer and employee share the cost of the healthcare insurance premium. The employer's share is larger than the employee's share; a few employers pay 100 percent of the premium for their employees. Thus, for beneficiaries, the costs of employer-based healthcare insurance are less than individual healthcare plans.

Analyses show that the number of employers offering the benefit of group healthcare insurance is declining. From 2000 to 2011, the percentage of workers covered by their employer's health plan dropped from 69.2 percent to 58.3 percent, a decline of almost 11 percent (Gould 2013, 606). Converting the percentages into numbers of people, this decline means that 11.7 million fewer nonelderly Americans had employer-based healthcare insurance in 2011 than in 2000. Finally, no demographic or socioeconomic group escaped the erosion of employer-based healthcare insurance from 2000 to 2011 (Gould 2013, 604).

Blue Cross and Blue Shield Plans

Blue Cross and Blue Shield is a national federation of 37 independent, locally operated plans united through membership in the Blue Cross and Blue Shield Association (BCBSA) (Blue Cross and Blue Shield 2014). Blue Cross and Blue Shield also has independent licensees in some geographic areas. The Blue Cross and Blue Shield plans are the second major category and the third classification of voluntary healthcare insurance (figure 3.1). The plans contract with hospitals, physicians, and other healthcare providers to offer services to their **subscribers** (policyholders).

Blue Cross and Blue Shield plans began in Dallas, Texas, in 1929, when Justin Ford Kimball established a health insurance plan for schoolteachers. In the plan, schoolteachers prepaid $6 per year for 21 days of hospitalization (Friedman 1998, 1863). Similar plans were also formed in Michigan and New Jersey (Koch 2002, 98). In 1934, the American Hospital Association (AHA) united the plans under its auspices (Koch 2002, 98). In 1939, the AHA adopted the symbol of the blue cross to indicate the health insurance plans that met specific criteria for covering hospital care. Also in 1939, Blue Shield was founded in California to cover physician services (Friedman 1998, 1863). In 1972, the AHA's sponsorship of Blue Cross ended. Blue Cross and Blue Shield merged in 1982 to form the Blue Cross and Blue Shield Association (Friedman 1998, 1865).

BCBSA is one of the most influential groups in healthcare (Hall and Conover 2006, 444). The Blue Companies insure nearly one in three Americans (Serota 2012, 50). More than 105 million Americans are enrolled in the Blue Companies in all 50 states, the District of Columbia, and Puerto Rico (Blue Cross Blue Shield Association 2014). The Blue Companies offer their subscribers a wide range of options, such as health maintenance organizations (HMOs), **point-of-service (POS) healthcare insurance** plans, preferred provider organizations, and indemnity plans. Blue Cross and Blue Shield also is contracted by the federal government to administer the Medicare program in some geographic areas and is contracted by some state governments to administer their Medicaid programs (Medicare and Medicaid are discussed in chapter 4).

Nonprofit versus Profit Status

Historically, the Blue Companies operated as nonprofits (also known as not-for-profit organizations). Blue Cross and Blue Shield plans were not-for-profit, and individual or commercial healthcare insurance companies were for-profit. Thus, traditionally, the nonprofit status of the Blue Companies differentiated them from the for-profit private or commercial healthcare insurance companies. However, this differentiation in status changed between 1993 and 2002. During those years, local Blue Cross and Blue Shield plans in 14 states converted to for-profit status from not-for-profit (Hall and Conover 2006, 444). Thus, more than one in four Blue Cross subscribers now belong to a for-profit plan (Hall and Conover 2006, 444). Meanwhile, commercial healthcare insurance companies maintained their for-profit status. The conversions of the Blue Companies blurred the distinction between the two types of health insurers.

Types of Blue Cross and Blue Shield Accounts

Blue Cross and Blue Shield have two types of accounts: geographic plans at the region, state, or substate level and the single plan associated with the federal employee program (FEP). Geographic plans cover subscribers (members) in a specific region, state, or area of a state. The FEP covers all enrolled federal government employees the world over.

Geographic Plans

Geographic plans cover specific geographic areas. Plans can operate at various levels:

- Multistate level, such as in the case of Wellpoint, Inc., an independent licensee of Blue Cross and Blue Shield

- State level, such as in the cases of Blue Cross of Alabama, Anthem Blue Cross and Blue Shield of Missouri, Regence Blue Cross and Blue Shield of Utah, and Blue Cross and Blue Shield of North Carolina

- Substate level, such as in the cases of Blue Cross and Blue Shield of Western New York, one of four Blue plans in New York state

The geographic plans are locally administered and have long-standing relationships with their local hospitals and medical communities (Hall and Conover 2003, 509).

Subscribers carry cards bearing the name of the plan, the subscribers' names, and contract and group numbers.

Federal Employee Program

Federal employees have health insurance through their employment in the federal government. These employees work throughout the nation. Therefore, on behalf of the 37 local Blue Cross plans, the BCBSA works with the federal Office of Personnel Management (OPM) to administer the employees' health insurance benefit. This government-wide health insurance is called the federal employee program (FEP) or the Service Benefit Plan. The FEP covers 5.3 million federal employees and retirees and their families. The notation "Government-Wide Service Benefit Plan" or "FEP" on an insured person's (insured's) cards identify the federal program.

State Healthcare Plans for the Medically Uninsurable

State legislatures in 35 states have established **state healthcare insurance plans** (Cauchi 2014, n.p.). The purpose of these state healthcare insurance plans was to provide access to healthcare insurance coverage to the medically uninsurable. These state healthcare insurance plans are often called **high-risk pools**.

People who are **medically uninsurable** have a pre-existing condition or a chronic disease or both (Gruber 2009, 2). Examples of conditions and diseases include acquired immunodeficiency syndrome (AIDS), cancer, chronic kidney failure, congestive heart failure, cystic fibrosis and other genetic disorders, diabetes, mental and emotional disorders, multiple sclerosis and other neurological disorders, obesity, quadriplegia, and spina bifida and other congenital disorders. As a result, these people need to use healthcare services more than healthy people, and their healthcare costs are higher.

Originally, under the Affordable Care Act (ACA), these high-risk pools were scheduled for elimination, because pre-existing conditions could not be a reason to deny healthcare insurance. The people would no longer be medically uninsurable. As a result of delays in the implementation of the ACA, some states have decided to continue their high-risk pools (Cauchi 2014, n.p.).

Check Your Understanding 3.1

1. True or False? When people purchase healthcare insurance for themselves and their dependents, they are purchasing single coverage.

2. True or False? In terms of healthcare insurance coverage, both children and spouses may be considered dependents.

3. In the healthcare insurance sector, which type of risk pool has the greatest diversity and the greatest ability to balance risks?

4. True or False? Individual (private) healthcare insurance is the most common means of coverage for the nonelderly in the United States.

5. What organization is one of the most influential in the healthcare sector? Why?

Provisions and Functioning of Healthcare Insurance Plans

Healthcare insurance companies assume the financial risk of the costs of individual and group healthcare. Healthcare insurance companies assume this risk because individuals or groups purchase the insurance companies' healthcare plans. Healthcare insurance companies issue policies to individuals or groups who purchase the healthcare plan.

A healthcare insurance **policy** is a formal contract between the healthcare insurance company and the individuals or groups for whom the company is assuming risk. This contract is called a **certificate of insurance**. This written document may also be known as a certificate of coverage, evidence of coverage, or summary plan description (PACER Family-to-Family Health Information Center 2011, n.p.). This contract is available upon request, free of charge.

The certificates of insurance (policies) stipulate all **covered conditions**, healthcare services related to covered conditions, and all other aspects of healthcare for which the healthcare plan will pay. Also important, a certificate of insurance discloses what the policy does *not* cover, the dollar limits, and the patients' responsibilities and obligations (PACER Family-to-Family Health Information Center 2011, n.p.). Thus, certificates of insurance detail all procedures that patients must follow and all conditions that patients must meet to receive full benefits under their healthcare insurance policies.

Per the ACA, healthcare insurers must also provide a **Summary of Benefits and Coverage (SBC)** to policyholders or certificate holders. The SBC is a document that, in plain language, concisely details information about a healthcare insurer's benefits and its coverage of health services. This information is presented in a simple, consistent, and uniform format. The SBC's purpose is to give consumers improved information about their coverage. The SBC is only a summary; it does not replace the policy, the certificate of insurance, or other formal insurance document that governs the contractual provisions of the coverage.

The purchasers of healthcare insurance policies (plans) are policyholders or insureds. If an employer or association purchases the healthcare insurance, the entity is the *group policyholder* and the employees or association members receive certificates of insurance coverage and, thus, are **certificate holders** or subscribers (also known as enrollees, **members**, **insureds**, and covered lives). To uniquely identify the certificate holders or subscribers, healthcare insurance companies issue **certificate numbers**, or subscriber (member) numbers. As stated previously, spouses and other family members of the policyholders are known as dependents.

Policyholders pay higher premiums for dependent coverage than for single, self-only coverage. In addition to premiums, policyholders also pay deductibles, coinsurance, and copayments as provided in the policy. To easily identify sets of policies with similar deductibles, coinsurance, and copayments, healthcare insurance companies issue group (plan) numbers.

Although the term *healthcare services* is used throughout this text, some sectors of the healthcare industry are more specific in their usage of terms. Medical services (care) include diagnostic and therapeutic measures provided to persons who are sick, injured, or concerned about their health status. Healthcare services expand medical services to include preventive care (Rowell 2000, 22).

Sections of a Healthcare Insurance Policy

Healthcare insurance policies are divided into sections. Typically, these sections include definitions (commonly used terms), eligibility and enrollment, benefits, limitations, exclusions, riders and endorsements, procedures, and appeals processes. The sections build upon one another, and one aspect of healthcare may be addressed in multiple sections. Because the sections interlock, reviewing multiple sections is often necessary to determine whether the healthcare insurance company will pay for (cover) a specific diagnostic procedure, treatment, or healthcare expense.

Definitions

Definitions are often in their own separate section, but they may also be incorporated into the benefits section. Definitions are important because they can affect healthcare insurance coverage and payment.

Example:

The healthcare plan of the state of North Carolina defines **medical necessity** as follows:

Those *covered services* or supplies that are

- Provided for the diagnosis, treatment, cure, or relief of a health condition, illness, injury, or disease; and, except for clinical trials as described under this health benefit plan, not for *experimental, investigational*, or *cosmetic* purposes

- Necessary for and appropriate to the diagnosis, treatment, cure, or relief of a health condition, illness, injury, disease, or its symptoms

- Within generally accepted standards of *medical care* in the community

- Not solely for the convenience of the insured, the insured's family, or the *provider* (North Carolina State Health Plan 2014, 78)

Thus, by definition, cosmetic services are not considered medically necessary and thus, would not be paid for by the healthcare insurance company. Terms often listed in definitions include the following:

- Accidental injury

- Medical emergency

- Medical necessity

- Prior approval

- Usual, customary, and reasonable (UCR)

Definitions sometimes are specific to the healthcare plan and may be more restrictive than those in everyday usage or dictionaries. For example, a dictionary definition of *emergency* is "an unexpected situation or sudden occurrence of a serious and urgent nature that demands immediate attention" (Pickett et al. 2000).

The healthcare insurance plan may define *emergency* as "life-threatening," a concept that is more extreme and less likely than demanding immediate attention.

Differences in the definition of **medical emergency** led to legal disputes between health insurance companies and their subscribers. Health insurance companies denied coverage for services that their subscribers perceived as emergencies. For example, a man entering an emergency room for chest pain could believe that he was having an acute myocardial infarction (heart attack). After diagnostic tests, the patient actually had reflux esophagitis (heartburn). Sometimes, based on the definition and the principal diagnosis, health insurance companies retrospectively denied this type of patient's emergency care. To address this situation, many states passed laws based on the **prudent layperson standard** (Hall 2004, 559). In prudent layperson laws, the decision whether symptoms required urgent or emergent treatment is based on an ordinary layperson's reasonable judgment (Hall 2004, 559). Moreover, the decision is based on the symptoms at the time, not the diagnosis after tests (Hall 2004, 559). The necessity for states' legal intervention highlights the importance of definitions for both health insurance companies and subscribers.

Eligibility and Enrollment

The **eligibility** section of a healthcare insurance policy specifies the persons who are eligible to apply for the healthcare insurance. The **enrollment** section specifies the procedures for obtaining healthcare insurance.

Eligibility is the set of stipulations that qualify a person to apply for healthcare insurance. For employer-based healthcare insurance, these stipulations often involve the percentage of the appointment or position. A common provision is that persons must be employed at least 50 percent of the time or half-time (0.5 full-time equivalent). People who are eligible include the subscribers or employees, themselves, and their dependents, if applicable. Eligible dependents include the following:

- Legally married spouses
- Children and young adults until they reach age 26. The definition of *children* includes natural children, legally adopted children, stepchildren, and children who are dependent during the waiting period before adoption. Effective

September 23, 2010, per the Affordable Care Act (ACA) (Title I, Part A, Subpart II, Sec. 2714), children and young adults were eligible *regardless* of any, or a combination of any, of the following factors: financial dependency, residency with parent, student status, employment, and marital status. The regulation applies to all individual (private) and employer-based (group) healthcare insurance plans created after the date of enactment of the ACA (March 23, 2010). For employer-based plans that were in existence before the date of enactment, young adults can qualify for dependent coverage only if they are ineligible for an employment-based health insurance plan.

- Dependents with disabilities. The age limit of 26 does not apply to dependents who are (1) incapable of self-sustaining employment by reason of a physically or mentally disabling injury, disease, or condition *and* (2) chiefly dependent on the policyholder or subscriber for support and maintenance

The ACA does *not* require that the spouse of a dependent or the dependent of a dependent (grandchild) be eligible for coverage. Reimbursement analysts should carefully review the definition of *eligible dependent* in their own state. Some states extend coverage more broadly than the ACA; for example, New Jersey extends the dependent age to 30 (Kaiser Family Foundation 2010, n.p.). The ACA does not supersede these states' expanded definitions of eligibility. The ACA does supersede states' narrower scopes of eligibility.

Under the **guaranteed issue** provision of the ACA, healthcare insurers are required to accept every qualified individual who applies for healthcare coverage, with two exceptions:

- Plans in existence before the ACA and that have not made significant changes since March 23, 2010 ("grandfathered" health plans)
- Individual healthcare policies renewed in 2013 under the transitional policy for expiring coverage (policy expires in 2017) (Giovannelli et al. 2014, 2, 9)

Group healthcare plans may require a general **waiting period** (also called a benefits eligibility waiting period). Waiting periods do not apply to individual healthcare insurance plans. A waiting period is the period that must pass before coverage for an employee or dependent who is *otherwise eligible* to enroll under the terms of a group health plan (including grandfathered plans) can become effective (Internal Revenue Service 2014, 35943). The waiting period cannot exceed 90 days, and all calendar days are counted, including weekends and holidays. Otherwise eligible means having met the plan's substantive eligibility conditions, such as achieving job-related licensure or satisfying a reasonable and bona fide employment-based orientation period (not exceeding one month) (Internal Revenue Service 2014, 35944).

Enrollment is the initial process by which new individuals apply for and are accepted as members (subscribers, enrollees, policyholders, certificate holders) of healthcare insurance plans. (Medicare uses the term *election* for enrollment.) During enrollment periods, insureds specify whether the coverage will be single (self-only) coverage or nonsingle (dependent) coverage, which includes employee-(purchaser)-plus-one coverage and family coverage. **Late enrollees** are people who apply *after* the earliest date on which coverage is available. Late enrollment is undesirable.

Open enrollment (election) periods are specific periods when applications are received and processed. Typical open enrollment periods are

- Within 30 days of hire for initial coverage

- During defined periods that occur annually (often between October and December)

During open enrollment, individuals may elect to enroll in, modify coverage under, or transfer between healthcare insurance plans. The selections individuals make during open enrollment are in effect for the upcoming calendar year and until the next open enrollment period.

Special enrollment (election) periods are unique (special) to certain circumstances and occur without regard to the healthcare insurance company's regularly scheduled, annual, open enrollment period. Timing of a special enrollment period is driven by specific events in the lives *of individuals* (not employers or health insurers). These specific events are called **qualifying life events (QLEs)**. Much as is the case with open enrollment periods, individuals may elect to enroll in, modify, or transfer between healthcare insurance plans

during special enrollment periods as a result of the QLEs. The QLEs that make an individual eligible for special enrollment are

- Loss of other healthcare coverage (self, spouse, or dependent)

- Marriage

- Divorce

- Birth

- Adoption

- Placement for adoption

Typically, individuals have 30 days after the event to request the special enrollment.

The enrollment is for the upcoming **benefit period** (also known as policy limit). The benefit period is the length of time for which the policy will pay benefits for the member (and family and dependents, if applicable). Often, in employer-based healthcare insurance, the benefit period is the entire next calendar year and until the next open enrollment period. This one-year period often occurs because each year employers renegotiate benefits and costs of health insurance. Self-insured people may also purchase their own health insurance annually; they, too, may vary their benefits depending on costs. However, some individual (private) health insurance policies have three-year benefit periods, five-year benefit periods, and lifetime (unlimited) benefit periods. In each case, the policies will provide coverage for the period as long as the members are qualified to receive the benefits.

Benefits

Benefits are the healthcare services for which the healthcare insurance company will pay (will cover). Benefits may include the following services:

- Healthcare services provided by physicians, allied health practitioners, and visiting nurses.

- Free preventive care for preventive services and immunizations recommended by the United States Preventive Services Task Force (A or B grade), routine immunizations, childhood preventive services, and women's preventive care services include well-woman visits; mammograms; screenings for cervical cancer, osteoporosis, colorectal cancer, and domestic violence; and other preventive healthcare services. Some services are linked to an age requirement or risk factor (Robertson and Collins 2011, 10). Free means that the preventive care services themselves are free and are exempt from cost-sharing. Grandfathered plans existing on March 23, 2010, may be exempt from some aspects.

- Confinement in an acute-care hospital, long-term care hospital, partial day center, specialty hospital, or nursing home, including necessary services, supplies, and medications.

- Inpatient and outpatient surgeries and associated anesthesia services.

- Emergency room, physician office visits, home healthcare, mental health and chemical dependency care, vision and dental care, laboratory tests, x-rays, and other radiological procedures and treatments.

- Rental or purchase of durable medical equipment (DME), prosthetic and orthotic appliances, prescriptions, medical supplies, and blood transfusions and administration.

- Emergency transport services.

- Stop–loss benefits.

For example, a stop–loss benefit is designed to provide coverage in the event of a catastrophic illness or injury. A **stop–loss benefit** is a specific amount, in a certain timeframe, such as one year, beyond which all covered healthcare services for that policyholder or dependent are paid at 100 percent by the healthcare insurance plan. This benefit is also known as the **maximum out-of-pocket cost** and the **catastrophic expense limit**. The total is the maximum amount that the policyholder will pay out of pocket for covered healthcare services in the specified period. Included in the total are deductibles, coinsurance, and copayments that the policyholder is responsible to pay out of pocket. Note that premiums are *not* included in the maximum out-of-pocket cost.

Benefits can be categorized into two broad classifications: core benefits for general healthcare services and special-limited benefits for specific situations. The core benefits are the types available in employer-based healthcare insurance and in individual healthcare insurance. Insureds may purchase differing levels of these benefits in policies. The levels vary widely in the range of services they cover. Premiums, deductibles, coinsurances, and copayments range accordingly. The deductible must be met before the healthcare insurance company will pay for any covered expenses. Coinsurance and copayments for all covered expenses must be paid until the maximum out-of-pocket cost is reached. Additional covered expenses are paid in full.

The core benefits include the following:

- Comprehensive policies: Providing coverage for most healthcare services, such as ambulatory patient services; emergency services; hospitalization; maternal and newborn care; surgery; diagnostic and therapeutic x-rays; laboratory services; mental health and substance use disorder services, including behavioral health treatment; prescription drugs; rehabilitative and habilitative services and devices; preventive services and chronic disease management; pediatric services, including oral and vision care; ambulance; durable medical equipment; hospice services; medical supplies; orthotic devices; private duty nursing; prosthetic appliances; and home health care.

- Essential health benefits (EHB) policies covering 10 categories, as required by the ACA: ambulatory patient services; emergency services; hospitalization; maternal and newborn care; mental health and substance use disorder services, including behavioral health treatment; prescription drugs; rehabilitative and habilitative services and devices; laboratory services; preventive services and chronic disease management; and pediatric services, including oral and vision care. Healthcare reform sets up four levels of cost sharing: bronze, in which the policyholder pays about 40 percent of costs; silver, in which the policyholder pays about 30 percent; gold, in which the policyholder pays about 20 percent; and platinum, in which the policyholder pays about 10 percent.

Special-limited benefits include the following:

- Hospital and surgical policies cover major expenses in the hospital and expenses related to surgeries, including outpatient surgery.

Healthcare insurance payments may be percentages or specific dollar amounts. Hospitalization policies typically have high deductibles and high coverage limits.

- Major medical (catastrophic) policies are designed to reduce risk associated with catastrophic illness or injury. A fixed amount is available during the lifetime of the policyholder or dependent. Major medical policies typically have high deductibles and high coverage limits.

- Hospital confinement indemnity policies pay a per diem for each day in the hospital. This policy is typically in addition to comprehensive policies, hospital and surgical policies, and major medical policies.

- Long-term (extended) care policies provide benefits for nursing home care and services.

- Disability income protection policies provide weekly or monthly payments during a lengthy illness or recovery from an injury. Disability income protection policies only begin to pay after a period established in the contract (30 days to six months). Contracts usually contain maximum payment limits based on a percentage of the policyholder's salary, such as 60 percent.

- Accidental death and dismemberment (loss) policies cover expenses arising from an accident that causes a loss such as death, amputation of a limb, or blindness. Benefits vary greatly depending on the specific policy.

- Specific condition, disease, or accident policies provide coverage for diseases or accidents listed in the policy. Common examples are vision care policies, dental policies, and cancer policies.

- Medicare supplemental health insurance **Medigap** policies which are designed to coordinate their payments with payments from Medicare. These policies "wrap around" the benefits of Medicare, filling in "gaps" in Medicare coverage, such as deductibles and coinsurance. Benefits vary by policy.

- Other **supplemental insurance (wraparound)** policies fill in or supplement the coverage in other policies. The policies "wrap around" the benefits in comprehensive policies, essential health benefits policies, hospital and surgical policies, and major medical policies, filling in their gaps. The previously listed long-term policies, disability income protection policies, accidental death or dismemberment policies, and specific disease or accident policies are common examples. Another example is a short-term health insurance policy purchased for the duration of a vacation, travel, or trip. Supplemental policies provide cash benefits; cover deductibles, coinsurances, and copayments; or provide other forms of payment. Patients and guarantors often use the additional funds to pay incidental costs associated with healthcare, such as travel, lodging, meals, and day care.

Limitations

Limitations are qualifications or other specifications that limit the extent of the benefits. Limitations can be placed on total dollar amount, timeframe, duration, and number. For example, purchases of durable medical equipment exceeding $500 require prior approval.

Cost-Sharing Provisions

Common limitations are the cost-sharing provisions of many policies. The extent and number of cost-sharing provisions have risen as the costs of healthcare have increased. Cost-sharing provisions require policyholders to bear some of the costs of healthcare that they consume. Making policyholders bear some of the financial burden of healthcare is a mechanism to control healthcare costs. Several types of cost-sharing provisions exist.

Coinsurance

Coinsurance is a preestablished percentage of eligible expenses after the deductible has been met. The percentage may vary by type or site of service.

Copayment

Copayment is a fixed dollar amount (flat fee). The fixed amount may vary by type of service, such as a visit or a prescription. For example, the healthcare plan may require that the policyholder pay $15 per visit to a primary care physician and $50 per visit to a specialist.

Tiered Benefits

Some health plans have **tiers** of benefits. A tier is a level of coverage. Specifically, in health insurance, tiers act as *limits*. Health insurers impose these limits to increase the certainty of their costs. The tiers limit their members' freedom of choice of providers, the amount of services allowed, and the types of drugs or other services. The number and types of tiers vary by the benefit being limited and by the health insurer. Common examples include the following:

- Tier by level of members' ability to freely choose their healthcare providers. In this type of tier, the health insurer has negotiated **contracted discount rates (discounts)** with a network of preferred providers (physicians, hospitals, other providers). Members' cost sharing increases with the tier of freedom in choice of provider. In an example from one health insurer,
  ○ Tier 1 is "**in-network**" and offers the lowest level of members' freedom of choice. In this tier, a member has *one* primary care physician, selected by the health insurer. This one primary care physician coordinates and authorizes all the member's healthcare services. Typically, the member pays the lowest premium of the tiers and is responsible for a small copayment.
  ○ Tier 2, a "contracted network" offers a little more freedom of choice than Tier 1. In Tier 2, the member elects to receive services from the health insurer's network of physicians (sometimes called preferred or select). These physicians do *not* coordinate the member's healthcare services. Typically, the member pays a mid-range premium, a deductible, and coinsurance.
  ○ Tier 3 is "**out-of-network**" and offers members the most freedom of choice. In this tier, members choose any provider that they want, including providers outside the health insurer's network. However, these members pay for that freedom with higher premiums, deductibles, coinsurance, copayments, or some combination of these cost shares than members who choose less freedom with Tier 1 and Tier 2.

Members elect Tier 1, Tier 2, or Tier 3 during their initial enrollment or during the annual enrollment period.

- Tier at point of service. Again, the health insurer has negotiated discounted rates with a set of providers (physicians, hospitals, other providers). However, unlike is the case with the previous type of tier, in a point-of-service tier, the type of care, provider, or healthcare service is made when the service is needed rather than during the enrollment period.

- Tier by amount of service. Health insurers may limit the number of visits. For example, patients may be limited to 30 chiropractic visits per benefit period (or visits for other types of rehabilitative services). In another example, a health insurer's three tiers of benefits for vision services vary by coverage for exam and materials.
  ○ Tier 1 Plan: Materials only ($5.14 per month for employee only and $12.72 per month for employee and family). Materials are corrective eyeglass lenses, frames, and contact lenses. The Tier 1 Plan pays up to $100 of cost of retail frames and offers a 20 percent discount on remainder.
  ○ Tier 2 Plan: Exam and materials ($6.84 per month for employee only and $17.38 per month for employee and family). Vision exam is on principal vision functions.
  ○ Tier 3 Plan: Exam and enhanced materials ($9.98 per month for employee only and $25.10 per month for employee and family). The Tier 3 Plan pays up to $150 of cost of retail frames plus 20 percent discount on remainder.

- Tiered benefits for prescription drugs. Most health plans have a **formulary**, or **preferred drug list**, a continually updated list of safe, effective, and cost-effective drugs that the healthcare plan prefers that insureds use. Formularies and preferred drug lists contain both generic and brand-name drugs approved by the US Food and Drug Administration (FDA). The term, formulary or preferred drug list, varies by health plan. A policy's prescription benefit covers the drugs in the formulary and may cover nonformulary drugs. Most health plans have multiple tiers, levels of coverage, for prescription drugs. A prescription drug's tier depends on its classification in the health plan's formulary, such as the following:

° Tier 1: Most cost-effective drugs, including most generic drugs
° Tier 2: Preferred brand-name drugs, including some high-cost generic drugs and specially compounded medications
° Tier 3 Nonpreferred brand-name drugs
° Tier 4: Preferred specialty drugs, which are drugs that are used to treat complex diseases; that require special administration, dosing, and handling; that are typically prescribed by specialists; and that are high-cost
° Tier 5: Nonpreferred specialty drugs

For prescription drug benefits, health plans use both copayments and coinsurance as policyholders' cost sharing. Table 3.1 shows one health plan's tiered prescription drug benefit. As shown in table 3.1, cost sharing is hierarchical, with Tier 1 drugs having the lowest cost sharing and Tier 5 drugs having the highest.

• Tiered benefit for services with high cost and high complexity. Health insurers may require patients that need high-cost, high-complexity services to obtain them at a **center of**

Table 3.1.   Example of limitations: Tiered prescription drug benefit

Prescription Drug Tier	Cost sharing per Prescription		
	Up to 30-Day Supply	31- to 60-Day Supply	61- to 90-Day Supply
Tier 1: Formulary (preferred) generic	$12	$24	$36
Tier 2: Formulary (preferred) brand name	$40	$80	$120
Tier 3: Nonformulary (nonpreferred) brand name	$64	$128	$192
Tier 4: Formulary (preferred) specialty drug	25% coinsurance up to $100 for each 30-day supply		
Tier 5: Nonformulary (nonpreferred) specialty drug	25% coinsurance up to $125 for each 30-day supply		

excellence. A center of excellence is a healthcare organization that performs high volumes of a service at a correspondingly high quality. Centers of excellence are often recognized by their medical peers for their expertise, cost-effectiveness, and superior outcomes.

Health insurers negotiate discounted rates at centers of excellence for the service. To receive full coverage for the service, health insurers may require their members to receive the service at the center of excellence. Centers of excellence date to the 1960s (Wess 1999, 28). The concept of center of excellence began with hospitals that specialized in organ transplantation (Coulter et al. 1998, 8). Hospitals that performed many transplants had better outcomes than hospitals that performed only a few transplants. An article in the *New England Journal of Medicine* showed that this effect could be applied to other complicated procedures and diseases, such as acute myocardial infarction (Thiemann et al. 1999, 1640). Since then, the concept of centers of excellence has been extended to other procedures and conditions, such as bariatric surgery and Alzheimer's disease. One analyst notes that the concept of "centers of excellence takes tiering to the max" (Haugh 2006, 42).

Benefit Cap

A **benefit cap** is an overarching limitation. A benefit cap is also known as a maximum dollar plan limit. A benefit cap is the total dollar amount that a healthcare insurance company will pay for a policyholder and each covered dependent for covered healthcare services during a specified period, such as a year or lifetime.

Exclusions

Exclusions are situations, instances, conditions, injuries, or treatments that the healthcare plan states will not be covered and for which the healthcare plan will pay no benefits. A synonym for exclusion is impairment rider. Specific and unique definitions may serve as exclusions. Typical exclusions include

• Experimental or investigational diagnostic and therapeutic procedures

- Medically unnecessary diagnostic or therapeutic procedures

- Cosmetic procedures, except when related to accidents, disease, or congenital defects, and source-of-injury treatments, such as for war-related injuries and injuries sustained in the course of risky recreational activities

For example, a healthcare plan may deny coverage for a prescription to remove wrinkles (tretinoin) because the purpose is cosmetic. Contraceptives are also sometimes excluded. Coverage for experimental or investigational services is also often denied. Examples of experimental or investigational procedures or therapies include face transplants, medications used to treat conditions for which the FDA has not issued approval, and active cold therapy units using mechanical pumps and portable refrigerators.

A **preexisting condition** (state) is a health condition, status, or injury that was diagnosed before the application for healthcare insurance. Under the ACA, a preexisting condition exclusion is a health plan's provision that limits benefits or excludes benefits or plan coverage based on the existence of a condition before the effective date of coverage. Only grandfathered individual healthcare insurers may deny coverage for costs related to preexisting conditions (Healthcare Reform Magazine 2014).

Riders and Endorsements

A rider is an additional document, and an **endorsement** is language or statements within the policy itself (see also carve-outs in chapter 5). Riders and endorsements are similar to limitations and exclusions. They provide additional details about coverage or noncoverage for special situations that are not usually included in standard policies.

Procedures

Procedures explain how policyholders obtain the healthcare benefit or qualify to receive the healthcare benefit. Healthcare plans may deny benefits because procedures are not followed. Moreover, the procedures can function as limitations and exclusions, even though they may be stated in the positive. For example, "all mental health and chemical dependency services must be rendered by an eligible provider." Therefore, if services were provided by an ineligible provider, they would not be covered (paid for).

A common procedure is obtaining **prior approval**. During this approval process, the healthcare plan determines medical necessity. Types of services often requiring prior approval include

- Outpatient surgeries

- Diagnostic, interventional, and therapeutic outpatient procedures

- Physical, occupational, and speech therapies

- Mental health and chemical dependency care

- Inpatient care, including surgery, home health, private nurses, and nursing homes

- Organ transplants

Therefore, if a policy requires prior approval for physical therapy services and the policyholder does not obtain the prior approval, the expenses related to the physical therapy services may be denied.

Coordination of Benefits and Other Party Liability

Other common procedures are **coordination of benefits (COB)** and determination of **other party liability (OPL)**. These procedures are used when multiple insurance companies are involved. The responsible insurance party must be determined through clauses of the policies and the circumstances of the case.

Coordination of benefits becomes necessary when people have multiple *healthcare* insurance carriers that are providing coverage. Multiple healthcare insurance carriers can occur in instances when both spouses or parents work and both employers provide healthcare insurance. The **primary insurer (payer)** is the healthcare insurance responsible for the greatest proportion or majority of the healthcare expenses. The **secondary insurer (payer)** is responsible for the remainder of the healthcare expenses. The two healthcare insurance companies are sharing the responsibility for the healthcare expenses. This integration of payments is known as coordination of benefits (Jones 2001, 495).

Determination of primary or secondary insurer can be complicated. Some common rules follow:

- Patient's healthcare insurance is primary over spouse's healthcare insurance.

- Dependent child's primary insurer is the insurance of the parent whose birthday comes first in the calendar year and is called the "birthday rule".

- A legal decree, such as divorce agreement, dictates determination.

In many instances, when policyholders enroll in a healthcare insurance plan, they are required to list all other healthcare insurance policies they may have. Often, clauses within the healthcare insurance policy state that the primary insurance will pay for the majority of the healthcare expenses and the secondary insurance for the remaining costs. Thus, the payments from all healthcare insurance companies do not exceed 100 percent of the covered healthcare expenses.

Other party liability is similar to coordination of benefits. OPL differs from COB in that the other party is totally responsible for paying the costs. The other insurance is typically nonhealth insurance. For example, should a person incur healthcare expenses related to an injury suffered in an automobile accident, the healthcare insurance may deny coverage because the other party, the automobile accident insurance, is liable (responsible) for these expenses. The two common examples of OPL are when an automobile insurance company or workers' compensation is paying for the treatment of injuries incurred during an automobile crash or during work-related activities, respectively.

Appeals Processes

An **appeal** is a request for reconsideration of denial of coverage for healthcare services or rejection of a **claim**. A claim is a bill for healthcare services submitted by a hospital, physician's office, or other healthcare provider facility. Claims are submitted for reimbursement to the healthcare insurance plan by either the policy or certificate holder or the provider. The appeals section of a policy describes the steps that policyholders must take to appeal a decision about coverage or payment of a claim. Typically, the appeal must be in writing and within a specific timeframe of the healthcare insurance company's decision concerning the issue.

Check Your Understanding 3.2

1. Who is included in a healthcare insurance policy offering dependent healthcare coverage?

2. Which two types of policies offer the widest ranging coverage but require the insured to pay coinsurance until the maximum out-of-pocket costs are met?

3. Which of the following is *not* a type of healthcare policy limitation?
   a. Benefit cap
   b. Cost-sharing provision
   c. Geographic plan
   d. Use of formulary

4. Which type of prescription drug, generic or nonformulary, is less costly for insureds using their drug benefit?

5. Describe the types of procedures and services that typically require prior approval.

6. Both parents carried healthcare insurance with dependent coverage through their employers. What procedure is used to determine which healthcare insurer is responsible for their child's health expenses?

Determination of Covered Services

Healthcare insurance policies must be studied in their entirety to determine covered services. All the sections of the policy operate together to delineate covered services and noncovered services. An example from a mental health and chemical dependency benefit illustrates the linkage of policy sections (figure 3.2). The benefit is inpatient care for a mental health condition or chemical dependency. In the definitions section of a policy, both **precertification** and prior approval are defined. These definitions detail how to properly complete the procedures of obtaining precertification and prior approval. The limitations section notes that there is a $100 copayment in addition to applicable deductibles and coinsurance. Moreover, the limitations for mental health facilities specify that patients must be in beds licensed as psychiatric or chemical dependency and that the eligible attending physician must have specialized credentials. Finally, the exclusions section specifies that care preceding precertification, delivered by a noneligible provider, or obtained at a noncontracting facility will be denied. This illustration demonstrates how intricately the sections of the policy integrate to define coverage.

Elements of Healthcare Insurance Identification Card

Health insurance identification (subscriber) cards have a common set of elements. The terms for these elements

Figure 3.2.   Illustration of linkage of policy sections for a mental health or chemical dependency benefit

Policy Sections	Language Demonstrating Linkage
Definitions	*Precertification for mental health and chemical dependency:* Process of calling the mental health claim management representative prior to receiving services and obtaining approval for *all* continuing care. (This requirement is different from prior approval and is not a guarantee of payment.) *Prior approval:* Review of request for coverage of services prior to services being rendered that ensures certain covered services are deemed medically necessary and appropriate in order to treat the patient's condition.
Benefits	Inpatient care
Limitations	$100 copayment in addition to deductible and coinsurance Inpatient mental health or psychiatric treatment must be in licensed psychiatric bed and have attending physician who is a psychiatrist Inpatient chemical dependency treatment must be in a licensed chemical dependency bed and have attending physician who is a psychiatrist or addictionologist Delivered by eligible provider listed on pages 61–62 of the benefits manual
Exclusions	Treatment preceding precertification Treatment provided by ineligible provider Treatment at a noncontracting facility
Procedures	Obtain prior approval Obtain precertification

Figure 3.3.   Sample healthcare insurance identification card

| XYZ Health Plan
Subscriber Name:
IAM A WORKER 01
Subscriber ID:
EDQY43211904

Options
Standard 80/20

Generic Rx $12 copay for 30-day supply
Preferred Brand Rx $40 copay for 30-day supply
Nonpreferred Brand Rx $64 copay for 30-day supply | The State Employees' Plan

Unknown State University
Group No: V730912
RX Bin/Group 150046
Date Issued: 10/01/**

In-Network Member Responsibility:
Primary $30
Specialist $70
PT/OT/ST/Chiro $52
MH, SA $52
Urgent Care $87*
ER $233* + 20%
*Same for out-of-network |

differ among health insurance companies and payers. However, these elements provide information about the benefits of that subscriber's policy. The following section reviews these elements.

Figure 3.3 is the front of a typical healthcare insurance identification card. Healthcare insurance identification (subscriber) cards contain information about patients' covered benefits and their cost sharing.

On the back of the card are details about requirements for prior approval, telephone numbers, addresses, and other important information. On the front of the card are the elements that provide details about coverage and the cost sharing:

- XYZ Health Plan: Name of the health insurer.

- IAM A WORKER: Name of the subscriber.

- 01: Dependent two-digit suffix. The suffix "01" means that Iam A. Worker is the subscriber. Suffixes for dependents are "02", "03", with the oldest dependent being 02, and 03 being the second oldest, continuing until all dependents have a suffix.

- Subscriber ID: EDQY43211904. Unique number that identifies the subscriber (holder, enrollee, member) of a healthcare insurance policy (also known as identification number, member number, policy number, certificate number).

- Options Standard 80/20: Type of plan determined by premium or other criteria. Standard 80/20 means that the health insurer pays 80 percent (after deductible, copayment, and other cost sharing) and the subscriber pays 20 percent. Other possible options include the Basic 70/30. Basic 70/30 means that the health insurer pays 70 percent (after deductible, copayment, and other cost sharing) and the subscriber pays 30 percent.

- Generic R_x, Preferred Brand R_x, and Nonpreferred Brand R_x: Identification of prescription drug benefit. For each prescription, the subscriber pays a copayment. The amount of the copayment is dependent on the tier of prescription (see table 3.1).

- Unknown State University: Name of employer.

- Group No. V730912: **Group number** identifies the set of benefits to which Iam A. Worker is entitled. Number identifies the employer, association, or other entity purchasing the healthcare insurance. Individuals within a group have the same set of healthcare benefits.

- RX Bin/Group 150046: Identification information for prescription coverage. RX (R_x) is the abbreviation for prescription. BIN (formerly bank identification number, though no banks are involved) identifies the payer who reimburses the pharmacy for the prescription.

- Date Issued 10/01/**: Effective date of the benefit period. This set of benefits was effective 10/01/**.

- In-Network Member Responsibility: Copayments for various types of providers.

The health insurance identification card conveys much information in this brief format. However, despite the abundance of information that the card provides, office and billing staff members must contact the health insurer for additional important data. Dependent on the specifics of the policy, these data may include

- Overall effective date (from initial coverage)
- Family effective date
- Dependent age limitations
- Detailed prior approval requirements
- Deductible amount met
- Maximum out-of-pocket cost
- Maximum out-of-pocket amount met

It is important to remember that complete details of the healthcare insurance coverage are found in the certificate of insurance.

Filing a Healthcare Insurance Claim

Claim submission is the process of transmitting claims data to payers for processing. Through claim submission, providers are requesting payment for the services that they rendered. Providers transmit (file or submit) healthcare insurance claims for their patients and clients in most instances. The process of filing claims is similar for voluntary healthcare insurance plans, government-sponsored healthcare programs (chapter 4), and managed care plans (chapter 5).

In 2012, under the Administrative Simplification Compliance section of HIPAA, all healthcare providers must use **electronic claims submission** (ECS) to transmit claims to Medicare (Department of Health and Human Services 2011). The transaction standard is the Accredited Standards Committee (ASC) X12N version of 5010, with the electronic formats being 837-I for facilities and 837-P for professionals. These electronic formats correspond to the paper formats of the Uniform Bill 2004 (UB04) and the Centers for Medicare and Medicaid Services 1500 (CMS 1500).

The electronic formats, 837-I and 837-P, standardize the format of health data. Paper claim submission is a nonstandardized format. Providers may send paper claims (nonstandardized health data) to **clearinghouses** for conversion into a standardized electronic format. Clearinghouses may also run software-based audits to verify the claims' compliance with payers' **edits** (internal consistency checks) and the claims' accuracy. The clearinghouses act as intermediaries between providers and payers. Providers pay fees for the services of clearinghouses.

Submitting **clean claims** speeds accurate and correct reimbursement (see also chapters 6 and 9). Clean claims are accurate and complete. Clean claims "have no defect or impropriety, including a lack of any required substantiating documentation and an absence of any particular circumstance that requires special treatment that impedes prompt payment" (Isenberg 2002, 88). **Editors** are software programs that detect inconsistencies and errors. Providers may use editors to help prevent the submission of **dirty claims**. Claims that are inaccurate, incomplete (missing data), defective, or improper are called dirty claims (or dingy claims or unclean claims). The processing of dirty claims is delayed. Ultimately, dirty claims may be rejected. Timely and correct reimbursement is dependent on clean claims. Table 3.2 lists and describes essential data required on clean claims.

At the third-party payer, the claims are adjudicated. **Adjudication** is the determination of the reimbursement payment based on the member's insurance benefits. When clean claims are submitted, auto-adjudication can occur. In auto-adjudication, computer software processes the claim automatically. Three outcomes may occur: auto-pay, auto-suspend, or auto-deny. In auto-suspend, a claims examiner or claims analyst must review the claim. Claims may be auto-suspended if they have **claim attachments**. In the adjudication of a claim, a claim attachment documents supplemental information

Table 3.2.   Essential data for healthcare insurance claims

Data Element	Description
Patient or client name	Patient or client's name. Patients and clients should strive to list their names consistently across sites of care and insurance policies (do not mix nicknames and given names or surnames).
Patient or client's health record number	Health record number that the provider uses to identify the patient or client's record across time.
Patient or client's account number	Identifier of specific episode of care, date of service, or hospitalization.
Patient or client's demographic data	Date of birth, sex, marital status, address, telephone number, relationship to subscriber, and circumstances of condition (such as related to automobile accident).
Subscriber (member, policyholder, certificate holder, or insured) name	Purchaser of the healthcare insurance or the member of group for which an employer or association has purchased insurance.
Subscriber's demographic data	Address and telephone number.
Subscriber (member) number (identifier)	Unique code used to identify the subscriber's policy.
Group or plan number (identifier)	Unique code used to identify a set of benefits of one group or type of plan.
Prior approval number (precertification or preauthorization number, if applicable)	Number indicating that the healthcare insurance company has been notified and has approved healthcare services prior to their receipt.
Provider name	Name of the hospital, physician, or other entity that rendered healthcare services.
National provider identifier (NPI)	Unique 10-digit code for healthcare providers (required by the Health Insurance Portability and Accountability Act of 1996).
Provider's address and telephone number	Address and telephone number of entity that rendered healthcare services and that will be reimbursed by the claim.
Date(s) of service	Date when the healthcare service was rendered.
Diagnosis code	*International Classification of Diseases* code representing the disease, condition, or status of the patient or client.
Procedure code	*International Classification of Diseases* code, Current Procedural Terminology code, or Healthcare Common Procedure Coding System code representing the procedure or service.
Revenue code	Four-digit code identifying specific accommodation, ancillary service, or billing calculation related to the services on the bill. Indicates where the service was performed and summarizes other services and supplies used for treatment.
Itemized charges for services	Detailed list of each service and its cost.
Number of services (or duration of time)	Details related to number of services or length of time service was rendered.
Secondary or other healthcare insurance information	Another entity that may be responsible to reimburse the provider for the healthcare services rendered (such as automobile insurance, workers' compensation).

that assists claims examiners in understanding specific services received by an individual and in determining payment. Examples of claim attachments include proof of prior authorization or documentation supporting medical necessity. In addition, claims examiners or claims analysts may resolve inconsistencies, if possible; may request additional supporting documentation; or may reject (deny) the claim. However, it must be emphasized that human intervention delays reimbursement. From the providers' viewpoint, delays in reimbursement occur when providers' staff must respond with the additional documentation requested by the payer. Auto-rejected and manually rejected claims waste time and further delay payment. The providers' staff must determine the cause of the rejection, resolve it (correct the claim or supply supporting documentation), and resubmit the claim. Thus, clean claims and auto-pay are the goals (see chapter 9 for more information).

Too often, the processing of claims, both in their submission by providers and in their adjudication by payers, is problematic. Common errors that providers make when submitting claims follow:

- Differences in patient name or name spelling, such as a nickname or hyphenation of last name

- Missing or invalid patient identification number

- Missing or invalid patient information, such as sex, date of birth, or Social Security number

- Missing or invalid subscriber (member) name

- Missing or invalid certificate or group number

- Lack of authorization or referral number

- Failure to check the box for **assignment of benefits** (contract in which the provider directly bills the payer and accepts the allowable charge as full payment, minus applicable cost sharing)

- Invalid dates of services

- Missing or invalid modifiers (see chapter 2)

- Missing or invalid provider information, such as tax identification number

- Incorrect place of service (Isenberg 2002, 88; Peregrin 2010, 838)

To address the problem of dirty claims, one solution is to use an electronic health record system that eliminates manual or duplicate entry of data and feeds directly into the computer software for claims submission (Jaspan 2008, 29). Additionally, before submitting claims, reimbursement analysts should audit claims' accuracy and compliance with edits (Isenberg 2002, 88) (see chapter 9).

Remittance Advice or Explanation of Benefits

Reimbursement payments are sent electronically to providers' banks through **electronic fund transfer (EFT)**. Usually, the payment includes reimbursements for several patients or clients and for several practitioners' services. Concurrently, two reports explaining the payments are generated. One report of the payment,

known as an **electronic remittance advice (ERA)**, is sent to the provider. For providers using clearinghouses, the RA is sent to the clearinghouse for conversion into paper (readable) format. A second, individualized, paper-based report of the payment is sent to the healthcare insurer's policyholder (certificate holder or subscriber).

Both of these reports show how the payment (or nonpayment) for the patients' healthcare services was determined. The report lists payments, rejections, denials, and **adjustments** (amounts deducted per contracted discount rates). The terms for these two reports are not standardized across third-party payers.

- Some third-party payers use the term **remittance advice** (RA) for the report sent to *all* providers.

- Other payers use the term **explanation of benefits (EOB)** for the report sent to *all* providers.

- Other payers use the term *RA* for facilities and the term *EOB* for professionals, such as physicians and audiologists.

- Many payers use the term EOB for the individualized reports sent to their policyholders.

Generally an RA is a report that is sent from a payer to a provider, and an EOB is a report that is sent from a healthcare insurer to its policyholder (certificate holder or subscriber).

RAs and EOBs both detail how the healthcare insurance company (payer) determined its payment for the healthcare service(s). Figure 3.4 is an example of an EOB, although many of its elements are also represented on RAs:

- Name of healthcare insurance company.

- Date of report (RA or EOB).

- Name of member (may also be known as subscriber or policyholder), identification number (also known as certificate number or member number), and group number.

- Name and address of provider (such as practice or durable medical equipment vendor).

- Patient's name (may or may not be the same as the subscriber).

Figure 3.4.   Explanation of benefits

XYZ Healthcare Insurance Company			Date: 07/02/201*		
Member's Name: Jane Green **ID Number:** 123-45-6789 **Date** MM/DD/YYYY					
Patient's Name: Jane Green (Member)					
Service	**Amount of Bill**	**Amount You Do Not Owe**	**Amount Paid by Plan**	**Your Balance**	**Explanation of Your Balance**
Surgicenter of Smith County 05-10-201* Ambulatory Surge	536.01	181.34	To Provider 150.00	204.67	**Your $150 wellness benefit maximum has been met.** 50.00 Outpatient services copay. 154.67 Applied to Plan year deductible.
City Physicians Group 05-10-201* Surgery	271.00	163.46	0.00	107.54	**Your $150 wellness benefit maximum has been met.** 107.54 Applied to Plan year deductible.
Smith County Hospital 05-16-201* X-Ray Services	450.63	72.10	To Provider 232.59	145.94	**Your $150 wellness benefit maximum has been met.** 58.15 Your 20 percent coinsurance. 87.79 Applied to Plan year deductible.
		TOTAL	382.59	458.15	
350 of 350 Deductible met for 07-01-201* to 06-30-201*		58.15 of 1,500.00 Coinsurance met for 07-01-201* to 06-30-201*			

- Healthcare service(s) with provider(s) and date(s).

- **Actual charge** (billed amount) of the healthcare service ("Amount of Bill" in figure 3.4). The actual charge is the amount that the provider charges for the healthcare service. This amount may or may not be equal to the **allowable charge**. The actual charge may be subject to discounts.

- Allowable charge (allowable fee; maximum fee; maximum allowable; usual-reasonable-customary, or UCR charge; or prevailing rate) is the amount that the healthcare insurer will cover. Allowable charges include discounted fees. The healthcare insurer negotiated these discounts with providers. The providers agree to accept the payment on the allowed charge as payment in full. Each healthcare insurer has its own schedule of allowed charges (also known as eligible charges). Allowable charges are subject to deductibles, copayments, and coinsurance. (In figure 3.4, subtract "Amount You Do Not Owe" from "Amount of Bill" to calculate)

- Adjustments, also known as **write-offs**, are the difference between the provider's actual charge and the allowable charge (see "Amount You Do Not Owe" in figure 3.4). Adjustments are deducted amounts that represent the contracted discount rates. They are often called write-offs because the provider has agreed to accept the payment on the allowable charge as payment in full (minus applicable deductible, copayment, and coinsurance) and, thus, writes off the excess amount.

- Applicable cost sharing, such as deductible, copayment, and coinsurance. Providers collect the cost sharing from the members or the **guarantors**. (In figure 3.4, see "Your Balance," which is the remainder of the costs and the policyholder's responsibility.)

- Rejections and denials (with reason or action code).

- Codes for reasons of adjustments, rejections, denials, and other actions.

Figure 3.4 illustrates how a Blue plan provides details about its determination of specific benefits for a subscriber (member). Upon receiving the EOB, the guarantor knows how much to pay the provider's billing office. Guarantors are the people responsible to pay the bill. Guarantors may be the member, the patient, or another responsible person, such as a parent of a child.

An RA contains the following additional information:

- Names of multiple patients and their account numbers (sometimes patient's date of birth as well). The subscriber's EOB was focused on one patient.

- Prior approval number (authorization or pre-certification number).

- Provider/practitioner number (in addition to name and address noted previously).

- Tax identification number.

- Check number and amount.

- Payment date.

- Service code and modifiers (HCPCS/CPT; see chapter 2; may also be on patient's EOB).

- Units of services.

- Claim status (paid, denied or rejected, reversed [correction], suspended).

- Rejections, reversals, denials, disallowed charges, allowances, reason codes, and other details for multiple patients.

From review and monitoring of the RAs, providers can determine the efficiency and effectiveness of their claims submission process. This topic is fully explained in chapter 9 on the revenue cycle. Subscribers also should review and monitor their EOBs. As discussed in the previous section, claims submission is an error-prone process. Patients should not assume that their healthcare services have been accurately submitted to and paid by their healthcare insurance company.

Check Your Understanding 3.3

1. When a patient's healthcare services are covered under a voluntary healthcare insurance plan, who pays the remainder of a healthcare bill *after* the healthcare insurance company has paid?

2. True or false? The patient and the guarantor are always the same person.

3. What is the term for the number that identifies the employer, association, or other entity purchasing the healthcare insurance and indicates a common set of healthcare benefits?

a. Subscriber
b. Standard
c. Group
d. Bin

4. True or false? The actual charge is the same as the allowable charge.

5. What is the term for the difference between the provider's actual charge and the allowable charge?

Trends

Related to voluntary health insurance, reimbursement analysts and other healthcare personnel should monitor two broad trends. The first trend is the ongoing implementation of the ACA (see chapter 1). Among its many aspects affecting the delivery of healthcare and healthcare quality, the ACA phases in reforms in the access to and coverage of healthcare insurance. However, the full implementation of the ACA depends on its not being repealed, on its withstanding constitutional challenges, and on its being funded. The other trend is ever-increasing private healthcare costs. Increasing healthcare costs affect patients, providers, and health insurance companies.

Implementation of Affordable Care Act

The purpose of the ACA is to achieve a high-performing healthcare system (Davis et al. 2010, viii). Accordingly, its many provisions attempt to address affordable and accessible healthcare insurance coverage, the efficiency of the delivery of healthcare, decreasing the costs and increasing the quality of healthcare, and improvements in outcomes and population health (Davis et al. 2010, viii). The provisions of Title I of the ACA particularly address issues related to this chapter's focus: voluntary healthcare insurance.

The ACA built upon the existing infrastructure of voluntary healthcare insurance. Employer-based healthcare insurance from large employers would experience few changes. For individual (private) healthcare plans and the small employer-based groups, benefits would be more comprehensive than in the past (Jost 2014, 7). The purpose of building on the existing infrastructure of voluntary healthcare insurance was to minimize disruption. However, building upon an existing structure is difficult and complex (Jost 2014, 7). Consequently, the implementation of the ACA was and continues to be complicated with waivers and delays (Jost 2014, 8–9).

Provisions Effective in 2014

Title I of the ACA requires most US citizens and legal residents to have health insurance.

- The requirement is enforced through tax penalties for noncoverage. This requirement becomes effective in 2014 (Kaiser Family Foundation 2011, 1). For eligible poor people, the law includes provisions subsidizing the costs of premiums. Update: Penalties for noncoverage were delayed until 2016 by actions of federal agencies (Redhead and Kinzer 2014, CRS-5).

- The law attempts to strengthen the system of employer-based health insurance by assessing penalties against employers with 50 or more full-time employees who do not offer health insurance benefits (Kaiser Family Foundation 2011, 1). Update: Penalties were delayed until 2015 by actions of federal agencies (Redhead and Kinzer 2014, 2).

- The law requires healthcare insurers to pay an annual fee, known as the health insurer fee, to fund provisions of the ACA, such as health premium subsidies. The fee amount is based on the insurer's market share of net premiums written for the previous year and the dollar value of its business (Kirchhoff 2013, 1–4). For example, the 2015 fee is based on 2014 premiums. After 2018, the fee will increase annually based on premium growth.

Provisions Effective Beyond 2015

In 2018, healthcare insurers with high annual premiums will pay a 40 percent excise tax, known as a Cadillac tax. The high-premium thresholds, indexed to inflation, are $10,200 for individual coverage or $27,500 for family coverage. In specific cases, such as retirees and high-risk industries, the thresholds for the premiums may be higher than $10,200 and $27,500 (Piotrowski 2013, 3). In 2020, for Medicare beneficiaries, the gap in prescription drug coverage ("donut hole") will be entirely closed (Congressional Budget Office 2012, 1).

Increasing Costs in Voluntary Healthcare Insurance

As discussed in chapter 1, costs in the US healthcare delivery system continue to increase. Five broad factors account for this increase: economy-wide inflation, medical-specific inflation, population change, shifts in the age and sex mix of the population, and other nonprice factors, such as increased greater utilization and intensity of healthcare services (Martin et al. 2014, 71). This section details how that general sector-level trend affects individual consumers, providers, and healthcare insurers.

Effects on Consumers

Consumers' expenditures on healthcare, in billions of dollars, are increasing (see table 3.4). Examples of consumers' expenditures are

- healthcare insurance premiums, including employer-based policies, private policies, and other supplemental policies

- out-of-pocket costs, including deductibles, coinsurance, copayments, and payments for noncovered services, such as dental services, nursing home services, and other costs not covered by healthcare insurance (Martin et al. 2014, 72)

This growth in consumers' healthcare spending is expected to continue (Sisko et al. 2014, 1848–1849.

Amounts in the billions of dollars are difficult to comprehend. The Kaiser Family Foundation and Health Research and Educational Trust (KFF/HRET) annually conducts a survey of employer-sponsored health benefits that puts these costs in terms of individuals and families. Selected key findings from these annual surveys are in tables 3.3 and 3.4.

Table 3.3 shows the average premiums that employers and employees contributed (paid) in selected years. As can be seen from table 3.3, the premiums represent substantial sums of money for both employees and employers. Generally, employees contribute 18 percent of the premium for single coverage and 29 percent of the premium for family coverage (KFF/HRET 2014, 92). Employees' contributions to premiums in one year increased about 8 percent for single coverage and about 6 percent for family coverage. In the long term, these increases result in significant amounts. Over the past five years, the accumulated increases totaled 39 percent for single coverage and 37 percent for family coverage (KFF/HRET 2014, 94). Employers' contributions are also substantial. To appreciate the size of the employers' contributions, the employers' contributions must be multiplied by the number of employees in the organization.

Table 3.3.   Health insurance premiums, selected representative years

Premium	2011		2012		2013		2014	
	Single Coverage	Family Coverage	Single Coverage	Family Coverage	Single Coverage	Family Coverage	Single Coverage	Family Coverage
Employee contribution	$921	$4,129	$951	$4,316	$999	$4,565	$1,081	$4,823
Employer contribution	$4,508	$10,944	$4,664	$11,429	$4,885	$11,786	$4,994	$12,011
Total	$5,429	$15,073	$5,615	$15,745	$5,884	$16,351	$6,025	$16,834

Source: Kaiser Family Foundation and Health Research and Educational Trust 2014, 97–98.

Table 3.4   Consumers' out-of-pocket healthcare expenditures

Out-of-pocket Cost Sharing	2011	2012	2013	2014
Annual Deductibles				
Single Coverage	$991	$1,097	$1,135	$1,217
Family Coverage	$2,136	$2,296	$2,624	$2,817
Average Copayments for In-Network Office Visits				
Primary Care	$22	$23	$23	$24
Specialty Care	$32	$33	$35	$36
Average Copayments for Tiered Drug Benefits				
Tier 1	$10	$10	$10	$11
Tier 2	$29	$29	$29	$31
Tier 3	$49	$51	$52	$53
Average Copayments for Inpatient Admissions	$246	$263	$278	$280
Average Copayments for Outpatient Surgeries	$145	$127	$140	$157

Source: Kaiser Family Foundation and Health Research and Educational Trust. 2011–2014.

Table 3.4 shows a few out-of-pocket costs. Over the past five years, the percentage of employees having deductibles exceeding $1,000 has nearly doubled, from 22 percent to 41 percent (KFF/HRET 2014, 126). It should be noted that today's healthcare plans have complex cost-sharing arrangements. Table 3.4 only includes representative out-of-pocket costs for consumers; excluded are cost-sharing requirements for ancillary services, such as durable medical equipment and physical therapy (KFF/HRET 2014, 124).

These healthcare expenditures can have long-term, catastrophic effects on individuals and families. Among individuals or couples who filed for bankruptcy, nearly eight of 10 stated that they had had medical expenses in the two years immediately before they filed (Jacoby and Holman 2010, 268). Of these filers, nearly 20 percent had more than $5,000 in medical expenses and 34 percent had $1,000 to $5,000 in medical expenses. In what has become known as "medical bankruptcy," individuals or couples meet one of the following criteria:

- Cite medical illness or medical bills as the specific cause of bankruptcy

- Report uncovered medical bills exceeding $5,000

- Lose at least two weeks of work-related income because of the illness

- Mortgage their home to pay medical bills (Himmelstein et al. 2011, 227–228)

Having healthcare insurance does not significantly change the number of medical bankruptcies (Himmelstein et al. 2011, 227). Instead, high premiums and substantial out-of-pocket costs still leave people exposed to financial crises and impoverishment (Himmelstein et al. 2011, 227–228).

Effects on Providers

For providers, increased out-of-pocket costs for patients and clients affect operations in their billing offices. Staff members must collect the out-of-pocket costs (private expenditures) from patients and clients. Staff members include physician practice managers, reimbursement specialists, and directors of accounts receivables. As the out-of-pocket costs increase, patients' and clients' ability to pay these costs decreases. Correspondingly, staff members' efforts to collect these out-of-pocket costs must become more demanding and time-consuming than in the past.

Effective collection procedures are critical to maintain cash flow. Experts advise healthcare organizations to develop the following (Redling 2007, 29):

- Policies and procedures

- Collection systems

- Front-office and checkout desk processes

Preparing billing offices of healthcare organizations for the increased share of healthcare costs that patients and clients must bear is essential to the financial welfare of the organization (figure 3.5).

Effects on Healthcare Insurers

In response to increasing healthcare costs, health insurance companies and employers have devised new or revised designs of health insurance plans.

Figure 3.5.   Preparing for increased out-of-pocket costs for patients and clients

Revamp cash collection processes	Collect deductibles, copayments, and coinsurances at front-desk or checkout desk
	Collect small deposit for other potential noncovered services (unless prohibited)
Revise policies and procedures	Institute minimum payments
	Implement discounts for full payment at time of service
	Offer extended payment plans
	Collect deductibles, copayments, and coinsurances at time of service
Equip staff	Preview appointments at least 24 hours in advance
	Obtain complete health insurance information from patients or clients prior to appointments
	Verify insurance coverage, deductibles, copayments, coinsurances, and allowable charges prior to appointments
	Create scripts for staff to use when they ask patients and clients for payments
Inform patients and clients	Educate patients and clients about organization's policies and procedures (website, statements, scripts for staff, and promotional and educational brochures and materials)
	Confirm with patients their covered and noncovered services, deductibles, copayments, coinsurances, and allowable charges
Communicate with payers	Obtain definitions, terms, and benefit structure
Update physicians and providers	Demonstrate effects of payments at time of service on cash flow

Source: Redling, B. 2007. Double exposure: Higher deductibles, uninsured patients add to administrators' challenges. *MGMA Connexion/Medical Group Management Association* 7(2):29–32.

Consumer-Directed Healthcare Plan

A **consumer-directed (consumer-driven) healthcare plan (CDHP)** is a form of healthcare insurance designed to reduce healthcare costs by providing subscribers and patients (consumers) with financial incentives to choose lower-priced packages of healthcare benefits (Fronstin et al. 2013, 1126). CDHPs are also known as **high-deductible health plans (HDHPs)**. The most common form of CDHP is the HDHP with a **health savings account** (HSA or HDHP/HSA) (Lo Sasso et al.

2010, 1043). The HDHP/HSA may also be known as an HDHP with a savings option (SO) or HDHP/SO or as an account-based health plan (ABHP).

CDHPs make consumers healthcare cost-conscious by exposing them more directly to healthcare costs than other types of healthcare insurance do. This cost-consciousness will influence consumers (subscribers and patients) to reduce their healthcare spending. CDHPs are attempting to decrease the effects of **moral hazard**. Moral hazard is "any change in behavior that occurs as a result of becoming insured" (Nyman 1998, 57). One change in behavior is that people spend the money of healthcare insurance companies differently than they would spend their own money (Robinson and Ginsburg 2009, W272). For example, potential moral hazards are undergoing an expensive procedure when a comparable inexpensive procedure exists or becoming an inpatient when outpatient services would have the same outcome (Nyman 1998, 57).

In consumer-directed healthcare, subscribers and patients are more involved in the design of their packages of health benefits than in traditional health plans. CDHPs give subscribers and patients flexibility and control in choosing how they spend their healthcare benefit dollars. CDHPs provide subscribers and patients with decision support tools and information so that they can make informed choices about the level of cost sharing appropriate for their health and their economic situation. In CDHPs, subscribers and patients are made more conscious of and sensitive to the costs of their healthcare than in fee-for-service or other types of reimbursement.

In CDHPs, premiums are lower and deductibles are higher than the overall averages of premiums and deductibles across all types of healthcare insurance.

- Average annual premium for single coverage in CDHPs with HSAs is $905, whereas the overall average annual premium for single coverage is $1,081 (Kaiser Family Foundation and Health Research and Educational Trust 2014, 92).

- Average annual deductible for single coverage in CDHPs with HSAs is $2,215, whereas the overall average annual deductible for single coverage is $1,217 (Kaiser Family Foundation and Health Research and Educational Trust 2014, 125, 136). This difference could be expected from the name "high-deductible."

Enrollment in CDHPs having HSAs continues to rise. In 2014, 20 percent of covered employees were in a CDHP having an HSA, up from 17 percent in 2011 and 8 percent in 2009 (Kaiser Family Foundation and Health Research and Educational Trust 2014, 170).

HSAs are special pretax savings accounts into which *both* employees and employers *may* contribute (not all employers do). Subscribers can withdraw the money to pay for qualified medical care and expenses. HSAs were enacted in January 2004 by the Medicare Prescription Drug, Improvement, and Modernization Act (MMA) of 2003 (Klug and Chianese 2010, 12). HSAs have the following tax benefits (Klug and Chianese 2010, 15):

- Pretax (untaxed) contributions can be made.

- Growth of assets (funds in account) is not taxed.

- Distribution (payment) for qualified medical expenses is tax-free.

HSAs are permanent and portable; they allow subscribers to save money over multiple years to pay for future medical expenses. HSAs expanded upon medical savings accounts (MSAs). A key expansion is that under HSAs, anyone under a qualified HDHP is eligible (all size employers and both self-employed people and people who are not self-employed). On the other hand, MSAs were limited to self-employed people and companies employing from 2 to 50 employees. HSAs require that the insured be covered under an HDHP.

Two other commonly encountered options are **flexible spending (saving) accounts (FSAs)** and **health reimbursement arrangements (HRAs)**. These options may appear very similar to HSAs, but key differences exist between HSAs and FSAs and between HSAs and HRAs.

- An FSA is a special account into which employers and employees may contribute. Employees determine the pretax deductions from their paychecks that are deposited into the accounts, up to the limit set by their employers. Funds from the account are used to pay qualified medical care and expenses. Unlike HSAs, funds from one FSA plan year *cannot* roll forward (carry over) to the next

FSA plan year. This requirement of FSAs is known as the "use-it-or-lose-it" rule (Klug and Chianese 2010, 13). One exception is the "grace period" that some employers' plans may have, which permits qualified medical expenses to be paid up to 2.5 months after the end of the plan year.

- An HRA is a special arrangement into which only employers may contribute (HSAs allow both employers and employees to contribute). HRAs are sometimes called health reimbursement accounts, but this name is a misnomer: An account is *not* required. The employer determines the eligible services. Money in the HRA belongs to the employer, so the HRA is not portable should the employee leave the company.

These three options attempt to increase consumers' consciousness of the costs of their healthcare.

For employers, CDHPs are a means to control the costs of their employees' health benefits. A 2011 study showed that CDHPs were effective in controlling costs. For both individual coverage and family coverage, the employers recorded that health benefits under CDHPs were less expensive than managed care plans (see chapter 5 for more details on managed care plans) (Towers Watson 2011, 5).

CDHPs are not without their critics. Critics are concerned that the low premiums and high deductibles do not benefit everyone. Forty-eight percent of families under a CDHP with members having chronic illnesses, such as hypertension, diabetes, and asthma, reported healthcare-related financial burdens, compared to 21 percent covered under traditional plans (Galbraith et al. 2011, 322). Critics are also concerned that patients and clients do not have the requisite education and information to choose needed medications and treatments when faced with high deductibles.

Value-Based Insurance Design

Value-based insurance design (VBID) is mandated under section 2713 of the ACA (Maciejewski et al. 2014, 301). VBID is the next generation of consumer-directed healthcare. VBID addresses a criticism of consumer-directed healthcare—that consumers do not have the necessary knowledge to choose needed medications and treatments when faced with high deductibles (Brennan and Reisman 2007, W205).

In value-based insurance design, copayments are set based on the value of the clinical services. Unlike traditional practices that focus only on costs of clinical services, VBID calculates both benefit and cost. There are two models of VBID (Chernew et al. 2007, W197):

- Targeting valuable interventions, such as beta blockers

- Targeting valuable interventions to patients having select diseases, such as beta blockers for patients with congestive heart failure

Typically, in VBID, healthcare insurers lower or eliminate the copayments for the drugs needed to treat chronic diseases, such as hypertension, hyperlipidemia, diabetes, and congestive heart failure (Choudhry et al. 2014, 493). Consequently, the belief is, patients will be more likely to buy their drugs and to adhere to their treatment plans. Thus, the business argument for VBID states that the higher drug and administration costs for the healthcare insurer will be offset by lower nonmedication costs, such as fewer hospitalizations and office visits that result from better disease control (Maciejewski et al. 2014, 305).

A small body of evidence is building about VBID. In one study, all patients' adherence to their prescription drug therapy rose 5 percent. Of note, by the third year of the study, cardiovascular patients' adherence to their drug therapy was 9.4 percent higher than at the beginning of the study. Moreover, patients' healthcare spending was reduced, and the program was cost-neutral for the employer (Gibson et al. 2011, 109). Another study had less dramatic results. For patients having cardiovascular diseases, improvements in medication adherence ranged between 2.7 and 3.4 percent, and the probability of an inpatient admission decreased slightly. However, the program was not cost-neutral; the healthcare insurer's drug expenditures were $6.4 million higher and its nonmedication expenditures only $5.7 million less (Maciejewski et al. 2014, 300). Finally, evidence from a literature review of the research showed improvements in quality but no cost savings (Lee et al. 2013, 1255).

Wellness Programs

Wellness programs promote health and fitness. Health insurance plans may offer wellness programs to their members; more often, employers offer them as an employee benefit. The number of wellness programs is increasing. Most US employers offer some type of wellness program (Towers Watson 2014, 22). Common activities include health risk appraisals, chronic diseases and weight management programs, smoking cessation, and promotion of physical activity (Towers Watson 2014, 22).

Typically, wellness programs offer incentives (or penalties) to encourage participation. Examples of incentives include discounts on premiums, cash rewards, and gym memberships. Examples of penalties are surcharges on premiums and lower-value health plan options. For instance, members who are smokers or who have a high body mass index (that is, who are of excessive weight) may be eligible only for the healthcare insurance plan with a 30 percent coinsurance. On the other hand, members who are nonsmokers and who have a body mass index within normal limits may be eligible for the healthcare insurance plan with a 20 percent coinsurance.

Little is known about the effects of wellness programs on health services utilization, outcomes, and cost (Gowrisankaran et al. 2013, 477). They were first introduced in the 1990s, with little evidence of return on investment (Greene 2011, 44). Moreover, as members change health insurers (and employers), the benefits of wellness do not accrue to the organization that paid the incentives. Research on wellness programs shows mixed results. The research has shown positive results for some employers. For example, Sentara Health System in Norfolk, Virginia, saved $3.4 million in healthcare costs over three years thanks to 80 percent participation among its eligible employees (Greene 2011, 41). On the other hand, the wellness program of BJC Healthcare in St. Louis, Missouri, resulted in no net change in the costs of health claims (Gowrisankaran et al. 2013, 482). Finally, though, a healthy workforce being a competitive edge, the prevalence of wellness programs will continue (Towers Watson 2014, 2–3).

Chapter 3 Review Quiz

1. Describe the health insurance plan that covers federal government employees.

2. What is the relationship between covered conditions and covered services in health insurance plans?

3. What type of insurance policy provides benefits to (a) a resident requiring nursing home care and services, (b) an insured who becomes blind, and (c) a homeowner who requires an eight-month recuperation after a fall down her basement stairs?

4. Name at least two of the three benefit terms that mean the amount beyond which all covered healthcare services for an insured or dependent are paid 100 percent by the insurance plan.

5. True or false? Copayments are cost-sharing provisions of policies that require insureds to pay a flat fee to healthcare service providers and suppliers.

6. Why can use of a formulary be considered a policy limitation?

7. List at least three typical exclusions found in insurance plan riders.

8. How does Blue Cross and Blue Shield notify insureds about the extent of payments made on a claim? What data elements does that notification include?

9. Why should providers submit clean claims to third-party payers?

10. True or false? Out-of-pocket costs for subscribers and patients are decreasing.

References

American Academy of Actuaries. 2006. Issue brief: Wading through medical insurance pools—A primer. http://www.actuary.org/pdf/health/pools_sep06.pdf.

Blue Cross Blue Shield Association. 2014. About the Blue Cross and Blue Shield Association. http://www.bcbs.com/about-the-association/.

Brennan, T., and L. Reisman. 2007. Value-based insurance design and the next generation of consumer-driven health care. *Health Affairs Suppl Web Exclusives* 26(2):W204–W207.

Cauchi, R.; National Conference of State Legislatures. 2014. Coverage of uninsurable pre-existing conditions: State and federal high-risk pools. http://www.ncsl.org/research/health/high-risk-pools-for-health-coverage.aspx.

Chernew, M.E., A.B. Rosen, and A.M. Fendrick. 2007. Value-based insurance design. *Health Affairs Suppl Web Exclusives* 26(2):W195–W203.

Choudhry, N.K., M.A. Fischer, B.F. Smith, G. Brill, C. Girdish, O.S. Matlin, T.A. Brennan, J. Avorn, and W.H. Shrank. 2014. Five features of value-based insurance design plans were associated with higher rates of medication adherence. *Health Affairs* 33(3):493–501.

Claxton, G., M. Rae, N. Panchal, A. Damico, H. Whitmore, N. Bostick, and K. Kenward. 2013. Health benefits in 2013: Moderate premium increases in employer-sponsored plans. *Health Affairs* 32(9):1667–1676.

Congressional Budget Office. 2012 (November). Offsetting effects of prescription drug use on Medicare's spending for medical services. Report No. 43741. http://www.cbo.gov/sites/default/files/cbofiles/attachments/43741-MedicalOffsets-11-29-12.pdf.

Coulter, C.H., R. Fabius, V. Hecksher, and H. Darling. 1998. Assessing HMO centers of excellence programs: One employer's experience. *Managed Care Quarterly* 6(1):8–15.

Davis, K., S. Guterman, S.R. Collins, K. Stremikis, S. Rustgi, and R. Nuzum. 2010. Starting on the path to a high-performance health system: Analysis of the payment and system reform provisions in the Patient Protection and Affordable Care Act of 2010. http://www.commonwealthfund.org/Publications/Fund-Reports/2010/Sep/Analysis-of-the-Payment-and-System-Reform-Provisions.aspx.

Department of Health and Human Services. 2011. Electronic billing and EDI transactions: 5010-D.0. https://www.cms.gov/electronicbillingeditrans/18_5010d0.asp.

Friedman, E. 1998. What price survival? The future of Blue Cross and Blue Shield. Journal of the American Medical Association 279(23):1863–1869.

Fronstin, P., M.J. Spelveda, and M.C. Roebuck. 2013. Consumer-directed health plans reduce the long-term use of outpatient physician visits and prescription drugs. *Health Affairs* 32(6):1126–1134.

Galbraith, A.A., D. Ross-Degnan, S.S. Soumerai, M.B. Rosenthal, C. Gay, and T.A. Lieu. 2011. Nearly half of families in high-deductible health plans whose members have chronic conditions face substantial financial burden. *Health Affairs* 30(2):322–331.

Gibson, T.B., S. Wang, E. Kelly, C. Brown, C. Turner, F. Frech-Tamas, J. Doyle, and E. Mauceri. 2011. A value-based insurance design program at a large company boosted medication adherence for employees with chronic disease. *Health Affairs* 30(1):109–117.

Giovannelli, J., K.W. Lucia, and S. Corlette. 2014. Implementing the Affordable Care Act: State Action to Reform the Individual Health Insurance Market. Commonwealth Fund Publication No. 1758. *Issue Brief* 15:1–15. http://www.commonwealthfund.org/~/media/files/publications/issue-brief/2014/jul/1758_giovannelli_implementing_aca_state_reform_individual_market_rb.pdf.

Gould, E. 2013. Employer-sponsored health insurance coverage continues to decline in a new decade. *International Journal of Health Services* 43(4):603–638.

Gowrisankaran, G., K. Norberg, S. Kymes, M.E. Chernew, D. Stwalley, L. Kemper, and W. Peck. 2013. A hospital system's wellness program linked to health plan enrollment cut hospitalizations but not overall costs. *Health Affairs* 32(3):477–485.

Greene, J. 2011. Employee wellness proves its worth. *Hospitals and Health Networks* 85(3):41–44.

Gruber., L.R.; National Association of State Comprehensive Health Insurance Plans (NASCHIP). 2009. How state health insurance pools are helping Americans: An important safety net for persons with chronic medical conditions. http://www.naschip.org/Position%20Paper%20NJRv25.pdf.

Hall, M.A. 2004. The impact and enforcement of prudent layperson laws. *Annals of Emergency Medicine* 43(5):558–566.

Hall, M.A., and C.J. Conover. 2003. The impact of Blue Cross conversions on accessibility, affordability, and the public interest. *The Milbank Quarterly* 81(4):509–542.

Hall, M.A., and C.J. Conover. 2006. For-profit conversion of Blue Cross plan: Public benefit or public harm? *American Review of Public Health* 27:443–463.

Haugh, R. 2006. Centers of excellence take tiering to the max. *Hospitals and Health Networks* 80(5):42–44.

Healthcare Reform Magazine. 2014 (January 23). Preexisting condition exclusions and the new health reform regulations. http://www.healthcarereformmagazine.com/issue-4/business-issue-4/preexisting-condition-exclusions-the-new-health-reform-regulations/.

Himmelstein, D.U., D. Thorne, and S. Woolhandler. 2011. Medical bankruptcy in Massachusetts: Has health reform made a difference? *American Journal of Medicine* 124(3):224–228.

Internal Revenue Service. 2014 (June 25). Ninety-day waiting period limitation; Final rule. *Federal Register* 79(122):35942–35948.

Isenberg, S.F. 2002. Clean claims are key to timely reimbursement, but be vigilant. *ENT—Ear, Nose & Throat Journal* 81(2):88.

Jacoby, M.B., and M. Holman. 2010. Managing medical bills on the brink of bankruptcy. *Yale Journal of Health Policy, Law, and Ethics* 10(2):239–298.

Jaspan, D.M. 2008. Before you give up, clean up your claims. *Medical Economics* 85(16):28–30.

Jones, L M., ed. 2001. Glossary. In *Reimbursement Methodologies for Healthcare Services* [CD-ROM]. Chicago: AHIMA.

Jost, T.S. 2014. Implementing health reform: Four years later. *Health Affairs* 33(1):7–10.

Kaiser Family Foundation. 2010. Explaining health care reform: Questions about extension of dependent coverage to age 26 [Publication #8065]. http://www.kff.org/healthreform/upload/8065.pdf.

Kaiser Family Foundation. 2011. Summary of new health reform law. http://www.kff.org/healthreform/upload/8061.pdf.

Kaiser Family Foundation and Health Research and Educational Trust. 2011. Employer health benefits: 2011 summary of findings. http://kff.org/health-costs/report/employer-health-benefits-annual-survey-archives/#2011.

Kaiser Family Foundation and Health Research and Educational Trust. 2012. Employer health benefits: 2012 annual survey. http://kff.org/private-insurance/report/employer-health-benefits-2012-annual-survey/.

Kaiser Family Foundation and Health Research and Educational Trust. 2013. Employer health benefits: 2013 annual survey. http://kff.org/private-insurance/report/2013-employer-health-benefits/.

Kaiser Family Foundation and Health Research and Educational Trust. 2014. Employer health benefits: 2014 annual survey. http://kaiserfamilyfoundation.files.wordpress.com/2014/09/8625-employer-health-benefits-2014-annual-survey4.pdf.

Kirchhoff, S.M. 2013 (December 12). Patient Protection and Affordable Care Act: Annual fee on health insurers. Congressional Research Service Report No. R43225. http://fas.org/sgp/crs/misc/R43225.pdf.

Klug, K., and L. Chianese. 2010. Health savings accounts: Back to the future. *Benefits Quarterly* 26(1):12–23.

Koch, A. L. 2002. Financing health services. In *Introduction to Health Services*, 6th ed. Edited by S.J. Williams and P.R. Torrens. Albany, NY: Delmar.

Lee, J.L., M.L. Maciejewski, S.S. Raju, W.H. Shrank, and N.K. Choudhry. 2013. Value-based insurance design: Quality improvement but no cost savings. *Health Affairs* 32(7):1251–1257.

Lo Sasso, A.T., M. Shah, and B.K. Frogner. 2010. Health savings accounts and health care spending. *Health Services Research* 45(4):1041–1060.

Maciejewski, M.L., D. Wansink, J.H. Lindquist, J.C. Parker, and J.F. Farley. 2014 (February). Value-based insurance design program in North Carolina increased medication adherence but was not cost neutral. *Health Affairs* 33(2):300–308.

Martin, A.B., H. Hartman, L. Whittle, A. Catlin, and the National Expenditure Accounts Team. 2014 (January). National health spending in 2012: Rate of health spending growth remained low for the fourth consecutive year. *Health Affairs* 33(1):67–77.

North Carolina State Health Plan. 2014. Consumer-directed health plan (CDHP) benefits booklet. http://www.shpnc.org/library/pdf/my-medical-benefits/benefits-booklets/cdhp-2014.pdf.

Nyman, J.A. 1998. Theory of health insurance. *Journal of Health Administration Education* 16(1):41–66.

PACER Family-to-Family Health Information Center. 2011. Understanding your health insurance certificate of coverage. Document No. HIAC-h9. http://www.pacer.org/health/pdfs/HIAC-h9.pdf.

Peregrin, T. 2010. From contracts to clean claims: Guidelines for getting paid. *Journal of the American Dietetic Association* 110(6):837–839.

Pickett, J.P., et al., eds. 2000. *American Heritage Dictionary of the English Language*, 4th ed. Boston, MA: Houghton Mifflin.

Piotrowski, J. 2013. Health policy brief: Excise tax on "Cadillac" plans. *Health Affairs* http://healthaffairs.org/healthpolicybriefs/brief_pdfs/healthpolicybrief_99.pdf.

Redhead, C.S., and J. Kinzer. 2014 (July 28). Implementing the Affordable Care Act: Delays, Extensions, and Other Actions Taken by the Administration. http://fas.org/sgp/crs/misc/R43474.pdf.

Redling, B. 2007. Double exposure: Higher deductibles, uninsured patients add to administrators' challenges. *MGMA Connexion/Medical Group Management Association* 7(2):28–32.

Robertson, R., and S. R. Collins. 2011. Realizing health reform's potential: Women at risk—Why increasing numbers of women are failing to get the health care they need and how the Affordable Care Act will help. Commonwealth Fund Publication No. 1502. *Issue Brief* 3:1–24. http://www.commonwealthfund.org/~/media/Files/Publications/Issue%20Brief/2011/May/1502_Robertson_women_at_risk_reform_brief_v3.pdf.

Robinson, J.C., and P.B. Ginsburg. 2009. Consumer-driven health care: Promise and performance. *Health Affairs* 28(Suppl 1):W272–W281.

Rowell, J.C. 2000. *Understanding Health Insurance: A Guide to Professional Billing*, 5th ed. Albany, NY: Delmar.

Serota, S. 2012. Blue Cross and Blue Shield healthier intelligence. *CIO* 25(8):50.

Sisko, A.M., S.P. Keehan, G.A. Cuckler, A.J. Madison, S.D. Smith, C.J. Wolfe, D.A. Stone, J.M. Lizonitz, and J.A. Poisal. 2014 (October). National health expenditure projections, 2013–23: Faster growth expected with expanded coverage and improving economy. *Health Affairs* 33(10):1841–1850.

Thiemann, D. R., J. Coresh, W.J. Oetgen, and N.R. Powe. 1999. The association between hospital volume and survival after acute myocardial infarction in elderly patients. *New England Journal of Medicine* 340(21):1640–1648.

Towers Watson/National Business Group on Health. 2011. The road ahead: Shaping health care strategy in a post-reform environment, 16th annual Towers Watson employer survey on purchasing value in health care. http://www.towerswatson.com/assets/pdf/3946/TowersWatson-NBGH-2011-NA-2010-18560.pdf.

Towers Watson/National Business Group on Health. 2014. 2013/2014 Staying@Work™ survey report: The business value of a healthy workforce. http://www.towerswatson.com/en-US/Insights/IC-Types/Survey-Research-Results/2013/12/stayingatwork-survey-report-2013-2014-us.

Wess, B.P. 1999. Defining "centers of excellence." *Health Management Technology* 20(7):28–30.

Additional Resources

National Association of State Comprehensive Health Insurance Plans (NASCHIP). http://www.naschip.org.

National Conference of State Legislatures (NCSL). http://www.ncsl.org/research/health/health-reform.aspx.

Chapter 4
Government-Sponsored
Healthcare Programs

Objectives

- To differentiate among and to identify the various government-sponsored healthcare programs

- To recall the history of the Medicare and Medicaid programs in America

- To describe the effect that government-sponsored healthcare programs have on the American healthcare system

Key Terms

Beneficiary
Civilian Health and Medical Program: Veterans Administration (CHAMPVA)
Federal Employees' Compensation Act (FECA) of 1916
Indian Health Service (IHS)
Medicaid
Medicare
Medicare Advantage
Medicare Modernization Act (MMA) of 2003
Medicare Part A

Medicare Part B
Medicare Part C
Medicare Part D
Programs of All-Inclusive Care for the Elderly (PACE)
Social Security Act
State Children's Health Insurance Program (CHIP)
Temporary Assistance for Needy Families (TANF)
TRICARE
Veterans Health Administration
Workers' compensation

Introduction

The various levels of government administer several health plans for various populations as mandated by laws and regulations. Perhaps the most well-known is Medicare, which serves persons who qualify for Social Security benefits and who are 65 years old or older. This chapter discusses Medicare and several other federal- and state-sponsored programs.

Medicare

The **Social Security Act** was amended by Public Law 89-97 on July 30, 1965, to create the Medicare program (Title XVIII). On July 1, 1966, Medicare's coverage took effect. **Medicare** is a national health insurance program that provides health services to elderly and other qualifying persons. Medicare benefits are available for

- Persons 65 years old or older who are eligible for Social Security or railroad retirement benefits

- Individuals entitled to Social Security or railroad retirement disability benefits for at least 24 months

- Government employees with Medicare coverage who have been disabled for more than 29 months

- Insured workers (and their spouses) who have end-stage renal disease

- Children who have end-stage renal disease

In 2010, two major laws passed that significantly affected the Medicare system. The Patient Protection and Affordable Care Act (P.L. 111-48) was enacted on March 23, 2010. In addition, the Health Care and Education Reconciliation Act of 2010 (P.L. 111-52) was passed on March 30, 2010. Together these two laws are known as the Affordable Care Act (ACA) of 2010. The ACA contains a number of provisions designed to do the following (HHS 2011a, 67803):

- Improve the quality of Medicare services

- Support innovation and the establishment of new payment models

- Better align Medicare payments with provider costs

- Strengthen program integrity within Medicare

- Put Medicare on a firmer financial footing

Several of the provisions included in this law are discussed through this textbook. Later in this chapter, the effects of the ACA provisions regarding Medicare payment system will be discussed. Prior to the ACA, the **Medicare Modernization Act (MMA) of 2003** called for significant changes to the Medicare system. MMA created an outpatient prescription drug benefit, provided beneficiaries with expanded coverage choices, and improved benefits.

Medicare is divided into four parts: Part A, Part B, Part C, and Part D.

Medicare Part A for Inpatients

Medicare Part A, inpatient hospital insurance, is provided with no premiums to most beneficiaries. Most services covered under this benefit require that an annual deductible and copayment be paid by the **beneficiary**. Services included in this benefit are

- Inpatient hospitalization

- Long-term care hospitalization

- Skilled nursing facility services

- Home health services

- Hospice care

Each site of service has specific limitations governing cost-sharing provisions per benefit period (table 4.1).

Medicare Part B

Medicare Part B, supplemental medical insurance, is an optional insurance package that beneficiaries may purchase. In 2015, the average monthly premium is $104.90 (http://www.Medicare.gov). Part B insurance covers physician services, medical services, and medical supplies not covered by Part A. Most of these services are provided on an outpatient basis. In addition to the monthly premium, beneficiaries are responsible for an annual deductible and for service copayments. Table 4.2 provides a summary of the services and cost-sharing provisions.

Medicare Part C

Several services are excluded from Part A and Part B Medicare coverage. Beneficiaries can purchase additional

Table 4.1. Part A services 2015

Site of Service	Benefit Period	Patient Responsibility
Hospital inpatient and long-term care hospital	First 60 days	$1,260 annual
	Days 61–90	$315 per day
	Days 91–150 (lifetime reserve days*)	$630 per day
	Beyond 150 (lifetime reserve days*)	All costs
Skilled nursing facility	First 20 days	Nothing
	Days 21–100	$157.50 per day
	Beyond 100 days	All costs
Home health	No time limit—based on medical necessity criteria	Nothing for services, 20 percent for durable medical equipment (DME)
Hospice	No time limit—based on physician certification	Limited costs for outpatient drugs and inpatient respite care

*Nonrenewable lifetime reserve of up to 60 additional days of inpatient hospital care.
Source: http://www.Medicare.gov.

Table 4.2. Part B services 2015

Site of Service	Benefit	Patient Responsibility
Medical services	Physician services, medical and surgical services and supplies, durable medical equipment (DME)	$147 annual deductible, plus 20 percent of approved amount (excludes hospital outpatient; see below)
	Mental health care	40 percent of most care
	Occupational, physical, and speech therapy	20 percent of approved amount
Clinical laboratory services	Blood tests, urinalysis, and more	Nothing
Home health	Intermittent skilled care, home health aide service, DME and supplies, and other services	Nothing for services, 20 percent for DME
Outpatient hospital services	Services for diagnosis and/or treatment of an illness or injury	$147 deductible, plus established copayment amount per covered service. No copayment for a single service can be higher than the hospital Part A deductible. 100 percent charges for noncovered services

Source: http://www.Medicare.gov.

coverage or choose **Medicare Part C** coverage, a managed care option known as **Medicare Advantage**, to gain insurance for these services. The Part A and Part B excluded services that are provided under Part C are

- Long-term nursing care
- Custodial care
- Dental services
- Vision services
- Routine examinations, except initial preventive medicine examination added by MMA
- Health and wellness education
- Acupuncture
- Hearing aids

Medicare Part C, Medicare Advantage, is available for beneficiaries participating in Part A, B, and D (drug benefit) coverage. In addition to the Part B premium, members of an approved Medicare Advantage program pay an additional premium for the full scope of services offered by the program that are not typically covered by Medicare.

Example:
Routine physical examinations and vision services are excluded from Medicare Parts A and B. However, these services are provided by Medicare Advantage programs.

MMA revised several components of the Medicare Advantage program, including a new process for determining beneficiary premiums. Monthly premiums range from $50 to $350, depending on the scope of service the beneficiary elects to purchase.

Medicare Part D

Medicare Part D, Medicare drug benefit, was created by the MMA of 2003. The benefit was fully implemented on January 1, 2006. The program offers outpatient drug coverage provided by private prescription drug plans and Medicare Advantage. Beneficiaries pay a monthly premium that varies by plan but that can be as low as $15 per month. In addition, beneficiaries have an annual deductible and make copayments for their prescriptions. Low-income beneficiary provisions are built into the program for seniors who cannot afford the standard copayment amounts. MMA also established improved access to pharmacies, an up-to-date formulary, and emergency access for Medicare beneficiaries.

Medigap

Medicare beneficiaries may elect to purchase private insurance policies to supplement their Medicare Part A or Part B coverage. This supplemental insurance, known as Medigap, covers most cost-sharing expenses, as shown in tables 4.1 and 4.2. Medigap policies must meet federal standards and are offered by various private insurance companies.

Medicare Market Basket Updates: Reductions and Productivity Adjustments

As mentioned previously, one of the goals of the ACA was to better align Medicare payments with provider costs. The various Medicare prospective payment systems currently in use are discussed in chapters 6 through 8 of this text. Each PPS has its own unique design, adjustments, and provisions. But one common theme through the payment systems is that Medicare used a market basket or another update factor on a yearly basis as a way to adjustment payments for input price inflation in the provision of medical services. Each year in the respective PPS final rule, the finalized market basket is published. It is through the market basket that Medicare will reduce facility payments. Based on section 3401 of the ACA, CMS must apply a reduction to the market basket for each PPS, as well as the execution of a productivity adjustment. The market basket adjustments are scheduled for 2011 through 2019. The amount of the reduction varies by year and by payment system. For example, the hospital market basket reduction for 2012 was −0.1 percent and for 2015 is −0.2 percent (HHS 2014, 49995).

The second adjustment is a productivity adjustment and as defined by the ACA as the 10-year moving average of changes in annual economy-wide, private nonfarm business multifactor productivity (MFP) (HHS 2011b, 51690). Currently, IHS Global Insight,

Inc. (IGI), an economic forecasting firm, calculates and releases the MFP. The finalized MFP adjustment percent to be used during a given rate year will be published in the respective PPS final rule. The MFP will vary by PPS due to timing and different medical services provided under the benefit packages. The MFP adjustment for hospital inpatient services (IPPS) for FY 2015 was −0.5 percent. To execute both provisions for the hospital inpatient setting (IPPS) for FY 2015, the market basket of 2.9 percent was reduced by 0.5 percent for the MFP adjustment and by 0.2 percent for the ACA reduction, leaving the update factor at 2.2 percent (HHS 2014, 49995).

CMS was expected to save $233 billion between 2010 and 2019 thanks to the execution of the market basket and productivity adjustments (Foster 2010, 8). This was a considerable savings to CMS and, ultimately, the Medicare Trust Fund. However, this provides a significant challenge for healthcare facilities. As payments are decreased each year, facility administrators are heavily incentivized to find ways to lower costs while still providing high-quality care as mandated by other sections of the ACA, as discussed further in chapter 10.

Medicaid

Originally known as the Medical Assistance Program, **Medicaid** (Title XIX) was added to the Social Security Act in 1965. Medicaid is a joint program between the federal and state governments to provide healthcare benefits to low-income persons and families. This program is designed to allow each individual state to develop and maintain a Medicaid program unique to its state. Each state determines specific eligibility requirements and services to be offered, so coverage varies greatly from state to state. A person qualifying for services in one state may not qualify in another state. Furthermore, coverage determination for services is state-specific. Federal funds allocated to each state are based on the average income per person for that state. However, for a state to qualify to receive Medicaid federal funds, the state's program must provide coverage to at least the following groups:

- Low-income families with children, including those who meet eligibility for Temporary Assistance for Needy Families (TANF)

- Supplemental Security Income recipients (or others who meet criteria in more restrictive states)

- Infants born to Medicaid-eligible pregnant women

- Children younger than 6 whose family income is at or below 133 percent of the federal poverty level

- Recipients of adoption assistance and foster care (Title IV-E of the Act)

- Certain Medicare beneficiaries

- Special protected groups

In addition, the state program must offer a designated set of services to members in order to receive federal matching funds (figure 4.1). Eligibility and services may be expanded by individual states based on that state's laws and regulations. For example, states may elect to provide members with optometry services and eyeglasses or dental services. States are also afforded the flexibility to determine cost-sharing (in terms of deductible and copayments) terms for their programs for certain services and members. For example, family planning services are exempt from cost sharing, as are services to pregnant women and children younger than 18. State programs may also offer managed care options. In 2010, 71.45 percent of all Medicaid enrollees chose the managed care option, up from 65.34 percent in 2006 and 56.82 percent in 2001 (CMS 2011a). Although there was a significant increase between 2001 and 2010, the penetration rate has been steady at around 70 percent since 2010 (CMS 2015a, n.p.).

Figure 4.1. Medicaid-required services

Inpatient hospital services	Rural health clinic services
Outpatient hospital services	Laboratory and x-ray services
Physician services	Pediatric and family nurse practitioner services
Medical and surgical dental services	Federally qualified health center services
Nursing facility services for individuals aged 21 or older	Nurse midwife services
Home health care for persons eligible for nursing facility services	Early and periodic screening, diagnosis, and treatment services for individuals younger than 21
Family planning services and supplies	

Other Government-Sponsored Healthcare Programs

Other government-sponsored healthcare programs include

- The TANF program
- Programs of All-Inclusive Care for the Elderly (PACE)
- The Children's Health Insurance Program (CHIP)
- TRICARE programs
- Veterans Health Administration (VHA)
- Civilian Health and Medical Program: Veterans Administration (CHAMPVA)
- Indian Health Services (IHS)
- Workers' compensation

Each of these programs serves a specific target group and has specific eligibility requirements, plan requirements, and participant benefits.

The Temporary Assistance for Needy Families Program

The Personal Responsibility and Work Opportunity Reconciliation Act of 1996 (also known as welfare reform) brought about many changes to Medicaid eligibility. For example, welfare reform repealed the Aid to Families with Dependent Children (AFDC) program.

AFDC was replaced with the **Temporary Assistance for Needy Families Program (TANF)**, which provides states with grant money designated to provide low-income families with case assistance. In 2006, under the Deficit Reduction Act of 2005, TANF became the TANF Bureau within the Office of Family Assistance (OFA). The mission of TANF is to help needy families achieve self-sufficiency (OFA 2011). By administering block grants, states support TANF goals by

- Assisting needy families so that children can be cared for in their own homes, reducing the dependency of needy parents by promoting job preparation, work, and marriage

- Preventing out-of-wedlock pregnancies

- Encouraging the formation and maintenance of two-parent families

The TANF Bureau is composed of several divisions, including State TANF Policy, State and Territory TANF Management, Data Collection and Analysis, and Tribal TANF Management.

Programs of All-Inclusive Care for the Elderly

The Balanced Budget Act (BBA) of 1997 authorized the creation of Programs of All-Inclusive Care for the Elderly (PACE). **PACE** is a joint Medicare–Medicaid venture that offers states the option of creating and administering this capitated managed care option for the frail elderly population (HHS 1999). PACE was designed to enhance the quality of life for the frail elderly population by enabling them to live in their own homes and communities and to preserve and support their family units.

States electing to administer PACE must be approved and provide designated services (figure 4.2). States must provide services in at least one facility in a geographic service area. The facilities must be accessible and offer adequate services to meet the needs of all participants in the programs. Additional facilities must be staffed and supply a full range of services when warranted by the growth of the PACE population in a service area. Participants may frequent the facility as determined by the multidisciplinary team and the patient's needs. Each facility must have in place a multidisciplinary team consisting of at least the following members (HHS 1999):

- Primary care physician

- Registered nurse

- Social worker

- Physical therapist

- Occupational therapist

- Recreation therapist or activity coordinator

- Dietician

- PACE center coordinator

- Home care coordinator

- Personal care attendants or representatives

- Drivers or representatives

Beneficiaries of PACE, frail elderly persons, must meet the following eligibility requirements:

- Minimum age of 55

- Resident in the PACE service area

- Assessed by the PACE multidisciplinary team

- Certified by the state Medicaid agency as eligible for nursing home level of care

PACE programs are not offered in all states, nor even in all service areas within states.

Children's Health Insurance Program

CHIP (formerly the State Children's Health Insurance Program [SCHIP]), or Title XXI of the Social Security Act, was created in 1997 by the BBA. **CHIP** is a state–federal partnership that targets the growing

Figure 4.2.   PACE-required services

Multidisciplinary assessment and treatment plan	Medical specialty services
Primary care services	Laboratory and x-ray services
Social work services	Drugs and biological agents
Physical, occupational, and speech therapies	Prosthetics and DME
Personal care and supportive services	Acute inpatient care
Nutritional counseling	Nursing facility care
Recreational therapy	All Medicaid-covered services
Transportation	
Meals	

number of children not covered by health insurance. CHIP was renewed and strengthened through the Children's Health Insurance Program Reauthorization Act (CHIPRA) of 2009. In addition, the ACA of 2010 maintains the CHIP eligibility standards in place as of enactment through 2019. At the time of signing CHIPRA, President Barack Obama stated, "In a decent society, there are certain obligations that are not subject to tradeoffs or negotiation—health care for our children is one of those obligations" (HHS 2010, 2). Currently CHIP provides healthcare coverage to more than eight million children. Since its inception, CHIP has provided healthcare services for more than 40 million children (HHS 2010, 5). It is designed to provide health insurance to children of families whose income level is too high to qualify for Medicaid but too low to afford private healthcare insurance. Specifically, to qualify for the program, the child must reside with a family whose income is at or below a specified percent of the federal poverty level. Most states offer coverage at 200 percent of the federal poverty level; other states offer coverage at 250 percent or 300 percent of the federal poverty level (CMS 2015b, n.p.).

CHIP varies from state to state. Each state may determine how it would like to deliver the healthcare benefit to qualifying persons. The state may elect to expand Medicaid eligibility to children who would qualify for CHIP. The state may design a separate program to provide the benefit, or the state may combine the Medicaid expansion and separate program concepts; regardless of the individual program design, state plans and revisions must be approved by the Centers for Medicare and Medicaid Services (CMS). By September 30, 1999, each state and territory had an approved CHIP plan in place (CMS 2011b). States must provide the following services to CHIP beneficiaries:

- Inpatient hospital services
- Outpatient hospital services
- Physicians' medical and surgical services
- Laboratory and radiology services
- Well-baby/child care services, including immunizations
- Dental services

States may impose cost-sharing provisions on individuals who are enrolled in the program. The cost sharing cannot exceed 5 percent of a family's gross or net income. States cannot impose cost sharing for preventive or immunization services. Furthermore, American Indian/Alaskan native children who are members of a federally recognized tribe may not be charged any cost-sharing fees.

TRICARE

The Department of Defense provides a healthcare program for active-duty and retired members of the seven uniformed services of the United States: the Air Force, Army, Coast Guard, Marine Corps, Navy, National Oceanic and Atmospheric Administration (NOAA) Commissioned Corps, and Public Health Service Commissioned Corps. In addition, coverage is provided for such members' families and survivors. The healthcare program is now titled **TRICARE**, replacing the Civilian Health and Medical Program of the Uniformed Services (CHAMPUS), which was enacted in 1966 by amendments to the Dependents Medical Care Act. TRICARE provides comprehensive coverage for all beneficiaries:

- Outpatient visits
- Hospitalization
- Preventive services
- Maternity care
- Immunizations
- Mental/behavioral health

TRICARE offers nine different health plan options to provide coverage for beneficiaries around the globe. Active-duty service members may enroll only in a TRICARE prime plan, but several additional plans are available for active-duty family members, retirees, and their family members and survivors.

TRICARE Prime Options

TRICARE Prime and TRICARE Prime Remote are the program's managed care options. All active-duty service members (ADSMs) and activated Guard or Reserve members are automatically covered by one of these programs, although the individual must complete an enrollment form and submit it to the regional contractor. TRICARE Prime is required when ADSMs live and work within 50 miles or less than an hour's drive from a military treatment facility.

TRICARE Prime Remote is required when ADSMs live and work in remote areas. By using this option, a member may access primary care from an out-of-network provider if network providers are unavailable in the area. There are no enrollment fees, deductibles, or copayments for authorized medical services and prescriptions with either TRICARE option.

TRICARE Prime Overseas and TRICARE Prime Remote Overseas follow the same concept as Prime and Prime Remote, but the ADSMs and active-duty family members (ADFMs), if applicable, are located overseas.

ADFMs may also enroll in TRICARE Prime, Prime Remote, Prime Overseas, and Prime Remote Overseas. This is the most economical program available for military families because there are no enrollment, deductible, or copayment fees for covered services. To participate in the managed care option, ADFMs must enroll during an open enrollment period.

The US Family Health Plan is a component of the TRICARE Prime plan that is available to all ADFMs, retirees, and retiree family members, including those 65 or older, regardless of whether they participate in Medicare Part B. The plan provides coverage in six geographic regions in the United States. After enrolling, beneficiaries will not access Medicare providers, military treatment facilities, or TRICARE network providers but instead receive care (including prescription drug coverage) from a primary care physician selected from a network of private physicians affiliated with one of the not-for-profit health care systems offering the plan. A primary care physician helps beneficiaries obtain appointments with specialists in the area and coordinates all care.

TRICARE Standard, TRICARE Standard Overseas, and TRICARE Extra

If ADFMs do not want to enroll in the managed care options, they can participate in TRICARE Standard, TRICARE Standard Overseas, or TRICARE Extra, which require members to pay an annual deductible as well as a cost share of allowed charges. The cost-sharing provisions require a 15 percent coinsurance for network providers and a 20 percent coinsurance for nonnetwork providers. In addition, there is a per-day coinsurance amount for inpatient hospitalizations. The ADFM need not enroll in either of these programs. Rather, each family member enrolls in the Defense

Enrollment Eligibility Reporting System (DEERS), which outlines eligibility dates. Service members are responsible for maintaining up-to-date information in DEERS. For TRICARE Standard Overseas, there is a 20 percent coinsurance amount for ADFMs.

Military retirees younger than 65, along with their families, may enroll in TRICARE Prime or participate in TRICARE Standard or TRICARE Extra. TRICARE Standard and TRICARE Extra require deductibles and copayments for covered services. Under TRICARE Standard and TRICARE Extra, enrollees have a 20 percent coinsurance for network providers and a 25 percent coinsurance for nonnetwork providers. In addition, in-network hospitalizations require the beneficiary to pay the lesser of the per-day copayment amount or 25 percent of the charges plus 20 percent of separately reportable professional charges (physician charges). Nonnetwork hospitalizations require the beneficiary to pay the lesser of the per-day copayment amount or 25 percent of charges plus 25 percent of separately reportable professional charges. For TRICARE Standard Overseas, there is a 25 percent coinsurance amount for military retirees and their families.

The National Defense Authorization Act for federal fiscal year 2005 expanded TRICARE coverage, making it available for Reserve Component (RC) members and their dependents when the RC member is called to active duty (on orders) for more than 30 consecutive days. RC dependents become eligible for TRICARE Standard or TRICARE Extra on the first day of the RC member's orders if the orders are for more than 30 days. RC dependents may choose to enroll in TRICARE Prime or TRICARE Prime Remote any time during the first month of the RC member's activation.

TRICARE Young Adult

This plan option is available for young adult children of ADSM, Reserve members, and military retirees. Young adults quality if they are a child of a qualified military member, 21 to 25 years old, unmarried, and not eligible to enroll in an employer-sponsored health plan based on their own employment. TRICARE Young Adult is a premium-based plan with additional cost sharing for outpatient and inpatient services. The Prime option allows for lower cost sharing per visit: free care at military treatment facilities, small copayment for network outpatient providers, and small per day copayment for network inpatient providers. The

Standard option allows great flexibility by allowing nonnetwork providers but requires a percentage coinsurance for network and nonnetwork visits.

TRICARE Reserve Select and TRICARE Retired Reserve

TRICARE Reserve Select is a premium-based health plan that qualified National Guard and Reserve members may purchase. There are individual plans and a family plan available. In addition to the monthly premium, there is a 15 percent coinsurance for outpatient network providers and a 20 percent coinsurance for nonnetwork providers. A per-day copayment for inpatient care is required as well. The Retired Reserve plan is similar but has higher premiums and higher coinsurance and copayment amounts for outpatient and inpatient services.

In addition to health services, TRICARE provides dental services for ADFMs and members of the Individual Ready and Selected Reserve and their families. There are single and family plans that consist of monthly premiums and copayments for covered services. In addition, TRICARE provides a dental program for retirees and their families. Single, two-party, and family plans are available that have monthly premiums, deductibles, and copayments for covered services.

TRICARE for Life

TRICARE for Life (TFL) is TRICARE's secondary coverage for TRICARE beneficiaries who become entitled to Medicare Part A. TRICARE becomes the secondary payer to Medicare. Members are required to participate in Medicare Part B and pay Medicare Part B premiums. TRICARE for Life minimizes out-of-pocket expenses such as coinsurance and deductibles for services that are covered by both Medicare and TRICARE.

Veterans Health Administration

The **Veterans Health Administration** (VA) is the nation's largest integrated health care system, with over 1,700 care sites serving over 8.76 million veterans each year (VA 2014, n.p.). The VA encourages all veterans to apply to determine eligibility for health benefits. Basic eligibility includes veterans who served in active military service and were separated under any condition other than dishonorable, as well as current and former members of Reserves or National Guard called to active

duty by federal order and having completed the full period for which they were called or ordered to active duty. The minimum duty requirement for most who enlisted after September 7, 1980, or entered active duty after October 16, 1981, is service of 24 continuous months or the full period for which they were called to active duty. There are however, many exceptions to the eligibility and minimum duty requirements, so all veterans are encouraged to apply. The VA program requires enrollment for participation in the program, but after enrolling, the member remains enrolled and has access to certain VA health benefits. Program members are placed into one of eight Priority Groups based on their individual service and circumstances. Figure 4.3 provides a sampling of the Priority Groups and those who qualify for each level.

The VA provides health care services at little or no cost to its members. There are copayments for treatment of nonservice-connection conditions. At time of enrollment, veterans complete a financial assessment that determines their level of copayment for services. The cost-sharing amounts are matched to the Priority Group for which the veteran is placed. For example, in 2015, a member in Priority Group 7 is responsible for 20 percent of the full inpatient copayment rate for the first ninety days of care, which is $252.00. Members in Priority Group 8 are responsible for the full inpatient

Figure 4.3. Sample of VHA Priority Groups

Priority Group 1
- Veterans with VA-rated service-connected disabilities 50% or more disabling.
- Veterans determined by VA to be unemployable due to service-connected conditions

Priority Group 2
- Veterans with VA-rated service-connected disabilities 30% or 40% disabling.

Priority Group 3
- Veterans who are Former Prisoners of War (POWs)
- Veterans awarded a Purple Heart medal
- Veterans whose discharge was for a disability that was incurred or aggravated in the line of duty
- Veterans with VA-rated service-connected disabilities 10% or 20% disabling
- Veterans awarded special eligibility classification under Title 38, U.S.C section 1151, "benefits for Individuals disabled by treatment or vocational rehabilitation"
- Veterans awarded the Medal of Honor (MOH)

Reference: Veterans Health Administration. 2014. Health Care Benefits Overview, page 4.

copayment rate for the first ninety days of care, which is $1,260 (VA 2014, n.p.). Having private insurance does not affect a veteran's eligibility for VA services. Veterans can choose to use their private insurance to supplement their VA benefits. For example, many private insurance plans will cover VA copayment requirements.

CHAMPVA

The Department of Veterans Affairs provides covered healthcare services and supplies to eligible beneficiaries through the **Civilian Health and Medical Program of the Department of Veterans Affairs (CHAMPVA).** This benefits program is available for the spouse or widow(er) and for the children of a veteran who meets one of the following criteria:

- Permanently and totally disabled due to a service-connected disability

- Was permanently and totally disabled due to a service-connected condition at time of death

- Died of a service-connected disability

- Died on active duty

Persons eligible for TRICARE benefits cannot participate in CHAMPVA. This program covers most healthcare services and supplies that are medically and psychologically necessary. CHAMPVA becomes a secondary payer when another health insurance benefit is available. For example, when a beneficiary reaches age 65, Medicare is the primary payer and CHAMPVA becomes the secondary payer.

The Indian Health Service

The **Indian Health Service (IHS)** was created to uphold the federal government's obligation to promote healthy American Indian and Alaskan Native people, communities, and cultures (IHS 2005). A government-to-government relationship between the United States and American Indian tribes was established in 1787 based on Article I, Section 8, of the US Constitution. From this relationship came the provision of health services for members of federally recognized tribes. Principal legislation for authorizing federal funds for Indian Health Services is the Snyder Act of 1921. The IHS is an agency within the Department of Health and Human Services.

Following are the functions of the IHS:

- Assist Indian tribes in the development of their own health programs

- Facilitate and assist Indian tribes in coordinating health planning

- Promote use of health resources available through federal, state, and local programs

- Provide comprehensive healthcare services

Healthcare services offered by the IHS include inpatient and outpatient care, preventive and rehabilitative services, and development of community sanitation facilities. The federal IHS healthcare delivery system consists of hospitals, health centers, health stations, and residential treatment centers.

Workers' Compensation

The **workers' compensation** benefit is provided to most employees to cover healthcare costs and lost income that results from a work-related injury or illness. Federal government employees are covered under the **Federal Employees' Compensation Act (FECA) of 1916**. Other employees are covered under state workers' compensation insurance funds if that program is established in the state in which the employees work.

FECA was established in 1916 and ensures that civilian employees of the federal government are provided medical, death, and income benefits for work-related injuries and illnesses. FECA is administered by the Office of Workers' Compensation Programs (OWCP), a division of the Department of Labor. OWCP also administered the Longshore and Harbor Workers' Compensation Act of 1927 and the Black Lung Benefits Reform Act of 1977.

State workers' compensation insurance funds are established by each state. Benefits may include burial, death, income, and medical. Rather than contracting individually with insurance companies for coverage, employers pay premiums into the nonprofit workers' compensation fund for their state. This allows the workers' compensation premiums to remain low and affordable for small-business owners.

In states where no fund is mandated for workers' compensation, employers must purchase insurance from private carriers or provide self-insurance coverage (LaTour and Eichenwald 2010, 382).

Check Your Understanding 4.2

1. Match each TRICARE program on the left with its description on the right:

a. ADFMs with deductible and 15 percent copay	____ TRICARE for Life (TFL)
b. ADFMs with deductible and 20 percent cost-share	____ TRICARE Prime
c. Managed care	____ TRICARE for ADSMs, Extra Nonnetwork
d. Secondary coverage for Medicare beneficiaries	____ TRICARE Standard Network

2. True or false? When a CHAMPVA beneficiary reaches age 65, Medicare becomes the primary payer, and CHAMPVA becomes the secondary payer.

3. Services offered by the IHS to Indian tribes include all of the following except
   a. Rehabilitative services
   b. Death benefits
   c. Outpatient care
   d. Development of sanitation facilities

4. Why was the PACE program created?

5. Which type of program is CHIP?
   a. Federal
   b. State
   c. Local
   d. Federal-State

Chapter 4 Review Quiz

1. Which program replaced Aid to Families with Dependent Children (AFDC)?

2. What recent legislation made a substantive change to Medicare benefits, and how did those benefits change?

3. List at least three types of Medicaid recipients required for states to qualify for federal matching funds.

4. How was the PACE venture designed to enhance the quality of life for the frail elderly population?

5. What is the target population of the State Children's Health Insurance Program (CHIP) (Title XXI)?

6. Which TRICARE program is the most economical program for military families, and why is it less expensive than the other options?

7. What program covers healthcare costs and lost income from work-related injuries or illness of federal government employees?

8. Individuals eligible for railroad retirement disability or retirement benefits are ineligible for Medicare. True or false?

9. Individuals who are eligible may choose between TRICARE benefits and CHAMPVA. True or false?

10. In states having no mandated workers' compensation fund, employers must purchase insurance from private carriers or provide self-insurance coverage. True or false?

References

Centers for Medicare and Medicaid Services. 2005. State requirements and options under Federal Medicaid law. http://www.cms.hhs.gov/medicaid/welfareref/welfare.asp#ch1State.

Centers for Medicare and Medicaid Services. 2011a. Medicaid managed care trends. http://www.cms.gov/MedicaidDataSourcesGenInfo/04_MdManCrEnrllRep.asp.

Centers for Medicare and Medicaid Services. 2011b. Children's Health Insurance Program (CHIP). http://www.medicaid.gov/Medicaid-CHIP-Program-Information/By-Topics/Childrens-Health-Insurance-Program-CHIP/Childrens-Health-Insurance-Program-CHIP.html.

Centers for Medicare and Medicaid Services. 2015a. Managed Care. http://www.Medicaid.gov.

Centers for Medicare and Medicaid Services. 2015b. CHIP Eligibility. http://www.Medicaid.gov/chip/eligibility-standards/chip-eligibility-standards.html.

Department of Health and Human Services. 1999. Medicare and Medicaid programs: Programs of all-inclusive care. *Federal Register* 64(226):66233–66304.

Department of Health and Human Services. 2010. The Department of Health and Human Services Children's Health Insurance Program Reauthorization Act annual report on the quality of care for children in Medicaid and CHIP. https://www.cms.gov/MedicaidCHIPQualPrac/Downloads/secrep.pdf.

Department of Health and Human Services. 2011a. Medicare program: Medicare shared saving program: Accountable care organizations; Final rule. *Federal Register* 76(212):67802–67990.

Department of Health and Human Services. 2011b. Medicare program: Hospital inpatient prospective payment systems for acute care hospitals and the long-term care hospital prospective payment system and FY 2012 Rates; Hospitals' FTE resident caps for graduate medical education payment; Final rule. *Federal Register* 76(160):51476–51846.

Department of Health and Human Services. 2014. Medicare program: Hospital inpatient prospective payment systems for acute care hospitals and the long-term care hospital prospective payment system and FY 2015 Rates; Final rule. *Federal Register* 79(163):49853-50536.

Foster, R.S. 2010. Estimated Financial Effects of the "Patient Protection and Affordable Care Act," as Amended. https://www .cms.gov/ActuarialStudies/Downloads/PPACA_2010-04-22.pdf.

Indian Health Service (IHS). 2005. http://www.ihs.gov.

LaTour, K., and S. Eichenwald, M., eds. 2010. *Health Information Management: Concepts, Principles, and Practice*. Chicago: AHIMA.

Office of Family Assistance. 2011. About TANF. http://www.acf .hhs.gov/programs/ofa/tanf/about.html.

Veterans Health Administration. 2014. Health Care Benefits Overview.

Additional Resources

Centers for Medicare and Medicaid Services. 2007. Fact sheet—Strong competition and beneficiary choices contribute to Medicare drug coverage with lower costs than predicted. http:// www.cms.gov/apps/files/FactSheetPartDBenchmark.pdf.

Centers for Medicare and Medicaid Services. 2007. Medicare and you 2008. http://www.medicare.gov.

Centers for Medicare and Medicaid Services. 2009. Medicare and you 2009. http://www.medicare.gov.

Centers for Medicare and Medicaid Services. 2015. Children's Health Insurance Program. http://www.medicaid.gov/chip/ chip-program-information.html.

TRICARE. 2012. TRICARE Plans. http://tricare.mil/mybenefit/ home/overview/LearnAboutPlansAndCosts.

Veterans Health Administration. 2014. Health Benefits. http:// www.va.gov/HEALTHBENEFITS/index.asp.

Chapter 5
Managed Care Plans

Objectives

- To define managed care

- To trace the origins of managed care

- To delineate characteristics of managed care in terms of quality and cost-effectiveness

- To describe common care management tools used in managed care

- To depict accreditation processes and performance improvement initiatives used in managed care

- To define cost controls used in managed care

- To discuss contract management and carve-outs

- To define types of managed care plans along a continuum of control

- To describe the use of managed care in states' Medicaid programs, Children's Health Insurance Program, and Medicare

- To discuss types of integrated delivery systems

- To define terms commonly used in managed care

Key Terms

Capitation
Carve-out
Case management
Cherry-picking
Closed panel
Community rating
Cost sharing
Disease management
Dual eligible (dual)
Enrollee
Episode-of-care reimbursement
Evidence-based clinical practice guidelines
Exclusive provider organization (EPO)
Fee-for-service reimbursement
Formulary
Gatekeeper
Global payment
Group practice model
Group (practice) (clinic) without walls (GWW, GPWW, CWW)
Health maintenance organization (HMO)
Independent practice association (IPA)
Integrated delivery system

Integrated provider organization
Managed care
Managed care organization (MCO)
Management service organization (MSO)
Medical foundation
Medical necessity
Medicare Advantage (MA)
Network
Network model
Open panel
Out-of-pocket
Per member per month (PMPM)
Pharmacy (prescription) benefit manager (PBM)
Physician-hospital organization
Point-of-service (POS) healthcare insurance plan
Preadmission certification
Preadmission review
Preauthorization
Preauthorization (pre-certification) number
Precertification
Preferred provider organization (PPO)
Prescription management
Primary care physician (PCP)

Primary care provider (PCP)
Prior approval (authorization)
Provider-sponsored organization (PSO)
Referral
Second opinion
Special needs plan (SNP)
Staff model

Subcapitation
Third opinion
Utilization management
Utilization review
Withhold
Withhold pool

Introduction to Managed Care

The purpose of **managed care** is to provide affordable, high-quality healthcare. Managed care systematically merges clinical, financial, and administrative processes to manage access, cost, and quality of healthcare.

Managed care traces its origins to the early 1900s. As early as 1906, Western Clinic in Tacoma, Washington, offered its members medical services for $0.50 per month (DeLeon et al. 1991, 15). The first Blue Cross plan, established in Dallas, Texas, was a form of managed care. In 1929, schoolteachers in this plan prepaid $6 per year for 21 days of hospitalization (Starr 1982, 295). In the 1930s, Kaiser Construction Company established a plan for its workers (DeLeon et al. 1991, 15). Today, as Kaiser Permanente, the healthcare plan has more than eight million enrolled members (Kaiser Permanente 2014).

In the United States between 1966 and the early 1970s, the costs of healthcare escalated quickly (Foster 2000). To control costs and provide affordable quality healthcare, federal legislation encouraged the growth of **health maintenance organizations (HMOs)**. The Health Maintenance Organization (HMO) Act of 1973 provided federal grants and loans for new HMOs.

Since the passage of the HMO Act, managed care has increased its share of the market, in part as a result of economic pressures. Plus, managed care evolved into numerous types in addition to HMOs. These multiple types emerged to meet the needs of consumers for freedom of choice and access to specialists and the need of employers to reduce their healthcare costs.

Managed Care Organizations

Managed care organizations (MCOs) are healthcare plans that attempt to manage care. In the Balanced Budget Act of 1997, these plans are termed coordinated care plans. MCOs implement provisions to manage both the costs and outcomes of healthcare. Managed care plans integrate the financing and delivery of specified healthcare services.

Benefits and Services of MCOs

MCOs offer differing levels of benefits, depending on the cost of their premiums and cost sharing:

- Physician services (inpatient and outpatient)

- Inpatient care
- Preventive care and wellness, such as immunizations, well-child examinations, adult periodic health maintenance examinations, and Pap smears
- Prenatal care
- Emergency services
- Diagnostic and laboratory tests
- Certain home health services

Enrollees (enrolled members) of MCOs have access to mental and behavioral health and specialty care through referral from their primary care provider (PCP).

Characteristics of MCOs

MCOs share characteristics associated with providing quality care and cost-effective care (tables 5.1 and 5.2). The lines between high-quality care and cost-effective care blur considerably. Moreover, these characteristics are not unique to MCOs; other payers also implement them. However, these characteristics are often associated with MCOs because of the characteristics' prevalence and extent of use in MCOs. MCOs coordinate and control healthcare services to improve quality and to contain expenditures.

Table 5.1. Managed care characteristics associated with quality care

Characteristic	Description
Selection criteria for providers	Criteria include quality, scope of services, cost, and location Credentialing and periodic recredentialing Procedural selection process at senior clinical staff level
Population	Responsible for delivery of healthcare services on continuum of care (prevention, wellness, acute, and chronic) Population receives recommended preventive care and appropriate care for chronic conditions Health and wellness management
Care management tools	Coordination of care by primary care provider Disease management Evidence-based clinical practice guidelines
Quality assessment and improvement	Entities are accredited and engage in performance improvement

Table 5.2.   Managed care characteristics associated with cost-effective care

Characteristic	Description
Service management tools	Medical necessity and utilization management Gatekeeper role of primary care provider Prior approval Second and third opinions Case management Prescription management
Episode-of-care reimbursement	Capitated reimbursement Global payment
Financial incentives	Providers to meet fiscal targets Members to use providers associated with the plan

Quality Patient Care

MCOs focus on providing high-quality patient care. They achieve this goal through careful selection of providers, an emphasis on the health of their populations of members, use of care management tools, and maintenance of accreditation or participation in quality improvement programs.

Selection of Providers

MCOs stress the use of criteria in their selection of providers. Senior clinicians in the upper echelons of the MCO select providers using preestablished procedures and standards. These criteria are based on quality, scope of services, cost, and location. Timelines for credentialing and recredentialing are followed. This emphasis ensures their members' access to superior and eminent providers throughout a geographic area.

Health of Populations

MCOs emphasize the health of their entire populations of members. These organizations are responsible for the delivery of healthcare services across the continuum of care in terms of setting and type. Examples of settings include the physicians' offices, home health agencies, and hospitals. Examples of types of care are preventive, wellness oriented, acute, and chronic. The MCO is clinically responsible for the health outcomes of its population. Members receive appropriate testing for preventive care, such as timely mammograms and Pap smears. Moreover, members with chronic conditions receive appropriate assessment and therapeutic procedures, as recommended by evidence-based clinical practice guidelines. In addition, MCOs often support their members' participation in health and wellness management. Wellness programs are one component of health and wellness management. These programs stress the habits of healthy lifestyles, such as exercise and proper nutrition. Other aspects of health and wellness management include smoking cessation, alcohol moderation, and harm reduction.

Care Management Tools

Care management tools include coordination of care, disease management, and the application of evidence-based clinical practice guidelines. Together, these tools foster continuity and accessibility of healthcare services and reduce fragmentation and misuse of resources and facilities.

Coordination of care is achieved through the use of PCPs. PCPs may be physicians, nurse practitioners, or physician assistants (Felt-Lisk 1996, 97–98). **Primary care physicians** often are family practitioners, general practitioners, internists, pediatricians, and obstetricians/gynecologists. In many MCOs, one PCP provides, supervises, or arranges for a patient or client's healthcare and makes necessary and appropriate **referrals**. A referral is a process in which a PCP makes a request to a managed care plan on behalf of a patient to send that patient to receive medical care from a specialist or provider outside the managed care plan.

Disease management focuses on preventing exacerbations of chronic diseases and promoting healthier lifestyles for patients and clients with chronic diseases. In disease management, patients are monitored to promote adherence to treatment plans and to detect early signs and symptoms of exacerbations. Disease management programs often focus on diabetes, congestive heart failure, coronary heart disease, chronic obstructive pulmonary disease, and asthma. Often the management of chronic diseases requires treatment plans and complex medication regimens involving multiple healthcare providers. Thus, disease management is closely aligned with coordination of care because the efforts of multiple providers must be synchronized.

Two literature reviews synthesized the results of research studies that reported the effects of disease management programs. One study focused on the outcomes of disease management programs for patients with both chronic obstructive pulmonary disease (COPD) and diabetes mellitus. The evidence from the review indicated that disease management programs could (1) improve health and the quality of life, (2) reduce hospital admissions, and (3) decrease hospital and total healthcare costs (Boland et al. 2013, 15). Specifically, the disease management programs tended to save costs when patients had severe COPD and had a history of exacerbations (flare-ups) (Boland et al. 2013, 1). Overall, however, the programs' outcomes were not consistent, varying by the type of research, the details of the interventions, and diseases' characteristics. The second review focused on disease management programs that used online tools to promote lifestyle changes for patients with Type 2 diabetes (Cotter et al. 2014, 243). In this review, successful disease management programs showed improvements in diet, physical activity, and control of blood sugar levels, or some combination of these improvements. These successful programs used interactive components, such as progress tracking tools and personalized feedback and provided opportunities for peer support (Cotter et al. 2014, 243).

Disease management programs have been overwhelmingly implemented across the US healthcare sector (Levy et al. 2007, 237). However, as the summaries of the two literature reviews show, multiple factors affect the effectiveness of disease management programs. Thus, despite the widespread implementation of disease management programs, healthcare administrators should inspect the programs' designs and features and should closely monitor the programs' achievement of their goals and objectives.

Evidence-based clinical practice guidelines are the foundation of members' care for specific clinical conditions. **Evidence-based clinical practice guidelines** are explicit statements that guide clinical decision making. They outline

- Key diagnostic indicators
- Timelines
- Alternatives in interventions and treatments
- Potential outcomes

They have been systematically developed from scientific evidence and clinical expertise to answer clinical questions. Other terms for these guidelines are *evidence-based guidelines, clinical practice guidelines, clinical guidelines, clinical pathways, clinical criteria,* and *medical protocols.* Sources of these guidelines are the US Preventive Services Task Force (USPSTF), the

Agency for Healthcare Research and Quality (AHRQ), the Centers for Disease Control and Prevention, and specialty organizations such as the American College of Cardiology, the American Academy of Family Physicians, the American Academy of Ophthalmology, and the American College of Obstetricians and Gynecologists. These guidelines are benchmarks of best practices in the care and treatment of patients and clients.

These guidelines are used to manage the wellness of members and to direct the care of acute illnesses and chronic conditions. The guidelines typically address the following:

- The entire plan of care across multiple delivery sites
- Appropriate diagnostic and therapeutic procedures for a disease or condition
- Reasons for referrals to specialists
- Clinical decision factors and decision points

Thus, evidence-based clinical practice guidelines serve as a means to standardize optimal care for all patients and to deliver comprehensive, coordinated care across multiple providers.

Quality Assessment and Improvement

MCOs participate in rigorous accreditation processes and in performance improvement initiatives. Organizations with accreditation standards for managed care include the following:

- National Committee for Quality Assurance (NCQA)
- URAC (formerly the Utilization Review Accreditation Commission)
- Accreditation Association for Ambulatory Health Care (AAAHC, also known as the Accreditation Association)

Plans also participate in performance improvement initiatives. Two common sets of measures to assess and improve quality follow:

- AHRQ's CAHPS® (formerly Consumer Assessment of Health Plans)
- NCQA's Healthcare Effectiveness Data and Information Set (HEDIS®)

Often as a part of these improvement initiatives, MCOs survey their members to obtain members' feedback on such issues as

- Satisfaction with administrative, clinical, and customer services

- Perceptions of the plan's strengths and weaknesses

- Suggestions for improvements

- Intentions regarding reenrollment

In addition to surveying members, MCOs conduct satisfaction surveys of patients, physicians, providers, customers, employers, and disenrolled members. Commitment to accreditation and performance improvement demonstrates MCOs' dedication to their members and to the delivery of quality healthcare.

Cost Controls

Managed care plans implement various forms of cost controls (table 5.2):

- Service management tools include medical necessity and utilization management, the gatekeeper role of the primary care provider, prior approval, second and third opinions, case management, and prescription management.

- Episode-of-care reimbursement includes capitation and global payment.

- Financial incentives include providers meeting fiscal targets and members using providers connected to the plan.

These forms of control will now be described.

Medical Necessity and Utilization Management

Several cost controls are related to medical necessity and utilization management. These cost controls contain and monitor use of healthcare services by evaluating the need for and intensity of the service prior to it being provided. Review of medical necessity and utilization review are often performed concurrently.

As stated in chapter 3, **medical necessity** can be defined as follows:

> A service or supply provided for the diagnosis, treatment, cure, or relief of a health condition, illness, injury, or disease. The service or supply must not be experimental,

investigational, or cosmetic in purpose. It must be necessary for and appropriate to the diagnosis, treatment, cure, or relief of a health condition, illness, injury, disease, or its symptoms. It must be within generally accepted standards of medical care in the community. It must not be solely for the convenience of the insured, the insured's family, or the provider. (North Carolina State Health Plan 2014, 78)

Utilization management is a program that evaluates the healthcare facility's overall efficiency in providing necessary care to patients in the most effective manner. Utilization management includes plans that define criteria, timelines, and other aspects of the overall program.

Utilization review, a component of utilization management, is a process that determines the medical necessity of a procedure and the appropriateness of the setting for the healthcare service in the continuum of care (inpatient or outpatient). Utilization review is a cost control because it answers the following two questions:

- Should this healthcare service occur?

- If so, then what setting is the most efficient in terms of delivery and cost?

Utilization review factors in patients' severity of illness and other medical conditions and illnesses. For example, utilization review assesses whether, in light of the patient's severity of illness, the services could be provided more efficiently and economically in an ambulatory setting rather than in the inpatient hospital.

MCOs and other insurers review medical necessity and utilization in a three-step process: initial clinical review, peer clinical review, and appeals consideration (table 5.3). Steps 2 and 3 are implemented only if the previous step results in a negative decision. If a step results in a positive decision, the process stops at that step.

Table 5.3.   Review of medical necessity and utilization

Step	Responsible Party	Activity or Resource
Clinical review	Licensed health professional	Review against established criteria
Peer clinical review	Peer clinician	Clinician qualified to render clinical opinion performs clinical review
Appeals consideration	Qualified, expert clinician in same specialty	Clinician not involved in initial decision but qualified to render clinical opinion performs clinical review

Medical necessity and utilization are reviewed using objective, clinical criteria. Multiple sets of criteria exist:

- Intensity of Service, Severity of Illness, and Discharge Screens (ISD)
- Appropriateness Evaluation Protocol (AEP)
- Making Care Appropriate to Patients (MCAP) (Oak Group 2014, n.p.)
- Indicia® for Utilization Review (MCG Health, LLC, 2014, n.p.)
- Truven (formerly Solucient) length-of-stay benchmarks (Truven Health Analytics 2014, n.p.)
- American Society of Addiction Medicine's Criteria (ASAM Criteria)
- Federal- and state-specific guidelines

Medical necessity and utilization are often reviewed for the following services:

- Confinement in acute-care hospital, long-term acute-care facility, long-term care facility psychiatric hospital, or partial-day hospital, or recipient of hospice or rehabilitation services
- Surgical procedures
- Emergency room services
- Emergent care received from out-of-**network** (out-of-plan) providers
- High-cost or high-risk diagnostic, interventional, or therapeutic outpatient procedures
- Physical, occupational, speech, and other rehabilitative therapies
- Mental health and chemical dependency care
- Home health services, private-duty nurses, and referrals to medical specialists
- Durable medical equipment, prosthetic and orthotic appliances, medical supplies, blood transfusions and administration, and medical transport

Generally, utilization review saves money through its prevention of overutilization. Overutilization is the unnecessary consumption of healthcare services or the consumption of unnecessarily expensive or sophisticated healthcare services.

Gatekeeper Role of Primary Care Provider

The **gatekeeper** role of the **primary care provider (PCP)** is a cost control. As the coordinator of all the healthcare services that a member may access, the PCP determines whether referrals are warranted. These referrals may be to (1) medical specialists, (2) other healthcare sites for diagnostic or therapeutic procedures, or (3) hospitals or other healthcare facilities. Gatekeepers determine the appropriateness of the healthcare service, the level of healthcare personnel, and the setting in the continuum of care.

Prior Approval

Prior approval (authorization) is also a cost control. Prior approval is the formal administrative process of obtaining prior approval for healthcare services. Alternative terms for this process are **preauthorization** and **precertification**. Terms for prior approval specific to inpatient services are **preadmission review** and **preadmission certification**. Inpatient admissions, surgeries, visits to medical specialists, elective procedures, and expensive or sophisticated diagnostic tests are all types of services requiring prior approval. Occasionally, for healthcare services such as mental or behavioral health, providers must submit entire treatment plans for prior approval. A **preauthorization** or **precertification number** is issued when the healthcare service is approved. MCOs may deny coverage, and third-party payers may deny payment for healthcare services for which required prior approval was not obtained. Policies identify the healthcare services for which prior approval must be obtained.

Second and Third Opinions

Second and **third opinions** are cost-containment measures to prevent unnecessary tests, treatments, medical devices, or surgical procedures. Second or third opinions are obtained from medical experts within the healthcare plan. They are particularly sought in the following circumstances:

- Test, treatment, medical device, or surgical procedure is high-risk or high-cost

- Diagnostic evidence is contradictory or equivocal

- Experts' opinions are mixed about efficacy

Case Management

Case management coordinates an individual's care, especially in complex and high-cost cases. Individuals are assigned case managers who are typically nurses or physicians. With patients or clients and their families, case managers coordinate the efforts of multiple healthcare providers at multiple sites over time. Consultants, specialists, PCPs, ancillary services, ambulatory care, inpatient services, and long-term care may all be involved. Case managers often are assigned to patients or clients with catastrophic illnesses or injuries, such as a severe head injury. Workers' compensation cases may involve a case manager. Goals of case management include continuity of care, cost-effectiveness, quality, and appropriate utilization.

Prescription Management

Prescription management is also a cost control measure. Prescription management expands the use of a **formulary** (see chapter 3) to a comprehensive approach to medications and their administration. This approach includes patient education; electronic screening, alert, and decision-support tools; expert and referent systems, especially related to drug–drug interactions, food–drug interactions, and cross-sensitivities; and criteria for drug utilization. Some electronic prescription management systems include point-of-service order entry, electronic transmission of the prescription to the pharmacy, and patient-specific medication profiles. As discussed in chapter 3, generic, less expensive drugs are preferred to brand-name, expensive drugs. However, the comprehensive approach also enhances quality patient care. Considering the cost of medications, prescription management is a powerful tool of cost containment.

Specialty management organizations exist to provide the comprehensive service of pharmacy (prescription) benefit management. These organizations are called **pharmacy (prescription) benefit managers (PBMs)**. PBMs administer healthcare insurance companies' prescription drug benefits. Administration encompasses the following (Hansen 1996, 3–4; Siracuse et al. 2008, 552; Slezak and Stine 2003, 38):

- Developing and managing formularies and preferred drug lists

- Negotiating contracts with drug manufacturers (pharmaceutical companies), including discounts and rebates, and with pharmacies, including payment levels

- Managing programs of prior authorization, drug utilization review, patient compliance, and cost-effective coordination of patients' drug regimens

- Processing and analyzing prescription claims

- Operating mail-order pharmacies

PBMs developed as a market force in the 1980s (Hansen 1996, 3). PBMs are "the predominant infrastructure for administration of prescription benefits in the United States" (Siracuse et al. 2008, 552). Understanding PBMs is essential because their widespread use affects millions of US citizens.

Episode-of-Care Reimbursement Method

MCOs use the episode-of-care reimbursement method. The purpose of the episode-of-care reimbursement method is to reduce the inflation of costs in a **fee-for-service reimbursement** environment.

Through the **episode-of-care reimbursement**, MCOs share the risks of costs of patients' care with providers. In the method, providers receive one predetermined amount for all the care a patient or client may receive during a period. The MCO does not increase payments for the complexity or extent of healthcare services, so the incentive to provide higher volumes of services to generate higher reimbursements is eliminated.

Episode-of-care reimbursement is based on averages. On average, the majority of enrolled members will rarely or never use healthcare services within a period. These low or nonusers offset the acutely or chronically ill members. In the aggregate, low users or nonusers balance out heavy users. MCOs most commonly use two of the episode-of-care payment methods: capitation and global payment.

Capitation

In **capitation**, providers are reimbursed a predetermined fixed amount per member per period. The common phrase is **per member per month (PMPM)**. The volume of services and their expense do not affect the reimbursement. Typically, capitation involves a group of physicians or an individual physician.

Global Payment

Global payment extends the scale of capitation. In global payment, providers in an integrated delivery system (IDS) or other type of network receive one fixed amount for members of the MCO. These providers include physicians, hospitals, and other care providers. The single payment is divided among all the providers. Therefore, in global payment, the scale of capitation is increased from the single group to an entire delivery system.

Financial Incentives

MCOs are fiscally accountable for the health outcomes of their populations. Thus, financial incentives exist for both providers and members. These incentives prevent the waste of financial resources through the provision of excessive or unnecessarily expensive healthcare services.

For providers, these incentives involve the provision of cost-efficient care. Incentives involve meeting targets for cost efficiency. The following types of healthcare services are the focus of incentives (Grumbach et al. 1998, 1517):

* Referrals to specialists

* Use of laboratory or other ancillary services

* Inpatient admissions or days

* Settings of care, such as office preferred to emergency room

* Productivity, in terms of number of visits per day

* Pharmaceuticals

For example, PCPs in MCOs may order less-expensive generic drugs rather than the more-expensive brand-name drugs. Medicaid MCOs also set targets, such as that "the number of emergency room visits for mental health or substance abuse treatment shall not exceed 8.5 visits per 1,000 enrollee months" (Carlson 2000, 13–14).

Incentives can be both positive and negative. As a positive incentive, providers may receive bonuses for meeting cost-containment targets. Conversely, a penalty

may be assessed as a negative incentive (disincentive). Examples of penalties include a percentage reduction of the PCP's salary if the provider does not meet the target or the loss of withholds (also known as physician contingency reserve [PCR]). A **withhold** is a part of the provider's capitated payment that the MCO deducts and holds to pay for excessive expenditures for expensive healthcare services, such as referrals to specialists. Withholds transfer risk to the providers. For a group practice, the withholds from individual providers are combined to form a **withhold pool**. At the end of period, surplus withheld funds are dispersed for meeting efficiency (utilization) or performance targets. Providers who do not meet targets do not receive their withholds at the end of the period.

It should be noted that since January 1, 1997, a federal rule has governed financial incentives in managed care Medicaid and Medicare plans (Gallagher et al. 1998, 409). This rule is titled Medicare and Medicaid Programs: Requirements for Physician Incentive Plans in Prepaid Health Care Organizations. The rule prohibits incentives that limit medically necessary referrals and requires MCOs to report information about financial incentives regarding referrals to the CMS and state Medicaid offices. Moreover, the rule mandates that MCOs disclose summaries about financial incentives to Medicare and Medicaid members who ask.

As financial incentives to members, MCOs set varying rates of **cost sharing**. Cost sharing is the portion that the patient or guarantor pays. For example, MCOs require higher **out-of-pocket** payments when members use out-of-plan providers than when they use in-plan providers. Other MCOs offer members levels of prescription drug benefits. The drug benefit with the most restrictive formulary is the least expensive, whereas the member's cost sharing increases with the liberality of the formulary. Incentives influence members' behavior without eliminating freedom of choice.

Contract Management

Contract management is critical in the episode-of-care reimbursement method. Providers and plans must be able to accurately project their expenditures in order to negotiate contracts that cover the costs of treating members. If a provider or plan underestimates the costs to treat plan members, the provider or plan loses money. Moreover, once the contract is established, entities must monitor and evaluate utilization and costs to assess whether projections align with reality.

If variances are detected, the plan or provider must implement corrective interventions on a timely basis.

Carve-outs are contracts that separate out (or "carve out") services or populations of patients or clients to decrease risk and costs. These services and populations are carved out of the global capitated payment. The types of services or populations that are carved out typically require long-term management, are high-cost, can be managed by one group of specialists, and are not usually managed by PCPs (figure 5.1). The use of carve-outs has been increasing since the mid-1980s. The provision of care for these services or to these populations is contracted out to vendors.

Contracts for carved-out services vary greatly. However, contracted functions may include

- Maintenance of a provider network

- Processing claims

- Utilization management and case management

- Operation of quality improvement programs

The payment methods for carved-out services and populations also vary greatly. A common payment for specialists' services is **subcapitation** (Alexander 1999, 9). Under subcapitation, the healthcare plan reimburses the specialists with a portion of the capitated rate. This portion is known as the subcapitation. Other methods of reimbursement for contracted vendors are administrative fees, prepayment (capitation based on per member per month), and fee-for-service. Given the variability in the diseases and their costs, healthcare plans often pay contracted vendors on a disease-by-disease or a population-by-population basis.

Advantages of carve-outs include reduction of **cherry-picking** (targeting the enrollment of healthy patients to minimize healthcare costs), increased quality resulting from volume of services, and increased cost savings resulting from economies of scale.

Potential disadvantages of carve-outs include fragmentation of care and decreased access. The benefits of managed care's coordination of care are negated without close synchronization between the gatekeeper and the provider of carved-out services. Care could become fragmented, as seen in fee-for-service. Moreover, the geographic dispersion of vendors of specialized services, such as behavioral health or substance abuse counseling, may be less widespread than that of PCPs. For example, vendors of behavioral health or substance

Figure 5.1.   Examples of carved-out services or populations

Chronically ill children
   Asthma
   Cancer
   Cerebral palsy
   Chromosomal and metabolic anomalies
   Congenital defects
   Cystic fibrosis
   Diabetes mellitus (Type 1)
   Down syndrome
   Epilepsy
   Hemophilia
   Muscular dystrophy
   Organ transplantation
   Rheumatoid arthritis
   Sickle cell disease and other hemoglobinopathies
   Spina bifida and other neural tube defects
Dental care
Diseases or conditions
   Acquired immunodeficiency syndrome/human immunodeficiency virus (AIDS/HIV)
   Alcoholism
   Behavioral health
   Cancer
   Chronic pain
   Congestive heart failure
   End-stage renal disease
   Mental health
   Quadriplegia or paraplegia
   Substance abuse
Prescription drug (pharmacy benefit)
Specialty services
   Cardiology
   Cardiovascular surgery
   Neurology
   Neurosurgery
   Occupational medicine
   Oncology
   Ophthalmology
   Orthopedics
   Physical therapy
   Radiology
   Rehabilitation
Vision care

abuse counseling may be clustered in large population centers rather than evenly distributed across urban and rural counties. Travel time and distance to these vendors may be increased for patients and clients who live in rural areas. Also, potential patients and clients who live on the opposite side of a very large city from the vendor may face problems related to travel. Moreover, the cost of travel may act as a barrier to services for these potential patients and clients. Thus, the lack of geographic dispersion may prevent utilization of specialized services by all persons who need them. Carve-outs that require use of specialized vendors may curtail access.

Types of MCOs

As managed care has evolved, lines have blurred among the types of MCOs. The blurring across types makes a continuum a better conceptualization of managed care than individual, separate categories. The different types of MCOs can be placed on a continuum of control. On this continuum, the HMOs represent the most controlled, and the **preferred provider organizations (PPOs)** represent the least controlled. This chapter discusses several managed care plans across the continuum of control.

Health Maintenance Organization

HMOs combine the provision of healthcare insurance and the delivery of healthcare services. The HMO Act of 1973 was an initiative to control healthcare costs. Subsequent amendments were enacted in 1976, 1978, and 1981 to implement regulations (42 CFR Part 417). Included in the act were conditions for becoming a federally qualified HMO. The conditions were a minimum benefits package, open enrollment, and **community rating**. In community rating, the rates for healthcare premiums are determined by geographic area (community) rather than by age, health status, or company size.

The act recognized three basic types of HMOs. These basic types are the **staff model**, the **group practice model**, and the **independent practice association (IPA)**. Since the 1970s, the **network model** HMO has developed. In some types of HMOs, the HMO hires the healthcare providers and owns the hospitals and other facilities. In other types of HMOs, the plans contract with providers, such as physicians, hospitals, and other healthcare professionals, to provide service. The negotiated payment rates in the contract are discounted. Providers accept the discounted rate because of the increased certainty of referrals and income. The different types of HMOs reflect these differing means of compensation.

HMOs share the following characteristics:

- Organized system of healthcare delivery to a geographic area

- Established set of basic and supplemental health maintenance and treatment services

- Voluntarily enrolled members

- Predetermined, fixed, and periodic prepayments for enrollees

HMOs emphasize preventive care in the belief that in the long term, preventive care saves money by preventing acute illness and chronic conditions. HMOs are the most restrictive form of managed care because they allow patients and clients the least freedom in choosing a provider. Offsetting this loss of freedom is the reduced out-of-pocket expenses and wide range of benefits.

Within HMOs, variation exists in the amount of freedom members have in selecting providers. For example, there are **closed panels** and **open panels**. A panel is a collection or a group. A panel can be a group of patients or a group of providers. In this case, the panel is a group of providers. "Closed" means that members of the HMO must seek care inside this group of providers or its contracted providers. The members are "closed" within this group of providers. Members must request referrals to use specialists or other providers outside the HMO. An open panel, on the other hand, uses incentives, such as increased cost sharing, to influence members to select providers within the plan. The members are "open" to seeking care outside this group of providers. Of the four types of HMOs, the staff model and the group practice model are closed panels. The other two types are open panels.

Staff Model

The staff model HMO provides hospitalization and physicians' services through its own staff. It owns its facility. Its physicians are employees of the HMO and paid on salary or on a capitated basis.

The staff model is the most controlled of the HMOs. Primary care physicians strictly control referrals to specialists within the HMO. Members who seek healthcare services outside the HMO receive no compensation for their healthcare costs.

Group Practice Model

In the group practice model, the HMO contracts with a medical group. The health professionals in this medical group provide services on a fee-for-service or capitation basis. An advantage for the HMO and a disadvantage for the medical group is that the medical group bears the risk. An advantage for the medical group is a guaranteed customer base.

Network Model

A network model is similar to the group practice model described in the immediately preceding paragraph. The difference between the network model and the group model is that a network model contracts with two or more independent group practices rather than just one medical group. It has the same advantages and disadvantages as the group practice model, with the added advantage of greater choice for members.

Independent Practice Model

The independent (individual) practice association (IPA) (or organization, IPO) is a type of MCO in which participating physicians maintain their private practices. In the independent practice model, the HMO contracts with the IPA. The IPA, in turn, contracts with individual health providers. The HMO reimburses the IPA on a capitated basis. However, the IPA may reimburse the physicians on a capitated basis or on a fee-for-service basis. The participating physicians have patients and clients who are members of the HMO as well as patients and clients who are not members. Existing facilities of the independent health professionals are used rather than a freestanding facility. Local, county, or state medical societies may sponsor this type of HMO.

Preferred Provider Organization

A preferred provider organization (PPO) is an entity that contracts with employers and insurers to render healthcare services to a group of members. Its common characteristics are as follows:

- Virtual rather than physical entity
- Decentralized
- Flexibility of choice for members
- Negotiated fees (may include discounts)
- Financial incentives to induce members to choose preferred option
- No prepaid capitation (retains aspects of fee-for-service)
- Not subject to regulatory requirements of HMOs
- Limited financial risk for providers

The PPO also contracts with providers for healthcare services at fixed or discounted rates. The providers are a network of physicians, hospitals, and other healthcare providers. Members can choose to use the healthcare services of any physician, hospital, or other healthcare provider. However, the PPO influences members to use the healthcare services of in-network (in-plan) providers. Members' out-of-pocket expenses are lower if they use in-network providers; members' out-of-pocket expenses are higher if they use the services of out-of-network (out-of-plan) providers. A PPO may be a separate legal entity, or it may be a functional unit of another MCO, such as an HMO. A PPO may also be a functional unit of a larger indemnity insurer. The PPO may be sponsored by the network of physicians, hospitals, and other healthcare providers. PPOs offer greater freedom of choice for patients and clients than HMOs. Because there is greater uncertainty about the number of referrals, PPOs typically reimburse providers at a higher rate than HMOs.

Point-of-Service Plan

A **point-of-service (POS) healthcare insurance plan** is one in which members choose how to receive services at the time they need them. For example, members can choose "at the point of service" whether they want an HMO, a PPO, or a fee-for-service plan. They do not need to make this decision during an open enrollment period. These healthcare insurance plans are also known as open-ended HMOs. Patients' out-of-pocket costs are increased if they receive services outside a referral network (out of network or out of plan).

Similar to a point-of-service plan is the **provider-sponsored organization (PSO)**. The PSO differs from the point-of-service plan in that the physicians who practice in a regional or community hospital organize the plan. Various levels of benefits are offered, including aggressiveness of gatekeeping, cost sharing for out-of-network healthcare services, and prescription drug benefits.

Exclusive Provider Organization

An **exclusive provider organization (EPO)** is an MCO that is sponsored by self-insured (self-funded) employers or associations. The EPO is very much a hybrid. Along a continuum of freedom of choice, EPOs feature characteristics of both HMOs and PPOs. Similar to operations of HMOs, a small network of primary care physicians frequently acts as a gatekeeper.

Similar to the system of PPOs, many EPOs reimburse providers on a discounted fee schedule. A few EPOs, however, do reimburse providers through capitation. Members are influenced to seek healthcare services from in-network providers. Patients or clients who choose to receive care outside the network receive lower, and in some cases, no, recompense. Contracts are created between the EPO and providers. Because they offer greater choice, EPOs ensure cost efficiency by aggressively reviewing medical necessity and utilization.

Managed Care and Medicaid and Children's Health Insurance Program

Medicaid and the Children's Health Insurance Program (CHIP) are joint federal and state healthcare programs (see chapter 4). These two programs finance healthcare coverage for 78 million people, almost one-quarter of the US population (Medicaid and CHIP Payment and Access Commission [MACPAC] 2014, xix). Medicaid finances healthcare services for people with low incomes, including children, seniors, and persons with disabilities (MACPAC 2014, xix). The Medicaid program accounts for approximately 15 percent of total US healthcare spending (MACPAC 2014, xix). CHIP, financing healthcare services for uninsured children, is much smaller than Medicaid, with approximately eight million enrollees (MACPAC 2014, xix).

States administer Medicaid and CHIP. Most states enroll their Medicaid and CHIP beneficiaries in managed care. As of July 2014, only three exceptions existed: Alaska, Connecticut, and Wyoming (Smith et al. 2014, 2).

States have three main purposes in enrolling their Medicaid and CHIP beneficiaries in managed care (MACPAC 2011, 13):

- Reduce spending
- Increase predictability of spending
- Improve quality of care and its coordination

Overall, spending on managed care accounts for 21 percent of total Medicaid spending. Thus, fee-for-service arrangements remain important in Medicaid (MACPAC 2011, 4).

The design and operation of Medicaid and CHIP managed care vary among states and vary from the private sector (MACPAC 2011, 2, 4). Across states, low-income children and low-income nondisabled adults younger than 65 are most likely to be enrolled in an MCO (about 60 percent and 44 percent, respectively) (MACPAC 2011, 2–3). However, the enrollment of low-income people with disabilities varies greatly among the states, from less than 1 percent to more than 90 percent (MACPAC 2011, 3). Moreover, Medicaid managed care is diverse in terms of both patients' characteristics and states' characteristics. For example, utilization of services varies greatly between primary care for children and complex care for people with disabilities. These differences affect how states use managed care to finance and deliver quality, cost-effective care to their Medicaid populations (MACPAC 2011, 2). Medicaid and CHIP managed care varies from managed care in the private sector in that it serves different populations and has a different history than managed care in the private sector (MACPAC 2011, 4). Medicaid and CHIP managed care is one more example of the wide range of types of managed care in the continuum of care.

Medicare Advantage

Medicare Advantage (MA, also known as Medicare Part C) is a form of managed care for Medicare beneficiaries. Managed care options for Medicare beneficiaries have existed since the 1970s (Kaiser Family Foundation 2014, n.p.). Types of plans available include HMOs, POSs, PPOs, and PSOs.

Deductibles and copayments are lower in Medicare Advantage. Other benefits may include

- Preventive care
- Prescription drug plan
- Eyeglasses and hearing aids
- Day care, respite care, assisted care, and long-term care insurance
- Health transport
- Education and health promotion programs

Because the elderly often present complex medical conditions, Medicare Advantage plans may incorporate case management and disease management.

Medicare beneficiaries who are entitled to Part A and enrolled in Part B have the option to switch to a Medicare Advantage plan, if a plan exists in their area. However, per federal law, a beneficiary's enrollment in managed care must be voluntary; a beneficiary cannot be mandated to enroll in MA (MACPAC 2011, 35). About 30 percent of Medicare beneficiaries are enrolled in MA; the majority are enrolled in fee-for-service plans (Kaiser Family Foundation 2014, n.p.). In the past decade, the number of beneficiaries enrolled in MA plans has almost tripled (Kaiser Family Foundation 2014, n.p.).

Special Needs Plan

Special needs plans (SNPs), a form of MA plan, were established by the Medicare Prescription Drug, Improvement, and Modernization Act (MMA) of 2003 (Gold et al. 2011, 1). Subsequently, in 2008, the Medicare Improvements for Patients and Providers Act (MIPPA) placed constraints on enrollments by restricting the chronic conditions that qualified beneficiaries for the plans (Gold et al. 2011, 2). Just as in other MA plans, federal law mandates that a beneficiary's enrollment in a SNP be voluntary.

There are three types of SNPs for three different groups of Medicare beneficiaries. The first type is for people who qualify for both Medicaid and Medicare. These people are known as **dual eligibles** or **duals** (US Government Accountability Office 2014, 1-2). The plan for *duals* is known as a D-SNP (US Government Accountability Office 2014, 1-2). Because of their history, some D-SNPs, known as disproportionate percentage SNPs, include some non-duals (Gold et al. 2011, 4). The second type of SNP is an I-SNP, which is for *institutionalized* Medicare beneficiaries. The third type is the C-SNP, which is for Medicare beneficiaries with severe *chronic* or disabling conditions (such as end-stage renal disease or amyotrophic lateral sclerosis) (MACPAC 2011, 36). Enrollments in D-SNPs of dual eligibles significantly exceed enrollments in the other two types, I-SNPs and C-CNPs, so the D-SNPs, for the dual eligibles, drive this subsector (Gold et al. 2011, 4).

Dual eligibles are Medicare beneficiaries whose low income also qualifies them for Medicaid benefits. State Medicaid programs provide varying levels of financial assistance depending on the lowness of the Medicare beneficiaries' incomes and assets.

Medicare is the primary payer. As the primary payer, Medicare covers

- Acute inpatient care
- Outpatient and ambulatory care
- Physician services
- Dialysis
- Prescription drugs
- Postacute care (such as home health and rehabilitation; see chapter 8)

State Medicaid programs are secondary payers to Medicare (see chapter 3, coordination of benefits). They provide assistance as a wraparound (see chapter 3). Thus, Medicaid fills in the gaps in what Medicare does not pay. There are three "pathways" of assistance based on the Medicare beneficiaries' incomes and assets (Kaiser Family Foundation 2011, n.p.):

- The first pathway is for the group of poor Medicare beneficiaries (specified low-income beneficiaries, SLMBs) who have the highest incomes and assets. For duals in the first pathway, Medicaid covers only their Medicare premiums.

- The second pathway is for the group of beneficiaries (qualified Medicare beneficiaries, QMBs) who are slightly poorer than those in the first pathway. For duals in the second pathway, Medicaid covers their Medicare premiums, deductibles, and coinsurance.

- The third pathway is for the group of beneficiaries who are the poorest. For the poorest duals, Medicaid pays Medicare premiums, deductibles, and coinsurance and also pays full Medicaid benefits, including
  - Long-term services and support (housing modification, assistive technologies, personal assistance services and transportation (Kaiser Family Foundation 2009, n.p.)
  - Behavioral health
  - Medical transportation (ground ambulance, air ambulance—fixed wing, air ambulance—rotary wing, wheelchair vans and coaches, etc.) (MACPAC 2011, 35)

Thus, Medicare beneficiaries with the lowest incomes and assets receive the greatest levels of assistance from their state Medicaid programs.

There are approximately nine million dual eligibles (Young et al. 2013, 3). Dual eligibles often have multiple chronic conditions. They are among "the sickest and poorest individuals" covered by either Medicare or Medicaid (Musumeci 2014, 3). Dual eligibles are also more likely to need mental health services or to live in nursing homes than other Medicare beneficiaries (Young et al. 2013, 2). Consequently, they have a much higher per capita cost than other Medicare and Medicaid beneficiaries (Young et al. 2013, 1). For example, Medicaid spending for each dual was more than six times higher than for each nondisabled adult (Centers for Medicare and Medicaid Services 2011, n.p.). Similarly, dual eligibles who are enrolled in SNPs tend to have the greatest medical and support needs. "As a result, they account for a disproportionate share of Medicare spending" (Jacobson et al. 2012, 2). Finally, though, fee-for-service Medicare and Medicaid pay for most healthcare costs of dual eligibles (Jacobson et al. 2012, 7).

Check Your Understanding 5.1

1. List three types of care delivered by MCOs.

2. How does a member of a staff model HMO obtain coverage for a specialist, such as an oncologist?

3. In terms of the health of populations, what type of program, supported by MCOs, stresses the habits of healthy lifestyles, such as exercise and proper nutrition?

4. What types of physicians are generally considered primary care physicians?

5. List at least three sources of evidence-based clinical practice guidelines.

Integrated Delivery Systems

Integrated delivery system (IDS) is a generic term referring to the collaborative integration of healthcare providers. Financial agreements or contracts or both underpin the legal entity. Formally, an IDS is defined as "a network of organizations that directly provides or arranges to provide a coordinated continuum of services to a defined population and is able and willing to be held accountable for the cost, quality, and outcomes of care and, (with others), the health status of the population served" (Shortell and McCurdy 2010, 370; Shortell et al. 1993, 20). The goal of the IDS is the seamless delivery of care along the continuum of care. Other terms for IDS are health delivery network, horizontally integrated system, integrated services network (ISN), and vertically integrated system.

Many types of IDSs exist along a continuum based on the number of different organizations in the IDS and on their economic or legal relationships (Shortell and McCurdy 2010, 370). Types along the continuum include the following:

- Hospitals, physicians, and healthcare plans are owned by or have exclusive contracts with each other, such as Kaiser Permanente and the Veterans Administration.

- Common ownership of hospitals and exclusive staff-model relationships with physicians (no healthcare plan), such as Geisinger Clinic and the Mayo Clinic.

- Hybrids with both employed physicians and non-employed physicians and with or without healthcare plans, such as Advocate Health Care and Intermountain Healthcare.

The existence of the healthcare plan alters the regulations under which the entity operates. These altered regulations include the following:

- An IDS with a healthcare plan is governed by applicable state and federal regulations for healthcare plans, insurance, or HMOs, as relevant.

- An IDS without a healthcare plan is governed by the regulations for each type of organization in the entity. Hospital regulations govern hospitals; clinic regulations govern clinics.

Two sorts of integration are important: process integration and functional integration (Shortell and McCurdy 2010, 370–371).

- Process integration, also known as clinical integration, is the coordination of direct patient care activities.

- Functional integration is the integration, across all units in the IDS, of the functions that support the delivery of direct patient care, such as financial management, information systems, human resources, and other support services.

Too often, IDSs have overemphasized functional integration and underemphasized process integration, producing disappointing results (Shortell and McCurdy 2010, 371).

Integrated Provider Organization

An **integrated provider organization (IPO)** is an entity that includes one or more hospitals, a large physician group practice, other healthcare organizations, or various configurations of these businesses. An IPO is the corporate umbrella for the management of an IDS.

Group (Practice) without Walls

A **group (practice) without walls (GWW, GPWW)** or **clinic without walls (CWW)** is a group practice in which the physicians have maintained their separate clinics and offices in a geographic area. The individual practices share administrative systems to form the group practice. The GWW is similar to an independent practice association. The purpose of the GWW is to gain bargaining power in the negotiation of managed care contracts. Economies of scale also accrue from the centralization of administrative systems.

Physician–Hospital Organization

A **physician–hospital organization (PHO)** is a legal entity formed by a hospital and a group of physicians. The single corporate umbrella gives the PHO bargaining power when the provider organization negotiates contracts with MCOs. The PHO also fosters the delivery of seamless healthcare to its patients and clients.

Management Service Organization

A **management service organization** or medical service organization (MSO) is a specialized entity that provides management services and administrative and information systems to one or more physician group practices or small hospitals. An MSO may be owned by a hospital, a physician group, a PHO, an IDS, or investors. The MSOs' services and systems are infrastructure for the smaller healthcare organizations. Patient billing and claims management are examples of services that an MSO provides.

Medical Foundation

A **medical foundation** is a nonprofit service organization. Members include physicians and other healthcare providers. Medical foundations are typically geographically based, such as a local organization or county organization. Medical foundations have many purposes other than serving as an MCO. For example, medical foundations may offer continuing medical education for their members. Medical foundations have, however, also involved themselves in some aspects of managed care. Medical foundations have established PPOs, EPOs, and MSOs. As physician-led organizations, their common characteristics are freedom of choice and preservation of the physician–patient relationship.

Consolidation

A current trend in the healthcare sector is its increasing consolidation. This trend includes activities such as hospital mergers; healthcare system mergers; agglomerations of physicians' practices; and hospitals' acquisitions of physicians' practices, nursing homes, and other providers (Sage 2014, 1076; Vladeck 2014). The consolidation is both horizontal and vertical:

- Horizontal consolidation: Hospitals merge with other hospitals

- Vertical consolidation: Hospitals merge with other health types of healthcare providers, such as home health agencies, nursing homes, physician practices, rehabilitation centers, and others (Cutler and Morton 2013, 1965)

Healthcare organizational leaders' purposes of consolidation are to increase economies of scale, to gain negotiating leverage, and to increase the diversity of business lines. In addition, the leaders hope to improve quality and reduce costs through standardization of care, negotiating power with suppliers, and investments in technology to augment providers' ability to coordinate care (Evans 2014, 20).

Policymakers have mixed views of consolidation. On the positive side, consolidation is believed to increase coordination of patients' care and efficiency in the delivery of services. Thus, consolidation could improve quality of patients' care and decrease costs. On the negative side, consolidation may create systems so large that they can eliminate competitors and increase prices. Thus, the outcome of consolidation may harm consumers and taxpayers (Cutler and Morton 2013, 1964).

As an example of vertical consolidation, hospitals are acquiring physician practices. Using national data, researchers studied the effects of hospitals owning physician practices and contracting with physician practices (Baker et al. 2014, 756). Their results reflected policymakers' mixed views—the consolidation had both negative and positive results. On the negative side, they found that as the level of hospital–physician integration increased, such as hospitals owning physician practices, hospital prices increased. However, on the positive side, for the entire healthcare system, the frequency of hospital admissions slightly decreased.

The American Medical Association (AMA) conducted a study that found that managed care plans were consolidating (2012, n.p.). The AMA's study showed that most areas of the US have a single health insurer—an MCO. Reflecting policymakers' concerns about consolidation, a single health insurer created anticompetitive market conditions in these areas with negative consequences for consumers. In the AMA's study, anticompetitive market conditions resulted in increased premiums and watered-down benefits (American Medical Association 2012, n.p.).

No decline in the rate of consolidation has been detected. The conflicting results of consolidation require that health professionals continue to monitor this trend.

Check Your Understanding 5.2

1. For what are integrated delivery systems willing to be held accountable?

2. True or false? For integrated delivery systems, process integration is more important than functional integration.

3. Name two ways that practices having integrated structures lower their overhead costs.

4. In which type of integrated delivery system do the physicians maintain their separate clinics, but share their administrative systems?

5. With which type of integrated delivery system would a small group practice contract for administrative and information systems?

Chapter 5 Review Quiz

1. Describe at least three ways in which MCOs work toward their goals of quality patient care.

2. From where do evidence-based clinical guidelines originate?

3. List at least two reasons that MCOs survey their members for feedback.

4. Name the three steps in medical necessity and utilization review.

5. Describe three types of cost controls used by MCOs.

6. Which type of HMO offers patients the least selection in referrals to specialists?

7. List at least five types of services or populations that are common examples of carve-outs.

8. True or false? Disease management is closely associated with coordination of care tools of MCOs because efforts of multiple providers must be synchronized in disease management.

9. True or false? By definition, integrated delivery systems must directly provide health services to their members.

10. True or false? Integrated delivery systems, as a result of strict federal regulation, have evolved into a single common type.

References

Alexander, J.M. 1999. Managed care contracting for specialists. *Healthcare Financial Management* 52(12 Suppl):S6–S10.

American Medical Association. 2012 (November 28). New AMA study finds anticompetitive market conditions are common across managed care plans. http://www.ama-assn.org/ama/pub/news/news/2012-11-28-study-finds-anticompetitive-market-conditions-common.page.

Baker, L.C., M.K. Bundorf, and D.P. Kessler. 2014. Vertical integration: Hospital ownership of physician practices is associated with higher prices and spending. *Health Affairs* 33(5):756–763.

Boland, M.R., A. Tsiachristas, A.L. Kruis, N.H. Chavannes, and M.P. Rutten-van Molken. 2013. The health economic impact of disease management programs for COPD: A systematic literature review and meta-analysis. BMC Pulmonary Medicine 13:40 (17 pages).

Carlson, B. 2000. Many state Medicaid agencies use financial incentives to boost quality. *Managed Care* 9(4):13–14.

Centers for Medicare and Medicaid Services. 2011 (August). Fact sheet: People enrolled in Medicare and Medicaid. https://www.cms.gov/Medicare-Medicaid-Coordination/Medicare-and-Medicaid-Coordination/Medicare-Medicaid-Coordination-Office/Downloads/MMCO_Factsheet.pdf.

Cotter, A.P., N. Durant, A.A. Agne, and A.L. Cherrington. 2014. Internet interventions to support lifestyle modification for diabetes management: A systematic review of the evidence. *Journal of Diabetes and Its Complications* 28(2):243–251.

Cutler, D.M., and F.S. Morton. 2013. Hospitals, market share, consolidation. *Journal of the American Medical Association* 310(18):1964–1970.

DeLeon, P.H., G.R. VandenBos, and E.Q. Bulatao. 1991. Managed mental health care: A history of the federal policy initiative. *Professional Psychology: Research and Practice* 22(1):15–25.

Evans, M. 2014. The big bulk up. Hospital systems grow through dealmaking as regulators fret about prices. *Modern Healthcare* 44(25):20–22, 24–25.

Felt-Lisk, S. 1996. How HMOs structure primary care delivery. *Managed Care Quarterly* 4(4):96–105.

Foster, R. S. 2000. Trends in Medicare expenditures and financial status, 1966–2000. *Health Care Financing Review* 22(1):35–49.

Gallagher, T., A. Alpers, and B. Lo. 1998. Health Care Financing Administration's new regulations for financial incentives in Medicaid and Medicare managed care: One step forward? *American Journal of Medicine* 105(5):409–415.

Gold, M., G. Jacobson, A. Damico, and T. Neuman. 2011. Special needs plans: Availability and enrollment. http://www.kff.org/medicare/upload/8229.pdf.

Grumbach, K., et al. 1998. Primary care physicians' experience of financial incentives in managed-care systems. *New England Journal of Medicine* 339(21):1516–1521.

Hansen, J.C. 1996. Pharmacy benefit managers: Early results on ventures with drug manufacturers. Testimony before the Committee on Insurance, California State Senate. Gaithersburg, MD: U.S. General Accounting Office. http://archive.gao.gov/papr2pdf/156151.pdf.

Jacobson, G., T. Neuman, and A. Damico. 2012 (April). Medicare's Role for Dual Eligible Beneficiaries. Kaiser Family Foundation Issue Brief 8138-02. http://kaiserfamilyfoundation.files.wordpress.com/2013/01/8138-02.pdf.

Kaiser Family Foundation. 2014 (May 1). Medicare Advantage Fact Sheet. http://kff.org/medicare/fact-sheet/medicare-advantage-fact-sheet/.

Kaiser Family Foundation. 2009. The Community Living Assistance Services and Supports (CLASS) Act. http://www.kff.org/healthreform/upload/7996.pdf.

Kaiser Family Foundation. 2011. Dual eligibles: Medicaid's role for low-income Medicare beneficiaries. http://www.kff.org/medicaid/upload/4091-08.pdf.

Kaiser Permanente. 2014. http://www.individual-health-plans.com/kaiserpermanente.htm.

Levy, P., R. Nocerini, and K. Grazier. 2007. Paying for disease management. *Disease Management* 10(4):235–244.

MCG Health, LLC. 2014. Indicia® for Utilization Review. http://www.mcg.com/provider/product/indicia-utilization-review.

Medicaid and CHIP Payment and Access Commission (MACPAC). 2011. Report to the Congress: The evolution of managed care in Medicaid. http://www.macpac.gov/reports.

Medicaid and CHIP Payment and Access Commission (MACPAC). 2014 (March). Report to the Congress on Medicaid and CHIP. http://www.macpac.gov/reports.

Musumeci, M. 2014. Financial and Administrative Alignment Demonstrations for Dual Eligible Beneficiaries Compared: States with Memoranda of Understanding Approved by CMS. Kaiser Family Foundation Issue Brief 8426-06. http://kaiserfamilyfoundation.files.wordpress.com/2014/07/8426-06-financial-alignment-demonstrations-for-dual-eligible-beneficiaries-compared.pdf.

North Carolina State Health Plan. 2014. Consumer-Directed Health Plan (CDHP) Benefits Booklet. http://www.shpnc.org/library/pdf/my-medical-benefits/benefits-booklets/cdhp-2014.pdf.

Oak Group. 2014. MCAP Clinical Review Criteria http://www.oakgroup.com/#!compnay-2/cmze.

Sage, W.M. 2014. Getting the product right: How competition policy can improve health care markets. *Health Affairs* 33(6):1076–1082.

Shortell, S.M., D.A. Anderson, R.R. Gillies, J.B. Mitchell, and K.L. Morgan. 1993. The holographic organization. *Healthcare Forum Journal* 36(2):20–26.

Shortell, S.M., and R.K. McCurdy. 2010. Integrated health systems. *Studies in Health Technology and Informatics* 153:369–382.

Siracuse, M.V., B.E. Clark, and R.I. Garis. 2008. Undocumented source of pharmacy benefit manager revenue. *American Journal of Health-System Pharmacy* 65(6):552–557.

Slezak, J., and N. Stine. 2003. The role of the PBM in the total health management strategies for individuals with chronic conditions. *Benefits Quarterly* 19(1):38–44.

Smith, V.K., K. Gifford, E. Ellis, R. Rudowitz, and L. Snyder 2014 (October 14). Medicaid in an Era of Health and Delivery System Reform: Results from a 50-State Medicaid Budget Survey for State Fiscal Years 2014 and 2015. http://kff.org/report-section/medicaid-in-an-era-of-health-delivery-system-reform-methodology/.

Starr, P. 1982. *The Social Transformation of American Medicine.* New York: Basic Books.

Truven Health Analytics. 2014. Length of stay benchmarks. http://truvenhealth.com/solutions/length-of-stay-benchmarks.

Vladeck, B.C. 2014. Paradigm lost: Provider concentration and the failure of market theory. *Health Affairs* 33(6):1083–1087.

U.S. Government Accountability Office. 2014 (August). Disabled Dual-Eligible Beneficiaries: Integration of Medicare and Medicaid Benefits May Not Lead to Expected Medicare Savings. Report GAO-14-523. http://www.gao.gov/assets/670/665491.pdf.

Young, K., R. Garfield, M. Musumeci, L. Clemans-Cope, and E. Lawton. 2013 (August). Medicaid's Role for Dual Eligible Beneficiaries. Kaiser Family Foundation Issue Brief 7846-04. http://kaiserfamilyfoundation.files.wordpress.com/2013/08/7846-04-medicaids-role-for-dual-eligible-beneficiaries.pdf.

Chapter 6
Medicare-Medicaid Prospective Payment Systems for Inpatients

Objectives

- To differentiate major types of Medicare and Medicaid prospective payment systems for inpatients

- To define basic language associated with reimbursement under Medicare and Medicaid prospective payment systems

- To explain common models and policies of payment for inpatient Medicare and Medicaid prospective payment systems

- To describe the elements of the inpatient prospective payment system

- To explain the elements of the inpatient psychiatric prospective payment system

Key Terms

Add-on
Arithmetic mean length of stay
Base payment rate
Case mix
Case-mix index
Code range
Complication/comorbidity (CC)
Cost-of-living adjustment (COLA)
Diagnosis-related group (DRG)
Disproportionate share hospital (DSH)
Encounter
Federal Register
Final rule
Fiscal intermediary (FI)
Fiscal year (FY)
Geometric mean length of stay (GMLOS)
Grouper
Indirect medical education (IME) adjustment
Inpatient psychiatric facility (IPF)

Labor-related share
Major complication/comorbidity (MCC)
Major diagnostic category (MDC)
Medicare-severity diagnosis-related group (MS-DRG)
New technology
Nonlabor share
Notice of proposed rulemaking
Outlier
Post-acute-care transfer (PACT)
Pricer
Proposed rule
Prospective payment system (PPS)
Rate year (RY)
Relative weight (RW)
Teaching hospital
Title
Transfer
Trim point

Introduction to Inpatient Prospective Payment Systems

Federal legislators are demanding that healthcare costs be controlled. These demands have led to federal healthcare reimbursement reform. Reform in the federal method of reimbursing providers for healthcare services resulted from three trends:

- Rising healthcare payments using the funds in the Medicare Trust at a rate faster than US workers were contributing dollars

- Fraud and abuse in the system, wasting funding

- Payment rules not uniformly applied across the nation

Federal analysts noted that the inpatient prospective payment system (IPPS), implemented in 1983, had successfully curbed payments for inpatient charges. In the first three years of the **prospective payment system (PPS)**, the rate of growth of Medicare Part A payments decreased from 7.3 percent in the five years before its implementation to 4 percent (Lave 1989, 152). Reporting on longer periods, the staff of the Office of the Inspector General wrote that Medicare hospital payments increased by 88 percent from 1970 to 1980 and that payment rates decreased by 52 percent from 1985 to 1990 and by 37 percent from 1990 to 1995 (Gottlober et al. 2001, 3).

This success of the IPPS prompted Congress to authorize the Department of Health and Human Services (HHS) to develop and implement PPSs across the continuum of care. Today, the original acute-care PPS has been augmented by PPSs for all types of patients, residents, and clients. This chapter describes the acute-care PPS and also the inpatient psychiatric facility (IPF) PPS. Chapter 7 describes reimbursement systems for ambulatory **encounters** and physicians. Chapter 8 finishes the descriptions of PPSs across the continuum of care with PPSs for postacute care.

The federal government issues information about its inpatient and ambulatory payment systems in the ***Federal Register***. Published every federal working day, the *Federal Register* is the official journal of the US government. It contains rules (regulations) and legal notices of federal administrative agencies, of departments of the executive branch, and of the president. The contents are organized alphabetically by agency. Rules and notices about federal payment systems are listed under Centers for Medicare and Medicaid Services (CMS).

Proposed changes to federal payment systems must be publicized in advance. Through a process known as **notice of proposed rulemaking**, federal agencies promulgate **proposed rules** in the *Federal Register*. In proposed rules, agencies publicize their intended rules and allow the public and interested organizations to comment and to provide relevant information. After the comment period has concluded, the agency reviews the comments and then publishes the final rule, also in the *Federal Register*, including its analysis of the comments and information. The final rule has the effect of law.

Each year, for the federal payment systems, CMS publishes proposed rules and final rules in the *Federal Register*. These proposed rules and final rules have vital details about the payment systems for the upcoming **rate year (RY)**. An RY is the 12-month period during which the payment rate is effective. Thus, reimbursement analysts and other healthcare personnel should monitor the *Federal Register* for changes to the federal payment systems.

Acute-Care Prospective Payment System

The IPPS is the Medicare reimbursement system for inpatient services provided in an acute-care setting. The system provides payment to facilities but does not include payment for professional services.

Conversion from Cost-Based Payment to Prospective Payment

From the implementation of the Medicare Program in 1966 until 1983, Medicare hospital inpatient claims were reimbursed based on the cost of services, reasonable cost, and/or per diem costs (LaTour et al. 2013, 387). This meant that a hospital was reimbursed for approximately 80 percent of its costs for treating Medicare beneficiaries. From the hospital's perspective, there was no incentive to reduce costs—if its costs associated with patient care increased, so did its payments. By the late 1970s, healthcare costs, hand in hand with Medicare reimbursement payments, were sharply on the rise. The steep increase in healthcare costs had a dramatic impact on the Medicare Program, as illustrated by the following (Averill et al. 2001, 105):

- Medicare payments to hospitals grew, on average, by 19 percent annually (three times the average overall rate of inflation).

- The Medicare hospital deductible expanded, creating a burden for Medicare beneficiaries.

- The solvency of the Medicare Trust Fund was endangered because of the increase of hospital costs.

- The increase in Medicare expenditures for hospital inpatient care jeopardized the ability of Medicare to fund other needed health programs.

- Under the variable cost-based payment system, Medicare paid up to sixfold differences across hospitals for comparable services.

- The reporting requirements of the cost-based system were some of the most burdensome in the federal government.

In response, Medicare administrators began to search for a different payment mechanism in the early 1970s to help control the rising healthcare costs.

Concept of Prospective Payment

The system that they began to investigate was based on the concept of prospective payment. In 1972, Congress authorized CMS (then the Health Care Financing Administration [HCFA]) to begin prospective payment demonstration projects (Averill et al. 2001, 83). The demonstration projects had to follow four guiding principles of prospective payment in their study (Averill et al. 2001, 106):

- Payment rates are to be established in advance and fixed for the fiscal period to which they apply.

- Payment rates are not automatically determined by the hospital's past or current actual cost.

- Prospective payment rates are considered to be payment in full.

- The hospital retains the profit or suffers a loss resulting from the difference between the payment rate and the hospital's cost, creating an incentive for cost control.

Prospective Payment Legislation

The Tax Equity and Fiscal Responsibility Act (TEFRA) of 1982 mandated extensive changes to the Medicare program. Many of the changes focused on controlling the rising costs of healthcare. TEFRA called for the implementation of a PPS for hospital inpatients (Johns 2007, 276). In 1983, P.L. 98–21 amended Sections 1886(d) and 1886(g) of the Social Security Act (the Act) and mandated Diagnosis Related Groups (DRGs) as the PPS for the operating and capital-related costs of acute-care hospital inpatient stays under Medicare Part A (HHS 2004a, 48920).

Diagnosis-Related Group Classification System

The DRG system takes into consideration the role that a hospital case mix plays in influencing costs (Averill et al. 2001, 83). Each DRG is assigned a **relative weight (RW)** that is intended to represent the resource intensity of the clinical group. It is also used to determine the payment level for the group. **Case-mix index** is a weighted average of the sum of the RWs of all patients treated during a specified time period. Notably, case mix is defined in many different ways, based on one's healthcare perspective. From a clinician's or physician's perspective, case-mix complexity or description of the patient population can refer to the severity of illness, risk for mortality, prognosis, treatment difficulty, or need for intervention. This viewpoint uses sickness as a proxy for resource consumption.

However, from the DRG perspective, the case-mix complexity is a direct measure of the resource consumption and, therefore, the cost of providing care. A high case mix in the DRG system means that patients are consuming more resources, so the cost of care is higher. However, it is a weak measure of the severity of illness, risk for mortality, prognosis, treatment difficulty, or need for intervention for the patient population (Averill et al. 2001, 84). Therefore, this case-mix complexity viewpoint allows DRGs to be an adequate system for hospital reimbursement because it measures the resources consumed for clinically similar patients.

Classification System Development

The hospital inpatient business is vast, with great variation in the types of diseases treated and procedures performed. Consequently, the task of creating a classification system to encompass the industry was, understandably, daunting. After statistical analysis and physician consultation, four guidelines were established as guiding principles for the DRG system's formation (Averill et al. 2001, 85):

- The patient characteristics used in the definition of the DRGs should be limited to information routinely collected on the hospital billing form.

- There should be a manageable number of DRGs, which encompass all patients seen on an inpatient basis.

- Each DRG should contain patients with a similar pattern of resource intensity.

- Each DRG should contain patients who are similar from a clinical perspective (that is, each class should be clinically coherent).

Medicare has been successful at implementing the DRG system because it strictly adheres to these guiding principles. All hospitals are able to compute a DRG because they routinely collect all data needed to calculate the DRG assignment. Version 32.0 (effective dates October 1, 2014 to September 30, 2015) of the DRG system includes 753 **Medicare-severity diagnosis-related groups (MS-DRGs)**, a reasonable number of groupings for hospitals to evaluate and manage. Linking like patients with like-resource consumption allows hospitals to perform cost management by DRG or DRG groupings. In addition, because DRGs were developed to monitor quality of care and resource use, hospitals can benchmark by DRG and continually improve on their quality and resource indicators.

Only one DRG can be assigned and reimbursed for a single admission. All hospital services performed during an admission are packaged into this single DRG payment. The payment provided for the DRG is intended to cover the costs of all hospital services performed during the patient stay, so individual tests, services, pharmaceuticals, and supply items are not paid separately from the DRG payment. One component of a PPS is that the predetermined payment for the clinical group is considered payment in full. Therefore, hospitals accept profit or loss based on their cost of providing services. The fully packaged concept drives facilities to practice cost management for inpatient services. Physician services are separately reimbursed

under resource-based relative value scales and are not included in the DRG reimbursement to the hospital.

Severity Refinement to Diagnosis-Related Groups

In **fiscal year (FY)** 2008 (October 1, 2007, through September 30, 2008), CMS adopted MS-DRGs for use in the IPPS. The Medicare Payment Advisory Commission (MedPAC) and the hospital community at large greatly influenced CMS to migrate to a severity-adjusted DRG system. Specifically, the 2005 MedPAC "Report to Congress on Physician Owned Specialty Hospitals" provided several recommendations regarding how CMS could add a severity component to IPPS. One of the biggest criticisms of the DRG system over the years was the lack of severity: Many believed the refinement was necessary for CMS to be able to adequately reimburse a facility for the more complex and resource-intensive cases.

Structure of the Diagnosis-Related Group System

The DRG system is hierarchal in design (figure 6.1). The highest level in the hierarchy is **major diagnostic categories (MDCs)**, which represent the body systems treated by medicine. There are 25 MDCs as displayed in table 6.1.

The next level in the hierarchy divides each MDC group into surgical and medical sections. The third and final level in the hierarchy divides the surgical or medical sections of the 25 MDC groups into DRGs. Table 6.2 presents the 10 MS-DRGs reported to Medicare most frequently in fiscal year (FY) 2013.

Each version of the DRG system defines the same components: **title, geometric mean length of stay (GMLOS), arithmetic mean length of stay**, RW, and the ICD **code range** that drives the DRG assignment (figure 6.2). The code range may consist of the principal diagnosis, operating room (OR) procedure, or a diagnosis and procedure combination.

Figure 6.1. Hierarchical DRG system

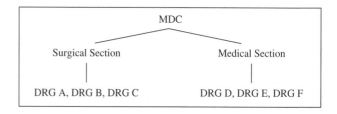

Table 6.1.   Major diagnostic categories

MDC	Title
	DRGs associated with all MDCs and the pre-MDC
1	Diseases and disorders of the nervous system
2	Diseases and disorders of the eye
3	Diseases and disorders of the ear, nose, mouth, and throat
4	Diseases and disorders of the respiratory system
5	Diseases and disorders of the circulatory system
6	Diseases and disorders of the digestive system
7	Diseases and disorders of the hepatobiliary system and pancreas
8	Diseases and disorders of the musculoskeletal system and connective tissue
9	Diseases and disorders of the skin, subcutaneous tissue, and breast
10	Endocrine, nutritional, and metabolic diseases and disorders
11	Diseases and disorders of the kidney and urinary tract
12	Diseases and disorders of the male reproductive system
13	Diseases and disorders of the female reproductive system
14	Pregnancy, childbirth, and the puerperium
15	Newborns and other neonates with conditions originating in the perinatal period
16	Diseases and disorders of the blood and blood-forming organs and immunological disorders
17	Myeloproliferative diseases and disorders and poorly differentiated neoplasms
18	Infectious and parasitic diseases
19	Mental diseases and disorders
20	Alcohol/drug use and alcohol/drug-induced organic mental disorders
21	Injury, poisoning, and toxic effects of drugs
22	Burns
23	Factors influencing health status and other contacts with health services
24	Multiple significant trauma
25	Human immunodeficiency virus infections

Table 6.2.   Medicare top 10 MS-DRGs based on FY 2013 data

MS-DRG	MS-DRG Title	Volume
470	Major Joint Replacement Or Reattachment Of Lower Extremity without MCC	606,028
871	Septicemia Or Severe Sepsis without MV 96+ Hours with MCC	520,702
885	Psychoses	475,026
945	Rehabilitation with CC/MCC	336,651
392	Esophagitis, Gastroenteritis & misc. Digestive Disorders without MCC	302,044
292	Heart Failure & Shock with CC	280,501
194	Simple Pneumonia & Pleurisy with CC	258,252
291	Heart Failure & Shock with MCC	258,161
690	Kidney & Urinary Tract Infections without MCC	249,253
683	Renal Failure with CC	209,455

Data taken from 2013 MedPAR data file. Provided by Health Policy Analytics, LLC.

Assigning Medicare-Severity Diagnosis-Related Groups

Computer programs that assign patients to case-mix groups are generically called **groupers**. Groupers have internal logic, or an algorithm, that determines the patients' groups. Although groupers are available and widely used for MS-DRG assignment, a good understanding of the assignment process is necessary to help coding and reimbursement professionals ensure proper payment for services communicated. A four-step process is used to assign MS-DRGs for hospital inpatient encounters (figure 6.3).

Step 1: Pre-MDC Assignment

The pre-MDC assignment step was added during the Version 8 revision of DRGs. A set of procedures was identified crossing all MDCs. The principal diagnosis is not considered for MS-DRG assignment; rather, the principal ICD procedure is used to assign the MS-DRG. These procedures, transplants, and tracheostomies can be performed for diagnoses from multiple MDCs. Once the encounter has been determined to qualify for pre-MDC assignment, the MS-DRG assignment is made and the process is complete. No other steps are

Figure 6.2. MS-DRG components

MS-DRG 293 FY 2015			
Title: Heart Failure and Shock without Complication/Comorbidity or Major Complication/Comorbidity			
Geometric Mean Length of Stay (GMLOS):		2.6	
Arithmetic Mean Length of Stay (AMLOS):		3.1	
Relative Weight:		0.6762	
Principal Diagnosis			
ICD-9-CM Codes		**ICD-10-CM Codes**	
398.91	404.13	I09.81	I50.31
402.01	404.91	I11.0	I50.32
402.11	404.93	I13.0	I50.33
402.91	*428	I13.2	I50.40
404.01	785.50	I50.1	I50.41
404.03	785.51	I50.20	I50.42
404.11		I50.21	I50.43
		I50.22	I50.9
		I50.23	R57.0
		I50.30	R57.9

*Entire code range is included.

taken to assign the payment group. The 15 MS-DRGs that qualify for pre-MDC assignment are displayed in table 6.3. If the MS-DRG assignment is made during step 1, all other steps are ignored.

Step 1 Example:

A pancreas transplant can be performed for a variety of clinical conditions, including diabetes with renal, ophthalmic, neurological, or peripheral circulatory manifestations (MDC 10); hypertensive renal disease (MDC 05); chronic pancreatitis (MDC 06); chronic renal failure (MDC 11); and complications of transplanted organs (MDC 21). The diagnoses that warrant a pancreas transplant can be found in multiple MDCs. There is only one MS-DRG for all pancreas transplants regardless of the principal diagnosis to maintain a manageable number of MS-DRGs and to adhere to the concept of like-resource consumption groupings. Thus, the patient who received a pancreas transplant would be assigned to MS-DRG 010 regardless of the principal diagnosis.

Step 2: Major Diagnostic Category Determination

The principal diagnosis assigned to an encounter is the reason "established after study to be chiefly responsible for occasioning the admission of the patient to the hospital for care" (Schraffenberger 2012, 64). The principal diagnosis is used to place the encounter into one of the 25 MDCs (see table 6.1). After the MDC is established for the encounter, step 2 is complete, and the case moves on to step 3.

Step 2 Example:

Patient A presents and is treated for pneumonia caused by Streptococcus, Group A. The ICD code for Group A Streptococcus pneumonia is assigned to MDC 04, Diseases and Disorders of the Respiratory System.

Step 3: Medical/Surgical Determination

The next step is to determine whether an OR procedure was performed. If a qualifying OR procedure was performed, the case is assigned a surgical status. The MS-DRG Definitions Manual identifies which procedures are valid/nonvalid OR procedures. Additionally, many ICD codebooks provide a flag or indicator for procedure codes that qualify as valid/nonvalid OR procedures. Minor procedures and testing are not qualifying procedures. If a qualifying OR procedure was not performed, the case is assigned a medical status.

Step 3 Example:

Patient A presents and is treated for an acute myocardial infarction of the anterolateral wall, initial episode (heart attack). The ICD code for this diagnosis is assigned to MDC 05, Diseases and Disorders of the Circulatory System (step 2). During the hospital stay, a percutaneous transluminal coronary angioplasty (PTCA) is performed on the right coronary artery. The PTCA code is a valid OR procedure. Thus, this case is a surgical case in MDC 05.

Like Patient A, Patient B is also evaluated for an acute myocardial infarction of the anterolateral wall, initial episode (heart attack). The ICD code for this diagnosis is assigned to MDC 05, Diseases and Disorders of the Circulatory System (step 2). However, no procedures were performed for this patient during the hospital stay. This case is a medical case in MDC 05.

Once the medical/surgical status is assigned, step 3 is complete, and the case proceeds to step 4.

Figure 6.3.   Excerpt of MS-DRG decision tree for surgical MDC 06

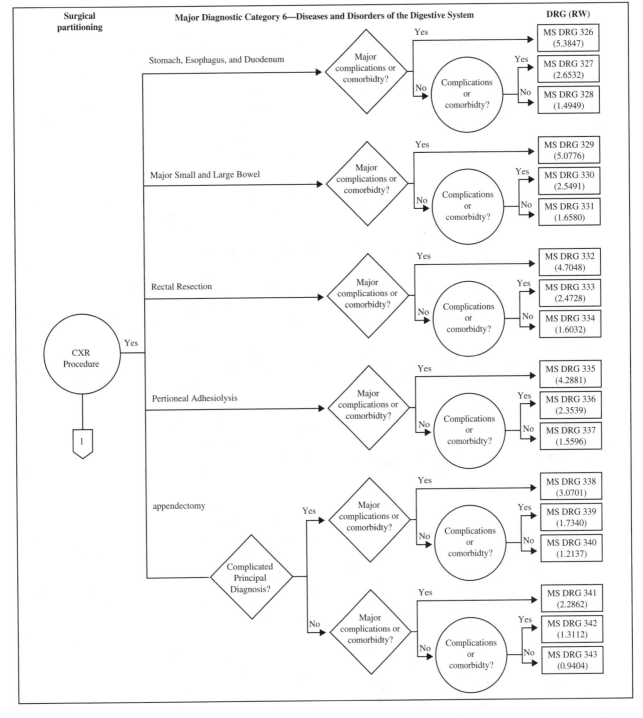

Step 4: Refinement

Step 4 uses various refinement questions to isolate the correct MS-DRG assignment. This refinement process allows for the MS-DRG system to group together like patients from the clinical perspective with like-resource consumption. The refinement questions group patients by like-resource consumption. The refinement questions are as follow:

- Is a major complication or comorbidity (MCC) present?

- Is a complication or comorbidity (CC) present?

- Is the principal diagnosis complicated?
- Is a major complication or complex diagnosis present?
- What is the patient's sex?
- What is the patient's discharge disposition (alive, expired, or against medical advice)?
- For neonates, what is the birth weight of the baby?

Step 4 examples illustrate how the refinement questions are utilized in the MS-DRG assignment process.

Step 4 Surgical Example:

Patient A is 67 years old and is admitted for a duodenum fistula closure procedure. The patient also has osteomyelitis of vertebra of the cervical region. The duodenum fistula code (principal diagnosis) is assigned to MDC 06, Diseases and Disorders of the Digestive System (step 2). The fistula closure procedure code is a valid OR procedure (step 3). Therefore, the case is a surgical MDC 06 case. There are two applicable pathway questions for this encounter. First, is there an MCC present? No, the osteomyelitis of vertebra is not on the MCC list (ICD-10-CM MS-DRGs v32). Second, is there a CC present? Yes, osteomyelitis of vertebra is a comorbidity. Now that all refinement questions have been answered, the MS-DRG assignment can be made. The MS-DRG assignment for this case is MS-DRG 327, Stomach, Esophageal, and Duodenal Procedures with CC.

Step 4 Medical Example:

Patient B is 68 years old and is admitted for cellulitis of the right ankle. Nonexcisional debridement is performed on the right ankle. The patient also has chronic obstructive pulmonary disease (COPD). The cellulitis (principal diagnosis) code is assigned to MDC 09, Diseases and Disorders of the Skin, Subcutaneous Tissue, and Breast (step 2). Nonexcisional debridement is not a valid OR procedure (step 3), so the case is a medical MDC 09 case.

There is one applicable pathway question for this encounter. Is an MCC present? No, COPD is not an MCC. Now that all refinement questions have been answered, the MS-DRG assignment can be made. The MS-DRG assignment for this case is MS-DRG 603, Cellulitis without MCC.

Invalid Coding and Data Abstraction

Accurate diagnosis/procedure coding and healthcare information abstracting are vital to MS-DRG

Table 6.3. Pre-MDC assignment for MS-DRGs

MS-DRG	Title
001	Heart transplant or implant of heart assist system with MCC
002	Heart transplant or implant of heart assist system without MCC
003	ECMO or tracheostomy with mechanical ventilation 96+ hours or principal diagnosis except face, mouth, and neck diagnoses with major OR procedure
004	Tracheostomy with mechanical ventilation 96+ hours or principal diagnosis except face, mouth, and neck diagnoses without major OR procedure
005	Liver transplant with MCC or intestinal transplant
006	Liver transplant without MCC
007	Lung transplant
008	Simultaneous pancreas/kidney transplant
010	Pancreas transplant
011	Tracheostomy for face, mouth, & neck diagnoses with MCC
012	Tracheostomy for face, mouth, & neck diagnoses with CC
013	Tracheostomy for face, mouth, & neck diagnoses without CC/MCC
014	Allogenic bone marrow transplant
016	Autologous bone marrow transplant with CC/MCC
017	Autologous bone marrow transplant without CC/MCC

assignment. When invalid codes or data are submitted on the patient claim form, one of two MS-DRGs is assigned. MS-DRG 998, Principal Diagnosis Invalid as Discharge Diagnosis, is assigned when the principal diagnosis reported is not specific enough for MS-DRG assignment. MS-DRG 999, Ungroupable, is assigned when an invalid diagnosis code, age, sex, or discharge status code is reported. Payment for each of these MS-DRGs is $0. The claim is returned to the provider and should be corrected, then resubmitted to Medicare.

Provisions of the Medicare-Severity Diagnosis-Related Group System

The MS-DRG system uses provisions to provide additional payments for specialized programs and unusual admissions that historically have added significant cost to patient care. Without the additional payments associated with these provisions, it may not be feasible for acute-care facilities to provide all services to Medicare beneficiaries.

Disproportionate Share Hospital

Effective for discharges occurring on or after May 1, 1986, **disproportionate share hospital (DSH)** status was enacted for facilities with a high percentage of low-income patients (CMS 2005, n.p.). Additional payment is provided for these hospitals because they experience a financial hardship by providing treatment for patients who are unable to pay for the services rendered. There are two methods of qualification for this provision. First, a hospital may qualify by exceeding 15 percent on the statutory formula. The statutory formula takes into consideration Medicare inpatient days for patients eligible for Medicare Part A, Medicare Advantage, and Supplemental Security Income (SSI), and total inpatient days for patients eligible for Medicaid but not Medicare Part A.

The second method for DSH qualification applies to large urban hospitals. If large urban hospitals are able to demonstrate that more than 30 percent of their total net inpatient care revenues come from state and local governments for indigent care (excluding Medicare and Medicaid), then they can be granted DSH status (CMS 2005). The DSH payment adjustment is hospital-specific and is based on a formula that incorporates the hospital bed size and hospital type (rural, sole-community, urban). The SSI/Medicare Part A Disproportionate Share Percentage File is updated once a year for the IPPS **final rule** and can be found on the Medicare website (CMS 2005, n.p.).

According to the Henry J. Kaiser Family Foundation, DSH payments equaled $11.6 billion in 2014 (Kaiser 2015, n.p.). With the implementation of the Affordable Care Act (ACA) many more Americans will have health insurance, so need for the DSH adjustment in IPPS is slowly diminishing. In accordance with the provisions of the ACA, DSH payments are reduced each year through 2022, when they are expected to no longer be provided.

Indirect Medical Education

Approved **teaching hospitals** are provided an **indirect medical education (IME) adjustment**. The hospitals must have residents in an approved graduate medical education program. Teaching hospitals experience an increased patient care cost in comparison with nonteaching hospitals. Thus, Medicare provides IME hospitals with additional reimbursement to help offset the costs of providing education to new physicians. The IME payment adjustment is hospital-specific. The adjustment factor is based on the hospital's ratio of residents to beds and a multiplier established by Congress. This formula is traditionally described as "a certain percentage increase in payment for every 10 percent increase in the resident-to-bed ratio" (CMS 2012, n.p.).

Several acts of Congress have decreased the percentage increase between 1997 and 2000. The Benefits Improvement and Protection Act of 2000 established the transition to a 5.5 percent increase that took effect in 2003. The percent increase of 5.5 percent in IME payment for every 10 percent increase in the resident-to-bed ratio was effective for FY 2003 and subsequent years.

High-Cost Outlier Cases

Because the Medicare payment for inpatient services is prospective, hospitals will experience profit or loss for individual cases whose reimbursements exceed or fall short of the cost incurred for a particular case. The payment provided to facilities is an average amount, meaning that some cases will result in a profit and some a loss. For the most part, costs are covered if reasonable cost management is performed. However, there are extreme cases, **outliers**, for which the costs are very high when compared with the average costs for cases in the same MS-DRG. The outlier payment provision provides some financial relief for those cases.

For an encounter to qualify for an outlier payment, the hospital's Medicare-approved charges reported on the claim are converted to costs using the cost-to-charge ratio (CCR) and are compared with the fixed-loss cost threshold. The fixed-loss cost threshold is the sum of the MS-DRG case rate, the IME **add-on**, the disproportionate share add-on, and the outlier threshold established for that FY. If the fixed-loss cost threshold is exceeded, additional payment is made. The payment is 80 percent of the difference between the hospital's entire cost for the stay and the fixed-loss cost threshold amount (CMS 2005, n.p.). Outlier payments for the Burn MS-DRGs (MS-DRGs 927–929 and 933–935) are 90 percent rather than 80 percent. The 2015 high cost outlier threshold is $24,758 (HHS 2014a).

New Medical Services and New Technologies

New medical services, new technologies, and innovative methods for treating patients are often very costly. A **new technology** is an advance in medical technology that substantially improves, relative to technologies previously available, the diagnosis or treatment of Medicare beneficiaries (CMS 2005, n.p.). Applicants for the status of new technology must submit a formal request, including a full description of the clinical applications of the technology and the results of any clinical evaluations demonstrating that the new technology represents a substantial clinical improvement, together with data to demonstrate the technology meets the high-cost threshold.

Providing these innovative services in a prospective system could, in many cases, lead to inadequate payments. These financial losses may prohibit a facility from offering new and innovative services to patients because they are simply not affordable, so to ensure that new and innovative services and technologies are provided to Medicare beneficiaries, the IPPS allows additional payments to be made for new medical services and new technologies. This payment provision allows for the full MS-DRG payment plus up to 50 percent of the cost for the new technology or service.

Transfer Cases

There are two types of **transfer** cases under the IPPS. The first category is a patient transfer between two IPPS hospitals. A type 1 transfer is when a patient is discharged from an acute IPPS hospital and is admitted to another acute IPPS hospital on the same day. If a patient leaves an acute IPPS hospital against medical advice and is admitted to another acute IPPS hospital on the same day, this situation is treated the same as a transfer between two IPPS hospitals.

Payment is altered for the transferring hospital and is based on a per diem rate methodology. The MS-DRG is established for the case and the full payment rate is calculated. This payment rate is divided by the GMLOS established for the MS-DRG, creating a per diem rate. The transferring facility receives double the per diem rate for the first day, plus the per diem rate for each day thereafter for the patient LOS. DHS, IME, and outlier add-ons are applied after the per diem rate is established. The receiving facility receives full PPS payment for the case. The one exception to this rule is MS-DRG 789, Neonates Died or Transferred to Another Acute Care Facility. The payment and GMLOS established for MS-DRG 789 are based on historical data; no reduction is necessary because it is a transfer-related MS-DRG.

A transfer that occurs from an IPPS hospital to a hospital or unit excluded from IPPS is known as a type 2 transfer. For this type of transfer case, the full PPS payment is made to the transferring hospital, and the receiving hospital or unit is paid on a reasonable cost basis or under prospective payment, whichever is applicable for that setting (CMS 2004, 1). However, there are exceptions to the payment policy, known as the **post-acute-care transfer (PACT)** policy, for type 2 transfer cases. Of the 278 MS-DRGs (Appendix 6A) that qualify for the PACT policy, a discharge from an acute IPPS hospital to an excluded IPPS hospital or unit is considered a type 1 transfer rather than a discharge.

The facilities excluded from IPPSs are

- Inpatient rehabilitation facilities or units

- Long-term care hospitals

- Psychiatric hospitals and units

- Children's hospitals

- Cancer hospitals

In addition, the case is considered a transfer instead of a discharge when a patient is discharged from an acute IPPS hospital and is admitted to a skilled nursing facility or is sent home with a written plan of care for home health services that will begin within three days after discharge from the IPPS hospital. In these three situations, the same transfer payment provision used for IPPS-to-IPPS transfer cases (type 1 transfer cases) is enacted and followed for 243 of the 278 qualifying MS-DRGs. For the remaining 35 MS-DRGs, there is a special payment policy that allows 50 percent of the full MS-DRG payment plus the per diem amount to be made for the first day of stay, then 50 percent of the per diem amount each day thereafter. These 35 MS-DRGs have significantly higher costs on admission. Creating this special payment policy better reimburses facilities in the post-acute-care transfer situation for these 35 MS-DRGs.

The post-acute-care transfer policy ensures that an incentive is not created for hospitals to discharge patients early to reduce costs while still receiving full MS-DRG payment. In addition, this concept allows for proper reimbursement levels when the full course of treatment is divided across two healthcare settings. Which MS-DRGs are included in the PACT policy are updated each year in the IPPS Final Rule.

IPPS Payment

Medicare provides a four-step methodology for calculating total MS-DRG payment (CMS 2005, n.p.). **Medicare Administrative Contractors (MACs)** use grouper and pricer software to calculate the MS-DRG and payment for each hospital encounter. Figure 6.4 shows the basic foundation for an IPPS payment. The payment steps reflect adjustments, provisions and add-on payments executed under IPPS.

Step 1: Establishment of Initial Payment Rate

A **base payment rate** is established for each Medicare-participating hospital for each FY. The base payment rate is a per-encounter rate that is based on historic claims data. The standardized amounts are derived from 1981 hospital costs per Medicare discharge figures. The 1981 costs established the base year amount that was adjusted to explain differences among facilities for case mix, wage rates, DSH status, IME status, and certain hospital costs. The base-year amount has been updated each year since 1981 by the **market basket**, an update factor established by Congress to account for inflation.

Each year, the standardized amount is divided into a labor-related portion and a nonlabor portion. The **labor-related share** is adjusted by the wage index for the hospital's geographic location based on core-based statistical areas (CBSAs). The **nonlabor share** is modified by a **cost-of-living adjustment (COLA)** if the hospital is located in Alaska or Hawaii. These adjustments establish the base payment rate for the effective FY. A listing of the wage index and COLA values can be found in the IPPS final rule released each year via the *Federal Register*. Past and current *Federal Register* publications can be located via the Government Printing Office (http://www.gpoaccess. gov). Current PPS rules are also posted on the Medicare website (CMS 2005, n.p.).

Step 2: Medicare-Severity Diagnosis-Related Group Assignment

Hospitals must submit a claim to Medicare for payment using an electronic claim to its designated MAC. The MAC performs electronic auditing of the claim to ensure that the claim contains correct information (also referred to as **clean claim**) based on edits found in the Medicare Code Editor. When the claim is deemed clean, the grouper software assigns an MS-DRG based on the demographic and coded data submitted. The base rate adjusted for geographic factors is multiplied by the MS-DRG relative weight.

Example:

Patient A was treated for congestive heart failure, and non-OR procedures were performed. MS-DRG 293 is assigned for the encounter. The RW for MS-DRG 293 is 0.6762. The base rate adjusted for geographic factors is $7,325. The RW is multiplied by the hospital base rate to calculate the initial payment rate. The initial payment rate for this case is $4,953.17 (0.6762 × $7,325).

Step 3: Policy Adjustments for Hospitals that Qualify

If the hospital has DSH status, the established percentage for that year for that facility is added into the hospital adjusted base payment rate. Likewise, if the hospital qualifies for IME payments, then the established percentage for that year for that facility is incorporated into the base rate value as well. Once the applicable adjustments have been made, the base rate is then considered to be fully adjusted, hospital-specific base payment rate.

Step 4: Add-on for High-Cost Outlier and New Medical Service and Technology

The costs incurred for providing services for the encounter are calculated and examined to determine whether the case qualifies for an outlier payment. If an outlier payment is warranted, the additional payment is added on during this step. Additionally, the encounter is reviewed to determine whether any qualifying new services or technology were used during the course of patient treatment. If a new service or technology was used, the costs are calculated for the service or supply. Fifty percent of the calculated costs are added on to the payment.

Pricer Software

The **pricer** software is used to complete steps 2 through 4. When the four steps are completed, payment is made to the facility, and the data from the encounter are included in the National Claims History File. The Medicare Provider Analysis Review (MedPAR) file, an extract from the National Claims History File, is used for statistical analysis and research.

Figure 6.4.   Foundation of acute care inpatient hospital prospective payment system

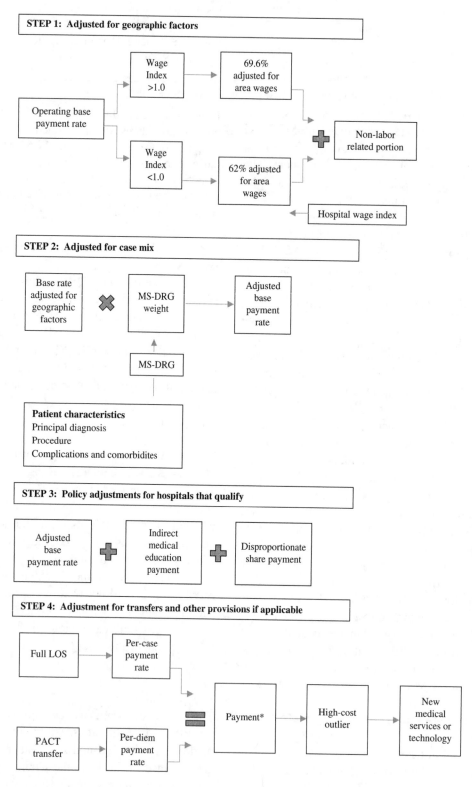

Note: Capital payments are determined by a similar system

*Additional payment made for certain rural hospitals

Adapted from Medicare Payment Advisory Commission (MedPAC). 2014a. Payment basics: Acute inpatient prospective payment system. P.2. http://www.medpac.gov.

Maintenance of the Medicare-Severity Diagnosis-Related Group System

CMS is responsible for updating the MS-DRG system. Each payment rate for each MS-DRG is intended to reimburse the costs for average resources required to care for encounters grouping to that MS-DRG, so adjustments are made to the MS-DRG system to account for changes in treatment patterns, technology, and other elements that influence resource cost. Section 1886(d)(4)(C) of the act requires that MS-DRG classifications and RWs be adjusted at least annually (HHS 2004a, 48925). Claims from the MedPAR file are used to evaluate possible changes to the system. Non-MedPAR issues are also considered. Interested parties (such as hospitals, supply companies, and national associations representing healthcare groups) can submit change requests to Medicare. Non-MedPAR issues should be submitted to CMS no later than December for consideration for the next federal FY, which begins annually on October 1. The group adjustments and recalibration of group weights are published in the *Federal Register* at least 45 days before the start of the new federal FY.

Check Your Understanding 6.1

1. Discuss two of the four guiding principles of prospective payment.

2. In the four-step MS-DRG assignment process, if a coder is able to assign the MS-DRG in step 1, the pre-MDC assignment, all subsequent steps in the process are _____.

3. List two refinement questions that help coders group together patients with like-resource consumption.

4. How are Medicare base payment rates increased to reflect inflation?

5. How is the discharge disposition used in the execution of PACT payment?

Inpatient Psychiatric Facility Prospective Payment System

The Medicare Program provides benefits for inpatient psychiatric care provided to its beneficiaries. Psychiatric hospitals and psychiatric units in acute-care hospitals, referred to as **inpatient psychiatric facilities (IPFs)** for payment purposes, were exempt from the IPPS from 1982 through 2004. Section 1886(ed)(1)(B) of the Social Security Act (the Act) created this exemption and established a reasonable cost payment scheme based on the TEFRA payment methodology (HHS 2004b, 66923).

The Balanced Budget Refinement Act (BBRA) of 1999 required the development of a per diem PPS for inpatient psychiatric services provided in IPFs. Specifically, the BBRA charged CMS with developing a classification system that would reflect the resource consumption and, thus, cost differences among various IPFs. The legislation gave CMS the authority to collect the hospital data necessary for the development of the new PPS. The system was mandated to maintain budget neutrality, and CMS was instructed to submit a report of the proposed system to Congress. The initial implementation date was set to be October 1, 2002 (HHS 2004b, 66923).

Prior to the BBRA, CMS had researched several PPS options for IPFs. However, its research focus was a by-discharge payment methodology similar to other established PPSs, such as the IPPS and the Hospital Outpatient Prospective Payment System (OPPS). The research showed that a per discharge system did not adequately explain the cost variations among psychiatric encounters (HHS 2004b, 66923). Thus, a new approach was necessary. The BBRA gave CMS a three-year period to research and develop a per diem system (HHS 2004b, 66923).

More than a year after the initial implementation date of October 1, 2002, the proposed rule for the IPF PPS was released on November 28, 2003 (HHS 2004b, 66920). The proposed rule outlined the new PPS based on a per diem rate with several add-on payments to provide reimbursement for cost variations. The new PPS called for major changes in how an IPF would be reimbursed for Medicare services and discussed complex cost issues. CMS received many comments on the proposed rule, and after the public requested an extended period of time to review the proposed PPS, the comment period was extended. On November 15, 2004, the final rule for the IPF PPS was released (HHS 2004b, 66922). The final rule established a new implementation date of April 1, 2005.

The IPF PPS is based on a federal per diem amount that represents the average daily operational, ancillary, and capital costs expended to care for Medicare beneficiaries. For FY 2015, the federal per diem amount is $728.31. Adjustments to the payment are made at the facility and patient levels, as described in table 6.4. Although the large number of payment modifications creates a complex system, the payment methodology

Table 6.4.   Facility- and patient-level adjustments

Facility-Level Adjustments	Patient-Level Adjustments
Wage index	Length of stay
Cost-of-living adjustment	MS-DRG with principal diagnosis of mental disorder
Rural location	Comorbid condition
Teaching status	Age of patient
Full-service emergency department	Electroconvulsive therapy

Table 6.5.   Length-of-stay adjustment schedule

Day of Stay	Variable Per Diem Payment Adjustment
Day 1	1.31/1.19*
Day 2	1.12
Day 3	1.08
Day 4	1.05
Day 5	1.04
Day 6	1.02
Day 7	1.01
Day 8	1.01
Day 9	1.00
Day 10	1.00
Day 11	0.99
Day 12	0.99
Day 13	0.99
Day 14	0.99
Day 15	0.98
Day 16	0.97
Day 17	0.97
Day 18	0.96
Day 19	0.95
Day 20	0.95
Day 21	0.95
Over 21	0.92

*The adjustment for day 1 would be 1.31 or 1.19, depending on whether the IPF has or is a psychiatric unit in an acute-care hospital with a qualifying emergency department.

Source: Department of Health and Human Services. 2014. *Federal Register* 79(151):45955.

is designed to adequately reimburse facilities for the services provided to Medicare beneficiaries.

CMS used a regression analysis model to determine the types and levels of adjustments that were necessary to create a payment system that would explain cost variation among IPFs. Regression analysis is a statistical methodology that uses an independent variable to predict the value of a dependent variable. In this case, patient demographics and length of stay (LOS; independent variables) were used to predict cost (dependent variable). The regression analysis performed for the IPF PPS proposed rule (2003) used data from the FY 1999 MedPAR file and the FY 1999 healthcare cost reporting information system (HCRIS). A revised regression analysis was performed for the final rule and used updated MedPAR data from 2002 and updated HCRIS data from 2001 and 2002.

Patient-Level Adjustments

Patient-level adjustments are made for LOS, DRGs containing a psychiatric ICD code, comorbidity conditions, treatment of older patients, and encounters including electroconvulsive therapy (ECT).

Length-of-Stay Adjustment

Cost regression, first based on 1999 claims data and then updated with 2002 data, showed that the per diem cost for psychiatric cases decreased as the LOS increased (HHS 2004b, 66949). Thus, the IPF PPS provides an LOS adjustment factor for each day of the patient encounter. Table 6.5 shows the adjustment schedule by day.

Medicare-Severity Diagnosis-Related Group Adjustment

The IPF PPS will provide reimbursement for MS-DRGs that contain a psychiatric ICD-9-CM code as identified

in chapter 5 of the codebook as principal diagnosis. However, a payment adjustment will be made only for 17 designated psychiatric MS-DRGs. Table 6.6 provides a listing of the 17 psychiatric MS-DRGs.

Comorbid Conditions

The regression analysis of 2002 cost data identified a need to provide a payment adjustment for some comorbid conditions. Table 6.7 provides a listing of the comorbidity groupings that warrant a payment

Table 6.6.   Psychiatric MS-DRGs that qualify for payment adjustment

DRG Title	MS-DRG Code	Adjustment Factor
Degenerative nervous system disorders w MCC	MS-DRG 056	1.05
Degenerative nervous system disorders w/o MCC	MS-DRG 057	1.05
Nontraumatic stupor & coma w MCC	MS-DRG 080	1.07
Nontraumatic stupor & coma w/o MCC	MS-DRG 081	1.07
O.R. procedure w principal diagnoses of mental illness	MS-DRG 876	1.22
Acute adjustment reaction & psychosocial dysfunction	MS-DRG 880	1.05
Depressive neuroses	MS-DRG 881	0.99
Neuroses except depressive	MS-DRG 882	1.02
Disorders of personality & impulse control	MS-DRG 883	1.02
Organic disturbances & mental retardation	MS-DRG 884	1.03
Psychoses	MS-DRG 885	1.00
Behavioral & developmental disorders	MS-DRG 886	0.99
Other mental disorder diagnoses	MS-DRG 887	0.92
Alcohol/drug abuse or dependence, left AMA	MS-DRG 894	0.97
Alcohol/drug abuse or dependence w rehabilitation therapy	MS-DRG 895	1.02
Alcohol/drug abuse or dependence w/o rehabilitation therapy w MCC	MS-DRG 896	0.88
Alcohol/drug abuse or dependence w/o rehabilitation therapy w/o MCC	MS-DRG 897	0.88

Source: Department of Health and Human Services. 2014. *Federal Register* 79(151):45946–45947.

adjustment in the IPF PPS system. This is not a complete list of comorbidities as used in the IPPS; rather, it is a listing of the conditions that were found to be more costly to treat for psychiatric patients in IPFs.

Older Patients

Reimbursement rates are altered to account for the additional costs incurred for treating older patients. Regression analysis showed that the cost per day increased with increasing patient age. Table 6.8 provides the age categories and adjustment factors used for the IPF PPS.

Electroconvulsive Therapy

Providing ECT to Medicare beneficiaries is costly. Regression analysis showed that an encounter that included ECT was twice as expensive as an encounter that did not include ECT. The cost is mostly associated with the increased LOS but is also a result of increased ancillary services (HHS 2004b, 66951). The IPF PPS provides a patient-level adjustment for this service. Facilities will receive additional payment for each ECT session performed. For FY 2015, the additional reimbursement equals $315.55. The ECT amount is subject to COLA and wage-index adjustments. ECT services should be reported with the CPT code 90870 and revenue code 901. The units of service must also be reported. ECT payments and charges are taken into account when MAC/FIs calculate the outlier threshold and outlier payment.

Facility-Level Adjustments

Payments are adjusted at the facility level to account for geographic variations such as wage differences, cost of living, and rural location. Adjustments are also made for teaching hospitals and facilities that provide emergency medical services. These adjustments are addressed in the following sections.

Wage-Index Adjustment

A facility-level adjustment is provided to account for wage differences among geographic areas. The labor portion of the federal per diem base rate is 69.294 percent. The unadjusted, prefloor, prereclassified IPPS hospital wage index using CBSA definitions is used to make the adjustment. Figure 6.5 provides the IPF wage-index adjustment formula. For example, the wage index for a hospital in Columbus, Ohio for 2015 is 0.9444. The federal per diem base rate for 2015 is $728.31. To wage index for this area, first multiply the

Table 6.7.   Comorbidity adjustment categories

Comorbidity Category	Applicable ICD-9-CM Codes	Adjustment Factor
Developmental disabilities	317, 318.0, 318.1, 318.2, and 319	1.04
Coagulation factor deficits	286.0 through 286.4	1.13
Tracheotomy	519.00 through 519.09 and V44.0	1.06
Renal failure, acute	584.5 through 584.9, 636.30, 636.31, 636.32, 637.30, 637.31, 637.32, 638.3, 639.3, 669.32, 669.34, and 958.5	1.11
Renal failure, chronic	403.01, 403.11, 403.91, 404.02, 404.12, 404.13, 404.92, 404.93, 585.3, 585.4, 585.5, 585.6, 585.9, 586, V45.11, V45.12, V56.0, V56.1, and V56.2	1.11
Oncology treatment	140.0 through 239.9 with either 92.21 through 92.29 or 99.25	1.07
Uncontrolled diabetes mellitus with or without complications	250.02, 250.03, 250.12, 250.13, 250.22, 250.23, 250.32, 250.33, 250.42, 250.43, 250.52, 250.53, 250.62, 250.63, 250.72, 250.73, 250.82, 250.83, 250.92, and 250.93	1.05
Severe protein calorie malnutrition	260 through 262	1.13
Eating and conduct disorders	307.1, 307.50, 312.03, 312.33, and 312.34	1.12
Infectious disease	010.00 through 041.10, 042, 045.00 through 053.19, 054.40 through 054.49, 055.0 through 077.0, 078.2 through 078.89, and 079.50 through 079.59	1.07
Drug- and/or alcohol-induced mental disorders	291.0, 292.0, 292.12, 292.2, 303.00, and 304.00	1.03
Cardiac conditions	391.0, 391.1, 391.2, 402.01, 404.03, 416.0, 421.0, 421.1, and 421.9	1.11
Gangrene	440.24 and 785.4	1.10
Chronic obstructive pulmonary disease	491.21, 494.1, 510.0, 518.83, 518.84, V46.11, V46.12, V46.13, and V46.14	1.12
Artificial openings—digestive and urinary	569.60 through 569.69, 997.5 and V44.1 through V44.6	1.08
Severe musculoskeletal and connective tissue diseases	696.0, 710.0, 730.00 through 730.09, 730.10 through 730.19, and 730.20 through 730.29	1.09
Poisoning	965.00 through 965.09, 965.4, 967.0 through 969.9, 977.0, 980.0 through 980.9, 983.0 through 983.9, 986 and 989.0 through 989.7	1.11

Source: Department of Health and Human Services. 2014. *Federal Register* 79(151):45952–45953.

*See the 2016 IPF PPS Final Rule, published in the Federal Register, for comorbidity adjustment categories converted to ICD-10-CM codes.

federal per diem base rate by the labor percent and the wage index amount ($728.31 × 0.69294 × 0.9444). Step 1 gives $475.62. The next step is to calculate the nonlabor amount. To do so, multiply the federal per diem base rate by the nonlabor percent ($728.31 × 0.30706). Step 2 gives $223.63. To calculate the wage index adjusted per diem amount, sum the results of steps 1 and 2 ($475.62 + $223.63). For this example, the wage index adjusted per diem amount equals $699.25. Because the wage index for Columbus, Ohio, is lower than 1.000, the wage indexed per diem amount is lower than the federal per diem amount. If the wage index was higher than 1.000, the wage index adjusted per diem amount would be higher than the federal per diem amount.

Cost-of-Living Adjustment

In addition to the wage-index adjustment, a COLA will be made for IPFs in Hawaii and Alaska. The nonlabor share portion (30.706 percent) of the federal per diem base rate will be adjusted by the adjustment factor provided for the county where the facility is located. Figure 6.6 provides the COLA formula. Table 6.9 provides a listing of the COLA adjustments.

Table 6.8.   Age-adjustment categories

Age	Adjustment Factor
<45	1.00
45 and under 50	1.01
50 and under 55	1.02
55 and under 60	1.04
60 and under 65	1.07
65 and under 70	1.10
70 and under 75	1.13
75 and under 80	1.15
≥80	1.17

Source: Department of Health and Human Services. 2014. *Federal Register* 79(151):45955.

For example, the COLA adjustment for a hospital in Anchorage, Alaska, for 2015 is 1.23. The federal per diem base rate for 2015 is $728.31. To COLA adjust for this area the first step is to multiply the federal per diem base rate by the labor percent ($728.31 × 0.69294). Step 1 gives $504.68. The next step is to calculate the nonlabor amount. To do so, multiply the federal per diem base rate by the nonlabor percent and the COLA adjustment ($728.31 × 0.30706 × 1.23). Step two gives $275.07. To calculate the COLA adjusted per diem amount, sum the results of steps 1 and 2 ($504.68 + $275.07). For this example, the COLA adjusted per diem amount equals $779.75. Because all the COLA adjustments are higher than 1.000 (see table 6.9), the COLA adjusted per diem amount will be higher than the federal per diem amount.

Figure 6.5.   Wage-index adjustment formula

(Federal per diem base rate × Labor percent × Wage index) + (Federal per diem base rate × Nonlabor percentage)

Figure 6.6.   COLA formula

(Federal per diem base rate × Labor percent) + (Federal per diem base rate × Nonlabor percent × COLA)

Rural Location Adjustment

Regression analysis showed that IPFs incurred costs 17 percent greater when treating patients in rural locations than when treating patients in urban locations. Many rural IPFs are small facilities that do not have the economy-of-scale advantages that larger facilities experience. Furthermore, providing psychiatric services requires a set of minimum fixed costs that cannot be avoided or decreased (HHS 2004b, 66954). Thus, the IPF PPS provides a rural location adjustment of 1.17.

Teaching Hospital Adjustment

IPFs are granted a teaching hospital adjustment similar to the adjustment made for IPPS facilities. The adjustment is based on the number of full-time residents at the facility. The coefficient value of 0.5150 will be used for FY 2015 in the teaching status adjustment.

Emergency Facility Adjustment

Patients who receive emergency department (ED) care before admission are more costly to treat than patients who do not receive such care, so CMS provides an adjustment to adequately reimburse facilities for this greater cost without creating an incentive to provide ED care when it is not medically necessary to receive additional payments. A facility-level adjustment is made for IPFs with full-service EDs. IPFs with qualifying EDs receive a greater per diem adjustment for the first day of each stay for all patients. (See table 6.5, Day 1.)

Provisions of the Inpatient Psychiatric Facility Prospective Payment System

The IPF PPS uses provisions to provide additional payments for unusual admissions that historically have added significant cost to patient care. Without the additional payments associated with these provisions, it might not be feasible for IPFs to provide all services to Medicare beneficiaries.

Outlier Payment Provision

The IPF PPS provides outlier payments for high-cost encounters. Outlier payments are projected by CMS to account for two percent of the total payment for the implementation year. The costs of an encounter must exceed the adjusted threshold amount to qualify for an outlier payment. Cost is determined by converting charges to cost using CCRs from the facility's most recent settled or tentatively settled Medicare

Table 6.9.   COLA areas

State	Location	COLA
Alaska	Anchorage	1.23
Alaska	Fairbanks	1.23
Alaska	Juneau	1.23
Alaska	All other areas	1.25
Hawaii	Honolulu County and City	1.25
Hawaii	Hawaii County	1.18
Hawaii	Kauai County	1.25
Hawaii	Maui County	1.25
Hawaii	Kalawao County	1.25

Source: Department of Health and Human Services. 2014. *Federal Register* 79(151):45958–45959.

cost report. Facilities that have CCRs outside of the designated **trim points** will be required to use national rural/urban CCRs. The adjusted threshold amount is calculated by applying wage index, rural location, and teaching status adjustments to the national amount. The unadjusted threshold amount for FY 2015 is $8,755. In addition to reimbursement for the encounter, facilities will receive 80 percent of the difference between the IPF's estimated cost and the adjusted threshold amount for days one through nine, as well as 60 percent for days thereafter (HHS 2004b, 66960).

Initial Stay and Readmission Provisions

The IPF PPS is designed to provide higher payment for initial days of a stay to adequately reimburse facilities for the higher costs associated with a new admission. CMS has expressed concern that this adjustment could provide an incentive for facilities to prematurely discharge patients and then subsequently readmit them to again receive the higher per diem rates associated with the first days of a stay. Therefore, an interrupted stay provision was created. Patients discharged from an IPF who are then admitted to the same or another IPF within three consecutive days (before midnight on the third day) of the discharge from the original facility stay would be treated as continuous for purposes of the variable per diem adjustment and outlier calculation (HHS 2004b, 66963).

A patient is admitted to IPF A on March 1. The patient is discharged on March 5 (LOS = four). The patient is then admitted to IPF B on March 7 and continues the hospital stay until March 10 (LOS = three). The admission to IPF B is considered a continuation of the initial stay at IPF A. Thus day 1 of the readmission will be considered day five of the combined stay for the purposes of the LOS adjustment and outlier calculation (see table 6.6).

Medical Necessity Provision

Medical necessity must be established for each patient on admission to the IPF. Physician recertification to establish continued need for inpatient psychiatric care is required on the 18th day after admission. Inpatient care requires more intense service than outpatient. Inpatient admissions or continued stays are necessary when care requires intensive comprehensive multimodal treatments such as 24-hour supervision, safety concerns, diagnostic evaluations, monitoring for side effects of psychotropic medications, and evaluation of behaviors.

Payment Steps

Medicare provides a four-step process for calculating the IPF payment. It is important to carefully review the encounter data to ensure that all applicable patient-level and facility-level adjustments are accurately applied and that all procedures are coded in order to determine the correct reimbursement amount. Figure 6.7 shows the basic foundation for an IPF PPS payment. The payment steps reflect adjustments, provisions and add-on payments executed under IPF PPS.

Check Your Understanding 6.2

1. Which piece of legislation charged CMS with creating a PPS for the inpatient psychiatric setting? What requirements were included in the law?

2. What type of reimbursement scheme is used in the IPF PPS?

3. What is the formula for the ECT adjustment for a facility with a wage index of .9812?

4. What are the two categories of adjustments in the IPF PPS?

5. List and discuss two of the provisions of the IPF PPS.

Figure 6.7.   Foundation of inpatient psychiatric hospital prospective payment system

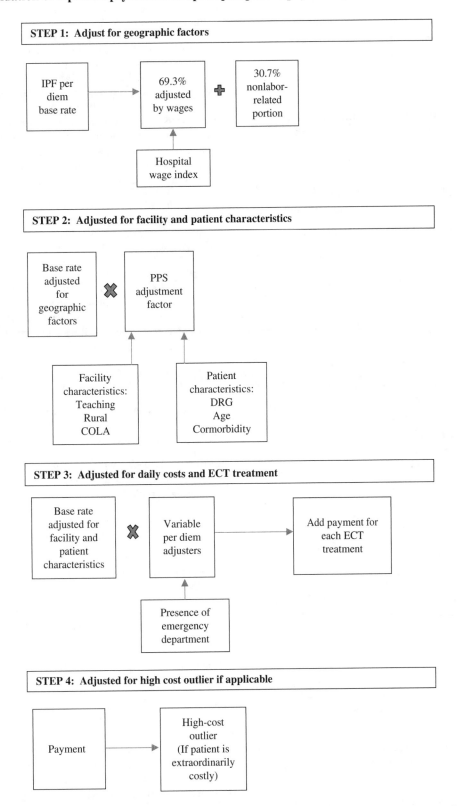

Adapted from Medicare Payment Advisory Commission (MedPAC). 2014b. Payment basics: Inpatient psychiatric facility prospective payment system. P.2. http://www.medpac.gov.

Chapter 6 Review Quiz

1. List at least two major reasons why Medicare administrators turned to the prospective payment concept for Medicare beneficiaries.

2. How do MS-DRGs encourage inpatient facilities to practice cost management?

3. Why was a severity of illness refinement performed on the DRG system? Was it supported by the healthcare community?

4. List the steps of MS-DRG assignment.

5. Why does the IPF PPS length-of-stay adjustment factor grow smaller during the patient encounter?

6. Describe at least two patient-level adjustments for IPF PPS claims and explain why they are used.

7. What is the labor portion of the IPF PPS per diem rate? What is the nonlabor portion of the IPF PPS per diem rate?

8. Why was the initial stay and readmission provision included in the IPF PPS?

9. Describe the medical necessity provision of the IPF PPS.

10. When performing the payment determination for IPF PPS admissions, which step comes first: wage-index adjustment, or application of the patient and facility-level adjustments?

References

Averill, R.F., N.I. Goldfield, J. Eisenhandler, J.S. Hughes, and J. Muldoon. 2001. Clinical risk groups and the future of healthcare reimbursement. In *Reimbursement methodologies for healthcare services* [CD-ROM]. Edited by L.M. Jones. Chicago: AHIMA.

Centers for Medicare and Medicaid Services (CMS). 2004. Expansion of transfer policy under inpatient prospective payment system. MedLearn Matters (MM2934), Medicare Learning Network. https://www.cms.gov/Outreach-and-Education/Medicare-Learning-Network-MLN/MLNMattersArticles/Downloads/MM2934.pdf.

Centers for Medicare and Medicaid Services (CMS). 2005. http://www.cms.hhs.gov.

Centers for Medicare and Medicaid Services (CMS). 2012. http://www.cms.gov/Medicare/Medicare-Fee-for-Service-Payment/AcuteInpatientPPS/Indirect-Medical-Education-IME.html.

Department of Health and Human Services (HHS). 2004a. Medicare program; Changes to the hospital inpatient prospective payment systems and fiscal year 2005 rates; Final rule. *Federal Register* 69(154):48915–48964.

Department of Health and Human Services (HHS). 2004b. Medicare program; Prospective payment system for inpatient psychiatric facilities; Final rule. *Federal Register* 69(219):66921–67015.

Department of Health and Human Services (HHS). 2011. Medicare program: Prospective payment system for inpatient psychiatric facilities; Final rule. *Federal Register* 76(88):26432–26487.

Department of Health and Human Services (HHS). 2014a. Medicare program: Prospective payment system for Acute Care Hospitals and the Long-Term Care Hospital Prospective Payment System and Fiscal Year 2015 Rates; Quality Reporting Requirements for Specific Providers; Reasonable Compensation Equivalents for Physician Services in Excluded Hospital and Certain Teaching Hospitals; Provider Administrative Appeals and Judicial Review; Enforcement Provisions for Organ Transplant Centers; and Electronic Health Record (EHR) Incentive Program; Final Rule. *Federal Register* 79(163):49853–50536.

Department of Health and Human Services (HHS). 2014b. Medicare program: Prospective payment system for inpatient psychiatric facilities; Final rule. *Federal Register* 79(151):45938–46009.

Gottlober, P., T. Brady, B. Robinson, T. Davis, S. Phillips, and A. Gruber. 2001. Medicare hospital prospective payment system: How DRG rates are calculated and updated. Publication No. OEI-09-00-00200. Office of Inspector General, Office of Evaluation and Inspections, Region IX. http://www.oig.hhs.gov/oei/reports/oei-09-00-00200.pdf.

Johns, M., ed. 2007. *Health information management technology: An applied approach*, 2nd ed. Chicago: AHIMA.

Kaiser Family Foundation. 2015. Federal Medicaid Disproportionate Share Hospital (DSH) Allotments. http://kff.org/medicaid/state-indicator/federal-dsh-allotments/.

LaTour, K., P. Oachs, and S. Eichenwald, eds. 2013 *Health information management: Concepts, principles, and practice*, 3rd ed. Chicago: AHIMA.

Lave, J.R. 1989. The effect of the Medicare prospective payment system. *Annual Review of Public Health* 10:141–161.

Medicare Payment Advisory Commission (MedPAC). 2014a. Payment basics: Hospital acute inpatient services payment system. http://www.medpac.gov.

Medicare Payment Advisory Commission (MedPAC). 2014b. Payment basics: Inpatient psychiatric facility services payment system. http://www.medpac.gov.

Schraffenberger, L. 2012. *Basic ICD-9-CM coding*, 2012 ed. Chicago: AHIMA.

Additional Resources

Centers for Medicare and Medicaid Services. 2003. Medicare prescription drug, improvement, and modernization act of 2003. Section 626(2)(B). http://www.gpo.gov/fdsys/pkg/BILLS-108hr1enr/pdf/BILLS-108hr1enr.pdf.

Department of Health and Human Services. 2003. Medicare program; Prospective payment system for inpatient psychiatric facilities; Proposed rule. *Federal Register* 68(229):66919–66978.

Department of Health and Human Services. 2007. Medicare program inpatient psychiatric facilities prospective payment system payment update for rate year beginning July 1, 2007 (RY 2008); Notice. *Federal Register* 72(86):25602–25673.

Department of Health and Human Services. 2007. Medicare program; Prospective payment system for long-term care hospitals RY 2008: Annual payment rate updates, and policy changes; and hospital direct and indirect graduate medical education policy changes; Final rule. *Federal Register* 72(91):26869–27029.

Department of Health and Human Services. 2007. Medicare program; Changes to the hospital inpatient prospective payment systems and fiscal year 2008 rates; Final rule. *Federal Register* 72(162):45768–48175.

Department of Health and Human Services. 2009. Medicare program; Inpatient psychiatric facilities prospective payment system payment update for rate year beginning July 1, 2009 (RY 2010); Notice. *Federal Register* 74(83):20362–20399.

Department of Health and Human Services. 2009. Medicare program: Changes to the hospital inpatient prospective payment system for acute care hospitals and fiscal year 2010 rates; and changes to long-term care hospitals prospective payment system and rate years 2010 and 2009 rates: Final rule. *Federal Register* 74(165):73754–74236.

Department of Health and Human Services. 2011. Medicare program: Hospital inpatient prospective payment systems for acute care hospitals and long term care hospital prospective payment system and fiscal year 2012 rates: Final rule. *Federal Register* 76(160):51476–51846.

Appendix 6A
Post-acute care transfer MS-DRGs for FY 2015

MS-DRG	PACT DRG	PACT Special Payment DRG	MS-DRG Title	Relative Weight	Geometric Mean LOS
003	Yes	No	ECMO OR TRACH W MV 96+ HRS OR PDX EXC FACE, MOUTH & NECK W MAJ O.R.	17.6399	26.2
004	Yes	No	TRACH W MV 96+ HRS OR PDX EXC FACE, MOUTH & NECK W/O MAJ O.R.	10.8533	20.2
023	Yes	No	CRANIO W MAJOR DEV IMPL/ACUTE COMPLEX CNS PDX W MCC OR CHEMO IMPLANT	5.2939	7.9
024	Yes	No	CRANIO W MAJOR DEV IMPL/ACUTE COMPLEX CNS PDX W/O MCC	3.7461	4.4
025	Yes	No	CRANIOTOMY & ENDOVASCULAR INTRACRANIAL PROCEDURES W MCC	4.3374	7.4
026	Yes	No	CRANIOTOMY & ENDOVASCULAR INTRACRANIAL PROCEDURES W CC	3.0011	4.7
027	Yes	No	CRANIOTOMY & ENDOVASCULAR INTRACRANIAL PROCEDURES W/O CC/MCC	2.2824	2.5
028	Yes	Yes	SPINAL PROCEDURES W MCC	5.3968	9.5
029	Yes	Yes	SPINAL PROCEDURES W CC OR SPINAL NEUROSTIMULATORS	3.1573	4.8
030	Yes	Yes	SPINAL PROCEDURES W/O CC/MCC	1.7835	2.6
031	Yes	No	VENTRICULAR SHUNT PROCEDURES W MCC	4.1493	7.7
032	Yes	No	VENTRICULAR SHUNT PROCEDURES W CC	2.0325	3.3
033	Yes	No	VENTRICULAR SHUNT PROCEDURES W/O CC/MCC	1.5602	2.0
040	Yes	Yes	PERIPH/CRANIAL NERVE & OTHER NERV SYST PROC W MCC	3.7960	8.1
041	Yes	Yes	PERIPH/CRANIAL NERVE & OTHER NERV SYST PROC W CC OR PERIPH NEUROSTIM	2.1267	4.7
042	Yes	Yes	PERIPH/CRANIAL NERVE & OTHER NERV SYST PROC W/O CC/MCC	1.8586	2.5
054	Yes	No	NERVOUS SYSTEM NEOPLASMS W MCC	1.3048	3.9
055	Yes	No	NERVOUS SYSTEM NEOPLASMS W/O MCC	1.0191	3.0
056	Yes	No	DEGENERATIVE NERVOUS SYSTEM DISORDERS W MCC	1.7615	5.2

Table   (Continued)

MS-DRG	PACT DRG	PACT Special Payment DRG	MS-DRG Title	Relative Weight	Geometric Mean LOS
057	Yes	No	DEGENERATIVE NERVOUS SYSTEM DISORDERS W/O MCC	1.0099	3.5
064	Yes	No	INTRACRANIAL HEMORRHAGE OR CEREBRAL INFARCTION W MCC	1.7381	4.6
065	Yes	No	INTRACRANIAL HEMORRHAGE OR CEREBRAL INFARCTION W CC OR TPA IN 24 HRS	1.0643	3.4
066	Yes	No	INTRACRANIAL HEMORRHAGE OR CEREBRAL INFARCTION W/O CC/MCC	0.7530	2.4
070	Yes	No	NONSPECIFIC CEREBROVASCULAR DISORDERS W MCC	1.6438	4.8
071	Yes	No	NONSPECIFIC CEREBROVASCULAR DISORDERS W CC	0.9748	3.4
072	Yes	No	NONSPECIFIC CEREBROVASCULAR DISORDERS W/O CC/MCC	0.6947	2.2
085	Yes	No	TRAUMATIC STUPOR & COMA, COMA <1 HR W MCC	1.9770	4.7
086	Yes	No	TRAUMATIC STUPOR & COMA, COMA <1 HR W CC	1.1181	3.2
087	Yes	No	TRAUMATIC STUPOR & COMA, COMA <1 HR W/O CC/MCC	0.7460	2.1
091	Yes	No	OTHER DISORDERS OF NERVOUS SYSTEM W MCC	1.5978	4.2
092	Yes	No	OTHER DISORDERS OF NERVOUS SYSTEM W CC	0.8989	3.0
093	Yes	No	OTHER DISORDERS OF NERVOUS SYSTEM W/O CC/MCC	0.6783	2.1
100	Yes	No	SEIZURES W MCC	1.5304	4.1
101	Yes	No	SEIZURES W/O MCC	0.7567	2.5
163	Yes	No	MAJOR CHEST PROCEDURES W MCC	5.0332	10.7
164	Yes	No	MAJOR CHEST PROCEDURES W CC	2.6010	5.4
165	Yes	No	MAJOR CHEST PROCEDURES W/O CC/MCC	1.8220	3.2
166	Yes	No	OTHER RESP SYSTEM O.R. PROCEDURES W MCC	3.6610	8.7
167	Yes	No	OTHER RESP SYSTEM O.R. PROCEDURES W CC	1.9818	5.1
168	Yes	No	OTHER RESP SYSTEM O.R. PROCEDURES W/O CC/MCC	1.3291	2.9
175	Yes	No	PULMONARY EMBOLISM W MCC	1.5271	5.2
176	Yes	No	PULMONARY EMBOLISM W/O MCC	0.9670	3.5
177	Yes	No	RESPIRATORY INFECTIONS & INFLAMMATIONS W MCC	1.9492	6.2

(*Continued on next page*)

Table   (Continued)

MS-DRG	PACT DRG	PACT Special Payment DRG	MS-DRG Title	Relative Weight	Geometric Mean LOS
178	Yes	No	RESPIRATORY INFECTIONS & INFLAMMATIONS W CC	1.3909	5.0
179	Yes	No	RESPIRATORY INFECTIONS & INFLAMMATIONS W/O CC/MCC	0.9693	3.6
186	Yes	No	PLEURAL EFFUSION W MCC	1.5452	4.8
187	Yes	No	PLEURAL EFFUSION W CC	1.0691	3.5
188	Yes	No	PLEURAL EFFUSION W/O CC/MCC	0.7609	2.5
190	Yes	No	CHRONIC OBSTRUCTIVE PULMONARY DISEASE W MCC	1.1743	4.2
191	Yes	No	CHRONIC OBSTRUCTIVE PULMONARY DISEASE W CC	0.9370	3.4
192	Yes	No	CHRONIC OBSTRUCTIVE PULMONARY DISEASE W/O CC/MCC	0.7190	2.7
193	Yes	No	SIMPLE PNEUMONIA & PLEURISY W MCC	1.4491	4.9
194	Yes	No	SIMPLE PNEUMONIA & PLEURISY W CC	0.9688	3.8
195	Yes	No	SIMPLE PNEUMONIA & PLEURISY W/O CC/MCC	0.7044	2.9
196	Yes	No	INTERSTITIAL LUNG DISEASE W MCC	1.6635	5.4
197	Yes	No	INTERSTITIAL LUNG DISEASE W CC	1.0615	3.7
198	Yes	No	INTERSTITIAL LUNG DISEASE W/O CC/MCC	0.8054	2.7
205	Yes	No	OTHER RESPIRATORY SYSTEM DIAGNOSES W MCC	1.3999	4.0
206	Yes	No	OTHER RESPIRATORY SYSTEM DIAGNOSES W/O MCC	0.7942	2.4
207	Yes	No	RESPIRATORY SYSTEM DIAGNOSIS W VENTILATOR SUPPORT 96+ HOURS	5.3425	12.4
216	Yes	Yes	CARDIAC VALVE & OTH MAJ CARDIOTHORACIC PROC W CARD CATH W MCC	9.5238	13.0
217	Yes	Yes	CARDIAC VALVE & OTH MAJ CARDIOTHORACIC PROC W CARD CATH W CC	6.3291	8.7
218	Yes	Yes	CARDIAC VALVE & OTH MAJ CARDIOTHORACIC PROC W CARD CATH W/O CC/MCC	5.5693	6.4
219	Yes	Yes	CARDIAC VALVE & OTH MAJ CARDIOTHORACIC PROC W/O CARD CATH W MCC	7.7067	9.8
220	Yes	Yes	CARDIAC VALVE & OTH MAJ CARDIOTHORACIC PROC W/O CARD CATH W CC	5.2056	6.6
221	Yes	Yes	CARDIAC VALVE & OTH MAJ CARDIOTHORACIC PROC W/O CARD CATH W/O CC/MCC	4.6347	4.9

Table   (Continued)

MS-DRG	PACT DRG	PACT Special Payment DRG	MS-DRG Title	Relative Weight	Geometric Mean LOS
233	Yes	No	CORONARY BYPASS W CARDIAC CATH W MCC	7.3493	11.8
234	Yes	No	CORONARY BYPASS W CARDIAC CATH W/O MCC	4.8816	8.0
235	Yes	No	CORONARY BYPASS W/O CARDIAC CATH W MCC	5.7089	9.0
236	Yes	No	CORONARY BYPASS W/O CARDIAC CATH W/O MCC	3.7952	6.0
239	Yes	No	AMPUTATION FOR CIRC SYS DISORDERS EXC UPPER LIMB & TOE W MCC	4.7590	10.6
240	Yes	No	AMPUTATION FOR CIRC SYS DISORDERS EXC UPPER LIMB & TOE W CC	2.7594	7.2
241	Yes	No	AMPUTATION FOR CIRC SYS DISORDERS EXC UPPER LIMB & TOE W/O CC/MCC	1.4111	4.4
242	Yes	No	PERMANENT CARDIAC PACEMAKER IMPLANT W MCC	3.7242	5.8
243	Yes	No	PERMANENT CARDIAC PACEMAKER IMPLANT W CC	2.6695	3.6
244	Yes	No	PERMANENT CARDIAC PACEMAKER IMPLANT W/O CC/MCC	2.1555	2.4
255	Yes	No	UPPER LIMB & TOE AMPUTATION FOR CIRC SYSTEM DISORDERS W MCC	2.6051	6.5
256	Yes	No	UPPER LIMB & TOE AMPUTATION FOR CIRC SYSTEM DISORDERS W CC	1.6986	5.3
257	Yes	No	UPPER LIMB & TOE AMPUTATION FOR CIRC SYSTEM DISORDERS W/O CC/MCC	1.0558	3.0
264	Yes	No	OTHER CIRCULATORY SYSTEM O.R. PROCEDURES	2.8292	5.4
266	Yes	Yes	ENDOVASCULAR CARDIAC VALVE REPLACEMENT W MCC	8.9920	8.4
267	Yes	Yes	ENDOVASCULAR CARDIAC VALVE REPLACEMENT W/O MCC	6.7517	5.0
280	Yes	No	ACUTE MYOCARDIAL INFARCTION, DISCHARGED ALIVE W MCC	1.7289	4.7
281	Yes	No	ACUTE MYOCARDIAL INFARCTION, DISCHARGED ALIVE W CC	1.0247	3.0
282	Yes	No	ACUTE MYOCARDIAL INFARCTION, DISCHARGED ALIVE W/O CC/MCC	0.7562	2.0
288	Yes	No	ACUTE & SUBACUTE ENDOCARDITIS W MCC	2.7138	7.6
289	Yes	No	ACUTE & SUBACUTE ENDOCARDITIS W CC	1.6991	5.8
290	Yes	No	ACUTE & SUBACUTE ENDOCARDITIS W/O CC/MCC	1.2476	3.9
291	Yes	No	HEART FAILURE & SHOCK W MCC	1.5097	4.6

(Continued on next page)

Table   (Continued)

MS-DRG	PACT DRG	PACT Special Payment DRG	MS-DRG Title	Relative Weight	Geometric Mean LOS
292	Yes	No	HEART FAILURE & SHOCK W CC	0.9824	3.6
293	Yes	No	HEART FAILURE & SHOCK W/O CC/MCC	0.6762	2.6
299	Yes	No	PERIPHERAL VASCULAR DISORDERS W MCC	1.4094	4.4
300	Yes	No	PERIPHERAL VASCULAR DISORDERS W CC	0.9770	3.5
301	Yes	No	PERIPHERAL VASCULAR DISORDERS W/O CC/MCC	0.6776	2.6
314	Yes	No	OTHER CIRCULATORY SYSTEM DIAGNOSES W MCC	1.9195	4.9
315	Yes	No	OTHER CIRCULATORY SYSTEM DIAGNOSES W CC	0.9613	3.0
316	Yes	No	OTHER CIRCULATORY SYSTEM DIAGNOSES W/O CC/MCC	0.6210	1.9
326	Yes	No	STOMACH, ESOPHAGEAL & DUODENAL PROC W MCC	5.3847	11.2
327	Yes	No	STOMACH, ESOPHAGEAL & DUODENAL PROC W CC	2.6532	5.8
328	Yes	No	STOMACH, ESOPHAGEAL & DUODENAL PROC W/O CC/MCC	1.4949	2.4
329	Yes	No	MAJOR SMALL & LARGE BOWEL PROCEDURES W MCC	5.0776	11.7
330	Yes	No	MAJOR SMALL & LARGE BOWEL PROCEDURES W CC	2.5491	7.1
331	Yes	No	MAJOR SMALL & LARGE BOWEL PROCEDURES W/O CC/MCC	1.6580	4.3
332	Yes	No	RECTAL RESECTION W MCC	4.7048	10.5
333	Yes	No	RECTAL RESECTION W CC	2.4728	6.3
334	Yes	No	RECTAL RESECTION W/O CC/MCC	1.6032	3.6
335	Yes	No	PERITONEAL ADHESIOLYSIS W MCC	4.2881	10.9
336	Yes	No	PERITONEAL ADHESIOLYSIS W CC	2.3539	6.8
337	Yes	No	PERITONEAL ADHESIOLYSIS W/O CC/MCC	1.5596	3.9
356	Yes	No	OTHER DIGESTIVE SYSTEM O.R. PROCEDURES W MCC	3.8573	8.4
357	Yes	No	OTHER DIGESTIVE SYSTEM O.R. PROCEDURES W CC	2.1072	5.1
358	Yes	No	OTHER DIGESTIVE SYSTEM O.R. PROCEDURES W/O CC/MCC	1.3737	2.9
371	Yes	No	MAJOR GASTROINTESTINAL DISORDERS & PERITONEAL INFECTIONS W MCC	1.8633	6.0
372	Yes	No	MAJOR GASTROINTESTINAL DISORDERS & PERITONEAL INFECTIONS W CC	1.1343	4.6

Table   (Continued)

MS-DRG	PACT DRG	PACT Special Payment DRG	MS-DRG Title	Relative Weight	Geometric Mean LOS
373	Yes	No	MAJOR GASTROINTESTINAL DISORDERS & PERITONEAL INFECTIONS W/O CC/MCC	0.8013	3.4
374	Yes	No	DIGESTIVE MALIGNANCY W MCC	2.0182	6.0
375	Yes	No	DIGESTIVE MALIGNANCY W CC	1.2429	4.1
376	Yes	No	DIGESTIVE MALIGNANCY W/O CC/MCC	0.9021	2.7
377	Yes	No	G.I. HEMORRHAGE W MCC	1.7775	4.7
378	Yes	No	G.I. HEMORRHAGE W CC	1.0021	3.2
379	Yes	No	G.I. HEMORRHAGE W/O CC/MCC	0.6776	2.3
380	Yes	No	COMPLICATED PEPTIC ULCER W MCC	1.9265	5.4
381	Yes	No	COMPLICATED PEPTIC ULCER W CC	1.0875	3.5
382	Yes	No	COMPLICATED PEPTIC ULCER W/O CC/MCC	0.7591	2.6
388	Yes	No	G.I. OBSTRUCTION W MCC	1.6100	5.3
389	Yes	No	G.I. OBSTRUCTION W CC	0.8717	3.5
390	Yes	No	G.I. OBSTRUCTION W/O CC/MCC	0.6034	2.6
405	Yes	No	PANCREAS, LIVER & SHUNT PROCEDURES W MCC	5.5387	10.7
406	Yes	No	PANCREAS, LIVER & SHUNT PROCEDURES W CC	2.8067	5.9
407	Yes	No	PANCREAS, LIVER & SHUNT PROCEDURES W/O CC/MCC	1.9472	3.9
414	Yes	No	CHOLECYSTECTOMY EXCEPT BY LAPAROSCOPE W/O C.D.E. W MCC	3.5545	8.7
415	Yes	No	CHOLECYSTECTOMY EXCEPT BY LAPAROSCOPE W/O C.D.E. W CC	2.0267	5.6
416	Yes	No	CHOLECYSTECTOMY EXCEPT BY LAPAROSCOPE W/O C.D.E. W/O CC/MCC	1.3465	3.6
441	Yes	No	DISORDERS OF LIVER EXCEPT MALIG,CIRR,ALC HEPA W MCC	1.8835	4.9
442	Yes	No	DISORDERS OF LIVER EXCEPT MALIG,CIRR,ALC HEPA W CC	0.9266	3.3
443	Yes	No	DISORDERS OF LIVER EXCEPT MALIG,CIRR,ALC HEPA W/O CC/MCC	0.6512	2.5
459	Yes	No	SPINAL FUSION EXCEPT CERVICAL W MCC	6.6686	6.8
460	Yes	No	SPINAL FUSION EXCEPT CERVICAL W/O MCC	3.9998	3.0
463	Yes	No	WND DEBRID & SKN GRFT EXC HAND, FOR MUSCULO-CONN TISS DIS W MCC	5.3345	10.6
464	Yes	No	WND DEBRID & SKN GRFT EXC HAND, FOR MUSCULO-CONN TISS DIS W CC	3.0085	6.2

(*Continued on next page*)

Table   (Continued)

MS-DRG	PACT DRG	PACT Special Payment DRG	MS-DRG Title	Relative Weight	Geometric Mean LOS
465	Yes	No	WND DEBRID & SKN GRFT EXC HAND, FOR MUSCULO-CONN TISS DIS W/O CC/MCC	1.9463	3.7
466	Yes	No	REVISION OF HIP OR KNEE REPLACEMENT W MCC	5.1513	6.7
467	Yes	No	REVISION OF HIP OR KNEE REPLACEMENT W CC	3.4231	3.8
468	Yes	No	REVISION OF HIP OR KNEE REPLACEMENT W/O CC/MCC	2.7652	2.9
469	Yes	No	MAJOR JOINT REPLACEMENT OR REATTACHMENT OF LOWER EXTREMITY W MCC	3.3905	6.1
470	Yes	No	MAJOR JOINT REPLACEMENT OR REATTACHMENT OF LOWER EXTREMITY W/O MCC	2.1137	3.0
474	Yes	No	AMPUTATION FOR MUSCULOSKELETAL SYS & CONN TISSUE DIS W MCC	3.5943	8.5
475	Yes	No	AMPUTATION FOR MUSCULOSKELETAL SYS & CONN TISSUE DIS W CC	2.0504	5.8
476	Yes	No	AMPUTATION FOR MUSCULOSKELETAL SYS & CONN TISSUE DIS W/O CC/MCC	1.1187	3.1
477	Yes	Yes	BIOPSIES OF MUSCULOSKELETAL SYSTEM & CONNECTIVE TISSUE W MCC	3.1638	8.5
478	Yes	Yes	BIOPSIES OF MUSCULOSKELETAL SYSTEM & CONNECTIVE TISSUE W CC	2.2441	5.4
479	Yes	Yes	BIOPSIES OF MUSCULOSKELETAL SYSTEM & CONNECTIVE TISSUE W/O CC/MCC	1.7312	3.2
480	Yes	Yes	HIP & FEMUR PROCEDURES EXCEPT MAJOR JOINT W MCC	3.0052	6.9
481	Yes	Yes	HIP & FEMUR PROCEDURES EXCEPT MAJOR JOINT W CC	1.9776	4.7
482	Yes	Yes	HIP & FEMUR PROCEDURES EXCEPT MAJOR JOINT W/O CC/MCC	1.6243	3.8
488	Yes	No	KNEE PROCEDURES W/O PDX OF INFECTION W CC/MCC	1.7225	3.4
489	Yes	No	KNEE PROCEDURES W/O PDX OF INFECTION W/O CC/MCC	1.3186	2.3
492	Yes	Yes	LOWER EXTREM & HUMER PROC EXCEPT HIP,FOOT,FEMUR W MCC	3.1873	6.4
493	Yes	Yes	LOWER EXTREM & HUMER PROC EXCEPT HIP,FOOT,FEMUR W CC	2.0354	3.9
494	Yes	Yes	LOWER EXTREM & HUMER PROC EXCEPT HIP,FOOT,FEMUR W/O CC/MCC	1.5397	2.6
495	Yes	Yes	LOCAL EXCISION & REMOVAL INT FIX DEVICES EXC HIP & FEMUR W MCC	3.0476	7.2

Table   (Continued)

MS-DRG	PACT DRG	PACT Special Payment DRG	MS-DRG Title	Relative Weight	Geometric Mean LOS
496	Yes	Yes	LOCAL EXCISION & REMOVAL INT FIX DEVICES EXC HIP & FEMUR W CC	1.7289	3.9
497	Yes	Yes	LOCAL EXCISION & REMOVAL INT FIX DEVICES EXC HIP & FEMUR W/O CC/MCC	1.2230	2.0
500	Yes	Yes	SOFT TISSUE PROCEDURES W MCC	3.2420	7.6
501	Yes	Yes	SOFT TISSUE PROCEDURES W CC	1.6474	4.2
502	Yes	Yes	SOFT TISSUE PROCEDURES W/O CC/MCC	1.1597	2.3
510	Yes	No	SHOULDER,ELBOW OR FOREARM PROC,EXC MAJOR JOINT PROC W MCC	2.2857	4.7
511	Yes	No	SHOULDER,ELBOW OR FOREARM PROC,EXC MAJOR JOINT PROC W CC	1.6509	3.2
512	Yes	No	SHOULDER,ELBOW OR FOREARM PROC,EXC MAJOR JOINT PROC W/O CC/MCC	1.2963	1.9
515	Yes	Yes	OTHER MUSCULOSKELET SYS & CONN TISS O.R. PROC W MCC	3.2235	7.1
516	Yes	Yes	OTHER MUSCULOSKELET SYS & CONN TISS O.R. PROC W CC	2.0434	4.3
517	Yes	Yes	OTHER MUSCULOSKELET SYS & CONN TISS O.R. PROC W/O CC/MCC	1.7251	2.6
518	Yes	Yes	BACK & NECK PROC EXC SPINAL FUSION W MCC OR DISC DEVICE/NEUROSTIM	3.0628	4.2
519	Yes	Yes	BACK & NECK PROC EXC SPINAL FUSION W CC	1.6468	3.0
520	Yes	Yes	BACK & NECK PROC EXC SPINAL FUSION W/O CC/MCC	1.1396	1.7
533	Yes	No	FRACTURES OF FEMUR W MCC	1.4495	4.3
534	Yes	No	FRACTURES OF FEMUR W/O MCC	0.7594	2.9
535	Yes	No	FRACTURES OF HIP & PELVIS W MCC	1.2410	4.1
536	Yes	No	FRACTURES OF HIP & PELVIS W/O MCC	0.7201	3.0
539	Yes	No	OSTEOMYELITIS W MCC	1.8276	6.1
540	Yes	No	OSTEOMYELITIS W CC	1.2967	4.7
541	Yes	No	OSTEOMYELITIS W/O CC/MCC	0.9218	3.5
542	Yes	No	PATHOLOGICAL FRACTURES & MUSCULOSKELET & CONN TISS MALIG W MCC	1.9472	6.0
543	Yes	No	PATHOLOGICAL FRACTURES & MUSCULOSKELET & CONN TISS MALIG W CC	1.1227	4.0
544	Yes	No	PATHOLOGICAL FRACTURES & MUSCULOSKELET & CONN TISS MALIG W/O CC/MCC	0.7936	3.1

(Continued on next page)

Table   (Continued)

MS-DRG	PACT DRG	PACT Special Payment DRG	MS-DRG Title	Relative Weight	Geometric Mean LOS
545	Yes	No	CONNECTIVE TISSUE DISORDERS W MCC	2.5341	6.0
546	Yes	No	CONNECTIVE TISSUE DISORDERS W CC	1.1711	3.9
547	Yes	No	CONNECTIVE TISSUE DISORDERS W/O CC/MCC	0.7985	2.8
551	Yes	No	MEDICAL BACK PROBLEMS W MCC	1.5556	4.7
552	Yes	No	MEDICAL BACK PROBLEMS W/O MCC	0.8698	3.0
557	Yes	No	TENDONITIS, MYOSITIS & BURSITIS W MCC	1.4269	5.0
558	Yes	No	TENDONITIS, MYOSITIS & BURSITIS W/O MCC	0.8522	3.4
559	Yes	No	AFTERCARE, MUSCULOSKELETAL SYSTEM & CONNECTIVE TISSUE W MCC	1.8555	4.9
560	Yes	No	AFTERCARE, MUSCULOSKELETAL SYSTEM & CONNECTIVE TISSUE W CC	1.0756	3.4
561	Yes	No	AFTERCARE, MUSCULOSKELETAL SYSTEM & CONNECTIVE TISSUE W/O CC/MCC	0.6688	2.0
562	Yes	No	FX, SPRN, STRN & DISL EXCEPT FEMUR, HIP, PELVIS & THIGH W MCC	1.3706	4.3
563	Yes	No	FX, SPRN, STRN & DISL EXCEPT FEMUR, HIP, PELVIS & THIGH W/O MCC	0.7756	2.9
570	Yes	No	SKIN DEBRIDEMENT W MCC	2.3952	7.1
571	Yes	No	SKIN DEBRIDEMENT W CC	1.4664	5.1
572	Yes	No	SKIN DEBRIDEMENT W/O CC/MCC	0.9919	3.7
573	Yes	No	SKIN GRAFT FOR SKIN ULCER OR CELLULITIS W MCC	3.7074	8.5
574	Yes	No	SKIN GRAFT FOR SKIN ULCER OR CELLULITIS W CC	2.6298	7.0
575	Yes	No	SKIN GRAFT FOR SKIN ULCER OR CELLULITIS W/O CC/MCC	1.4926	4.2
579	Yes	No	OTHER SKIN, SUBCUT TISS & BREAST PROC W MCC	2.7263	6.9
580	Yes	No	OTHER SKIN, SUBCUT TISS & BREAST PROC W CC	1.5727	3.8
581	Yes	No	OTHER SKIN, SUBCUT TISS & BREAST PROC W/O CC/MCC	1.1338	2.0
592	Yes	No	SKIN ULCERS W MCC	1.4249	5.1
593	Yes	No	SKIN ULCERS W CC	1.0196	4.2
594	Yes	No	SKIN ULCERS W/O CC/MCC	0.7124	3.0
602	Yes	No	CELLULITIS W MCC	1.4557	5.0
603	Yes	No	CELLULITIS W/O MCC	0.8447	3.5

Table   (Continued)

MS-DRG	PACT DRG	PACT Special Payment DRG	MS-DRG Title	Relative Weight	Geometric Mean LOS
616	Yes	No	AMPUTAT OF LOWER LIMB FOR ENDOCRINE, NUTRIT, & METABOL DIS W MCC	4.1611	10.7
617	Yes	No	AMPUTAT OF LOWER LIMB FOR ENDOCRINE, NUTRIT, & METABOL DIS W CC	1.9956	6.0
618	Yes	No	AMPUTAT OF LOWER LIMB FOR ENDOCRINE, NUTRIT, & METABOL DIS W/O CC/MCC	1.3512	4.0
622	Yes	No	SKIN GRAFTS & WOUND DEBRID FOR ENDOC, NUTRIT, & METAB DIS W MCC	3.8047	9.1
623	Yes	No	SKIN GRAFTS & WOUND DEBRID FOR ENDOC, NUTRIT, & METAB DIS W CC	1.8308	5.6
624	Yes	No	SKIN GRAFTS & WOUND DEBRID FOR ENDOC, NUTRIT & METAB DIS W/O CC/MCC	1.1314	3.6
628	Yes	No	OTHER ENDOCRINE, NUTRIT & METAB O.R. PROC W MCC	3.2935	6.6
629	Yes	No	OTHER ENDOCRINE, NUTRIT & METAB O.R. PROC W CC	2.2471	6.1
630	Yes	No	OTHER ENDOCRINE, NUTRIT & METAB O.R. PROC W/O CC/MCC	1.4305	3.1
637	Yes	No	DIABETES W MCC	1.3944	4.1
638	Yes	No	DIABETES W CC	0.8261	3.0
639	Yes	No	DIABETES W/O CC/MCC	0.6068	2.2
640	Yes	No	MISC DISORDERS OF NUTRITION, METABOLISM, FLUIDS/ ELECTROLYTES W MCC	1.1044	3.2
641	Yes	No	MISC DISORDERS OF NUTRITION, METABOLISM, FLUIDS/ ELECTROLYTES W/O MCC	0.7051	2.6
643	Yes	No	ENDOCRINE DISORDERS W MCC	1.6460	5.4
644	Yes	No	ENDOCRINE DISORDERS W CC	1.0199	3.8
645	Yes	No	ENDOCRINE DISORDERS W/O CC/MCC	0.7180	2.7
653	Yes	No	MAJOR BLADDER PROCEDURES W MCC	5.7958	12.1
654	Yes	No	MAJOR BLADDER PROCEDURES W CC	3.0973	7.6
655	Yes	No	MAJOR BLADDER PROCEDURES W/O CC/MCC	2.2590	4.8
659	Yes	No	KIDNEY & URETER PROCEDURES FOR NON-NEOPLASM W MCC	3.3813	7.5
660	Yes	No	KIDNEY & URETER PROCEDURES FOR NON-NEOPLASM W CC	1.8888	4.1
661	Yes	No	KIDNEY & URETER PROCEDURES FOR NON-NEOPLASM W/O CC/MCC	1.3494	2.2

(Continued on next page)

Table   (Continued)

MS-DRG	PACT DRG	PACT Special Payment DRG	MS-DRG Title	Relative Weight	Geometric Mean LOS
682	Yes	No	RENAL FAILURE W MCC	1.5194	4.6
683	Yes	No	RENAL FAILURE W CC	0.9512	3.5
684	Yes	No	RENAL FAILURE W/O CC/MCC	0.6085	2.4
689	Yes	No	KIDNEY & URINARY TRACT INFECTIONS W MCC	1.1172	4.2
690	Yes	No	KIDNEY & URINARY TRACT INFECTIONS W/O MCC	0.7794	3.1
698	Yes	No	OTHER KIDNEY & URINARY TRACT DIAGNOSES W MCC	1.5625	5.1
699	Yes	No	OTHER KIDNEY & URINARY TRACT DIAGNOSES W CC	1.0170	3.5
700	Yes	No	OTHER KIDNEY & URINARY TRACT DIAGNOSES W/O CC/MCC	0.7110	2.6
840	Yes	No	LYMPHOMA & NON-ACUTE LEUKEMIA W MCC	3.1058	7.6
841	Yes	No	LYMPHOMA & NON-ACUTE LEUKEMIA W CC	1.6226	4.7
842	Yes	No	LYMPHOMA & NON-ACUTE LEUKEMIA W/O CC/MCC	1.0777	2.9
853	Yes	No	INFECTIOUS & PARASITIC DISEASES W O.R. PROCEDURE W MCC	5.2068	10.8
854	Yes	No	INFECTIOUS & PARASITIC DISEASES W O.R. PROCEDURE W CC	2.3877	6.7
855	Yes	No	INFECTIOUS & PARASITIC DISEASES W O.R. PROCEDURE W/O CC/MCC	1.7057	3.3
856	Yes	No	POSTOPERATIVE OR POST-TRAUMATIC INFECTIONS W O.R. PROC W MCC	4.8177	10.0
857	Yes	No	POSTOPERATIVE OR POST-TRAUMATIC INFECTIONS W O.R. PROC W CC	2.0500	5.6
858	Yes	No	POSTOPERATIVE OR POST-TRAUMATIC INFECTIONS W O.R. PROC W/O CC/MCC	1.3390	3.7
862	Yes	No	POSTOPERATIVE & POST-TRAUMATIC INFECTIONS W MCC	1.8506	5.5
863	Yes	No	POSTOPERATIVE & POST-TRAUMATIC INFECTIONS W/O MCC	0.9836	3.7
867	Yes	No	OTHER INFECTIOUS & PARASITIC DISEASES DIAGNOSES W MCC	2.7245	7.0
868	Yes	No	OTHER INFECTIOUS & PARASITIC DISEASES DIAGNOSES W CC	1.0897	3.9
869	Yes	No	OTHER INFECTIOUS & PARASITIC DISEASES DIAGNOSES W/O CC/MCC	0.6877	2.7
870	Yes	No	SEPTICEMIA OR SEVERE SEPSIS W MV 96+ HOURS	5.8698	12.6

Table   (Continued)

MS-DRG	PACT DRG	PACT Special Payment DRG	MS-DRG Title	Relative Weight	Geometric Mean LOS
871	Yes	No	SEPTICEMIA OR SEVERE SEPSIS W/O MV 96+ HOURS W MCC	1.8072	5.1
872	Yes	No	SEPTICEMIA OR SEVERE SEPSIS W/O MV 96+ HOURS W/O MCC	1.0528	4.0
884	Yes	No	ORGANIC DISTURBANCES & MENTAL RETARDATION	1.0783	4.1
896	Yes	No	ALCOHOL/DRUG ABUSE OR DEPENDENCE W/O REHABILITATION THERAPY W MCC	1.5244	4.7
897	Yes	No	ALCOHOL/DRUG ABUSE OR DEPENDENCE W/O REHABILITATION THERAPY W/O MCC	0.6905	3.2
907	Yes	No	OTHER O.R. PROCEDURES FOR INJURIES W MCC	3.7873	7.4
908	Yes	No	OTHER O.R. PROCEDURES FOR INJURIES W CC	1.9575	4.2
909	Yes	No	OTHER O.R. PROCEDURES FOR INJURIES W/O CC/MCC	1.2556	2.5
917	Yes	No	POISONING & TOXIC EFFECTS OF DRUGS W MCC	1.4051	3.4
918	Yes	No	POISONING & TOXIC EFFECTS OF DRUGS W/O MCC	0.6412	2.1
945	Yes	No	REHABILITATION W CC/MCC	1.2709	8.5
946	Yes	No	REHABILITATION W/O CC/MCC	1.0662	6.5
947	Yes	No	SIGNS & SYMPTOMS W MCC	1.1368	3.5
948	Yes	No	SIGNS & SYMPTOMS W/O MCC	0.7131	2.6
956	Yes	No	LIMB REATTACHMENT, HIP & FEMUR PROC FOR MULTIPLE SIGNIFICANT TRAUMA	3.6692	6.6
981	Yes	No	EXTENSIVE O.R. PROCEDURE UNRELATED TO PRINCIPAL DIAGNOSIS W MCC	4.9968	9.9
982	Yes	No	EXTENSIVE O.R. PROCEDURE UNRELATED TO PRINCIPAL DIAGNOSIS W CC	2.8150	5.7
983	Yes	No	EXTENSIVE O.R. PROCEDURE UNRELATED TO PRINCIPAL DIAGNOSIS W/O CC/MCC	1.8039	2.7
987	Yes	No	NON-EXTENSIVE O.R. PROC UNRELATED TO PRINCIPAL DIAGNOSIS W MCC	3.3008	8.3
988	Yes	No	NON-EXTENSIVE O.R. PROC UNRELATED TO PRINCIPAL DIAGNOSIS W CC	1.7643	4.7
989	Yes	No	NON-EXTENSIVE O.R. PROC UNRELATED TO PRINCIPAL DIAGNOSIS W/O CC/MCC	1.0454	2.2

Chapter 7
Ambulatory and Other Medicare-Medicaid Reimbursement Systems

Objectives

- To differentiate major types of Medicare and Medicaid reimbursement systems for beneficiaries

- To define basic language associated with reimbursement under Medicare and Medicaid healthcare payment systems

- To explain common models and policies of payment for Medicare and Medicaid healthcare payment systems for physicians and outpatient settings

- To identify the elements of the relative value unit and the major components of the resource-based relative value scale payment system.

- To describe the elements of the ambulance fee schedule.

- To explain the elements of the outpatient prospective payment system and the ambulatory surgical center payment system

- To describe the end-stage renal disease prospective payment system

- To describe the elements of the payment systems for federally qualified health centers and rural health clinics.

- To explain the elements of the hospice services payment system

Key Terms

All-inclusive rate (AIR)
Ambulatory payment classification (APC)
Ambulatory surgical center (ASC)
Ambulatory surgery center list of covered procedures (ASC list)
Assignment of benefits
Budget neutrality (budget-neutral)
Budget neutrality adjustor (BN adjustor)
Bundling
Calendar year (CY)
Carrier
Conversion factor (CF)
Critical care services
Discounted fee-for-service
Electronic prescribing (e-prescribing or eRx)
Electronic Prescribing (E-Prescribing) Incentive Program

Eligible professional (EP)
Episode of care
Federally qualified health center (FQHC)
Federally qualified health center prospective payment system (FQHC PPS)
Geographic practice cost index (GPCI)
Hold-harmless status
Hospice
Locality
Malpractice (MP)
Market basket
Medicare physician (provider) fee schedule (MPFS)
National unadjusted payment
Nonparticipating physician
Observation
Packaging
Palliative care

Partial hospitalization
Participating physician (PAR)
Pass-through
Payment status indicator
Physician (provider) fee schedule (PFS)
Physician Quality Reporting System (PQRS)
Physician work (WORK)
Practice expense (PE)
Professional liability insurance (PLI)
Relative value scale
Relative value unit (RVU)

Resource-based relative value scale (RBRVS)
Respite care
Revenue code
Rural area
Rural health clinic (RHC)
Safety-net provider
Sliding scale
Sustainable growth rate (SGR) system
Underserved area
Urban area

Introduction to Reimbursement Systems for Physicians and Ambulatory Settings

The first prospective payment system (PPS), the acute-care PPS, was a successful initiative for Medicare reimbursement reform. However, as the rate of growth of Medicare inpatient payments was effectively curbed, the rate of growth of Medicare payments for ambulatory patients and to physicians escalated sharply. For example, in the 1980s, the average rate of growth for Medicare spending on physicians grew at an average rate of more than 12 percent (Scanlon 2002, 2). Thus, Congress authorized the Department of Health and Human Services (HHS) to develop and implement reformed fee systems and PPSs across the continuum of care for Medicare beneficiaries. These payment systems include the resource-based relative value scale (RBRVS) for physician services, the ambulance fee schedule, the hospital outpatient payment system, the ambulatory surgical center (ASC) payment system, the end-stage renal disease payment system, safety-net provider payments, and the hospice services payment system.

Resource-Based Relative Value Scale for Physician and Professional Payments

A **resource-based relative value scale (RBRVS)** is a system of classifying health services based on the cost of furnishing physician services in different settings, the skill and training levels required to perform the services, and the time and risk involved. The **relative value scale** permits comparisons of the resources needed or appropriate prices for various units of service. It takes into account labor, skill, supplies, equipment, space, and other costs for each procedure or service. The RBRVS is the federal government's payment system for physicians and some other health professionals. For health personnel, it is important to understand the RBRVS because 77 percent of public and private payers, including Medicaid, have adopted its various components (American Academy of Pediatrics 2014, 1).

Background

The services of physicians and other health professionals to Medicare beneficiaries are covered under Part B Medicare. These services include office visits, diagnostic and surgical procedures, and other therapies. These services may be delivered in a wide range of settings, such as in offices, ambulatory surgery centers, inpatient acute-care hospitals, outpatient dialysis facilities, skilled nursing facilities, and hospice.

Providers of these services are physicians and other health professionals, such as audiologists, chiropractors, clinical social workers, optometrists, podiatrists, psychologists, nurse midwives, nurse practitioners, nutritionists, physician assistants, physical and occupational therapists, and speech-language pathologists. Approximately half of the clinicians in Medicare's registry are physicians; the remainder are health professionals practicing either independently or under the supervision of a physician (Medicare Payment Advisory Commission [MedPAC] 2014a, 1). In this chapter about payments to physicians and other health professionals, the term *physician* includes the other health professionals. Any differences in the payment system based on type of profession are noted when needed.

Medicare beneficiaries pay premiums and have cost-sharing for these professional services. Cost sharing includes annual deductibles, coinsurance for medical and health services, and co-payments for prescription drugs (see chapter 4).

In 1985, under a grant from the Centers for Medicare and Medicaid Services (CMS) (formerly the Health Care Financing Administration [HCFA]), Dr. William Hsiao of Harvard University devised a system of classifying health services using resource-based relative values. Congress authorized the implementation of the RBRVS in the Omnibus Budget Reconciliation Acts (OBRA) of 1989 and 1990. The RBRVS became effective January 1, 1992. The RBRVS is a fee-for-service system of payment; however, the reimbursement is based on Centers for Medicare and Medicaid Services' (CMS's) estimation of the value of a physician's service. The fees in the payment system are based on the CMS's estimation of the value of a physician's service. While the fees are predetermined, the RBRVS is *not* a prospective payment system. A physician and other health professionals can increase reimbursements by increasing the volume of services provided to a patient.

Structure of Payment

Payments to physicians are based on three components: a relative value unit (RVU), its geographic adjustment, and a conversion factor (CF). These basic components may be further adjusted for provider characteristics, additional geographic considerations, and other factors (figure 7.1).

Relative Value Unit and Geographic Practice Cost Index

The RBRVS is based on the Healthcare Common Procedure Coding System (HCPCS, including Current Procedural Terminology [CPT], Level I codes). Each HCPCS/CPT code has been assigned an RVU (see chapter 2). A **relative value unit (RVU)** is a unit of measure designed to permit comparison of the amounts of resources required to perform various provider services by assigning weights to such factors as personnel time, level of skill, and sophistication of equipment required to render service.

Each RVU is subdivided into three elements. Each element has a unique weight. The weights of these three elements are summed to calculate the total RVU weight:

- Physician work (WORK)

- Physician practice expense (PE)

- Professional liability insurance (PLI) or Malpractice (MP)

Figure 7.1. Foundation of resource-based relative value scale payment system

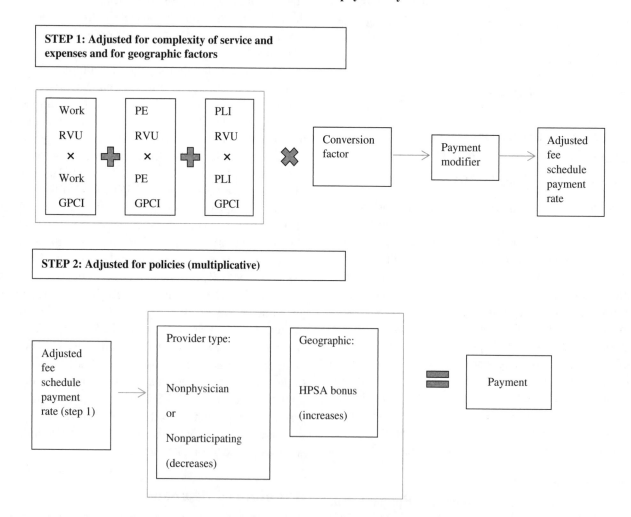

Source: Adapted from Medicare Payment Advisory Commission (MedPAC). 2014a. Payment basics: Physician and other health professional payment system. Pg. 2. http://www.medpac.gov.

National averages for these three elements are available on the CMS website.

Physician work (WORK) is the element that covers the physician's salary. This work is the time the physician spends providing a service and the intensity with which that time is spent. The four aspects of intensity are

- Mental effort and judgment

- Technical skill

- Physical effort

- Psychological stress

Professional **practice expense (PE)** is the overhead costs of the practice. CMS conducts a survey entitled the Socioeconomic Monitoring System (SMS) to obtain data to calculate the overhead costs of a practice. The SMS includes six categories of PE costs:

- Clinical payroll (including fringe benefits) for nonphysician clinical personnel (such as physician assistants, nurse practitioners, among others)

- Administrative payroll (including fringe benefits) for nonphysician administrative personnel (for example, administrators, secretaries, and clerks)

- Office expenses for rent, mortgage interest, depreciation on medical buildings, utilities, telephones, and other related costs

- Medical material and supply expenses for drugs, x-ray films, disposable medical products, and other related costs

- Medical equipment expenses, including depreciation, leases, and rentals for medical equipment used in the diagnosis or treatment of patients

- All other expenses, such as legal services, accounting, office management, professional association memberships, and any professional expenses

PE is categorized as either facility or nonfacility (table 7.1). According to CMS experts, practice expenses differ for physicians when they perform services in facilities, such as hospitals, than when they

Table 7.1. Facility and nonfacility settings for physician practice expenses (PE)

Facility	Nonfacility
Ambulance (land, air, or water)	Clinic
Ambulatory surgical center	Dialysis center
Community mental health center	Independent laboratory
Comprehensive inpatient rehabilitation facility	Nonskilled nursing facility
Emergency department	Patient's home
Inpatient hospital setting	Physician's office
Inpatient psychiatric facility	All other settings
Military treatment facility	
Outpatient hospital setting	
Psychiatric facility partial hospital	
Psychiatric resort treatment center	
Skilled nursing facility	

perform services in nonfacilities, such as their own offices and clinics.

- Facilities: Organization incurs the overhead costs of personnel, supplies, and equipment, among other costs.

- Nonfacilities: Physician incurs the overhead costs of personnel, supplies, and equipment, among other costs.

Thus, the PE is generally higher for nonfacilities than for facilities because the physician in nonfacilities is incurring more costs. Some procedural codes do not have separate facility and nonfacility PEs. In these procedural codes, the description includes the setting (evaluation and management, initial hospital care), or the nature of the procedure restricts it to a particular site (major surgical procedures in hospitals).

Physicians can provide services in these multiple settings. Factors in choice of setting include the following (MedPAC 2004, 19):

- Patient's medical condition

- Type of procedure

- Patient's preference

- Geographic location

- Technology

- Regulation or healthcare insurance policies

The final decision of setting is a blend of the factors.

Professional liability insurance (PLI) or **Malpractice (MP)** is the cost of the premiums for malpractice (MP) or professional liability insurance (PLI). CMS bases the MP element of the RVU on the premiums for malpractice insurance. CMS collects data from both commercial and physician-owned malpractice insurance carriers from all 50 states, the District of Columbia, and Puerto Rico. Because the services of nonphysicians may also be reimbursed under the RBRVS, this element may also be called PLI.

RVUs are routinely maintained to keep them up-to-date. Annually, as new health services are implemented or existing health services are revised, the Relative Value Scale Update Committee (RUC) of the American Medical Association makes recommendations to the CMS on appropriate RVUs for these health services. In addition, CMS analysts must review the RVUs at least every five years to ensure the accuracy of the weights. The update includes a review of changes in medical practice, coding changes, and new data (MedPAC 2014a, 3).

Each of the three elements is adjusted to local costs through the **geographic practice cost indexes (GPCIs)**. A geographic adjustment is necessary because costs vary in different areas of the country. To reflect local costs, CMS defines about 90 payment areas, known as **localities**. Localities reflect differences in the cost of resources (HHS 2013, 74230). Localities can be large metropolitan areas, such as Boston or San Francisco, portions of states ("rest-of-state areas"), or entire states. The GPCI for the locality is based on relative variations in the cost of a **market basket** of goods across different geographic areas. In that way, different localities have GPCIs that match the costs in that geographic area. Each element of the RVU—WORK, PE, and MP—has its own unique GPCI. The GPCIs can be found on the CMS website. Through the GPCIs, each element of an RVU is adjusted for the geographic cost differences.

Conversion Factor

The **conversion factor (CF)** is an across-the-board multiplier. Unlike the GPCIs, the CF is a constant that applies to the entire RVU. The CF transforms the geographic-adjusted RVU into a **Medicare physician (provider) fee schedule (MPFS** or simply **PFS)** payment amount. The CF is the government's most direct control on Medicare payments to physicians and other professionals. CMS raises or lowers the CF to raise or lower physician and professional payments. CMS updates the CF annually and publishes the amount in the *Federal Register* (table 7.2).

The amount of the update is calculated using a formula known as the **sustainable growth rate (SGR) system**. The SGR formula is used because the RBRVS is a fee-for-service system. Therefore, the RBRVS is susceptible to increases solely based on falsely inflated volumes (see the chapter 1 discussion of fee-for-service reimbursement). The purpose of the SGR is to match updates in physician reimbursement to growth in the national economy. Thus, growth in federal spending on physician reimbursement does not exceed growth in the economy.

CMS estimates the growth of the national economy to create a target for Medicare spending on physician services. The SGR formula is CMS's way of creating the target. The SGR formula sets the yearly targets for controlled growth in aggregate Medicare expenditures for physicians' services. The SGR formula takes into account changes in physicians' fees for services, number of beneficiaries enrolled in fee-for-service Medicare, the 10-year average change in the gross domestic product (economic growth), and differences in expenditures because of laws or regulations (MedPAC 2014b, 97). Updates in the CF are intended to keep the growth in spending within the target. Therefore, based on the SGR formula, CMS has proposed negative updates. A negative update sets the CF to *less* than the previous year's value. However, for several years, through specific legislation, Congress has overridden CMS's proposals and set its own updated CF. Thus, Congress averted the

Table 7.2.   Conversion factors over time

2004	2006	2008	2010	2012	2014
$37.3374	$37.8975	$38.0870	$36.8729	$34.0376	$35.8228

Conversion factors have four decimal places rather than two decimal places.
Source: CMS 2015.

formula's negative updates in the CF. Consequently, for several years, MedPAC has recommended that the SGR be repealed (MedPAC 2014b, xv). The outcome of this ongoing issue is a critical concern to providers reimbursed under the RBRVS.

Calculation

Medicare reimbursements under the RBRVS are on the MPFS. The MPFS is the maximum amount of reimbursement that Medicare will allow for a service. The MPFS consists of a list of payments (fees) for services in HCPCS. The MPFS is calculated by the following formula:

$$[(\text{WORK RVU})(\text{WORK GPCI}) + (\text{PE RVU})(\text{PE GPCI}) + (\text{MP RVU})(\text{MP GPCI})] = (\text{SUM}) \times \text{CF} = \text{MPFS}$$

Figure 7.1 shows the calculations of the general RBRVS formula, and table 7.3 shows the formula in action for a sample CPT/HCPCS code. Reimbursement specialists should understand the generic formula to determine how proposed changes in components of the formula will affect the revenues of their healthcare entity.

Finally, as previously stated, for covered services, the actual Medicare beneficiary is responsible for an annual deductible and a 20 percent coinsurance (see chapter 4). After the beneficiary has met the deductible, the provider receives 80 percent of the PFS amount.

Potential Adjustments

Reimbursement under the RBRVS may be adjusted for various reasons, such as requirements for budget neutrality, the type of clinician providing the service, special circumstances, additional geographic considerations, and other factors.

Budget Neutrality

A provision of Section 1848 in the law establishing the RBRVS stipulates that refinements to RVUs must maintain **budget neutrality**. Budget neutrality requires that refinements to federal payment systems do not result in significant differences in expenditures. Generally, upcoming expenditures must equal past expenditures, accounting for inflation. Specifically, for refinements to the RVUs, payments for physicians' services cannot differ by more than $20 million (HHS 2014c, 67550). Thus, a **budget neutrality (BN) adjustor** may be applied to a component of the generic formula to maintain budget neutrality. An adjustor is not applied every year, and the exact procedures and amount have varied in the years when an adjustor was applied. Thus, reimbursement specialists should be aware of the BN adjustor, be familiar with its functioning, and recognize the importance of monitoring the *Federal Register*.

Clinician Type

Medicare's reimbursement may be adjusted by the type or characteristics of the provider. Three types of providers for whom the RBRVS payment system makes adjustments are participating and nonparticipating physicians, anesthesiologists, and nonphysician providers (NPPs).

Participating Physician versus Nonparticipating Physician

Physicians may participate in Medicare (**participating physicians**) or they can opt out of participation

Table 7.3. Example of calculation of nonfacility payment under resource-based relative value scale

Element	RVU	GPCI*	Geographic adjustment (RVU × GPCI)*	Adjusted payment [Adjusted RVU × Conversion factor ($35.8228)]
CPT code = 99202 (Office visit, new patient, expanded problem-focused)				
Work value (WORK)	0.93	1.00	0.93	
Practice expense (PE)	1.08	0.925	1.00322	
Malpractice (MP)	0.07	0.634	0.05124	
Sum			1.98456	
Adjusted allowance				$71.09

*North Carolina payment locality (1150200).
Data source: Centers for Medicare and Medicaid Services. 2014a. Physician Fee Schedule Search. http://www.cms.hhs.gov/pfslookup/.

(**nonparticipating physicians**). Participating physicians have signed a contract with Medicare to accept an **assignment of benefits**. Assignment of benefits is a contract between a physician and Medicare in which the physician agrees to bill Medicare directly for covered services, to bill the beneficiary only for any coinsurance or deductible that may be applicable, and to accept the Medicare payment as payment in full. Medicare pays the physician directly rather than sending the check to the Medicare beneficiary. Physicians who do not accept assignment are nonparticipating physicians. Medicare payments to nonparticipating physicians are reduced by 5 percent (95 percent of what a participating physician receives).

Anesthesiologists

Anesthesia services have a separate payment method. The following elements are used to calculate a payment for anesthesia services:

- Base units for anesthesia services from a uniform relative value guide based on anesthesia CPT codes (RVUs)

- Base units for CPT anesthesia codes range from 3 (anesthesia services for needle biopsy of thyroid) to 30 (anesthesia services for liver transplant)

- Time units in 15-minute intervals (personal performance of anesthesia services) or in 30-minute intervals (medically directing the performance of others, such as certified nurse anesthetists) and reduced for the number of concurrent procedures

- Separate CF adjusted for locality (because there is no GPCI) (table 7.4)

The generic formula is

[Base Unit + Time (in units)] × CF = MPFS

Nonphysician Providers

Providers of covered Medicare services practicing within their scope of practice and within state laws may receive payment under the RBRVS. NPPs reimbursed under the RBRVS include audiologists; certified nurse midwives; certified registered nurse anesthetists; clinical nurse specialists; clinical psychologists;

Table 7.4. Anesthesia services: Representative conversion factors over time by locality in dollars

	2010	2012	2014
Montana	20.91	21.71	22.99
Manhattan, NY	23.40	23.56	25.21
Rest of New York	20.62	20.50	21.84

clinical social workers; nurse practitioners; physician assistants; registered dieticians; occupational, physical, and speech therapists; and others. For the purposes of Medicare payment, these NPPs generally receive 85 percent of the full MPFS amount. NPPs may only submit claims for reimbursement when their services are neither "incidental to" nor under the direct supervision of a physician. If the services are "incidental to" or under the physician's direct supervision, Medicare pays the full MPFS amount to the physician.

Special Circumstances

Medicare can adjust payments for special circumstances through the use of modifiers. Sometimes services or procedures are altered some way (see chapter 2). Modifiers provide information about this alteration so that Medicare and other payers can process the claim. Following are examples (MedPAC 2014a, 2):

- Bilateral procedures. For bilateral procedures, Medicare will pay the lower of (a) the total actual charge for both sides or (b) 150 percent of the PFS amount for the single code.

- Multiple procedures. When multiple procedures are performed on the same day, Medicare reimburses the physician for the first procedure at 100 percent; subsequent procedures through the fifth procedure are reimbursed at 50 percent (sixth and more require review).

- Physicians assisting in surgery. When physicians assist in surgery, they are reimbursed at 16 percent of the PFS amount for the primary surgeon.

Other common modifiers represent preoperative or postoperative management only or surgery only.

Underserved Area

Through the RBRVS payment system, CMS provides an incentive for physicians to render services in underserved areas. The purpose of the incentive is to attract physicians to these areas (MedPAC 2014a, 3). CMS makes bonus payments to physicians who render medical care services in underserved areas.

The US Health Resources and Services Administration (HRSA) designates certain geographic areas as health professional shortage areas (HPSAs). These areas have a shortage of providers in medical care, dental, or mental health or some combination of these.

Eligibility for the bonus depends on the location where the service is rendered. The service must be rendered in a HPSA. Eligibility is *not* based on the address of the beneficiary or the address of the physician's office. In addition, psychiatrists who render services in mental health HPSAs are also eligible to receive bonus payments. Moreover, to be considered for the bonus payment, physicians and psychiatrists must include the name, address, and zip code of the location where the service was rendered on all electronic and paper claim submissions. In some instances, zip code areas do not fall entirely within a full- or partial-county HPSA. In such instances, physicians and psychiatrists must enter the AQ modifier on their claims to receive the bonus. Quarterly, physicians who render services in these areas receive a 10 percent bonus. The CMS website has information about the HPSAs and about the zip codes that qualify for the bonus (CMS 2014d).

Quality

The Tax Relief and Health Care Act (TRHCA) of 2006 (P.L. 109-432) required the establishment of a system to report physician quality. This system is the **Physician Quality Reporting System (PQRS)**. Although participation in the PQRS is voluntary, **eligible professionals (EPs)**, such as physicians, practitioners, and therapists, who do not satisfactorily report quality data under the PQRS are subject to a two percent reduction in their MPFS (CMS 2011b, 3). The PQRS is only one component of a much broader and more influential federal initiative called value-based purchasing. Chapter 10 explains the CMS's vision and comprehensive framework for value-based purchasing that spans its multiple payment systems.

Technology

The federal government encourages the use of technology through the use of penalties. CMS reduces the payments of EPs who do not successfully use technology. Medicare has two programs:

- **Electronic Prescribing (e-Prescribing or eRx) Incentive Program**: The eRx Incentive Program was authorized by Section 132 of the Medicare Improvements for Patients and Providers Act (MIPPA) of 2008. This incentive program is for EPs who successfully use electronic prescribing (e-prescribing or eRx) systems as defined by MIPPA. Payments of unsuccessful EPs are negatively adjusted by 2.0 percent, although "hardship" exceptions exist (CMS 2011b, 3).

- Electronic Health Record (EHR) Incentive Program: The EHR Incentive Program was authorized by the American Recovery and Reinvestment Act (ARRA) of 2009 under the Health Information Technology for Economic and Clinical Health (HITECH) Act. Payments of EPs who cannot demonstrate meaningful use are progressively negatively adjusted from by 2.0 percent to 5.0 between 2016 and 2020 and from 3.0 percent to 5.0 after 2020 (CMS 2014c, 1-2).

The EP's services must be paid under the MPFS and not under some other fee schedule or reimbursement method.

Operational Issues

Many physician offices in the United States are solo or two-person practices (Morra et al. 2011, 1443). Close management of operations is critical in these small offices, which have little margin. Two important issues are processes to ensure full, accurate reimbursement and the impact of unnecessary administrative costs.

Coding and Documentation

Poor coding and inadequate documentation negatively affect RBRVS reimbursement. For example, overlooking the removal of a polyp or lesion during an esophagoscopy can significantly reduce payment (table 7.5).

Table 7.5.   Comparison of impact of coding on nonfacility reimbursement under resource-based relative value scale*

	CPT 43200, Esophagoscopy			CPT 43217, Esophagoscopy, with removal of tumor(s), polyp(s), or other lesion(s) by snare technique		
	RVU ×	GPCI*	=	RVU ×	GPCI	=
Work value (WORK)	1.50	1.000	1.50	2.9	1.000	2.9
Practice expense (PE)	5.96	0.929	5.53684	9.36	0.929	8.69544
Malpractice (MP)	0.21	0.732	0.15372	0.47	0.732	0.34404
Sum			7.19056			11.93948
× Conversion factor			$35.8228			$35.8228
Total			$257.29			$427.71
Loss because of incomplete coding			$170.12			

*North Carolina payment locality (1150200).

Based on Centers for Medicare and Medicaid Services. 2014. Physician fee schedule search. Medicare physician fee schedule. http://www.cms.hhs.gov/pfslookup/.

Other examples illustrate the difference documentation and accurate coding make (tables 7.6 and 7.7). The column Lost Payment in table 7.6 shows the effects of inadequate documentation or inaccurate coding or both. Table 7.7 shows the effect on fees of the accurate selection of the site: nonfacility versus facility.

Unnecessary Administrative Costs

Time spent on administrative details is adding unnecessary costs to the US healthcare delivery system. An Institute of Medicine (IOM) report estimated that excess administrative costs totaled $190 billion in 2009 (2013, 13). These costs were related to extra paperwork, insurers' administrative inefficiencies, and inefficiencies arising from required care documentation of care (IOM 2013, 13).

One example of administrative waste is time spent in dealing with multiple health plans (Morra et al. 2011, 1443). Physician practices must contact multiple health plans for prior authorizations, billing requirements, claim submission and adjudication procedures, and formularies. Furthermore, each health plan has its own unique policies and rules with which the physician practices must be familiar. One study assessed the potential time savings that could be accrued from reduced interactions with health plans (Morra et al. 2011, 1443). The study compared the time that Canadian physician practices spent interacting with the *single payer* in Ontario, Canada, with the time that US physician practices spent interacting with *multiple payers*. The

study captured data on four roles in the two sets of physician practices: physicians, nurses, clerical staff, and senior administrators (Morra et al. 2011, 1446).

- Ontario, Canada, physicians spent 2.2 hours per week, whereas US physicians spent 3.4 hours per week.

- Ontario, Canada, nurses spent 2.5 hours per week, whereas US nurses spent 20.6 hours per week.

- Ontario, Canada, clerical staff spent 15.9 hours per week, whereas US clerical staff spent 53.1 hours per week.

- Ontario, Canada, senior administrators spent 24.6 hours per year, whereas US senior administrators spent 163.2 hours per year.

The researchers noted that much of the time differential was related to obtaining prior authorizations and to billing (Morra et al. 2011, 1446). When time is converted into dollars (adjusted for exchange rate), US physician practices spent four times as much money interacting with health plans as Ontario physician practices (Morra et al. 2011, 1445). In terms of the entire healthcare delivery system, if US physician practices had costs similar to the Ontario practices, total savings would be approximately $27.6 billion per year (Morra et al. 2011, 1446). Widespread agreement exists that these interactions could be more

Table 7.6. Examples of lost nonfacility revenue from poor coding or inadequate documentation under resource-based relative value scale*

Careless Coding or Incomplete Documentation			Accurate Coding with Complete Documentation			Lost Payment
Code	**Description**	**$**	**Code**	**Description**	**$**	**$**
10060	Incision and drainage of abscess; simple or single	$110.48	10061	Incision and drainage of abscess; complicated or multiple	$196.54	$86.92
11400	Excision benign lesion; excised diameter 0.5 cm or less	$115.43	11406	Excision benign lesion; excised diameter more than 4.0 cm	$295.96	$180.63
19100	Biopsy of breast; percutaneous, needle core, not using imaging guidance	$141.90	19101	Biopsy of breast; open, incisional	$320.85	$178.95
45378	Colonoscopy	$372.50	45382	Colonoscopy with control of bleeding	$576.55	$204.05

*North Carolina payment locality (1150200).

Source: Based on Centers for Medicare and Medicaid Services. 2014a. Physician fee schedule search. Medicare physician fee schedule. http://www.cms.hhs.gov/pfslookup/.

Table 7.7. Selected codes: Comparison of Medicare allowables by category of site and by selected years

Code	Description	2009		2014	
		Nonfacility Fee, $*	Facility Fee, $*	Nonfacility Fee, $*	Facility Fee, $*
99202	Office/outpatient visit, new patient	60.57	43.56	71.09	48.80
99211	Office/outpatient visit, established patient	17.70	8.36	19.02	9.04
99213	Office/outpatient visit, established patient	58.89	43.54	69.86	49.90
33533	Coronary artery bypass, using arterial graft; single	NA	1,793.29	NA	1,848.06
43239	Upper gastrointestinal endoscopy, biopsy	304.37	158.58	380.61	145.32
66984	Extracapsular cataract removal with insertion of intraocular lens prosthesis (one-stage procedure)	NA	614.76	NA	637.96
71020	Chest x-ray	29.43	NA	29.37	NA
93000	Electrocardiogram, routine ECG with at least 12 leads; with interpretation and report	19.49	NA	15.93	NA

*North Carolina payment locality (1150200).

Based on Centers for Medicare and Medicaid Services. 2009a and 2014a. Physician fee schedule search. http://www.cms.hhs.gov/pfslookup/.

efficient than they currently are (Morra et al. 2011, 1447). Efficiency has the potential to reduce these unnecessary costs.

Check Your Understanding 7.1

1. What is the name of the researcher who developed a system of classifying health services using resource-based relative values? With which university is this researcher associated?

2. In the RBRVS, what is another term for the element that represents the cost of malpractice insurance?

3. In the RBRVS, what is the term for the across-the-board multiplier that transforms the geographically adjusted RVU into an MPFS payment amount?

4. What does GPCI stand for?

5. True or false? Payments under the RBRVS are unaffected by the clinician's type.

Ambulance Fee Schedule

Section 1861(s)(7) of the Social Security Act under Medicare Part B provides beneficiary coverage for ambulance services. The benefit is intended to provide transportation services only if other means are inadvisable based on the beneficiary's medical condition. Transportation services are provided to the nearest facility able to provide services for the patient's condition. Beneficiaries may be transported from one hospital to another, to home, or to an extended-care facility (HHS 2002, 9100). There are two types of entities that provide ambulance services; providers and suppliers. Providers are ambulance service entities associated with a medical facility such as a hospital, critical access hospital (CAH), skilled nursing facility, or home health agency.

Suppliers are ambulance service entities not associated with any medical facility.

The Balanced Budget Act (BBA) of 1997 added a new section, 1834(l), to the act. The section required the creation of a fee schedule to establish prospective payment rates for ambulance services. The implementation date for the ambulance fee schedule was April 1, 2002.

Reimbursement for Ambulance Services

Reimbursement for ambulance services is based on the level of service provided to the beneficiary. The seven levels of service are defined in table 7.8. Each level specifies the EMT skill set necessary to provide services and care. The EMT skill sets are based on the National Emergency Medical Services Education and Practice Blueprint (table 7.9).

The fee schedule consists of two types of transports (ground and air) and is divided into nine payment levels as shown in table 7.10. It is important to note that ground transports and air transports have different conversion factors, as shown in table 7.10.

Nonemergency Transport

Medical necessity must be established for nonemergency transport provided to Medicare beneficiaries. There are two categories of nonemergency transport: repetitive and nonrepetitive. For repetitive nonemergency transports, the ambulance provider or supplier may attain physician certification in advance for the transportation service. The certification should be obtained no earlier than 60 days before transport.

Table 7.8.   Levels of ambulance services

Service	Acronym	Description
Basic Life Support	BLS	Service level of an Emergency Medical Technician (EMT)-Basic, including the establishment of a peripheral intravenous line.
Advanced Life Support, Level 1	ALS1	In emergency cases, an assessment provided by an EMT-Intermediate or Paramedic (ALS crew) to determine patient needs and the furnishing of one or more ALS interventions. An ALS intervention is a procedure beyond the scope of an EMT-Basic.
Advanced Life Support, Level 2	ALS2	The administration of at least three different medications or the provision of one or more ALS procedures.
Specialty Care Transport	SCT	For critically injured or ill patient, the level of interhospital service furnished is beyond the scope of a paramedic. Ongoing care must be furnished by one or more health professionals in an appropriate specialty area.
Paramedic ALS Intercept	PI	ALS services furnished by an entity that does not provide the ambulance transport.
Fixed Wing Air Ambulance	FW	Destination is inaccessible by land vehicle or great distances or other obstacles (heavy traffic) and the patient's condition is not appropriate for BLS or ALS ground transportation.
Rotary Wing Air Ambulance	RW	Helicopter transport. Destination is inaccessible by land vehicle or great distances or other obstacles (heavy traffic) and the patient's condition is not appropriate for BLS or ALS ground transportation.

Source: Department of Health and Human Services. 2002. *Federal Register* 67(39):9106.

Table 7.9. National Emergency Medical Services (EMS) education and practice blueprint

EMS Provider	Skill Set
First Responder Level	Personnel use a limited amount of equipment to perform initial assessments and interventions.
EMT-Basic	Has the knowledge and skill of the First Responder, but is also qualified to function as the minimum staff for an ambulance.
EMT-Intermediate	Knowledge and skills identified at the First Responder and EMT-Basic levels, but is also qualified to perform essential advanced techniques and to administer a limited number of medications.
EMT-Paramedic	In addition to having competencies of an EMT-Intermediate, has enhanced skills and can administer additional interventions and medications.

Source: Department of Health and Human Services. 2002. *Federal Register* 67(39):9106.

Table 7.10. Ambulance fee schedule payment levels

Ambulance Service Level	Relative Value Units	Conversion Factor
Ground Transports		
BLS nonemergency	1.00	$218.35
BLS emergency	1.60	$218.35
ALS nonemergency	1.20	$218.35
ALS emergency level 1	1.90	$218.35
ALS emergency level 2	2.75	$218.35
Specialty care transport	3.25	$218.35
Paramedic ALS intercept	1.75	$218.35
Air Transports		
Fixed wing	1.00	$2,963.12
Rotary wing	1.00	$3,445.07

Source: Adapted from Medicare Payment Advisory Commission (MedPAC). 2015. Payment Basics: Ambulance Services Payment System. Pg.3. http://www.medpac.gov.

For reimbursement of nonrepetitive nonemergency transports, the ambulance provider or supplier must provide physician certification within 21 days after the service was provided. The physician certification is ideally collected from the attending physician.

However, the certification may be provided by a physician assistant, nurse practitioner, clinical nurse specialist, registered nurse, or discharge planner who is employed by the facility, hospital, or physician. The service provider should have personal knowledge of the beneficiary's case. If the certification cannot be obtained from the physician or other service provider, the ambulance supplier or provider may submit a claim with documentation (that is, a signed return receipt from the US Postal Service or similar delivery service) that shows all the attempts by the ambulance service to obtain certification (HHS 2002, 9111).

Immediate Response Payment

Additional payment is made to ambulance providers and suppliers who furnish immediate response services in emergency situations. An emergency response involves responding immediately at the Basic Life Support (BLS) or Advanced Life Support Level 1 (ALS-1) level of service to a 911 or 911-type call. Immediate response is one in which the ambulance supplier/provider begins as quickly as possible to take the steps necessary to respond to a call (HHS 2002, 9108). The additional payment is provided to compensate those providers/suppliers the extra overhead expenses that are incurred to stay prepared at all times for emergency services. Ambulance suppliers and providers indicate that an emergency response service was provided by selecting the appropriate HCPCS Level II ambulance code (see table 7.11 for examples).

Payment Adjustment for Regional Variations

The ambulance fee schedule provides a payment adjustment to account for regional variations. Based on the point of beneficiary pickup (as indicated by zip code), a geographic adjustment factor is applied. The adjustment factor used for this payment system is equal to the practice expense portion of the GPCI established and maintained for the MPFS. For ground transport services, 70 percent of the payment rate is adjusted by the GPCI. For air ambulance services, 50 percent of the payment rate is adjusted by the GPCI (HHS 2002). Payments for mileage are not adjusted.

Multiple-Patient Transport

An ambulance supplier or provider may encounter a situation in which multiple patients must be transported (for example, in a traffic accident). In these situations,

Table 7.11.   Sample of emergency response HCPCS Level II ambulance codes

HCPCS Code	Description
A0427	Ambulance service, ALS, emergency transport, level 1 (ALS 1—emergency)
A0429	Ambulance service, BLS, emergency transport, (BLS—emergency)

Table 7.12.   Ambulance-specific modifiers

Modifier	Definition
D	Diagnostic or therapeutic site other than "P" or "H" when these are used as origin codes
E	Residential, domiciliary, custodial facility (other than an 1819 facility, SNF)
H	Hospital
I	Site of transfer (for example, airport or helicopter pad) between modes of ambulance transport
J	Non–hospital-based dialysis facility
N	Skilled nursing facility (1819 facility)
P	Physician's office (includes HMO nonhospital facility, clinic, and so on)
R	Residence
S	Scene of accident or acute event
X	Intermediate stop at physician's office en route to the hospital (includes HMO nonhospital facility, clinic, and so on); destination code only

Source: Centers for Medicare and Medicaid Services. 2005. Revisions and corrections to the Medicare Claims Processing Manual, Chapter 6, Section 30 and various sections in Chapter 15. Pub 100-04 Medicare Claims Processing. CMS Transmittal 437. http://www.cms.gov/Regulations-and-Guidance/Guidance/Transmittals/downloads/R437CP.pdf.

CMS prorates the payment rate for the ambulance service for each Medicare beneficiary. If two or more patients are transported, the payment rate for each Medicare beneficiary is 75 percent of the base rate for the level of service provided. If three or more patients are transported, the payment rate for each Medicare beneficiary is 60 percent of the base rate for the level of service provided. A single payment is made for the mileage (HHS 2002, 9113). HCPCS Level II modifier GM, multiple patients on one ambulance trip, must be reported with the ambulance level of service code.

Transport of Deceased Patients

Specific rules exist for transport cases in which a Medicare beneficiary is pronounced dead. When a beneficiary is pronounced dead by an individual who is licensed to pronounce death in that state, the following rules apply (HHS 2002, 9113):

- When a patient is pronounced dead before the ambulance is called, no payment is made to the ambulance supplier/provider.

- When a patient is pronounced dead after the ambulance has been called but before the ambulance arrives, a BLS base rate (for ground transport) or air ambulance base rate payment will be paid. Mileage will not be reimbursed.

- When a patient is pronounced dead during the ambulance transport, payment rules are followed as if the patient were alive.

HCPCS Level II modifier QL, patient pronounced dead after ambulance called, should be reported with the ambulance level of service code.

Use of HCPCS Level II Modifiers

Providers must report HCPCS level II modifiers for services provided to Medicare beneficiaries. An origin and destination modifier must be reported for each ambulance trip. A two-character alpha code is designated for each line item on the claim. The first character of the modifier represents the origin of the trip. The second digit represents the destination of the trip. Table 7.12 provides a listing of the alpha characters.

In addition, a modifier must be reported to indicate whether the service was provided under arrangement by a provider of services (QM) or whether the service was furnished directly by a provider of services (QN). Figure 7.2 displays example line items from an ambulance claim with correct use of origin/destination modifiers and service modifiers.

Payment Steps

The ambulance conversion factor is adjusted for geographic variations and for the trip mileage as shown in figure 7.3. Other factors such as status of the patient (deceased) and number of patients transported should also be considered prior to the final payment determination.

The following example provided in figure 7.4 illustrates the reimbursement calculation for a 15-mile BLS transport in Ohio.

Figure 7.2.   Ambulance origin and destination modifier example

Record Type	Revenue Code	HCPCS Code	Modifier		Date of Service	Units	Total Charges
			#1	#2			
61	0540	A0428	RH	QN	082714	1 (trip)	$450.00
61	0540	A0425	RH	QN	082714	4 (mileage)	$25.00

Figure 7.3.   Ambulance fee schedule equation

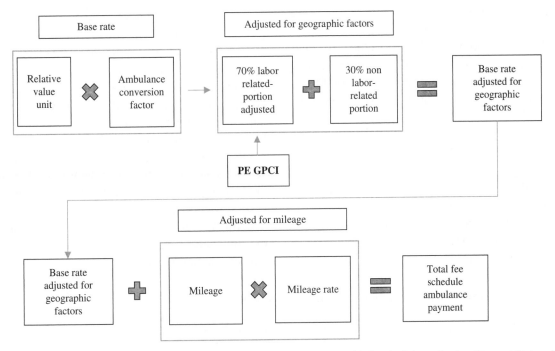

Source: Adapted from Medicare Payment Advisory Commission (MedPAC). 2014d. Payment Basics: Ambulance Services Payment System. Pg.2. http://www.medpac.gov.

Office of Inspector General Report

In January 2006, the Office of Inspector General (OIG) released the "Medicare Payments for Ambulance Transports" report. In this study, the OIG evaluated whether claims for ambulance transports met Medicare billing requirements and evaluated the effectiveness of safety measures used by fiscal intermediaries and carriers to identify improper payments (OIG 2006, i).

Prior OIG studies identified that the ambulance transport benefit was susceptible to fraud and abuse (OIG 2006, i):

- A 1994 report indicated that 70 percent of sampled dialysis-related ambulance transport claims did not meet CMS coverage requirements.

- A 1998 report indicated that two-thirds of sampled ambulance transports did not meet CMS coverage requirements.

The 2006 report included 720 ambulance transport claims from 2002. Interestingly enough, 2002 was the first year of the Ambulance Fee Schedule implementation. The study found that 25 percent of the ambulance transport claims did not meet CMS program requirements. These deficient claims resulted in $401 million of improper payments (OIG 2006, i). The breakout of error or deficient claims is as follows:

- 13 percent of transport claims did not meet coverage criteria based on the patient's condition ($220 million).

- 9 percent of transport claims did not meet level of service criteria, and a lower-level ambulance transport should have been reported ($31 million).

- 5 percent of transport claims were categorized as error claims because the supplier did not respond to the OIG request for documentation ($150 million).

Dialysis and nonemergency transport claims (27 and 20 percent, respectively) were found to have larger error rates than emergency transport claims (7 percent). However, more disturbing than the error rates for ambulance transport claims is the finding regarding contractors' safeguards for fraud and abuse monitoring. The report identifies several areas of weakness (OIG 2006, ii):

- Contractors use few prepayment edits consistently.

- Less than half of the contractors conducted postpayment reviews; of those contractors who did administer postpayment reviews, most conducted only one or two postpayment reviews in **calendar years (CYs)** 2001 and 2002.

- CMS does not provide any uniform requirements regarding the kind of documentation contractors should review to determine the appropriateness of ambulance transports.

- Contractors make minimal effort to educate healthcare providers regarding coverage and level of service criteria for ambulance transports.

The OIG provided CMS with three main recommendations to improve program integrity for the ambulance transport benefit. First, CMS should consider requiring all Medicare contractors, including Medicare Administrative Contractors (MACs), to implement prepayment edits. The OIG specifically suggests that dialysis and nonemergency transport claims should be highlighted in the edit set. Establishing this safeguard would provide consistency in claims processing activities, similar to the Outpatient Code Editor (OCE) used under OPPS. Second, the OIG recommends that CMS provide instructions for postpayment reviews. Specifically, documentation should be obtained from the ambulance supplier and third-party providers before a determination regarding coverage is made. Third, the

Figure 7.4. Specific example of calculation of ambulance fee schedule payment

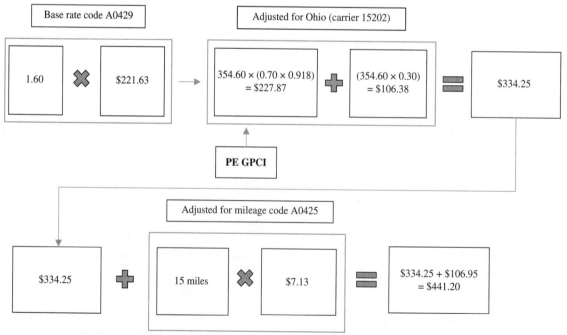

Data Source: Ambulance Fee Schedule Public Use Files. http://www.cms.gov/Medicare/Medicare-Fee-for-Service-Payment/AmbulanceFeeSchedule/afspuf.html.

OIG stressed that education must be provided to the ambulance and the third-party communities regarding the appropriate use of the Medicare ambulance benefit. The education should focus attention on the coverage guidelines for nonemergency transports. Once education is provided, CMS should monitor progress and take administrative action where necessary.

Clearly, the ambulance transport benefit needs greater attention from the A/B MACs and Part B carriers. However, increased education is necessary for the provider community as well. Recent improvements to the ambulance fee schedule area appear to be a move in the right direction.

Medical Conditions List

A major area of concern for many providers and suppliers has been the determination of level of service. Many providers and suppliers have called for the use of medical condition lists to aid in determining the level of service required to transport patients. The proposed medical condition lists were broad in topic and did not use the mandated *International Classification of Diseases, Ninth Revision, Clinical Modification* (ICD-9-CM) coding system as required by the Health Insurance Portability and Accountability Act (HIPAA) of 1996. In response to the numerous requests for level of service guidance, CMS provided an updated Medical Conditions List to be used in conjunction with

the Ambulance Fee Schedule in February 2007 (CMS 2007). The Medical Conditions List is intended to be an educational tool for providers, suppliers, and A/B MACs. There are two parts to the Medical Conditions List. The first part is the Conditions List, which provides ICD-9-CM codes for use with ambulance claims. The Conditions List provides one set of codes for novice coders or providers with little ICD-9-CM coding experience (ICD-9 Primary Code) and a second, more specific set of codes for experienced coders (ICD-9 Alternative Specific Code). Figure 7.5 provides an extract from section one of the Medical Conditions List.

The provider/supplier is instructed to choose a code from the Conditions List that most accurately reflects the on-site condition of the patient and that is the reason for the transport. The ICD-9-CM code is reported on the claim form and should be used by the MAC to understand why the level of service reported was chosen by the provider/supplier. The MAC can then determine whether a prepayment or postpayment review is necessary. The ICD codes on the conditions list do not guarantee that payment will be provided for the ambulance service reported; however, it is a guideline for providers and suppliers to use when determining the level of service for individual cases in conjunction with other documentation from the transport. At the time of this textbook's publication, an ICD-10-CM–based Medical Conditions List has

Figure 7.5.   Excerpt of ambulance medical conditions list

ICD-9-CM Primary Code	ICD-9-CM Alternative Specific Code	Condition (General)	Condition (Specific)	Service Level	Comments and Examples (not all-inclusive)	HCPCS Crosswalk
		Emergency Conditions—Nontraumatic				
535.50	458.9 780.2 787.01 787.02 787.03 789.01 789.02 789.03 789.04 789.05 789.06 789.07 789.09 789.60 through 789.69 or 789.40 through 789.49 PLUS any other code from 780 through 799 except 793, 794, and 795	Severe abdominal pain	With other signs or symptoms	ALS	Nausea, vomiting, fainting, pulsatile mass, distention, rigid tenderness on exam, guarding	A0427 A0433

Source: Centers for Medicare and Medicaid Services. 2007. CR 1442. Transmittal R1185CP. Ambulance Fee Schedule—Medical Revisions List. Manualization Revisions, 11.

yet to be released by CMS. However, after the implementation of ICD-10-CM/PCS takes place, users should refer to chapter 15, Ambulance, of the *Medicare Claims Processing Manual* for ICD-10-CM updates to the Medical Conditions List.

Part two of the conditions list provides a listing of Transportation Indicators. These indicators should be reported by the supplier/provider to communicate why it was necessary for the patient to be transported in a particular way. Figure 7.6 provides the Transportation Indicator list. The Medical Conditions List is provided by CMS to foster and improve communication between the provider/suppliers and the MACs. In addition, this education tool should be used by MACs in their program integrity safeguards as a way to identify potentially fraudulent claims.

Future Updates

Few enhancements or changes have been made to the Ambulance Fee Schedule since its implementation. However, CMS notified the provider community on November 25, 2011, that providers may begin to submit "no-pay bills" for statutorily excluded ambulance transport services beginning on January 1, 2012. This is an important feature because it allows providers to submit an excluded service bill to Medicare, to obtain the appropriate denial from Medicare, and then to be able to bill the patient's secondary insurance carrier for the portion of the service that was not covered by Medicare. Providers must submit "no-pay bills" to the A/B MAC with services reported in revenue codes 541, 542, 544, 547, or 549 and with modifier GY applied.

Section 1834(I)(3)(B) of the Social Security Act provides for payment updates that are equal to the urban consumer price index (CPI-U) for the 12-month period ending with June of the previous year (Medicare Learning Network 2008, 2). The percentage of the update is referred to as the ambulance inflation factor (AIF). The CPI-U for 2015 is 2.10 percent. However, the multifactor productivity adjustment (MFP) implemented by the Affordable Care Act (see chapter 4) is 0.60 percent for CY 2015. Therefore, the CY 2015 AIF is 1.50 percent (MLN 2014a). To identify the AIF for future years, visit the AFS Regulations and Notices and Ambulance Services Transmittals section of the Ambulance Fee Schedule page of the CMS website (http://www.cms.hhs.gov).

Hospital Outpatient Prospective Payment System

In 1983, Medicare moved to a PPS for hospital inpatient services to help control increasing healthcare costs and Medicare expenditures. As CMS experienced savings by reducing Medicare expenditures for inpatient care by $17 billion per year from the payment system change, the program's administrators made efforts to incorporate prospective payment concepts into other healthcare settings (Averill et al. 2001, 108). After more than 13 years, CMS implemented the outpatient prospective payment system (OPPS) on August 1, 2000.

Hospital Outpatient Prospective Payment Methodology

Before the implementation of OPPS, Medicare payment for hospital outpatient services was based on cost. The cost of services was calculated by converting total charges for each encounter to cost by using department-specific CCRs developed from cost report statistics. However, as healthcare costs continued to rise, CMS moved toward a PPS to help encourage a more efficient delivery of care for outpatient beneficiaries (HHS 2004a, 50450).

Reimbursement for Hospital Outpatient Services

CMS uses a variety of models to reimburse facilities for hospital outpatient services. The system uses three reimbursement methods: fee schedules, prospective payment, and cost-based. The primary standard that distinguishes a PPS from a fee schedule system is that, in the PPS, the costs for certain items and secondary services associated with a primary procedure are packaged into the payment for that procedure. A fee schedule system establishes a separate payment amount for each item or service and no packaging occurs (HHS 2004a, 50505). Certain items and services, such as acquisition of corneal tissue and influenza and pneumococcal pneumonia vaccines, continue to be paid on a reasonable cost basis.

Most procedures and services are reimbursed under APCs. Ambulance transportation, physical therapy, occupational therapy, and speech-language pathology are reimbursed via various fee schedules. Molecular pathology and surgical pathology laboratory services are paid via the clinical diagnostic laboratory fee schedule. End-stage renal disease (ESRD) services are reimbursed under their own PPS, as discussed the ESRD PPS section later in this chapter. Physician and nonphysician practitioners are paid under the MPFS (see Resource-Based Relative Value Scale for Physician and Professional Payments section earlier in this chapter) (HHS 2004a, 50451).

Reporting of Services and Supplies under Hospital Outpatient Prospective Payment System
OPPS requires that facilities use Levels I and II HCPCS codes to report services/procedures performed and items/supplies provided for beneficiaries. Each code in HCPCS has been assigned a **payment status indicator**.

Figure 7.6.   Ambulance Transportation Indicator List

Transportation Indicators Air and Ground	Transport Category	Transportation Indicator Description		Service Level	Comments and Examples (not all-inclusive)	HCPCS Crosswalk
C1	Interfacility transport	EMTALA-certified interfacility transfer to a higher level of care	Beneficiary requires higher level of care.	BLS, ALS, SCT, FW, RW	Excludes patient-requested EMTALA transfer.	A0428 A0429 A0426 A0427 A0433 A0434
C2	Interfacility transport	Service not available at originating facility and must meet one or more emergency or nonemergency conditions		BLS, ALS, SCT, FW, RW		A0428 A0429 A0426 A0427 A0433 A0434
C3	Emergency Trauma Dispatch Condition Code	Major incident or mechanism of injury	Major incident—this transportation indicator is to be used ONLY as a secondary code when the on-scene encounter is BLS-level patient.	ALS	Trapped in machinery, close proximity to explosion, building fire with persons reported inside, major incident involving aircraft, bus, subway, metro, train and watercraft. Victim entrapped in vehicle.	A0427 A0433
C4	Medically necessary transport, but not to the nearest facility	BLS or ALS response	Indicates to carrier/intermediary that an ambulance provided a medically necessary transport, but that the number of miles on the Medicare claim form may be excessive.	BLS/ALS	This should occur if the facility is on divert status or the particular service is not available at the time of transport only. In these instances, the ambulance units should clearly document why the beneficiary was not transported to the nearest facility.	Based on transport level
C5	BLS transport of ALS-level patient	ALS-level condition treated and transported by a BLS-level ambulance	This transportation indicator is used for ALL situations where a BLS-level ambulance treats and transports a patient that presents an ALS-level condition. No ALS-level assessment or intervention occurs at all during the patient encounter.	BLS		A0429

(Continued on next page)

Figure 7.6.   (Continued)

Transportation Indicators Air and Ground	Transport Category	Transportation Indicator Description		Service Level	Comments and Examples (not all-inclusive)	HCPCS Crosswalk
C6	ALS-level response to BLS-level patient	ALS response required based on appropriate dispatch protocols—BLS-level patient transport	Indicates to carrier/ intermediary that an ALS-level ambulance responded appropriately based on the information received at the time the call was received in dispatch, and after a clinically appropriate ALS assessment was performed on scene, it was determined that the condition of the patient was at a BLS level. These claims, properly documented, should be reimbursed at an ALS-1 level based on coverage guidelines under the Medicare Ambulance Fee Schedule.	ALS		A0427
C7		Intravenous (IV) medications required en route	This transportation indicator is used for patients who require an ALS-level transport in a nonemergent situation primarily because the patient requires monitoring of ongoing medications administered intravenously. Does not apply to self-administered medications. Does not include administration of crystalloid IV fluids. The patient's conditions should also be reported on the claim with a code selected from the list.	ALS	Does not apply to self-administered IV medications	A0426

Air Ambulance Transportation Indicators						
Transportation Indicators Air and Ground	Transport Category	Transportation Indicator Description		Service Level	Comments and Examples (not all-inclusive)	HCPCS Crosswalk
D1		Long distance—patient's condition requires rapid transportation over a long distance		FW, RW	Only if the patient's condition warrants	A0430 A0431
D2		Under rare and exceptional circumstances, traffic patterns preclude ground transport at the time the response is required.		FW, RW		A0430 A0431
D3		Time to get the closest appropriate hospital because the patient's condition precludes transport by ground ambulance. Unstable patient with need to minimize out-of-hospital time to maximize clinical benefits for the patient.		FW, RW		A0430 A0431
D4		Pickup point not accessible by ground ambulance.		FW, RW		A0430 A0431

Source: Centers for Medicare and Medicaid Services. 2007. CR 1442. Transmittal R1185CP. Ambulance fee schedule—Medical Revisions List. Manualization Revisions, 32.

The payment status indicator establishes how that service, procedure, or item is paid (that is, fee schedule, APC, reasonable cost, unpaid). Table 7.13 provides a listing of the payment status indicators and their definitions for CY 2015.

Because Level I HCPCS codes (CPT codes) were originally designed to report physician services, the system contains codes for inpatient and outpatient procedures. OPPS covers only outpatient services. Each year, the secretary of the HHS reviews claims

Table 7.13. Payment status indicators for calendar year 2015

Payment Status Indicator	Reimbursement Method	Procedure or Service Example
A	Fee schedule payment	Ambulance, separately payable clinical diagnostic laboratory, physical, occupational, and speech therapy, durable medical equipment, prosthetics, orthotics, and supplies (DMEPOS)
B	Not reimbursed under hospital outpatient prospective payment system (OPPS)	Service not appropriate for Part B claim
C	Not reimbursed under OPPS	Inpatient-only services
D	Not reimbursed under OPPS	Code is discontinued
E	Not reimbursed under OPPS	Service not covered by Medicare
F	Reasonable cost payment	Acquisition of corneal tissue, certain certified registered nurse anesthetist (CRNA) services, and hepatitis B vaccines
G	Pass-through ambulatory payment classification (APC) payment	Drugs and biologicals
H	Pass-through APC payment	Devices
J1	Comprehensive APC payment	All services are packaged with the primary J1 service
K	APC payment	Non-pass-through drugs and nonimplantable biological agent, including therapeutic radiopharmaceuticals
L	Reasonable cost payment with no copayment or deductible amount	Influenza and pneumococcal immunizations
M	Services not billable to the Medicare Administrative Contractor (MAC) and not payable under OPPS	Pharmacy dispensing fee, chemo assessment of nausea, pain, fatigue, and such
N	Not reimbursed under OPPS	Packaged into APC payment
P	Only reimbursed in partial hospitalization programs	Partial hospitalization
Q1	APC payment when criteria are met	STVX conditionally packaged services
Q2	APC payment when criteria are met	T conditionally packaged services
Q3	APC payment when criteria are met	Services that may be paid through a composite APC
R	APC payment	Blood and blood products
S	APC payment	Significant procedures, multiple procedure reduction does not apply
T	APC payment	Surgical procedures, multiple procedure reduction applies
U	APC payment	Brachytherapy sources
V	APC payment	Clinic or emergency department visits
Y	Not reimbursed under OPPS	Non-implanted durable medical equipment that must be billed directly to the durable medical equipment (DME) regional carrier

Source: Department of Health and Human Services. 2014d. Addendum D1.

data and determines which procedures are inpatient-only procedures and creates the "inpatient-only list" (payment status indicator C). To move off of the inpatient-only list, a procedure must be performed in outpatient settings at least 60 percent of the time. To be reimbursed, procedures indicated as inpatient only must be provided to Medicare beneficiaries in an inpatient setting, and payment is made under the IPPS.

Excluded Facilities

Excluded from OPPS are Maryland hospital services that are part of a cost containment waiver; CAHs; hospitals outside the 50 states, District of Columbia, and Puerto Rico; and the Indian Health Service, as different reimbursement systems are used for these types of facilities or areas.

Maintenance of the Hospital Outpatient Prospective Payment System

CMS maintains OPPS. As mandated by the BBRA, CMS must perform an annual review of the APC groups and relative weights. The wage index amounts adjusted for the current IPPS must also be incorporated into OPPS each year. In addition, the payment amounts are updated each year via an adjustment to the CF. The CF update amount is based on the same market-basket percentage amount that is applied to the IPPS standardized amount. The market basket reflects the input price inflation encountered by facilities for providing goods and services to patients (CMS 2011a, 1). For CY 2015, the market basket amount is 2.9 percent. However, because of the provisions of the Affordable Care Act (discussed in chapter 4), this amount was reduced by 0.5 for the MFP and 0.2 for the additional required adjustment for CY 2015. The result is an adjustment of 2.2 percent to the OPPS CF (HHS 2014d).

BBRA also established the APC Advisory Panel to assist with the maintenance of OPPS. The APC Advisory Panel is composed of 15 experts from various healthcare settings. The panel is technical in nature and provides analysis and recommendations to CMS. CMS considers and addresses all panel recommendations but does not have to accept them. CMS makes the final ruling for updates and changes to OPPS. The panel has three subcommittees that focus on data issues, observation issues, and packaging issues.

In addition, the MedPAC provides Congress and CMS with recommendations to improve OPPS.

Again, CMS considers and responds to all MedPAC recommendations but does not have to accept or implement them. CMS has the final ruling for updates and changes to OPPS. Revisions to OPPS are released in the *Federal Register* within 45 days of the start of the CY.

Ambulatory Payment Classification System

Each APC group comprises procedures or services that are clinically comparable with respect to resource use. All procedures and/or services assigned to an APC group must meet the "two-times rule," which establishes that the median cost of the most expensive item or service within a group cannot be more than two times greater than the median cost of the least expensive item or service within the same group (HHS 2004a, 50454). CMS can propose exceptions to the two-times rule based on the following criteria (HHS 2004a, 50463):

- Resource homogeneity
- Clinical homogeneity
- Hospital concentration
- Frequency of service (volume)
- Opportunity for upcoding and code fragments

Violations of the two-times rule are reviewed by the APC Advisory Panel. After analysis of each situation, the panel makes recommendations for each group that violated the rule. CMS uses the recommendations proposed by the panel and makes the final determination.

Partially Packaged System Methodology

Packaging and **bundling** concepts are used in OPPS as a way to combine payment for multiple services. In the CY 2008 outpatient prospective payment system (OPPS) final rule, CMS defines packaging and bundling. Packaging occurs when reimbursement for minor ancillary services associated with a significant procedure are combined into a single payment for the procedure. Bundling occurs when payment for multiple significant procedures or multiple units of the same procedure related to an outpatient encounter or to an episode of care is combined into a single unit of payment. The logic of groupers in the APC system includes ancillary packaging and bundling.

By using packaging and bundling concepts, CMS is providing incentives for healthcare facilities to improve their efficiency by avoiding unnecessary ancillary services, supplies, and pharmaceuticals, and by substituting less expensive, but equally effective, options.

In ancillary packaging, many ancillary service APC groups will automatically combine into a significant procedure APC group or a surgical service APC group, if one is present. The packaging of ancillary and supportive services continues to be expanded. CMS moved several procedures in the following categories to packaged or conditionally packaged status:

- Guidance services

- Image processing services

- Intraoperative services

- Imaging supervision and interpretation services

- Diagnostic radiopharmaceuticals

- Contrast media

- Observation services

- Drugs, biologicals, and radiopharmaceuticals that function as supplies when used in a diagnostic test or procedure

- Drugs and biologicals that function as supplies when used in a surgical procedure

- Certain clinical diagnostic laboratory tests

- Certain procedures described by add-on codes

- Device removal procedures

The majority of services included in these categories are assigned payment status indicator N, meaning that the service is always packaged and separate reimbursement is not provided. However, some of the services are assigned payment status indicators Q1–Q3, meaning that the services are conditionally packaged or packaged only when certain criteria are met. There are three types of conditionally packaged services. First are Q1 or STVX-packaged codes. When an ancillary service with payment status indicator Q1 is performed on the same date of service as a service with an S, T, V, or X payment status indicator, then the ancillary service is packaged and has a payment rate of $0.00. But if the ancillary service is performed without any S, T, V, or X services, then payment is provided for the ancillary service. The second type is Q2 or T-packaged codes. The concept is similar to the STVX-packaged codes, but only payment status indicator T affects whether the ancillary service is separately paid or not. The third type is codes that may be paid through a composite APC. Composite APCs are discussed later in this chapter.

Example:

A patient is admitted to the emergency department (ED) for a possible hip dislocation. A hip x-ray with contrast is performed and shows that the hip is dislocated. Therefore, treatment is provided to return the hip to proper alignment. The hip x-ray is assigned to APC group 0275 and has a payment status indicator of Q2. The dislocation treatment is assigned to APC group 0129, which has a payment status indicator of T. Because the hip x-ray is conditionally packaged and performed with a T procedure, payment is made only for APC group 0129.

Bundling combines supply and pharmaceutical costs or medical visits with associated procedures or services. APC systems have two methods of bundling:

- Supply and pharmaceutical cost bundling

- Medical visit bundling

Supply and pharmaceutical cost bundling involves supplies and drugs, except certain expensive chemotherapy drugs. Medical visits may also be bundled in some situations. For example, if a simple laceration repair occurs during an encounter that also includes extensive medical and diagnostic services, the medical visit would be bundled into the laceration repair.

The APC system uses a partially packaged system methodology. Services or items, such as recovery room, anesthesia, and some pharmaceuticals, are packaged into the APC payment for the service or procedure with which they are associated. Bundled services that are reported with a HCPCS code have the payment status indicator N. Some services and items have not been assigned a HCPCS code and, therefore, are reported by revenue code. Table 7.14 provides a list of services that are bundled into APC payment by revenue code. Although some services are packaged, many others are not. Ancillary services, such as x-rays, and magnetic resonance imaging (MRI) and minor

Table 7.14.   CY 2015 packaged revenue codes

Revenue Code	Description
0250	Pharmacy; General Classification
0251	Pharmacy; Generic Drugs
0252	Pharmacy; Non-Generic Drugs
0254	Pharmacy; Drugs Incident to Other Diagnostic Services
0255	Pharmacy; Drugs Incident to Radiology
0257	Pharmacy; Non-Prescription
0258	Pharmacy; IV Solutions
0259	Pharmacy; Other Pharmacy
0260	IV Therapy; General Classification
0261	IV Therapy; Infusion Pump
0262	IV Therapy; IV Therapy/Pharmacy Svcs
0263	IV Therapy; IV Therapy/Drug/Supply Delivery
0264	IV Therapy; IV Therapy/Supplies
0269	IV Therapy; Other IV Therapy
0270	Medical/Surgical Supplies and Devices; General Classification
0271	Medical/Surgical Supplies and Devices; Non-sterile Supply
0272	Medical/Surgical Supplies and Devices; Sterile Supply
0275	Medical/Surgical Supplies and Devices; Pacemaker
0276	Medical/Surgical Supplies and Devices; Intraocular Lens
0278	Medical/Surgical Supplies and Devices; Other Implants
0279	Medical/Surgical Supplies and Devices; Other Supplies/Devices
0280	Oncology; General Classification
0289	Oncology; Other Oncology
0331	Radiology—Therapeutic and/or Chemotherapy Administration; Injected
0332	Radiology—Therapeutic and/or Chemotherapy Administration; Oral
0335	Radiology—Therapeutic and/or Chemotherapy Administration; IV
0343	Nuclear Medicine; Diagnostic Radiopharmaceuticals
0344	Nuclear Medicine; Therapeutic Radiopharmaceuticals
0360	Operating Room Services; General
0361	Operating Room Services; Minor Surgery
0362	Operating Room Services; Organ Transplant, other than kidney
0369	Operating Room Services; Other OR Services
0370	Anesthesia; General Classification

Table 7.14.   (Continued)

Revenue Code	Description
0371	Anesthesia; Anesthesia Incident to Radiology
0372	Anesthesia; Anesthesia Incident to Other DX Services
0379	Anesthesia; Other Anesthesia
0390	Administration, Processing and Storage for Blood and Blood Components; General Classification
0392	Administration, Processing and Storage for Blood and Blood Components; Processing and Storage
0399	Administration, Processing and Storage for Blood and Blood Components; Other Blood Handling
0410	Respiratory Services; General
0412	Respiratory Services; Inhalation Services
0413	Respiratory Services; Hyperbaric Oxygen Therapy
0419	Respiratory Services; Other
0621	Medical Surgical Supplies—Extension of 027X; Supplies Incident to Radiology
0622	Medical Surgical Supplies—Extension of 027X; Supplies Incident to Other DX Services
0623	Medical Supplies—Extension of 027X, Surgical Dressings
0624	Medical Surgical Supplies—Extension of 027X; FDA Investigational Devices
0630	Pharmacy—Extension of 025X; Reserved
0631	Pharmacy—Extension of 025X; Single Source Drug
0632	Pharmacy—Extension of 025X; Multiple Source Drug
0633	Pharmacy—Extension of 025X; Restrictive Prescription
0681	Trauma Response; Level I Trauma
0682	Trauma Response; Level II Trauma
0683	Trauma Response; Level III Trauma
0684	Trauma Response; Level IV Trauma
0689	Trauma Response; Other
0700	Cast Room; General Classification
0710	Recovery Room; General Classification
0720	Labor Room/Delivery; General Classification
0721	Labor Room/Delivery; Labor
0722	Labor Room/Delivery; Delivery Room
0724	Labor Room/Delivery; Birthing Center
0729	Labor Room/Delivery; Other
0732	EKG/ECG (Electrocardiogram); Telemetry
0760	Specialty services; General

(Continued on next page)

Table 7.14.   (Continued)

Revenue Code	Description
0761	Specialty services; Treatment Room
0762	Specialty services; Observation Hours
0769	Specialty services; Other
0770	Preventive Care Services, General
0801	Inpatient Renal Dialysis; Inpatient Hemodialysis
0802	Inpatient Renal Dialysis; Inpatient Peritoneal Dialysis (Non-CAPD)
0803	Inpatient Renal Dialysis; Inpatient Continuous Ambulatory Peritoneal Dialysis (CAPD)
0804	Inpatient Renal Dialysis; Inpatient Continuous Cycling Peritoneal Dialysis (CCPD)
0809	Inpatient Renal Dialysis; Other Inpatient Dialysis
0810	Acquisition of Body Components; General Classification
0819	Inpatient Renal Dialysis; Other Donor
0821	Hemodialysis-Outpatient or Home; Hemodialysis Composite or Other Rate
0824	Hemodialysis-Outpatient or Home; Maintenance—100%
0825	Hemodialysis-Outpatient or Home; Support Services
0829	Hemodialysis-Outpatient or Home; Other OP Hemodialysis
0942	Other Therapeutic Services (also see 095X, an extension of 094x); Education/Training
0943	Other Therapeutic Services (also see 095X, an extension of 094X), Cardiac Rehabilitation
0948	Other Therapeutic Services (also see 095X, an extension of 094X), Pulmonary Rehabilitation

Source: HHS 2014d. Pp. 66791–66792.

procedures, such as injections, are not packaged, but rather paid separately via APC groups. For the inpatient setting, it is easier to predict which resources a patient will consume for a given clinical issue. However, in the outpatient setting, treatment pathways greatly vary from patient to patient, making it much more difficult to determine the resources that will be consumed for a clinical issue. Consequently, average cost for a "typical" outpatient encounter cannot be accurately forecasted. Therefore, a partially packaged system provides adequate reimbursement and allows the treatment flexibility that is needed to appropriately care for patients in the outpatient setting.

Structure of the Ambulatory Payment Classification System

In the APC system, there are nine types of APCs. The type for any APC can be identified by the payment status indicator assigned to the APC and the procedures and/or services in the group. All procedures or services in an APC have the same payment status indicator. The nine types are as follow:

- Clinic or emergency department visit (payment status indicator V)

- Significant procedure, multiple reduction applies (payment status indicator T)

- Significant procedure, not discounted when multiple (payment status indicator S)

- Non-pass-through drugs and nonimplantable biological agents, including therapeutic radiopharmaceuticals (payment status indicator K)

- Pass-through drugs or biological agents (payment status indicator G)

- Pass-through device categories (payment status indicator H)

- Partial hospitalization (payment status indicator P)

- Blood and blood products (payment status indicator R)

- Brachytherapy sources (payment status indicator U)

Each HCPCS code is assigned to one and only one APC. The APC assignment for a procedure or service does not change based on the patient's medical condition or the severity of illness. There may be an unlimited number of APCs per encounter for a single patient. The number of APC assignments is based on the number of reimbursable procedures or services provided for that patient.

Each APC contains the same components that drive the APC assignment (figure 7.7):

- Title

- Payment status indicator

- Relative weight

- **National unadjusted payment** amount

- National unadjusted copayment amount

- Code range

The relative weight is a measure of the resource intensity of a particular procedure or service. The national unadjusted payment amount is the total amount a hospital will receive for a procedure or service in that APC. Hospital outpatient claims data from 1996 were used to determine the APC payment rates for implementation

Figure 7.7. APC components

APC 0609 Title: Level 1 Type A Emergency Visits	
Payment Status Indicator	V
Relative Weight	0.8155
National Unadjusted Payment Amount	$60.49
National Unadjusted Copayment Amount	$12.10
Minimum Copayment Amount	$12.10
HCPCS Procedure Code 99281 Emergency Department Visit	

in 2000. The national unadjusted payment amount is divided into two components: Medicare facility amount and beneficiary copayment amount.

Copayment

CMS wanted to move to a PPS to ensure that the beneficiary copayment amount from hospital to hospital is consistent. Prior to PPS, beneficiaries were responsible for 20 percent of total charges, and charges for procedures varied from hospital to hospital. Therefore, if Hospital A charged $3,000 for a colonoscopy, the beneficiary amount would be $600, but if Hospital B charged $3,500 for the same colonoscopy, the beneficiary would be responsible for $700.

Again using 1996 data, CMS established the historical average copayment amount as the starting copayment amount in the APC system. However, the intent of the OPPS is for all copayment amounts to be only 20 percent of the total APC payment amount. Section 1833(t)(8)(C)(ii) of the Social Security Act requires CMS to reduce the national unadjusted copayment amount to meet reduction requirements mandated in BIPA (HHS 2004a, 50544). For CY 2008, the national unadjusted copayment amount cannot exceed 40 percent of the total APC payment. Any newly created APCs (those added to the system after August 1, 2000) must be added with a copayment amount equal to 20 percent of the total APC payment. The copayment amount may be collected from the beneficiary at the time of service or on a retrospective basis.

Both the Medicare facility component and the beneficiary copayment components are adjusted for differences in wage indexes. This is the only adjustment made to APC payment rates to account for differences among hospitals. Sixty percent of the facility amount is wage index adjusted. The wage index amount for the facility location based on core-based statistical area (CBSA) is determined in the IPPS update for the corresponding federal fiscal year.

New Technology Ambulatory Payment Classifications

New technology APCs were created to allow new procedures and services to enter OPPS quickly, even though their complete cost and payment information is not known. New technology APCs house modern procedures and services until enough data are collected to properly place the new procedure in an existing APC or to create a new APC for the service/procedure. A procedure/service can remain in a new technology APC for an indefinite amount of time.

The APC system contains 82 new technology APCs. Forty-one groups have payment status indicator S and are not subject to multiple-procedure discounting. The remaining 41 groups have payment status indicator T and are subject to the multiple-procedure discount provision. Placement into new technology APCs is based on cost bands. For example, APC 1491, New Technology–Level IA, contains procedures whose average cost is $0 to $10. The payment for the group is $5.

Composite Ambulatory Payment Classifications

In CY 2008, CMS began to add the concept of composite APCs to OPPS. In an effort to move toward an episode-of-payment-based payment system, the creation of composite APCs allows for multiple services that are typically performed together to be reimbursed by one APC rather than multiple APCs. There are several composite APCs; following is a list of those valid for CY 2015:

- Mental health services composite APC 0034
- Cardiac electrophysiological evaluation and ablation composite APC 8000
- Low-dose rate prostate brachytherapy composite APC 8001
- Level I Extended assessment and management composite APC 8002
- Level II Extended assessment and management composite APC 8003
- Ultrasound composite APC 8004
- CT and CTA without contrast composite APC 8005
- CT and CTA with contrast composite APC 8006
- MRI and MRA without contrast composite APC 8007
- MRI and MRA with contrast composite APC 8008

For each composite APC, a code set is established. This code set represents the services that are almost always performed together. When the codes in this code set are reported together on the same date of service, the composite APC is activated and one reimbursement amount is released. It is important to note that these services are *almost* always performed together. Therefore, the payment will still be made if only one of the services is performed, but at a reduced regular APC rate. For example, composite APC 8001 is activated when transperineal placement of needles or catheters into prostate (55875) and the interstitial radiation source application procedures (77778) are performed together on the same date of service. However, if code 55875 is performed during a different admission than 77778, then only APC 0163 is reimbursed. The opposite situation occurs if code 77778 is performed on a different date of service than code 55875, in which case only APC 651 is reimbursed. Notably, no financial incentive exists to report these two procedures together or separately; the payments are almost identical either way. Thus, hospitals should continue to follow correct coding guidelines and report these services as warranted by health record documentation.

Observation Services

With the inception of OPPS, the APC system bundled costs for observation services into the APC payment for the procedure or visit with which the observation was associated. However, the CY 2002 revision added APC 0339 to pay separately for certain observation services associated with clinic visits, emergency department visits, or critical care services. Three clinical conditions qualified as an observation service for APC 0339: chest pain, congestive heart failure, and asthma. However, CMS moved to a composite APC payment for observation services in CY 2008. The clinical and ancillary requirements have been removed, and separate observation services reimbursement is open to all cases that meet the new criteria. Two composite APCs are provided for observation services: Level I extended assessment and management composite, and Level II extended assessment and management composite. Observation services (G0378) must be provided for at least eight hours and provided on the same date of service as a high-level clinic visit (99205 or 99215) or a direct admission to the facility (G0379) to activate the Level I composite APC (8002). In addition, a surgical procedure (payment status indicator T) may not be performed on the same day as, or the day before, the observation services. The Level II composite APC (8003) criteria are very similar. Observation services

(G0378) must be provided for at least eight hours and provided on the same date of service as a high-level emergency department visit (99284 or 99285) or a critical care service (99291). In addition, a surgical procedure (payment status indicator T) may not be performed on the same day as, or the day before, the observation services. All observation services that do not meet the composite APC criteria are bundled and do not receive separate reimbursement.

Partial Hospitalization

Partial hospitalization is an intensive outpatient program of psychiatric services provided to patients who have an acute mental illness as an alternative to inpatient psychiatric care (HHS 2004a, 50543). Partial hospitalization may be provided by hospital outpatient departments and Medicare-certified community mental health centers. Patients who receive psychiatric services and who have a diagnosis of an acute mental health disorder are grouped to APC 0034, Mental health services composite. The unit of service for partial hospitalization is one day. Therefore, the APC payment for APC 0034 is based on a per diem amount. For CY 2015, the APC payment rate for APC 0034 is $195.70, of which $39.14 is the beneficiary copayment amount (HHS 2014b).

Provisions of the Ambulatory Payment Classification System

The APC system uses provisions to provide additional payments for high-cost items and unusual admissions that historically have added significant cost to patient care. Without the additional payments associated with these provisions, it may not be feasible for hospital outpatient facilities to provide all services to Medicare beneficiaries.

Discounting

Multiple surgical procedures with payment status indicator T performed during the same operative session are **discounted**. The highest-weighted procedure is fully reimbursed. All other procedures with payment status indicator T are reimbursed at 50 percent (figure 7.8). This reduction is made to account for resource saving that hospitals experience by performing multiple procedures together. For example, operating room surgical instruments are prepped only once, anesthesia is administered once, and recovery room is used once for all of the procedures performed.

Figure 7.8.   Discounting provision illustration for OPPS

APC	Payment Status Indicator	Payment Rate
1	T	100%
2	T	50%
3	T	50%
4	S	100%
5	S	100%

Interrupted Services

Interrupted services are reported with modifiers. When modifiers are applied to the surgical codes, a reduction in payment may be applied. Procedures reported with modifier 73, surgery discontinued for a patient who has been prepared for surgery (that requires anesthesia) and taken to the operating room but before the administration of anesthesia, will be reduced by 50 percent. A procedure reported with modifier 74, surgery discontinued after administration of anesthesia or initiation of the procedure, will be reimbursed at 100 percent of the APC rate. Procedures and services that do not require anesthesia but that are reduced or discontinued at the physician's discretion should be reported with modifier 52. For these procedures, the payment rate will be reduced by 50 percent.

High-Cost Outlier

This provision is intended to provide financial assistance for unusually high-cost services. The equations for case qualification and additional payment levels are adjusted each year. Medicare limits the percentage of total payments that can be attributed to outlier payments to two percent. For CY 2015, two requirements must be met for costs to be eligible for outlier payment. The cost for a service must exceed 1.75 times the APC payment. The cost must also exceed the APC payment plus a fixed dollar threshold of $2,775 (HHS 2014d). If these two conditions are met, the outlier payment is 50 percent of the cost that exceeds 1.75 times the APC payment. Some separately paid drugs and biological agents (payment status indicator G) and cost-based services and supplies are excluded from the outlier calculation.

Rural Adjustment

P.L. 108-173, better known as the Medicare Modernization Act of 2003, allowed for a rural adjustment to be applied if warranted after study. CMS presented the results of its study in the CY 2006 final rule. Regression analysis showed that overall, rural hospital costs were only 2.4 percent greater than urban hospital costs and did not warrant an adjustment. However, further analysis showed that rural sole-community hospitals' (SCHs') cost was 7.1 percent greater than that of urban hospitals and, thus, warranted an adjustment. Therefore, beginning in CY 2006 OPPS, a rural adjustment of 7.1 percent was provided to SCHs, including essential access community hospitals. For CY 2015, the adjustment of 7.1 percent continues to be provided to these select rural facilities.

Cancer Hospital Adjustment

The Affordable Care Act of 2010 (P.L. 111-148) provides for an adjustment to dedicated cancer hospitals to address the higher costs incurred by this type of facility. For CY 2015, there are 11 IPPS-exempt dedicated cancer hospitals. CMS first proposed an adjustment in the 2011 proposed rule, but the proposed methodology was disputed by many in the healthcare community. One of the major issues with the proposed methodology was that the copayment amounts for beneficiaries would be significantly higher at the cancer hospitals. Based on the numerous comments received by CMS, the proposed methodology was not adopted.

In the 2012 final rule, a new methodology was adopted by the CMS for the cancer hospital adjustment. This methodology allows for aggregate payments to be made to each cancer hospital at cost report settlement rather than at the APC level on each claim. This allows the adjustment to be provided to the cancer hospitals without negatively impacting the beneficiary copayments.

The adjustment is facility-specific. CMS compares each facility's payment-to-cost ratio (PCR) with the target PCR for the given year. Additional payment will be provided to the facility so that the facility's PCR will be equal to the target PCR. The target PCR is the weighted average PCR for all other hospitals that furnish services under OPPS (noncancer hospitals). For CY 2015, the target PCR is 0.89. Table 7.15 provides the 11 cancer hospitals and the estimated payment increase under this new adjustment. The actual payment increases will be calculated at the time of the final cost report settlement for each facility.

Pass-through Payments

Pass-throughs are exceptions to the Medicare PPSs. These exceptions exist for high-cost services. Pass-throughs are not included in the packaging component of PPS and are passed through to other payment mechanisms that attempt to adjust for the high cost of pass-throughs. Therefore, pass-throughs minimize the negative financial effect of combining all services into one lump-sum payment. Pass-throughs occur in both IPPS and OPPS.

Table 7.15. Estimated cancer hospital adjustment for CY 2015

Provider Number	Hospital Name	Estimated Percentage Increase in OPPS payments for CY 2015
050146	City of Hope Comprehensive Cancer Center	15.8%
050660	USC Kenneth Norris Jr. Cancer Hospital	32.8%
100079	Sylvester Comprehensive Cancer Center	28.4%
100271	H. Lee Moffitt Cancer Center & Research Institute	22.4%
220162	Dana-Farber Cancer Institute	44.8%
330154	Memorial Sloan-Kettering Cancer Center	39.4%
330354	Roswell Park Cancer Institute	25.2%
360242	James Cancer Hospital & Solove Research Institute	30.9%
390196	Fox Chase Cancer Center	16.0%
450076	M. D. Anderson Cancer Center	39.4%
500138	Seattle Cancer Care Alliance	44.7%

Pass-through payments were established by the BBRA to provide hospitals with additional payment for high-cost drugs, biological agents, and devices. This specification was added to ensure the use of new and innovative drugs and supplies for Medicare beneficiaries when medically appropriate. Such drugs and supplies are often costly. If cost exceeds the payment for a new and innovative drug, a hospital might be motivated by cost containment practices to use a less expensive and potentially less effective drug for Medicare beneficiaries.

Pass-through payments cannot exceed two percent of the total payments for the year. CMS uses historical claims data to project whether pass-through payments will exceed this limit. If so, CMS can put a pro rata reduction in place for that CY. The pro rata reduction decreases all pass-through payments by a selected percentage so that the total pass-through payments will not exceed two percent for the year.

Drugs, biological agents, and devices qualify for pass-through status if they were not being paid for as a hospital outpatient drug as of December 31, 1996, and their cost is "not insignificant" in relation to the OPPS payment for the procedures or services associated with their use (HHS 2004a, 50502). An item can have pass-through status for at least two years, but not more than three years. After three years, the cost of the item will be bundled into the APC payment for the procedure in which the item is used or be transitioned into an individual APC group. The pass-through status application process is described on the CMS website (CMS 2009b).

Pass-through device APCs (payment status indicator H) are paid on a reasonable cost basis less the device offset amount. The device offset amount is the portion of the APC payment amount that CMS has determined is associated with the cost of the device (HHS 2004a, 50501). This amount is deducted from the pass-through payment because it is already reimbursed as part of the surgical APC payment. Drug and biological pass-through APCs (payment status indicator G) are reimbursed by using an average sales price (ASP) methodology. The ASP is equivalent to the dollar amount at which these drugs and biological agents would be reimbursed in the physician office setting (HHS 2004a, 50503). From this amount the portion of the applicable fee schedule amount (APC payment rate) is subtracted. The result is the pass-through payment.

Transitional Outpatient Payments (TOPs) and Hold-Harmless Payments

The BBRA provided a mechanism for hospitals to decrease the financial burden of the implementation of OPPS. This phase-in period provided the transitional outpatient payments. Transitional outpatient payments were provided beginning in 2000 and were discontinued December 31, 2003. However, hold-harmless payments are permanent for IPPS-exempt cancer centers and children's hospitals.

Eligible facilities receive a quarterly interim hold-harmless payment that provides additional reimbursement when the payment received under OPPS is less than the payment the facility would have received for the same services under the prior reasonable cost-based system in 1996 (HHS 2004a, 50530). The interim payment is based on CCRs from their most recently closed Medicare cost report and their assigned pre-BBRA PCR determined from their 1996 cost report. PCRs average around 80 percent. Figure 7.9 displays the formula for hold-harmless payment calculation. The final hold-harmless amount is determined at the settlement of the cost report for that facility's fiscal year.

Ambulatory Payment Classification Assignment

The APC system is primarily based on the HCPCS code(s) assigned for each service or procedure performed and for devices, drugs, and reimbursable items provided to the patient. The first step in APC assignment is to code the encounter accurately and completely. The APC system is a partially packaged system and several items/services are separately reimbursed, so failure to capture all reimbursable charges with HCPCS codes will result in lost revenue for the facility. After all HCPCS codes have been assigned, the payment status indicator is identified for

Figure 7.9.   Hold-harmless formula for OPPS

For specified quarter:

Department charges × Department-specific ratios of cost-to-charge = Department cost

Sum department cost for all departments = Total cost

Total cost × Payment to cost ratio from 1996 = Pre-OPPS reimbursement

OPPS reimbursement from current quarter − Pre-OPPS reimbursement = Hold-harmless payment

When current OPPS exceeds Pre-OPPS reimbursement, no hold-harmless payment is made.

each code. Payment status indicators that are assigned to an APC and indicate APC payment are G, H, K, P, R, S, T, U, and V. There may be multiple APCs with the same or different payment status indicator per claim.

There is one exception to this process. For partial hospitalization services, the ICD diagnosis code assignment is crucial. In partial hospitalizations (APC 0034), an acute mental health disorder diagnosis must be assigned with an ICD code. If the appropriate ICD diagnosis code is not assigned, the procedure/service will not group to the correct APC and may result in incorrect reimbursement.

Payment Determination

Hospitals submit a claim to Medicare for payment. Claims are sent electronically to the designated MAC. Each claim contains visit information, patient information, facility information, detailed charges by procedure code, and diagnosis codes. The MAC performs an audit of the claim to ensure that the claim contains complete and accurate information based on the edits found in the OCE. During the editing process, APC(s) are assigned using grouper software as appropriate, based on the HCPCS codes submitted. The foundation of OPPS payment is displayed in figure 7.10.

During step one, the OPPS conversion factor is adjusted to account for geographic differences. The formula for wage-index adjustment under OPPS is provided in figure 7.11. The CF for 2015 is $74.17. The pricer software completes steps necessary to calculate the claim payment. When the payment steps are completed, payment is made to the facility, and the data from the encounter is included in the national claims history file. The outpatient standard analytical file and the OPPS file, extracted from the national claims history file, are used for statistical analysis and research. Figure 7.12 provides an example of a payment calculation for a level II emergency department visit provided in Columbus, Ohio.

Check Your Understanding 7.2

1. Define packaging and bundling as it pertains to OPPS.

2. Name the two reimbursement methods used by OPPS.

3. True or false? Procedures in OPPS with a status indicator of C are indicated as inpatient-only; they must be provided to Medicare beneficiaries in an inpatient setting and are reimbursed under the IPPS.

4. List three of the nine APC types, providing the applicable payment status indicator(s).

5. Why did CMS establish new technology APCs?

Ambulatory Surgical Center Prospective Payment System

Designated surgical services may be provided to Medicare beneficiaries in the outpatient setting at Ambulatory Surgical Centers (ASCs) under the Medicare supplementary medical insurance program (Part B). In an effort to control healthcare costs, CMS introduced a PPS for ambulatory surgery centers in 1982. Section 934 of the Omnibus Budget Reconciliation Act (OBRA) of 1980 amended sections 1832(a)(2) and 1833 of the Social Security Act (the Act) to specify procedures that would be covered under the PPS, called the **ASC List of Covered Procedures (ASC list)**. The ASC list was in effect from 1982 to 2007. In 2003, the MMA required that CMS revise the ASC PPS and implement the modified system between 2006 and 2008. Therefore, on January 1, 2008, CMS implemented the APC system for use in the ASC PPS.

Medicare Certification Standards

ASCs that choose to treat Medicare beneficiaries must be state-licensed and Medicare-certified and are considered a supplier of services rather than a provider. Several standards must be met to qualify as a Medicare-certified ASC. The surgical center must (Jones 2001, 13)

- Be a separate entity distinguishable from any other entity or type of facility.

- Have its own national identifier or supplier number under Medicare.

- Maintain its own licensure, accreditation, governance, professional supervision, administrative functions, clinical services, recordkeeping, and financial and accounting systems.

- Have a sole purpose of delivering services in connection with surgical procedures that do not require inpatient hospitalization.

Figure 7.10. Foundation of hospital outpatient prospective payment system

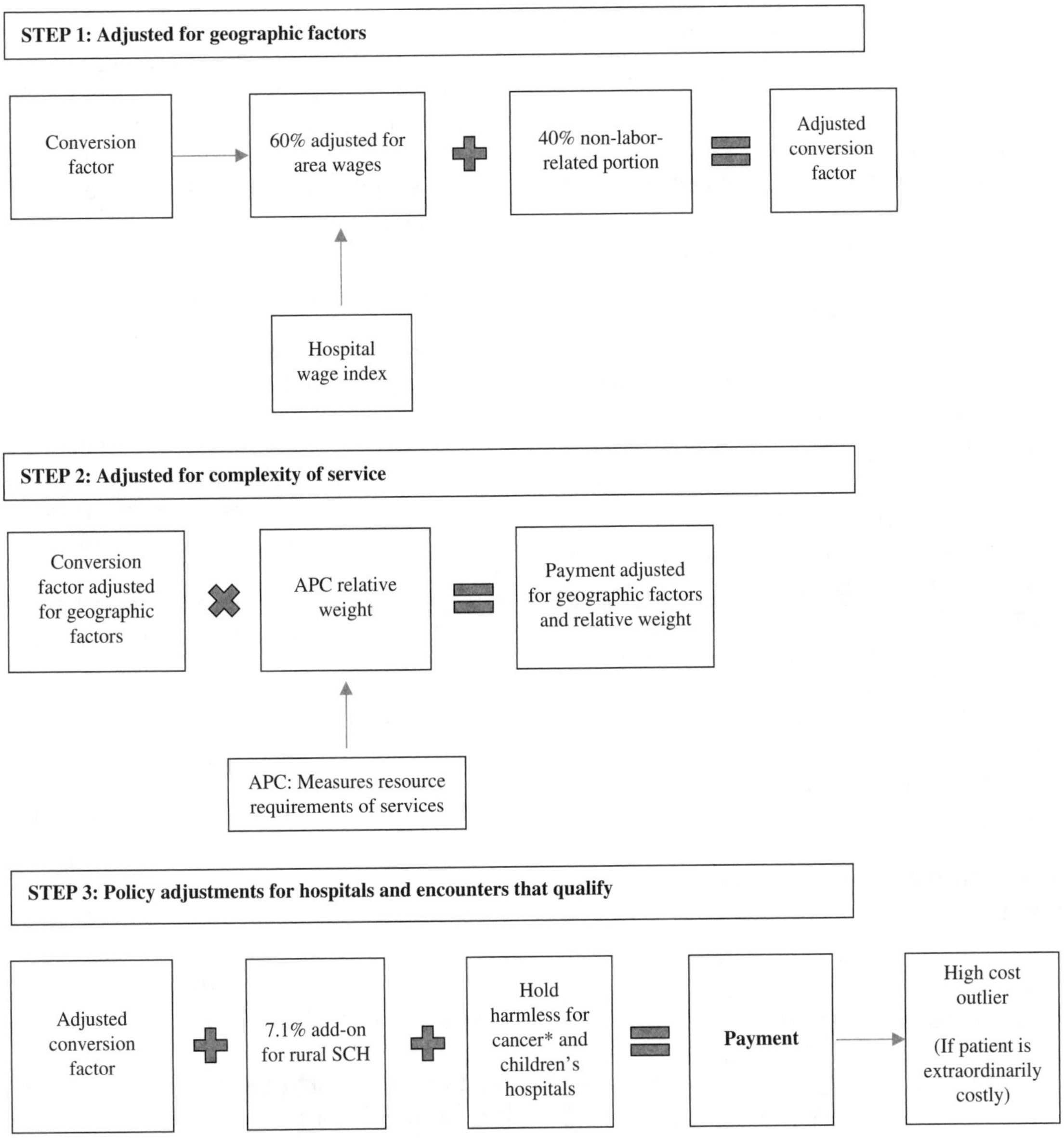

*Medicare adjusts outpatient prospective payment system payment rates for 11 cancer hospitals so that the payment-to-cost ration (PCR) for each cancer hospital is equal to the average PCR for all hospitals.

Source: Adapted from Medicare Payment Advisory Commission (MedPAC). 2014e. Payment Basics: Outpatient Hospital Services Payment System. p.2. http://www.medpac.gov.

• Meet all conditions and requirements set forth in Section 1832(a)(2)(F)(i) of the Act, in 42 CFR 416, Subpart B and Subpart C in the *Federal Register*.

Payment for Ambulatory Surgical Center Services

As a Medicare-certified ASC, the facility must accept Medicare reimbursement as payment in full for the services supplied to Medicare beneficiaries. The MMA established a lesser of provision for the revised ASC PPS. Therefore, beginning January 1, 2008, the Medicare program payment will equal 80 percent of the lesser of the actual charge for the services or the payment amount under APCs for the ASC PPS (HHS 2007a, 42473).

Medicare payment equals 80 percent of the total reimbursement for services provided. Beneficiaries are

Figure 7.11. Wage index adjustment formula for OPPS

[(National unadjusted payment amount × 60%) × Wage index]
+ (National unadjusted payment amount × 40%)
= Locality payment

responsible for the 20 percent copayment of the total payment and any deductible that is required. There are two exceptions to the copayment percentage. Screening flexible sigmoidoscopy and screening colonoscopy procedures are subject to a 25 percent coinsurance rate. However, there is no deductible requirement for these two types of services under the ASC PPS. In addition, beneficiaries are responsible for ASC charges associated with noncovered services furnished in the ASC setting (HHS 2007b, 42792).

Payment for the procedures allowed in the ASC setting is intended to reimburse ASCs for the facility resources extended to provide surgical services in that locality. The costs of the physician's professional services are excluded from the ASC payment. Professional services must be reported separately and are reimbursed via the MPFS. The payment rate is wage index adjusted to account for regional differences among providers. The labor portion for CY 2015 is 50 percent. The urban and rural wage index tables are used from the applicable year.

Criteria for Ambulatory Surgical Center Procedures

With the adoption of APCs for the ASC setting, CMS moved from an inclusion methodology for approved ASC services to an exclusion methodology. Using a payment indicator system similar to the one used in OPPS, CMS identifies each year in the *Federal Register* which services can and cannot be performed for Medicare beneficiaries in the ASC setting. Beginning in CY 2008, the scope of services dramatically increased when CMS added more than 800 procedures to the ASC scope of services.

By creating a list of appropriate outpatient surgery procedures, CMS influences the site of service for certain procedures. The ASC list of approved procedures creates a motivation for surgical procedures to migrate from the more expensive inpatient setting to the less expensive outpatient surgery setting without creating a motivation to shift procedures from the less expensive physician office setting to the more expensive outpatient surgery setting (HHS 2004b, 69179). The procedures

and services covered under the ASC PPS are reported using Levels I and II HCPCS codes. The ASC scope of services criteria was modified with the adoption of APCs as well. To identify procedures eligible for the revised ASC PPS, CMS excluded the following types of procedures (HHS 2007b, 42778):

- Surgical procedures that are on the OPPS inpatient list

- Procedures that are packaged under the OPPS CPT unlisted surgical procedure codes

- Surgical procedures that are not recognized for payment under the OPPS

In addition, CMS followed established criteria to determine whether a procedure could pose a significant safety risk to beneficiaries when performed in the ASC setting. The criteria identified procedures that (HHS 2007b, 42778)

- Generally result in extensive blood loss

- Require major or prolonged invasion of body cavities

- Directly involve major blood vessels

- Are emergent or life-threatening in nature

- Commonly require systemic thrombolytic therapy

These criteria for evaluating surgical procedures are included in section 416.166(c) of the Act. These services are excluded from the ASC PPS.

Ambulatory Payment Classifications and Payment Rates

The Medicare Prescription Drug, Improvement and Modernization Act (MMA) of 2003 required CMS to implement a revised PPS for ASC services between January 1, 2006, and January 1, 2008. On August 2, 2007, CMS released the final rule for the revised ASC payment system. The rule solidified that APCs would be implemented for ASC PPS on January 1, 2008. The ASC PPS is based on the OPPS APC system. The APC system is updated yearly to account for changes in the HCPCS; each year codes are added, deleted, and modified to account for changes in healthcare delivery practices. These updates are applicable to the ASC PPS as well.

Figure 7.12.   Specific example of calculation of OPPS payment

2015 APC CF	Wage index adjusted CF	Service/RW	Adjusted CF × RW	Total Payment
$74.17	(74.17 × .60 × .9444) + (74.17 × .40) 42.02 + 29.67 = 71.69	99282 / 1.5206	$71.69 × 1.5206	$109.01

Data source: January 2015 Addendum B. http://www.cms.gov/Medicare/Medicare-Fee-for-Service-Payment/HospitalOutpatientPPS/Addendum-A-and-Addendum-B-Updates.html.

Even though the ASC PPS is very similar to OPPS, the payment rates are adjusted to reflect the lower cost setting that ASCs provide. Reimbursement for the procedures performed in the ASC equals approximately 59 percent of the OPPS APC payment rate for CY 2015, which results in a CF of $44.07.

Separately Payable Services

Like the OPPS, the ASC PPS allows for separate payment of certain ancillary services and supplies.

Radiology Services

ASCs will receive separate payment for ancillary radiology procedures designated as separately payable under the OPPS when the services are integral to the performance of a covered surgical procedure provided on the same day. No separate payment will be made for radiology procedures packaged under OPPS (payment status indicator N).

Brachytherapy Sources

ASCs will receive separate payment for brachytherapy sources when they are implanted in conjunction with covered surgical procedures. The ASC brachytherapy source payment rate is the same as the OPPS payment rate for a given year. Brachytherapy sources are considered a supply and potentially cost the same if purchased by a hospital outpatient department facility or by an ASC; therefore, the payment rate is not reduced by 41 percent. If OPPS prospective payment rates are unavailable, ASC payments will be contractor-priced by the MAC in that region. In addition, brachytherapy reimbursement is not subject to the geographic adjustment (wage index adjustment).

Drugs and Biological Agents

Separate payment will be made when certain drugs and biological agents are provided integral to a covered surgical procedure. The ASC payment for these items is equal to the OPPS payment rates for the same year without application of the ASC budget neutrality adjustment. ASC payments for these items are not subject to the geographic adjustment.

Implantable Devices with Pass-Through Status under OPPS

Pass-through devices will be reimbursed at a contractor-priced rate. The device must be provided in the ASC immediately before, during, or immediately following the covered surgical procedure and is billed by the ASC on the same day as the covered surgical procedure. Pass-through devices are not subject to the geographic adjustment.

Corneal Tissue Acquisition

The cost of acquiring corneal tissue varies by geographic location, so corneal tissue acquisition is reported with HCPCS Level II code V2785, and reimbursement is based on invoice costs. This allows facilities to avoid a financial loss when obtaining this supply.

Device-Intensive Procedures

Payment methodology is modified for certain device-intensive procedures. Each year a list of device-intensive procedures is published in the *Federal Register*. The list consists of those procedures for which the device offset percentage is greater than 50 percent of the median cost under OPPS, meaning that the cost of the device is a significant amount of the cost of providing the service. Then, the intent of the modified methodology is to ensure that ASCs are adequately reimbursed for the supply cost associated with these device-intensive procedures.

The modified methodology divides the unadjusted OPPS national payment rate into two portions: a device portion and a service portion. The ASC CF is applied only to the service portion of the payment rate. The device portion is not modified by the CF. Both portions are subject to the geographic adjustment. Figure 7.13 provides the device-intensive formula for the ASC PPS.

Multiple and Bilateral Procedures

When multiple procedures are performed during the same surgical session, a payment reduction is applied. Each year services applicable for the discounting provision are identified in the *Federal Register*. The procedure in the highest-weighted APC group is reimbursed at 100 percent, and all remaining procedures eligible for discounting are reimbursed at 50 percent. Bilateral procedures are reimbursed at 150 percent of the payment rate for their group.

Interrupted Procedures

Procedures reported with modifier 73, surgery discontinued for a patient who has been prepared for surgery (that requires anesthesia) and taken to the operating room but before the administration of anesthesia, will be reduced by 50 percent. A procedure reported with modifier 74, surgery discontinued after administration of anesthesia or initiation of the procedure, will be reimbursed at 100 percent of the ASC rate. Procedures and services that do not require anesthesia but are reduced or discontinued at the physician's discretion should be reported with modifier 52. For these procedures, the payment rate will be reduced by 50 percent.

ASC PPS Payment

The ASC PPS does not follow the same provisions as the OPPS. Therefore, the foundation for the ASC PPS is a streamlined equation. Figure 7.14 provides the foundation for ASC PPS payment determination. It is important to remember to adjust the payment for applied modifiers when determining the final payment amount. As previously discussed, multiple and bilateral

Figure 7.13.   Device-intensive formula for the ASC PPS

National unadjusted OPPS payment rate × device offset percentage
∇ device portion

National unadjusted OPPS payment rate − device portion
= service portion

Service portion × ASC CF = adjusted service portion

Adjusted service portion + unadjusted device portion
∇ ASC payment rate for device-intensive APC

procedure modifiers, as well as interrupted procedure modifiers, affect the payment amount.

Check Your Understanding 7.3

1.   True or false? Medicare-certified ASCs may share recordkeeping and financial and accounting systems with hospitals in the same parent corporation.

2.   CMS created a motivation for surgical procedures to migrate from the more expensive inpatient setting to the less expensive outpatient surgery setting without creating a motivation to shift procedures from the less expensive physician office setting to the more expensive outpatient surgery setting by creating _____.

3.   How are multiple and bilateral procedures adjusted in the ASC PPS?

4.   Which three modifiers are utilized for interrupted procedures in the ASC setting?

5.   True or False? Because the ASC PPS uses the same APCs groups as the OPPS, the payment rates for the ASC setting are the same as the hospital outpatient setting.

End-Stage Renal Disease Prospective Payment System

Benefits for end-stage renal disease (ESRD) patients have been included under Medicare since 1972 (HHS 2010, 49031). Benefits are provided for persons who have permanent kidney failure, requiring either dialysis or kidney transplantation to maintain life, and meet other eligibility requirements, regardless of their age. Thus, coverage under this section of Medicare is unique because it is extended to patients of all ages. The other Medicare payment systems discussed in this text have been designed based on the point of care location (that is, inpatient setting, outpatient setting, home health), but this payment system has been designed to provide services for a particular condition. Rather than breaking non-inpatient ESRD services out by service area (outpatient, home health), all non-inpatient services for ESRD are included in this payment system. Why did Medicare create a payment system specific to a medical condition? In CY 2012, CMS spending for ESRD dialysis services totaled $10.7 billion. Clearly, this is a high-cost service area for CMS, so considerable attention is warranted to

Figure 7.14.   Foundation of ambulatory surgical center prospective payment system

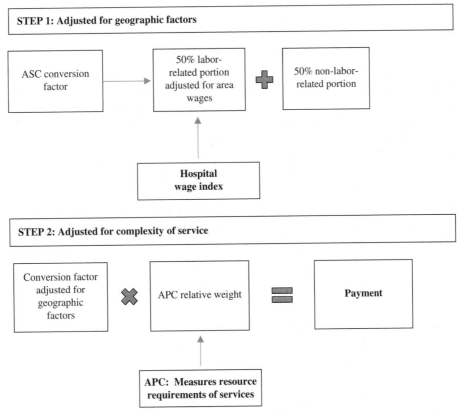

Source: Adapted from Medicare Payment Advisory Commission (MedPAC). 2014f. Payment Basics: Ambulatory Surgical Center Services Payment System. Pg. 2. http://www.medpac.gov.

ensure that the Medicare Trust Fund remains intact so that continued access to care is sustained.

Legislative Background

Medicare began covering ESRD under Medicare in 1972. The OBRA of 1981 required Medicare to make changes to the payment system for ESRD services. Prior to OBRA, services were reimbursed on a cost-based payment system. OBRA required Medicare to establish prospective payments for dialysis services whether services are provided at a dedicated facility or at the patient's home (HHS 2010, 49032). Therefore, on August 1, 1983, Medicare established a payment system for outpatient dialysis services; this system is known as the composite rate. At the time, the composite rate system was comprehensive for dialysis services, meaning that all services were reimbursed under the composite rate. However, over time, a significant portion

of the services, such as erythropoiesis-stimulating agents (ESA) drugs, associated with dialysis that were excluded from the composite rate and that were paid separately from the composite rate grew to approximately 40 percent of the total expenditures (HHS 2010, 49032). Thus, instead of having a purely PPS, Medicare was reimbursing dialysis services under a mix of prospective payment, fee-for-service, and other payment mechanisms and rules.

Congress twice required Medicare to conduct studies on the ESRD composite rate system—once under the Medicare, Medicaid, and SCHIP BIPA, and again under the MMA of 2003. Along with the study, the MMA required Medicare to submit a new PPS design for a bundled ESRD system. The intent of the bundled ESRD system was to combine the services paid under the composite rate and the separately payable services, drugs, and supplies into one unit of payment. In addition, the MMA required Medicare to make a basic case-mix adjustment to the current composite rate which reflected a limited number of patient characteristics. On April 1, 2005, Medicare implemented a basic case-mix-adjusted composite payment system that was developed from research conducted by the University of Michigan Kidney Epidemiology and Cost Center (UM-KECC) (HHS 2010, 49033). This system adjusted the composite rate for a limited set of patient characteristics such as age and body mass index (BMI). This system is important in this timeline because the basic case-mix-adjusted composite payment system is the foundation for the system that is in place today.

MIPPA mandated that a bundled payment system for ESRD be designed and implemented by January 2011 and referred to it as ESRD PPS (HHS 2010, 49033). Specifically, the law required CMS to do the following:

- Implement a payment system under which a single payment is made for renal dialysis services, including home dialysis and self-care home dialysis support.

- Create a definition for renal dialysis services that details all of the services included in the payment bundle.

- Estimate the total amount of payments for 2011 under the new payment system. The total payments must be equal to 98 percent of the total amount that would have been paid in 2011 if the payment mechanisms were unchanged.

- The ESRD PPS must include adjustments for case-mix variables, high-cost outlier payments, and low-volume facilities and provide for a four-year transition period. ESRD facilities must be able to elect to opt out of the transition period.

- The ESRD PPS may include other payment adjustments as determined by the Secretary of the HHS.

- The ESRD PPS payments must be increased on an annual basis based on the ESRD bundled market basket beginning in 2012.

By creating a single payment system, CMS is able to make one bundled payment for all services associated with the renal dialysis treatment. However, there is significant variation in the resources required in providing renal dialysis services among patients. The resources, and hence cost, are affected by several patient characteristics. Thus, it was extremely important for Medicare to design a PPS that extended the basic case-mix adjustments so that facilities that treat a greater proportion of resource-intensive patients would be adequately reimbursed under the ESRD PPS. By using the research provided by UM-KECC, Medicare was able to provide payment adjustments that were based on objective quantifiable criteria (HHS 2010, 49034).

The foundation of the ESRD PPS is a base rate that is a national per treatment amount that is based on the average cost or Medicare allowable payment (MAP) for providing one dialysis treatment when it is part of a three per week treatment plan. The base rate was developed from CY 2007 claims data. For 2015, the ESRD PPS base rate is $239.43 (HHS 2014e). The ESRD PPS allows for several adjustments to the base rate, both at the facility level and patient level, as described in tables 7.16 and 7.17. In addition to the adjustments, there are provisions for high-cost outlier payments and self-dialysis training.

Definition of Renal Dialysis Services

As part of the ESRD PPS, CMS had to define which services would be included in the ESRD base rate. These services are known as renal dialysis services and are bundled into the single per treatment payment rate. This new definition of renal dialysis services is

Table 7.16. Facility- and patient-level adjustments for adults

Facility-Level Adjustments	Patient-Level Adjustments
Wage index Low-volume facility	Patient age Body surface area Low body mass index New patient (onset of dialysis) Specified comorbidities

Table 7.17. Facility- and patient-level adjustments for pediatrics

Facility-Level Adjustments	Patient-Level Adjustments
Wage index Low-volume facility	Patient age Treatment modality

expanded from previous ESRD payment mechanisms. The new definition, effective January 1, 2011, includes all services historically known as renal dialysis services included in the composite rate and expands to incorporate drugs, laboratory tests, and supplies that were previously separately billable and reimbursed outside of the composite rate. This was a significant change for facilities. Of significant issue is the inclusion of ESAs, which are typically high-cost drugs that were previously paid under Medicare Part B. In 2007, approximately 23 percent of all ESRD payments were for ESAs (HHS 2010, 49075). Because these drugs are now included in the payment bundle, facilities are incentivized to pay close attention to the utilization and cost of these drugs. The categories that are defined as renal dialysis services under the ESRD PPS are as follows (HHS 2010, 49036):

- Composite rate services: maintenance dialysis treatments and all associated services, including historically defined dialysis-related drugs, laboratory tests, equipment, supplies, and staff time

- ESAs and any oral form of such agents furnished to individuals for the treatment of ESRD

- Other drugs and biological agents furnished to individuals for the treatment of ESRD and for which payment was (before application of the ESRD PPS) made separately under the ESRD benefit and any oral equivalent form of such drug or biological agent

- Diagnostic laboratory tests and other items and services furnished to individuals for the treatment of ESRD

The base rate under the ESRD PPS is based on the average per treatment cost for renal dialysis services. Several adjustments are provided at the facility and patient levels to adequately reimburse facilities that have a patient population of high resource intensity. The adjustment is made by applying the applicable multipliers, also referred to as patient multipliers (PM), to the ESRD PPS base rate. Although one may mistake PM as patient-level adjustments only, in fact, one facility-level adjustment, low-volume facility, is also considered a PM in this system. In addition, the order of application of the various adjustments is important.

A later section in this chapter outlines the payment determination steps.

Facility-Level Adjustments

Payments are adjusted at the facility level to account for geographic wage variations and for those facilities that have a consistently low volume of ESRD patients and treatments per year.

Wage Index Adjustment

A facility-level adjustment is provided to account for wage differences among geographic areas. The labor portion of the base rate amount is 50.673 percent for CY 2015. The Office of Budget and Management's CBSA-based geographic area to define urban and rural facilities. In addition, CMS is utilizing a wage index floor as a substitute wage index amount for those facilities that have extremely low wage index values. The CY 2015 wage index floor is 0.40. Figure 7.15 provides the ESRD PPS wage index adjustment formula.

Low-Volume Adjustment

A low-volume facility adjustment is included in the ESRD PPS to allow for adequate access to care for Medicare beneficiaries. The adjustment allows for small ESRD facilities to continue providing renal dialysis services even though their unit costs (per service costs) are typically much higher than those of facilities that have a greater patient volume.

Two requirements must be met to qualify as a low-volume facility. First, the facility has to have furnished less than 4,000 treatments in each of the three years preceding the payment year. When determining the number of treatments per year, facilities that are under common ownership and within 25 road miles or less from each other must combine the treatment volumes (HHS 2010, 49124). This condition prevents a healthcare system from opening separate facilities in close proximity to each other and to distribute treatment volume among facilities to qualify for the low-volume adjustment. The second criteria is that the facility has not opened, closed, or received a new Medicare provider number because of a change

Figure 7.15. Wage index adjustment formula for ESRD PPS

(National base rate × Labor percentage × wage index)
+ (National base rate × Nonlabor percentage)

in ownership during the three years preceding the payment year (HHS 2010, 49118).

MIPPA mandated that the low-volume adjustment must be equal or greater than 10 percent. After analysis using 2006 through 2008 data, CMS determined that the appropriate adjustment for low-volume facilities is 18.9 percent. If a facility qualifies for the low-volume adjustment, but during the current payment year determines that it has furnished more than 4,000 treatments, the facility must notify the MAC and request to no longer have the adjustment applied to its treatments (HHS 2010, 49122). To add some perspective, furnishing 4,000 treatments in a year equates to approximately 25 patients per year receiving three dialysis treatments a week (HHS 2011, 70236). Although 4,000 treatments may seem like a lot of treatments, 25 patients are really not very many patients to be treated for a whole CY.

Patient-Level Adjustments

The ESRD PPS allows for multiple patient-level adjustments. The adjustments vary for adult and pediatric patients. Not all adjustments are made for each patient; rather, only the applicable adjustments are activated based on the data reported on the ESRD claim form.

Patient Age

The regression analysis used to develop the ESRD PPS indicated that age explains a significant portion of the variation in the resource intensity of renal dialysis services. There is a parabolic or U-shaped relationship between age and cost, with the youngest and oldest categories being the most resource-intensive groups. The patient age adjustments are shown in table 7.18.

Table 7.18.   Patient age adjustment for adult

Variable	Multiplier
Ages 18–44	1.171
Ages 45–59	1.013
Ages 60–69	1.000
Ages 70–79	1.011
Ages 80≦	1.016

Source: Department of Health and Human Services. 2010 (August 12). *Federal Register* 75(155):49088, Table 21.

Body Surface Area and Body Mass Index

MIPPA required that the ESRD PPS take into account a patient's weight, BMI, and other appropriate physical factors. During analysis, CMS evaluated patient's height and weight as predictors of resource intensity. Using the measures of body surface area (BSA) and BMI as independent variables in regression analysis, CMS determined that body size measures are strong predictors of resource consumption (HHS 2010, 49090). Accordingly, two adjustments are made for body size under the ESRD PPS: BSA and low BMI.

For CY 2015, a BSA adjustment of 1.020 is made per 0.1m2 difference in BSA between the patient's value and the national average BSA. The national BSA that is in effect for a particular payment year is provided in the ESRD PPS final rule. The CY 2015 national average BSA is 1.87. The formula for calculating the PM for the BSA adjustment is provided in figure 7.16.

Calculating the BSA PM requires the use of a scientific calculator or the use of the exponential function in a spreadsheet program because the change in BSA is compounded rather than additive. Figure 7.17 provides an example of a BSA PM calculation.

Analysis showed that only low BMI has a significant effect on the resource consumption for renal dialysis services, so an adjustment is provided when the patient's BMI is less than 18.5. The adjustment multiplier for CY 2015 is 1.025.

New Patient Adjustment (Onset of Dialysis)

MIPPA required the CMS consider an adjustment based on the length of time a patient is on dialysis. The studies showed that during the first four months of dialysis treatment, the costs of providing services are significantly higher. Therefore, an adjustment is provided for all treatments during the first four months

Figure 7.16.   BSA patient multiplier formula

$$PM_{BSA} = 1.020^{(\text{patient BSA} \,''\, \text{national average BSA})/0.1}$$

Figure 7.17.   BSA patient multiplier example

Patient A's BSA is 2.2161
National average BSA is 1.87

$$PM_{BSA} = 1.020^{(2.2161 - 1.87)/0.1}$$
$$PM_{BSA} = 1.020^{3.461}$$
$$PM_{BSA} = 1.0709$$

of treatment. However, the individual must be eligible for the Medicare ESRD benefit at the time of the treatment delivery (HHS 2010, 49090). For example, if a patient is covered by a non-Medicare insurer (private insurance) during the first six months of dialysis and then at month seven is eligible for Medicare coverage, the new patient adjustment would not be applied to treatments provided in month seven. To receive the adjustment, the patient must be Medicare ESRD eligible at the onset of dialysis. Therefore, this adjustment is also referred to as the onset of dialysis adjustment. For CY 2015, the adjustment is 1.510 for in-facility and home dialysis patients.

This adjustment has one caveat. If a patient is eligible for and receives the onset of dialysis adjustment for a treatment, then the application of that adjustment cancels out the activation of the comorbidity adjustment and the home training add-on provision (HHS 2010, 49094).

Comorbidity Adjustment

ICD diagnosis codes for all documented comorbid conditions should be reported on the ESRD claim form (bill type 72x). The codes must be reported in compliance with the official ICD coding guidelines, which can be found at http://www.cdc.gov/nchs/icd.htm. All conditions should be reported regardless of whether the condition is on the comorbidity adjustment list. Reporting all comorbid conditions allows for claims data to be used for future enhancements to the ESRD PPS.

Under the ESRD PPS, there are six comorbidity diagnostic categories for which a payment adjustment is provided. The six categories are provided in table 7.19. The specific ICD diagnosis codes for each of the categories are published in the appendices of the ESRD PPS final rule, which is available for download from the CMS website at http://www.cms.gov.

When a patient has multiple comorbid conditions that are in multiple comorbid categories, the condition in the comorbid category with highest multiplier is used for the payment calculation. Furthermore, if a patient has an acute condition, the comorbid adjustment is applicable for four consecutive months from when the condition was reported. For example, if gastrointestinal (GI) bleeding is documented and reported in May, the adjustment multiplier for GI bleeding (1.183) will be applied for treatments in May through August. Chronic conditions do not have the four-month limitation (HHS 2010, 49148).

Table 7.19. Comorbidity diagnostic categories recognized for a payment adjustment under the ESRD PPS

Diagnostic Category	Multiplier
Pericarditis (acute)	1.114
Bacterial Pneumonia (acute)	1.135
Gastrointestinal Tract Bleeding with Hemorrhage (acute)	1.183
Hemolytic Anemia with Sickle Cell Anemia (chronic)	1.072
Myelodysplastic Syndrome (chronic)	1.099
Monoclonal Gammopathy (chronic)	1.024

Source: Department of Health and Human Services. 2010 (August 12). *Federal Register* 75(155):49100, Table 22.

Pediatric Patients

Under the previous basic case-mix-adjusted composite payment system, an adjustment was provided for pediatric patients. This concept is continued in the ESRD PPS, but it has a more detailed approach. Under ESRD PPS, CMS provides for a pediatric adjustment that combines age and modality. There are two modality categories: peritoneal dialysis (PD) and hemodialysis (HD). The pediatric adjustments are provided in table 7.20. Based on the multipliers provided, it is clear that HD treatments are more resource-intensive than PD services for pediatric patients.

Outlier Policy

The outlier policy for ESRD PPS is a rather complicated policy, even though it does in some ways parallel the outlier policies adopted under other Medicare PPSs. The policy states that an ESRD facility is eligible for outlier payment when its imputed Medicare allowable payments (MAP) amount per treatment for outlier

Table 7.20. Pediatric adjustments under ESRD PPS

Patient Characteristics		Payment Multiplier
Age	Modality	
<13	PD	1.033
<13	HD	1.219
13–17	PD	1.067
13–17	HD	1.277

Source: Department of Health and Human Services. 2010 (August 12). *Federal Register* 75(155):49133, Table 27.

services exceeds the outlier threshold. The outlier threshold is equal to the facility's predicted MAP amount per treatment for the outlier services plus the fixed dollar loss amount established for the rate year. The outlier payment is equal to 80 percent of the amount by which the facility's imputed costs (imputed MAP) exceeds the outlier threshold. Several components of this policy require definition to be executable by a facility.

First, the outlier policy specifies that outlier services are eligible for outlier payment. Outlier services are not all renal dialysis services, but rather a subset of services. Outlier services are as follows (HHS 2010, 49138):

- ESRD-related drugs and biological agents that were or would have been, prior to January 2, 2011, separately billable under Medicare Part B

- ESRD-related laboratory tests that were or would have been, prior to January 1, 2011, separately billable under Medicare part B

- Medical/surgical supplies, including syringes, used to administer ESRD-related drugs that were or would have been, prior to January 1, 2011, separately billable under Medicare part B

- Renal dialysis service drugs that were or would have been, prior to January 1, 2011, covered under Medicare Part D

A listing of eligible outlier services by CPT, HCPCS, or national drug code (NDC) code is available from the ESRD PPS Medicare page at http://www.cms.gov. Only the services provided on this list are eligible for outlier payment.

Two types of MAP figures are included in the policy: imputed MAP and predicted MAP. The predicted MAP is provided by Medicare. There are two predicted MAP amounts: The adult predicted MAP is $51.29, and the pediatric predicted MAP is $43.57 for CY 2015 (HHS 2014e). The imputed MAP is a facility-specific amount that is calculated for each claim. CMS elected not to use ESRD facility CCRs to determine cost because it appears as if ESRD-related drugs and biological agents were underreported in the historical data sets. Instead of CCRs, CMS is using a variety of methods to calculate the facility's cost required to calculate the imputed MAP for the outlier calculation. The bases for pricing are as follows:

- Part B drugs that were or would have been separately billable prior to January 1, 2011, will be priced based on the most current average sale price (ASP) pricing plus six percent.

- Laboratory tests that were or would have been separately billable prior to January 1, 2011, will be priced based on the most current laboratory fee schedule amount.

- ESRD-related supplies used to administer separately billable Part B drugs that prior to January 1, 2011, were or would have been separately billable are priced from the MAC elected options such as the Drug Topics Red Book, Med-Span, or First Data Bank.

- Renal dialysis drugs and biological agents that prior to January 1, 2011, were or would have been separately covered under Medicare Part D will be priced by NDC code based on the national average pricing data retrieved from the Medicare Prescription Drug Plan Finder.

To calculate the imputed MAP amount, the MAC will apply one of the pricing methods described earlier for each service or supply on the claim that is outlier eligible. Notably, ESRD services are reported on a monthly claim. The imputed outlier services MAP amounts for each of the services or supplies would be summed and then divided by the corresponding number of treatments identified on the claim (for the entire month) to yield the imputed outlier services MAP amount per treatment.

The last piece of data that is required is the fixed dollar loss amount, which is provided by Medicare on a yearly basis. It is updated each year in the final rule of the ESRD PPS, published in the *Federal Register*. For CY 2015, the fixed dollar loss amount for adults is $86.19 and for pediatric patients is $54.35 (HHS 2014e).

Outlier payments are estimated to equal 1 percent of the total payments for the ESRD PPS. Each year the predicted MAP values and fixed dollar loss amounts are updated with the most current claims data available and published with the ESRD final rule. Please see the workbook that accompanies this text to examine an outlier example.

Self-Dialysis Training

When developing the ESRD PPS base rate, CMS included the cost of training home dialysis patients into the analysis. However, during the proposed rule-making period, CMS received numerous comments from the provider community related to training. The arguments were compelling, and CMS agreed that an add-on payment for self-dialysis training on a per treatment basis was warranted. In addition to there being an enhanced quality of life via home dialysis, CMS also agreed with comments about the required staff expertise necessary to provide adequate training. A registered nurse is required to provide one-on-one focused home dialysis training treatments in accordance with ESRD Conditions for Coverage requirements (HHS 2010, 49062–49063). The self-dialysis training add-on is provided for treatments during which training is provided by a registered nurse. The national add-on amount is wage index adjusted to account for variations in nurse wages by geographic area.

There are, however, some caveats for this adjustment. First, the training add-on is not provided for patients who are receiving the onset of dialysis adjustment. It is expected that a significant amount of training is provided during the beginning dialysis treatments, so the add-on is not provided in addition to the adjustment, as this would be duplicative. Second, there is a cap on training treatments for ESRD. The PD cap is 15 and the HD cap is 25. For CY 2015, the national unadjusted training add-on amount is $50.16 per applicable treatment session (HHS 2014e).

Payment Steps

A three step process is used to determine the ESRD PPS final payment per session. Figure 7.18 provides the foundation for the ESRD PPS payment. It is critical to review all medical record document to ensure that all facility and patient-level adjustments are taken into consideration when determining payment. The following example illustrates the important of including all adjustments.

Example: Patient with ESRD with Multiple Comorbidities

The following example is taken from Example 3 (eight examples were provided in total) in the ESRD PPS 2011 Final Rule (HHS 2010, 49149–49150). The example has been modified slightly to include applicable payment methodology updates for CY 2015.

Mary, a 66-year-old woman, is 167.64 cm in height and weighs 105 kg. She has diabetes mellitus and cirrhosis of the liver. Mary was diagnosed with ESRD in 2006 and has been receiving HD since that time. Mary was admitted for a two-week hospitalization from January 2–16, 2015 because of GI tract bleeding, a diagnosis confirmed on discharge. Mary's hemorrhaging caused by her GI bleeding ceased during her hospitalization. While in the hospital, Mary received inpatient dialysis. Mary was also discharged with a diagnosis of monoclonal gammopathy. After convalescing at home for three days, she resumed HD at an ESRD facility on January 20, 2015. The facility records the GI bleeding and monoclonal gammopathy diagnoses using the relevant ICD-9-CM codes for treatments received during the month of January. For claims submitted beginning with the month of February and continuing thereafter, the facility reports only the monoclonal gammopathy diagnosis, a chronic condition. Mary's BMI = 37.3626, and she does not qualify for the low BMI adjustment.

The PM that must be considered for this example includes GI tract bleeding, monoclonal gammopathy, age, and BSA. Although Mary has diabetes and cirrhosis of the liver, these comorbidities are not used in determining the case-mix adjusters under the ESRD PPS. Mary's BSA = 2.1284. The PM for her BSA is 1.0525.

Although Mary has both an acute comorbidity (GI bleeding) and a chronic comorbidity (monoclonal gammopathy) for the month of January, the facility may only be paid using the condition with the higher adjustment factor for the maximum number of four consecutive claim months in which payment for both comorbidities must be considered. Because the case-mix adjustment for GI bleeding (1.183) exceeds that for monoclonal gammopathy (1.024), Mary's case-mix adjustment for comorbidities will reflect GI bleeding only for treatments received in January 2015 through April 2015. Therefore, for these treatments, Mary's PM may be expressed as

$$PM_{Mary} = PM_{age} \times PM_{BSA} \times PM_{GIBleed}$$

$$PM_{Mary} = 1.000 \times 1.0525 \times 1.183$$

$$PM_{Mary} = 1.2451$$

For treatments received from January 20, 2015, through April 2015, Mary's payment rate per treatment is $239.43 \times 1.2541 = 300.27.

Figure 7.18.   Foundation of end-stage renal disease payment system

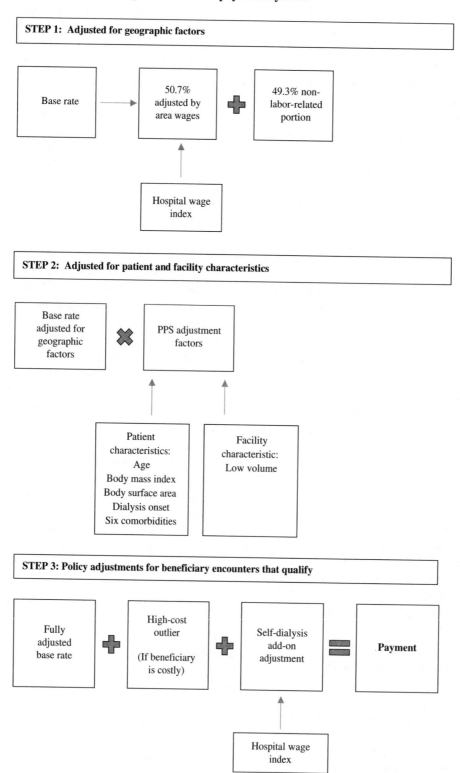

Source: Adapted from Medicare Payment Advisory Commission (MedPAC). 2014g. Payment Basics: Outpatient Dialysis Services Payment System. Pg. 2. http://www.medpac.gov.

Payment for Safety-Net Providers

Safety-net providers are also known as "essential community providers" and "providers of last resort" (Lewin and Altman 2000, 54). The Institute of Medicine has defined "core safety net provider" as a set of

> providers that organize and deliver a significant level of healthcare and other health-related services. These providers have two distinguishing characteristics: (1) by legal mandate or explicitly adopted mission they maintain an "open door," offering services to patients regardless of their ability to pay; and (2) a substantial share of their patient mix is uninsured, Medicaid, and other vulnerable patients. (Lewin and Altman 2000, 21)

Examples of core ambulatory safety-net providers are federally qualified health centers (FQHCs; community health centers), rural health clinics (RHCs), migrant clinics, free clinics, public health department clinics, and emergency departments of public and teaching hospitals. Two of the ambulatory safety-net providers are the focus of this section: FQHCs and RHCs. FQHCs and RHCs have a 50-year history in the US healthcare system.

Background

Early roots of FQHCs are in the Migrant Health Act of 1962 and the Economic Opportunity Act of 1964 (Bureau of Primary Health Care 2008, 1; Lefkowitz 2005, 297). These acts provided federal support for medical care delivered in what were then known as migrant health centers and neighborhood health centers. In the mid-1970s, neighborhood health centers became known as community health centers (Bureau of Primary Health Care 2008, 2). In the 1980s and 1990s, Congress expanded the concept of community health centers to cover healthcare provided to homeless people and residents of public housing under the McKinney Homeless Assistance Act of 1987 and the Disadvantaged Minority Health Improvement Act of 1990, respectively (Bureau of Primary Health Care 2008, 2). The FQHC program was established under the OBRA of 1989 and expanded under the OBRA of 1990. The Health Centers Consolidation Act of 1996 consolidated four federal primary care programs (community, migrant, homeless, and public housing) under section 330 of the Public Health Service Act (Bureau of Primary Health Care 2008, 2).

Federally qualified health centers (FQHCs) are nonprofit, patient-governed, and community-directed healthcare entities (HHS 2014a, 25439). FQHCs are located in both urban and rural areas. The purpose of FQHCs is to increase access to comprehensive basic healthcare services. Providing care to 21 million people at more than 9,000 sites, FQHCs are one of the largest networks of primary care providers in the United States (HHS 2014a, 25439; Health Resources and Services Administration 2013).

Two additional types of FQHCs exist. Look-Alikes are healthcare organizations that are similar to FQHCs in terms of eligibility requirements and benefits but that do not receive the section 330 grant funding (see next section). Also qualifying as FQHCs are outpatient health programs/facilities operated by tribal organizations or urban Indian organizations under the Indian Self-Determination Act and Indian Health Care Improvement Act, respectively (HHS 2014a, 25433).

Rural health clinics (RHCs) are a federal category of health provider that is unique to **rural areas**. RHCs were established under the Rural Health Clinic Services Act of 1977. The purpose of RHCs is to increase access to primary and preventive healthcare services in rural areas. RHCs must be located in nonurbanized areas with health professional shortages (HPSA or governor-designated). There are approximately 4,000 RHCs in the United States (Medicare Learning Network 2014c, 1-2). RHCs may be public or private, for-profit or not-for-profit, and provider-based or independent. Provider-based clinics are owned and operated as integral and subordinate parts of a larger healthcare organization, such as s hospital, nursing home, or home health agency. Provider-based RHCs operate under the licensure, governance, and professional supervision of the larger organization. Most provider-based RHCs are hospital-owned. Independent clinics are free standing clinics or office-based practices not owned or operated by a larger healthcare organization. More than half of independent clinics are owned by clinicians (George Washington University 2012, 47).

Characteristics of Federally Qualified Health Centers and Rural Health Clinics

The majority of the patients of FQHCs and RHCs have limited access to healthcare services. Most of the patients have low incomes. They are often members of medically **underserved areas/populations** (MUA/Ps;

also known as medically underserved patients). HRSA defines MUA/Ps as areas or populations with one, or some combination, of the following statuses:

- HPSAs (see earlier section in RBRVS)

- Residents with shortages of personal health services

- High infant mortality

- High poverty

- High elderly population

MUAs may be whole counties, groups of contiguous counties or other civil divisions, or groups of urban census tracts. MUPs may include groups of persons who face economic, cultural, or linguistic barriers to healthcare. Included in medically underserved populations are migratory and seasonal agricultural workers, the homeless, and residents of public housing.

Community health centers are not automatically FQHCs. They must apply for the designation of federally qualified and must meet criteria to maintain the designation. Benefits of the FQHC designation include

- Start-up grant funding up to $650,000

- Federal grant funding under section 330 (not available to Look-Alikes)

- Medical malpractice coverage through the Federal Tort Claims Act

- Eligibility to purchase prescription and nonprescription medications for outpatients at reduced cost through the 340B Drug Pricing Program (20 to 40 percent of average wholesale price on open market) (HHS 2014a, 25439)

- Access to Vaccine for Children Program

- Eligibility for various other federal grants and programs

Generally, similarities exist between FQHCs and RHCs in terms of eligibility requirements and benefits. Key differences for RHCs follow (Medicare Learning Network 2014c, 2):

- Must be in nonurbanized areas (unlike FQHCs, which may be in **urban areas**)

- Have narrower scopes of services

- Must have at least one midlevel practitioner (nurse practitioner, physician assistant, or nurse midwife) on-site and available to see patients 50 percent of the time

- Cannot be FQHCs, rehabilitation agencies, or facilities primarily for the treatment of mental disease

FQHCs and RHCs both provide outpatient primary care services. FQHCs, in addition to primary care services and laboratory services, provide dental, mental health, substance abuse, and transportation services. These services may be provided on site or through an arrangement with another provider. RHCs, on the other hand, are only required to provide outpatient primary care services and basic laboratory services (Health Resources and Services Administration n.d., n.p.). For both FQHCs and RHCs, similar services that are covered under Medicare and Medicaid include:

- Physician services

- Services and supplies incident to the services of physicians

- Services of nurse practitioners (NPs), physician assistants (PAs), certified nurse midwives (CNMs), clinical psychologists (CPs), and clinical social workers (CSWs)

- Services and supplies incident to the services of NPs, PAs, CNMS, CPs, and CSWs

- Visiting nurse services to the homebound where CMS has determined a shortage of home health agencies

- Medicare Part B–covered drugs furnished by and incident to services of FQHC/RHC provider (Medicare Learning Network 2014c, 2; HHS 2014a, 25439)

Reimbursement

Medicare and Medicaid are key payers for FQHCs and RHCs. Medicare beneficiaries account for approximately 8 percent of the patients of FQHCs and approximately 31 percent of the patients of RHCs. Medicaid recipients account for approximately 41 percent of the patients of FQHCs and 25 percent of the patients of RHCs (HHS 2014a, 25439; George Washington University 2012, 13).

Medicare

Medicare reimburses FQHCs and RHCs for medically necessary covered services. However, CMS has different payment methods for the two types of healthcare organizations. The different payment methods reflect the varying intensity and scope of services between the two types of healthcare organizations (MedPAC 2011, 149). Moreover, physicians and nonphysicians providing care at FQHCs and RHCs are not reimbursed under the RBRVS. Instead, the FQHCs and RHCs where the clinicians provided services receive facility-based reimbursements (George Washington University 2012, 26).

Federally Qualified Health Center Prospective Payment System

Medicare reimburses FQHCs under the FQHC prospective payment system (PPS). The FQHC PPS was effective October 1, 2014, as required by the Affordable Care Act of 2010. The FQHC PPS is a single, encounter-based per diem rate. The unit of payment is the single, face-to-face encounter between a patient and an FQHC practitioner. Medicare pays for all medically-necessary, FQHC services furnished to a patient on the same day during a face-to-face FQHC visit. The FQHC is paid the *lesser* of its actual charges or the PPS rate.

The FQHC PPS consists of the following three elements: base rate, geographic adjustment factor (GAF), and, if applicable, a risk-adjustment factor (Figure 7.19).

The base rate is adjusted for differences in costs in various geographic areas by a geographic adjustment factor (GAF) based on the locality of the center. The geographically adjusted base rate is then risk-adjusted, if applicable, for the following patient characteristics:

- New patient
- Initial preventive physical exam (IPPE)
- Annual wellness visit (AWV) initial or subsequent

The base rate, GAF, and the risk adjustment are determined annually and published in the *Federal Register*. Table 7.21 shows the calculation of a FQHC PPS payment for a new patient. If the patient had been a returning patient who was not having an annual wellness visit, the payment would have no risk adjustment and the amount is seen in Cell D3. The actual payment that the FQHC receives is 80 percent of the calculated payment, with the beneficiary paying a 20 percent coinsurance.

Figure 7.19. Foundation of federally qualified health center prospective payment system

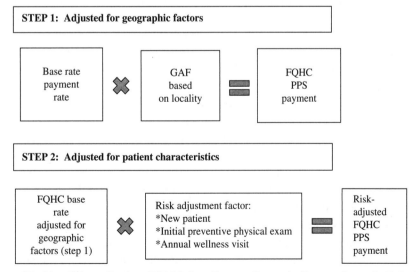

Source of content: Department of Health and Human Services. 2014. Medicare Program; Prospective Payment System for Federally Qualified Health Centers; Changes to Contracting Policies for Rural Health Clinics; and Changes to Clinical Laboratory Improvement Amendments of 1988 Enforcement Actions for Proficiency Testing Referral; Final Rule. *Federal Register* 79(85):25454–25455.

Table 7.21.   Example of risk-adjusted payment under the federally qualified health center prospective payment system

	A	B	C	D	E	F
1	Year	Base payment rate	Locality GAF*	Geographic-adjusted payment (base payment rate x GAF)	Risk-adjustment, if applicable	Geographic and risk adjusted payment (geog.-adjusted pymt x risk adj. amt.)
2				B x C		D x E
3	2015	$158.85	0.953	151.3841	1.3416	$203.10

*North Carolina payment locality (60).

Source: Department of Health and Human Services. 2014 (May 2). Medicare Program; Prospective Payment System for Federally Qualified Health Centers; Changes to Contracting Policies for Rural Health Clinics; and Changes to Clinical Laboratory Improvement Amendments of 1988 Enforcement Actions for Proficiency Testing Referral; Final Rule. *Federal Register* 79(85):25481–25482.

Exceptions to the single, encounter-based per diem are:

- Occurrence of an illness or injury subsequent to the initial medical visit that requires another subsequent encounter on the same day

- Mental health visit is furnished on the same day as the medical visit

- Services not paid at the encounter rate, such as lab tests and technical components, that are billed separately to Medicare Part B using a professional claim

- Flu and pneumonia vaccines, which will continue to be reimbursed at 100 percent of reasonable costs through the cost report process (CMS 2014b)

CMS has established five specific payment G-codes to be used by FQHCs submitting claims under the PPS (Table 7.22).

These G-codes are HCPCS Level II codes. The G-codes require specific revenue codes and qualifying HCPCS/CPT Level I codes (see chapter 2). **Revenue codes** are three- or four-digit billing codes that categorize charges based on type of service, supply, procedure, or location of service. FQHCs report the G-code that represents the type of encounter. FQHCs also report a single charge for the G-code that bundles (aggregates) the regular rates charged for services that typically would be furnished during the encounter.

FQHCs must also provide Medicare with line-by-line reports of all healthcare services rendered for each patient visit. Each line must contain the appropriate HCPCS/CPT code, revenue code, and charge (see chapters 2 and 9, respectively) (Medicare Learning Network 2014b, 4).

Rural Health Clinic (RHC) All-Inclusive Rate

Medicare reimburses RHCs under an **all-inclusive rate (AIR)** for each visit. A visit is defined as a face-to-face encounter between the patient and a physician, physician assistant, nurse practitioner, nurse midwife, clinical psychologist, or clinical social worker during which an *RHC covered service is rendered* (Medicare Learning Network 2014c, 2). RHC visits may take place in the RCH or in the patient's home. The AIR pays for healthcare services defined as RHC covered services (see previous section). Examples of RHC noncovered services are ambulance services, durable medical equipment, and services delivered at an inpatient hospital.

The RHC receives the AIR as reimbursement for each face-to-face encounter that its practitioners provide. For each visit, the rate is the same regardless of the number or type of covered services provided during the visit (all-inclusive) and the type of provider, physician or midlevel provider.

The AIR is based on reasonable costs as reported on the cost report. For each RHC, the AIR is calculated by dividing the total allowable costs of the RHC by the total number of visits of all its patients. The AIR is also subject to annual reconciliation (resolution of differences between estimates and actual costs) and to a national maximum payment per visit (cap or upper limit). The national upper payment limit is set annually and is updated for inflation based on the Medicare

Table 7.22. G-codes used by federally qualified health centers to submit claims under the Medicare prospective payment system

G-code	Brief title	Description	Revenue Code	Representative Qualifying HCPCS/ CPT codes
G0466	FQHC visit, new patient	A medically necessary, face-to-face encounter (one-on-one) between a new patient and a FQHC practitioner during which time one or more FQHC services are rendered and includes a typical bundle of Medicare-covered services that would be furnished per diem to a patient receiving a FQHC visit.	052X or 0519*	92002 99201 99202 99203 99204 99205
G0467	FQHC visit, established patient	A medically necessary, face-to-face encounter (one-on-one) between an established patient and a FQHC practitioner during which time one or more FQHC services are rendered and includes a typical bundle of Medicare-covered services that would be furnished per diem to a patient receiving a FQHC visit.	052X or 0519	92012 99211 99212 99213 99214 99215
G0468	FQHC visit, IPPE or AWV	A FQHC visit that includes an IPPE or AWV and includes a typical bundle of Medicare-covered services that would be furnished per diem to a patient receiving an IPPE or AWV.	052X or 0519	G0402 G0438 G0439
G0469	FQHC visit, mental health, new patient	A medically necessary, face-to-face mental health encounter (one-on-one) between a new patient and a FQHC practitioner during which time one or more FQHC services are rendered and includes a typical bundle of Medicare-covered services that would be furnished per diem to a patient receiving a mental health visit.	0900 or 0519	90791 90792 90832 90845
G0470	FQHC visit, mental health, established patient	A medically necessary, face-to-face mental health encounter (one-on-one) between an established patient and a FQHC practitioner during which time one or more FQHC services are rendered and includes a typical bundle of Medicare-covered services that would be furnished per diem to a patient receiving a mental health visit.	0900 or 0519	90791 90792 90832 90845

*0519 only used with Medicare Advantage (MA) Supplemental claims

Source: Centers for Medicare and Medicaid Services. 2014b. CMS Manual System. Pub 100-20 One-Time Notification. Transmittal 1395. Change Request 8743. Attachment A. Specific Payment Codes for the FQHC PPS:1-6. http://www.cms.gov/Regulations-and-Guidance/Guidance/Transmittals/downloads/R1395OTN.pdf.

Economic Index (MEI). As a reference point, the upper payment limit in 2015 was $80.44 (Medicare Learning Network 2015, 2).

Medicare Cost Sharing

Cost sharing for Medicare beneficiaries varies between FQHCs and RHCs:

- No annual deductible for FQHC services
- Annual deductible for RHC services
- 20 percent coinsurance of the usual and customary charge (FQHCs and RHCs) except for certain preventive services (such as initial preventive physical examination; annual wellness visit; mammography, pelvic, Pap smear, prostate, glaucoma, abdominal aortic aneurysm screening exams; and diabetes self-management training services)
- Vaccines (influenza, pneumococcal, hepatitis B) have no cost sharing (FQHCs and RHCs) (Medicare Learning Network 2014b, 6; Medicare Learning Network 2014c, 3)

In addition, FQHCs must offer services using a **sliding scale** (fee adjusted to ability to pay). No requirement of a sliding scale exists for RHCs, though many choose to offer the option (MedPAC 2011, 149).

Medicaid

The Medicare, Medicaid, and SCHIP Benefits Improvement and Protection Act (BIPA) of 2000 established a Medicaid PPS. FQHCs and RHCs share this Medicaid payment method (Mann 2010, 1). The payment rate is specific to individual FQHCs and RHCs because the PPS is based on the historical reasonable costs of each FQHC or RHC (Mann 2010, 2). State Medicaid programs make payments calculated on a per-visit basis equal to the reasonable cost of such services as documented in a baseline period. Adjustment factors in the PPS take into account inflation and changes in the FQHC's or RHC's scope of services during the fiscal year (Mann 2010, 2). State Medicaid programs may also choose to continue under a reasonable cost methodology or may choose an alternative payment methodology (APM) as long as the alternative methodology does not pay less than the PPS and the affected center agrees to the APM (Mann 2010, 3).

Hospice Services Payment System

Hospice is a comprehensive, holistic approach to healthcare that recognizes patients' impending deaths. Hospice "uses an interdisciplinary approach to deliver medical, nursing, social, psychological, emotional, and spiritual services through use of a broad spectrum of professional and other caregivers" (HHS 2014b, 50454). Hospice services are provided to terminally ill patients and their families. The services are **palliative**, meaning that they are designed to relieve patients' pain and suffering; they are not designed to cure patients' underlying conditions. Hospice patients have decided to forego curative treatments for their diseases. Covered services include the following (MedPAC 2014c, 1):

- Physicians' services
- Skilled nursing care
- Drugs and biological agents for pain control and symptom management
- Medical equipment (such as wheelchairs or walkers)
- Medical supplies (such as bandages and catheters)
- Physical, occupational, and speech therapy

- Counseling (dietary, spiritual, family bereavement, and other services)
- Home health aide and homemaker services
- Short-term inpatient acute care
- Inpatient **respite care** (relief for caregivers; up to five days per inpatient hospitalization)
- Other services necessary for palliation and management of terminal illness

The goal of hospice is to make patients as physically and emotionally comfortable as possible. The broad spectrum of professional and other caregivers includes

- Physicians
- Nurses
- Counselors
- Social workers
- Physical, occupational, and speech therapists
- Hospice aides and homemakers
- Volunteers

In addition, the patient and family members have important roles in hospice. Finally, a hospice nurse and a physician are available 24 hours per day, 7 days a week to provide care to the patient and support to the family as needed.

Typically, hospice services are delivered in patients' homes; however, hospice services may also be provided in inpatient settings. Providers of hospice services may be free-standing healthcare entities, or the providers may be based in acute-care inpatient hospitals, skilled nursing facilities, or home health agencies. Medicare beneficiaries' use of hospice is rapidly increasing, with Medicare's payments for hospice services exceeding $15 billion (MedPAC 2014c, 1).

Background

Hospice is covered under Medicare Part A. The hospice benefit began in 1983 as authorized by the Tax Equity and Fiscal Responsibility Act of 1982 (TEFRA). Coverage requirements include the following:

- Two physicians (beneficiary's attending physician and a hospice physician) must certify that the patient is terminally ill and has six months or fewer to live based on the normal progression of the patient's illness.

- Beneficiary has "elected" (formally selected or enrolled in) the Medicare hospice benefit in writing, thereby agreeing to forgo Medicare coverage for intensive, conventional, curative treatment of the terminal illness.

- Written plan of care has been established and is maintained by the attending physician, the medical director, or another hospice physician and by an interdisciplinary group. The plan of care identifies the services to be provided (including management of discomfort and symptom relief) and describes the scope and frequency of services needed to meet the needs of the beneficiary and the family.

Beneficiaries elect hospice for defined benefit periods. The first hospice benefit period is 90 days, and as stated previously, two physicians must certify that the patient is likely to die within six months. *Only the hospice physician* may recertify the patient for another 90 days if the patient's death is likely within the next six months. Before the patient's 180-day recertification (for a third benefit period), a hospice physician or nurse practitioner must have a face-to-face encounter with the patient. The encounter must occur no more than 30 calendar days prior to the start of the hospice patient's third benefit period. After the 180-day recertification, the patient can be recertified for an unlimited number of 60-day periods. Each subsequent recertification also requires a face-to-face encounter. Beneficiaries can transfer from one hospice to another once during a hospice election period and can disenroll from hospice at any time. *Note: Should the patient live longer than six months, the Medicare hospice benefit continues to cover the cost of services until the patient's death or disenrollment from hospice.*

Beneficiaries' cost sharing for hospice services is minimal (see chapter 4). There is no deductible. For prescriptions, hospices may charge 5 percent coinsurance (not to exceed $5) for each prescription furnished outside the inpatient setting. For inpatient respite care, beneficiaries may be charged 5 percent of Medicare's respite care payment per day (not to exceed the Part A inpatient hospital deductible, approximately $1,200) (MedPAC 2014c, 3).

Reimbursement

Hospices are reimbursed under a prospective payment system (PPS) in which the Medicare payment is made based on a predetermined, fixed per diem for each day of hospice care. Four levels of hospice care exist. The per diem rate based on four levels of care was established in 1983 as authorized by TEFRA. This four-level payment structure remains essentially the same today as when initially established. The unit of payment is the enrolled day.

Structure of Payment

The hospice PPS consists of the following two elements: category standard daily base payment rate and geographic adjustment factors (Figure 7.20). Figure 7.20 shows the four steps of calculating a payment.

Category Standard Daily Base Payment Rate

Medicare pays a standard daily base payment rate to hospice providers for each day a beneficiary is enrolled in hospice. The daily rate (or per diem) is all-inclusive. The daily rate is based on the location and intensity of services. All costs and services related to the patient's terminal illness are included in the daily rate. The daily rate takes into account the cost of:

- Professionals' and other caregivers' visits to their patients

- Other costs hospices incurred, such as on-call services, care planning, drugs and medical equipment, supplies related to the patient's terminal condition, and patient transportation between sites of care specified in the plan of care

The daily rate is *not* related to the amount of services the hospice provides. The rate for a day with no visit and no services is the same as the rate for a day with a visit and many services (MedPAC 2014c, 1). Services and items unrelated to the terminal illness (such as from an accident) are not included in the daily rate and are covered under the beneficiary's Medicare Part A and Medicare Part B as applicable and with appropriate deductibles and coinsurance.

Based on the location and intensity of services, care of hospice patients is divided into four categories of daily base payment rates. Following are the four categories of care and their representative daily rates:

- Routine home care (RHC): home care provided during a typical day ($159)

- Continuous home care (CHC): home care provided during periods of patient crisis ($930)

- Inpatient respite care (IRC): inpatient care for a short period to provide relief for the primary caregiver ($165)

- General inpatient care (GIC): inpatient care to treat symptoms that cannot be managed in another setting ($709) (MedPAC 2014c, 2)

During a benefit period, patients may vary among the four categories based on their needs. Each day is

Figure 7.20. Foundation of hospice prospective payment system

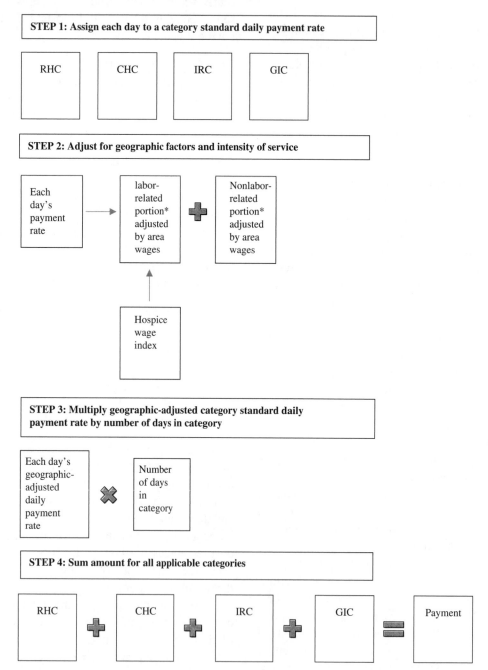

*Labor-related portions for each category: RHC=69%, CHC=69%, IRC=54%, GIC=64%

Source: Adapted from Medicare Payment Advisory Commission (MedPAC). 2014c. Payment basics: Hospice services payment system. p. 2. http://www.medpac.gov.

assigned to the appropriate category. Routine home care accounts for more than 95 percent of hospice care days. The Medicare daily payment rates for hospice are updated annually by the inpatient hospital market basket index (relative measure that averages the costs of a mix of goods and services).

Geographic Adjustment Factors

The categories' base payment rates are adjusted for geographic factors and intensity of human resources. For the geographic location, the hospice PPS uses urban and nonurban core based statistical areas (CBSAs, federally designated geographic locations). The geographic adjustment is necessary to account for differences in two types of expenses:

- Labor portion: varying wage rates across US urban and nonurban CBSAs. The labor portion is adjusted by the hospice wage index for the CBSA where care is furnished.

- Nonlabor portion: costs of goods and services, such as supplies, equipment, and other services, in various parts of the United States.

Additionally, the intensity of human resources varies across the four categories. For example, the intensity of human resources is higher for routine home care (RHC) than for inpatient respite care (IRC). Therefore, each category of care's base rate has its own labor portion (ranging from 54 to 69 percent) to account for differing labor costs among the categories. Correspondingly, each category of care's base rate has its own nonlabor portion (ranging from 46 to 31 percent). The adjusted labor portion and the nonlabor portion are added together for the total geographic adjustment.

Calculation

Figure 7.20 and table 7.23 show the calculation of a hospice payment for a patient who had a total of 19 days of hospice care with 16 days in the most common category, routine home care (RHC), and three days in general inpatient care (GIC).

Table 7.23 shows the following steps to calculate payment:

Step 1: Each day of hospice care is assigned to one of the four categories. The assignment of the daily base payment rate is based on the location and intensity of services *for that day*. The hospice provider is paid the daily base payment for that day. Thus, on various days,

Table 7.23.   Example of calculation of hospice prospective payment

	A	B	C	D	E	F	G	H	I	J	K
1	Category	No. of Days	Standard Base Payment Rate	Labor-related portion	Nonlabor-related portion	Local wage index*	Adj labor portion (labor related portion × local wage index × standard reate)	Adj nonlabor portion (nonlabor-related portion × standard rate)	Per diem geographic adj standard rate (adj labor portion plus non labor portion)	Total per diem geographic adj standard rate (No. of days × adj rate)	Total payment (SUM all categories)
2							D × F × C	E × C	G + H	B × I	J3 + J4
3	RHC	16	$159	69%	31%	0.9430	$103.46	$49.29	$152.75	$2,443.94	
4	GIC	13	$709	64%	36%	0.9430	$427.90	$255.24	$683.14	$2,049.41	
5	All Categories										$4,493.35

*Urban CBSA: Greenville, NC; 24780

Source: Centers for Medicare and Medicaid Services. n.d. Addendum B: Final hospice wage index for FY 2015. http://www.cms.gov/Medicare/Medicare-Fee-for-Service-Payment/Hospice/Downloads/FY2015-Hospice-Wage-Index-Counties.pdf.

different daily base payment rates may be paid for one patient's care.

Step 2: The categories' base payments are adjusted for geographic factors and intensity of human resources. The hospice daily payment rates are adjusted geographically to account for differences in wage rates among local markets. The labor portion is adjusted by the hospice wage index for the location where care is furnished. The adjusted labor portion is added to the nonlabor portion.

Step 3: Payment is calculated as the number of days in each category multiplied by categories' base daily payment amount and adjusted for geographic factors and labor intensity.

Step 4: All the categories' geographically adjusted base daily payment amounts are summed.

In the calculation shown in Table 7.23, it should be noted that the geographically adjusted standard base payment rates for the categories, RHC and GIC (cells I3 and I4), are *less* than the original standard base payment rate because the CBSA's wage index is *less* than one.

Implementation

Two limits or "caps" on hospice provider services exist.

- Number of days of inpatient care. The number of days of inpatient care (GIC) that a hospice provider renders may not exceed 20 percent of its total patient care days.

- Hospice aggregate cap amount. Medicare aggregates all the payments to a hospice provider. The total payments cannot exceed this aggregate cap amount. The aggregate cap amount is a dollar limit based on the average annual payment per beneficiary. The hospice cannot receive payments exceeding this amount. This aggregate cap amount is updated annually. To calculate the hospice provider's compliance, this average payment amount is multiplied by the total number of the hospice's beneficiaries. Currently, the average payment per beneficiary is about $25,000. Thus, if Hospice Provider A rendered care to 100 beneficiaries, the amount cannot exceed $2,500,000 ($25,000 × 100). If the total payments to Hospice Provider A exceed $2,500,000, Hospice Provider A must repay the overpayment.

These caps limit the amount and cost of care that any one hospice provider renders in a single year (MedPAC 2014c, 3).

Check Your Understanding 7.4

1. True or false? Medicare payments made under the ESRD PPS can cover dialysis services rendered to children.

2. True or false? In the ESRD PPS, a patient-level adjustment for adults is high body mass index.

3. True or false? The federal 340B drug pricing program makes prescription drugs available to eligible providers at reduced cost.

4. True or false? FQHCs, similar to RHCs, must be established in nonurban areas.

5. True or false? Medicare payments for a Medicare beneficiary's hospice services terminate at six months or the beneficiary's death, whichever comes first.

6. In the hospice PPS, which category of care has the lowest per diem rate of reimbursement?

Chapter 7 Review Quiz

1. In the RBRVS, which codes have associated RVUs?

2. What are the three elements of the RVU?

3. How can physician payments be adjusted for the price differences among various parts of the country?

4. What is the control mechanism the government uses on Medicare payments to physicians, and how is it applied?

5. What are the bases for the seven levels of service used in the ambulance services fee schedule?

6. True or false? When a patient is pronounced dead during ambulance transport, Medicare payment rules are followed as if the patient were alive.

7. How is the "two-times rule" applied to APC groups?

8. True or false? CMS, not the APC Advisory Panel or MedPAC, makes the final ruling for updates and changes to OPPS.

9. True or false? The number of APCs per encounter for a single patient is limited to 10.

10. Describe how observation services are currently reimbursed under OPPS.

11. What adjustments, if any, are used under OPPS to account for cost differences among facilities under OPPS?

12. Describe how the ASC PPS conversion factor is different from the OPPS conversion factor.

13. Why are device-intensive procedure APCs payments adjusted for ASCs?

14. Which federal law mandated the current bundled payment system for ESRD?

15. In the ESRD payment system, list two facility-level adjustments.

16. What law consolidated the four federal primary care programs?

17. True or false? Both FQHCs and RHCs must offer services using a sliding scale.

18. What law established the Medicare hospice benefit?

19. True or false? In the hospice PPS, palliative care provides relief for caregivers.

References

American Academy of Pediatrics. 2014. 2014 RBRVS: What is it and how does it affect pediatrics? http://www.aap.org/en-us/professional-resources/practice-support/Coding-at-the-AAP/Documents/rbrvsbrochure.pdf.

Averill, R.F., N.I. Goldfield, J. Eisenhandler, J.S. Hughes, and J. Muldoon, 2001. Clinical risk groups and the future of healthcare reimbursement. In *Reimbursement methodologies for healthcare services* [CD-ROM]. Edited by L.M. Jones. Chicago: AHIMA.

Bureau of Primary Health Care. 2008. Health centers: America's primary care safety net, reflections on success, 2002–2007. http://www.hrsa.gov/ourstories/healthcenter/reflectionsonsuccess.pdf.

Centers for Medicare and Medicaid Services. n.d. Addendum B: Final hospice wage index for FY 2015. http://www.cms.gov/Medicare/Medicare-Fee-for-Service-Payment/Hospice/Downloads/FY2015-Hospice-Wage-Index-Counties.pdf.

Centers for Medicare and Medicaid Services. 2015. Estimated Sustainable Growth Rate and Conversion Factor, for Medicare Payments to Physicians in 2015. http://www.cms.gov/Medicare/Medicare-Fee-for-Service-Payment/SustainableGRatesConFact/Downloads/SGR2015f.pdf.

Centers for Medicare and Medicaid Services. 2005. Revisions and corrections to the *Medicare Claims Processing Manual*, Chapter 6, Section 30, and various sections in Chapter 15. Pub 100-04 Medicare claims processing. CMS Transmittal 437. http://www.cms.gov/Regulations-and-Guidance/Guidance/Transmittals/downloads/R437CP.pdf.

Centers for Medicare and Medicaid Services. 2007. Ambulance fee schedule—Medical conditions list: Manualization. CR 5442: Transmittal R1185CP. Pub. 100-4. https://www.cms.gov/Regulations-and-Guidance/Guidance/Transmittals/Downloads/R1185CP.pdf.

Centers for Medicare and Medicaid Services. 2009a. Physician fee schedule search. http://www.cms.hhs.gov/pfslookup/.

Centers for Medicare and Medicaid Services. 2009b Process and information required to apply for additional device categories for traditional pass-through payment status under the Hospital Outpatient Prospective Payment System. http://www.cms.hhs.gov/HospitalOutpatientPPS/Downloads/catapp.pdf.

Centers for Medicare and Medicaid Services. 2011a. Market basket definitions and general information. http://www.cms.gov/MedicareProgramRatesStats/downloads/info.pdf.

Centers for Medicare and Medicaid Services. 2011b. Medicare EHR incentive program, physician quality reporting system and e-prescribing comparison. ICN no. 903691. https://www.cms.gov/MLNProducts/downloads/EHRIncentivePayments-ICN903691.pdf.

Centers for Medicare and Medicaid Services. 2014a. Physician Fee Schedule Search. http://www.cms.hhs.gov/pfslookup/.

Centers for Medicare and Medicaid Services. 2014b. CMS Manual System. Pub 100-20 One-Time Notification. Transmittal 1395. Change Request 8743. Attachment A. Specific Payment Codes for the FQHC PPS. http://www.cms.gov/Regulations-and-Guidance/Guidance/Transmittals/downloads/R1395OTN.pdf

Centers for Medicare and Medicaid Services. 2014c. EHR Incentive Program: Payment adjustments & hardship exceptions tipsheet for eligible professionals. http://www.cms.gov/Regulations-and-Guidance/Legislation/EHRIncentivePrograms/Downloads/PaymentAdj_HardshipExcepTipSheetforEP.pdf.

Centers for Medicare and Medicaid Services. 2014d. Physician bonuses. http://www.cms.gov/Medicare/Medicare-Fee-for-Service-Payment/HPSAPSAPhysicianBonuses/index.html?redirect=/HPSAPSAPhysicianBonuses/.

Department of Health and Human Services. 2002. Medicare program; Fee schedule for payment of ambulance services and revisions to the physician certification requirements for coverage of nonemergency ambulance services; Final rule. *Federal Register* 67(39):9099–9135.

Department of Health and Human Services. 2004a. Medicare program; Proposed changes to the Hospital Outpatient Prospective Payment System and calendar year 2005 payment rates; Proposed rule. *Federal Register* 69(157):50447–50546.

Department of Health and Human Services. 2004b. Medicare program; Update of ambulatory surgical center list of covered procedures; Proposed rule. *Federal Register* 69(227):69178–69180.

Department of Health and Human Services. 2007a. Medicare program; Revised payment system policies for services furnished in ambulatory surgical centers (ASCs) beginning in CY 2008; Final rule. *Federal Register* 72(148):42470–42626.

Department of Health and Human Services. 2007b. Medicare program; Proposed changes to the Hospital Outpatient Prospective Payment System and CY 2008 payment rates; Proposed changes to the ambulatory surgical center payment system CY 2008 payment rates; Proposed rule. *Federal Register* 72(148):42628–43129.

Department of Health and Human Services. 2009. Medicare program: Changes to the hospital outpatient prospective payment system and CY 2010 payment rates: Changes to the ambulatory surgical center payment system and CY 2010 payment rates. *Federal Register*. 74(223):60592–60594.

Department of Health and Human Services. 2010. Medicare program; End-stage renal disease prospective payment system; Final rule and proposed rule. *Federal Register* 75(155):49030–49214.

Department of Health and Human Services. 2011. Medicare program; End-stage renal disease prospective payment system and quality incentive program; ambulance fee schedule; durable medical equipment and competitive acquisition of certain durable medical equipment, prosthetics, orthotics and supplies. *Federal Register* 76(218):70228–70316.

Department of Health and Human Services. 2013 (December 10). Medicare Program; Revisions to Payment Policies under the Physician Fee Schedule, Clinical Laboratory Fee Schedule & Other Revisions to Part B for CY 2014; Final Rule. Federal Register 78(237):74229–74823.

Department of Health and Human Services. 2014a (May 2).Medicare Program; Prospective Payment System for Federally Qualified Health Centers; Changes to Contracting Policies for Rural Health Clinics; and Changes to Clinical Laboratory Improvement Amendments of 1988 Enforcement Actions for Proficiency Testing Referral; Final Rule. *Federal Register* 79(85):25435–25482.

Department of Health and Human Services. 2014b (August 22). Medicare Program; FY 2015 Hospice Wage Index and Payment Rate Update; Hospice Quality Reporting Requirements and Process and Appeals for Part D Payment for Drugs for Beneficiaries Enrolled in Hospice; Final Rule. Federal Register 79(163):50451–50510.

Department of Health and Human Services. 2014c (November 13). Medicare Program; Revisions to Payment Policies Under the Physician Fee Schedule, Clinical Laboratory Fee Schedule, Access to Identifiable Data for the Center for Medicare and Medicaid Innovation Models & Other Revisions to Part B for CY 2014; Final Rule. *Federal Register* 79(219):67547–68010.

Department of Health and Human Services. 2014d (November 10). Medicare Program: Hospital Outpatient Prospective Payment and Ambulatory Surgical Center Payment Systems and Quality Reporting Programs; Physician-Owned Hospitals: Data Sources

for Expansion Exception; Physician Certification of Inpatient Hospital Services; Medicare Advantage Organizations and Part D Sponsors: CMS-Identified Overpayments Associated with Submitted Payment Data; Final Rule. *Federal Register* 79(217):66770–67034.

Department of Health and Human Services. 2014e (November 6). Medicare Program; End-Stage Renal Disease Prospective Payment System, Quality Incentive Program, and Durable Medical Equipment, Prosthetics, Orthotics, and Supplies; Final Rule. *Federal Register* 79(215):66120–66265.

George Washington University. 2012 (January 23). Department of Health Policy, School of Public Health and Health Services. Quality incentives for federally qualified health centers, rural health clinics and free clinics: A report to Congress. http://www.healthit.gov/sites/default/files/pdf/quality-incentives-final-report-1-23-12.pdf.

Health Resources and Services Administration. n.d. What are rural health clinics (RHCs)? http://www.hrsa.gov/healthit/toolbox/RuralHealthITtoolbox/Introduction/ruralclinics.html.

Health Resources and Services Administration. 2013. The Affordable Care Act and Health Centers. http://bphc.hrsa.gov/about/healthcenterfactsheet.pdf.

Institute of Medicine (IOM). 2013. Best care at lower cost: The path to continuously learning health care in America. *Washington, DC: National Academies Press.*

Jones, L.M., ed. 2001. Ambulatory payment classifications for freestanding ambulatory surgery centers. In *Reimbursement methodologies for healthcare services* [CD-ROM]. Chicago: AHIMA.

Lefkowitz, B. 2005. The health center story: Forty years of commitment. *Journal of Ambulatory Care Management.* 28(4):295–303.

Lewin, M.E., and S. Altman, eds. 2000. *America's health care safety net: Intact but endangered.* Washington, DC: National Academy Press.

Mann, C. 2010 (February 4). Dear State Health Official: Prospective payment system for FQHCs and RHCs. http://www.medicaid.gov/Federal-Policy-Guidance/downloads/SHO10004.pdf.

Medicare Learning Network. 2008. Ambulance inflation factor (AIF) for CY 2009. *MLN Matters* MM 6113. http://www.cms.hhs.gov/MLNMattersArticles/downloads/mm6113.pdf.

Medicare Learning Network. 2014a. Ambulance inflation factor for CY 2015 and productivity adjustment. http://www.cms.gov/Outreach-and-Education/Medicare-Learning-Network-MLN/MLNMattersArticles/downloads/MM8895.pdf.

Medicare Learning Network. 2014b (July 18). Implementation of a prospective payment system (PPS) for federally qualified health centers (FQHCs). *MLN Matters* Number MM 8743 (Revised). http://www.cms.gov/Outreach-and-Education/Medicare-Learning-Network-MLN/MLNMattersArticles/downloads/MM8743.pdf.

Medicare Learning Network. 2014c (August). Rural health fact sheet series: Rural health clinic. ICN 006398. https://www.cms.gov/MLNProducts/downloads/RuralHlthClinfctsht.pdf.

Medicare Learning Network. 2015 (January). Calendar Year (CY) 2015 Rural Health Clinic (RHC) and Federally Qualified Health Centers (FQHC) Updates: Payment Rate Increases for RHCs and FQHCs Billing Under the All-Inclusive Rate System (AIR), and Urban and Rural Designations for FQHCs Billing Under the AIR. MM8980. http://www.cms.gov/Outreach-and-Education/Medicare-Learning-Network-MLN/MLNMattersArticles/downloads/MM8980.pdf.

Medicare Payment Advisory Commission. 2004 (December). Report to the Congress: Growth in the volume of physician services. http://www.medpac.gov/publications/congressional_reports/Dec04_PhysVolume.pdf.

Medicare Payment Advisory Commission (MedPAC). 2011(June). Report to the Congress: Medicare and the health care delivery system. http://www.medpac.gov.

Medicare Payment Advisory Commission (MedPAC). 2014a. Payment basics: Physician and other health professional payment system. http://www.medpac.gov.

Medicare Payment Advisory Commission (MedPAC). 2014b (March). Report to the Congress: Medicare and the health care delivery system. http://www.medpac.gov.

Medicare Payment Advisory Commission (MedPAC). 2014c. Payment basics: Hospice services payment system. http://www.medpac.gov.

Medicare Payment Advisory Commission (MedPAC). 2014d. Payment basics: Ambulance services payment system. http://www.medpac.gov.

Medicare Payment Advisory Commission (MedPAC). 2014e. Payment basics: Outpatient hospital services payment system. http://www.medpac.gov.

Medicare Payment Advisory Commission (MedPAC). 2014f. Payment basics: Ambulatory surgical center services payment system. http://www.medpac.gov.

Medicare Payment Advisory Commission (MedPAC). 2014g. Payment basics: Outpatient dialysis services payment system. http://www.medpac.gov.

Morra, D., S. Nicholson, W. Levinson, D.N. Gans, T. Hammons, and L.P. Casalino. 2011. US physician practices versus Canadians: Spending nearly four times as much money interacting with payers. Health Affairs 30(8):1443–1450.

Office of Inspector General. 2006 (January). Medicare payments for ambulance transports. http://oig.hhs.gov/oei/reports/oei-05-02-00590.pdf.

Scanlon, W.J. 2002. Medicare physician payments: Spending targets encourage fiscal discipline, modifications could stabilize fees. Publication No. GAO-02-441T. Government Accounting Office. http://www.gao.gov/cgi-bin/getrpt?GAO-02-441T.pdf.

Additional Resources

Centers for Medicare and Medicaid Services. 2008. Pub. 100-04 Transmittal 1067. Ambulance inflation factor for CY 2009. http://www.cms.hhs.gov/AmbulanceFeeSchedule/.

Department of Health and Human Services. 2003. Payments for procedures in outpatient departments and ambulatory surgical centers. Report of a study from the Office of the Inspector General. http://www.oig.hhs.gov/oei/reports/oei-05-00-00340.pdf.

Department of Health and Human Services. 2006. Office of Inspector General; Medicare payments for ambulance transports. OEI-05-02-00590. http://oig.hhs.gov/oei/reports/oei-05-02-00590.pdf.

Department of Health and Human Services. 2007. Medicare program; Changes to the Hospital Outpatient Prospective Payment System and CY 2008 payment rates, the ambulatory surgical center payment system and CY 2008 payment rates, the hospital IPPS and FY 2008 payment pates; and payments for graduate medical education for affiliated teaching hospitals in certain emergency situations; Medicare and Medicaid programs: Hospital conditions of participation; Necessary provider designations of critical access hospitals; interim and final rule. Federal Register 72(227):66580–67225.

Department of Health and Human Services. 2009. Medicare program; Changes to the Hospital Outpatient Prospective Payment System and CY 2010 payment rates; Changes to the ambulatory surgical center payment system and CY 2010 payment rates; Final rule. Federal Register 74(223):60315–61012.

Department of Health and Human Services. 2011. Medicare and Medicaid programs: Hospital outpatient prospective payment; Ambulatory surgical center payment; Hospital value-based purchasing program; Physician self-referral; and Patient notification requirements in provider agreements; Final rule. Federal Register 76(230):74122–74584.

Medicare Learning Network. 2011. MLN Matters Number MM7489—Instructions to accept and process all ambulance transportation Healthcare Common Procedure Coding System (HCPCS) codes. http://www.cms.gov/AmbulanceFeeSchedule/ASTrans/list.asp#TopOfPage.

Medicare Learning Network. 2014 (April). How to use the searchable Medicare Physician Fee Schedule (MPFS) (ICN 901344). http://www.cms.gov/Outreach-and-Education/Medicare-Learning-Network-MLN/MLNProducts/downloads/How_to_MPFS_Booklet_ICN901344.pdf

Medicare Payment Advisory Commission (MedPAC). 2014 (June). Report to the Congress: Medicare and the health care delivery system. http://www.medpac.gov.

Chapter 8
Medicare-Medicaid Prospective Payment Systems for Postacute Care

Objectives

- To define the postacute care settings
- To differentiate Medicare and Medicaid prospective payment systems for healthcare services delivered to patients in postacute care
- To describe Medicare's all-inclusive per diem rate for skilled nursing facilities
- To describe Medicare's prospective payment systems for long-term care hospitals and inpatient rehabilitation facilities
- To describe Medicare's per-episode payment system for home health agencies
- To differentiate the specialized collection instruments, standardized base rates, and case-mix groups that exist in postacute care
- To define basic language associated with reimbursement under Medicare and Medicaid prospective payment systems in postacute care
- To explain the grouping models and payment formulae associated with reimbursement under Medicare and Medicaid prospective payment systems in postacute care

Key Terms

Activities of daily living (ADLs)
Average length of stay (ALOS)
Base rate
Base year
Budget neutrality factor
Case mix
Case-mix diagnosis
Case-mix group (CMG)
Certification
Cognitive
Compliance percentage
Concurrent therapy
Confined to the home
Consolidated billing (CB)
Core-based statistical area (CBSA)
Cost report
Durable medical equipment (DME)
Episode of care
Etiologic diagnosis
Functional independence assessment tool

Functional status
Group therapy
Health Insurance Prospective Payment System (HIPPS) codes
High-cost outlier
Home assistance validation and entry (jHAVEN/ HAVEN)
Home health agency (HHA)
Home health resource group (HHRG)
Hospital within hospital (HwH)
Impairment group code (IGC)
Individual therapy
Inpatient rehabilitation facility (IRF)
Inpatient rehabilitation facility patient assessment instrument (IRF PAI)
Inpatient Rehabilitation Validation and Entry (IRVEN)
Interrupted stay
Length of stay (LOS)
Long-term care hospital (LTCH)

Long-term care hospital Continuity Assessment and
  Record Evaluation (CARE) Data Set
Low-utilization payment adjustment (LUPA)
Market basket
Market basket (price) index
Medicare-severity long-term care diagnosis-related
  group (MS-LTC-DRG)
Minimum Data Set (MDS)
Motor
National standardized episode rate
Non-case-mix-adjusted component
Non-case-mix component
Non-case-mix therapy component
Nonroutine medical supply (NRS)
Normalization
Nursing component
Nursing index

Nursing per diem amount
Outcome Assessment Information Set (OASIS)
Postacute care (PAC)
Quintile
Regression analysis
Rehabilitation impairment category (RIC)
Request for Anticipated Payment (RAP)
Resource utilization group (RUG)
Short-stay outlier
Site neutral payment
Skilled nursing facility (SNF)
Standard federal rate
Standard payment conversion factor
Therapy component
Therapy index
Therapy per diem amount
Wage index

Introduction to Prospective Payment Systems in Postacute Care

Postacute care (PAC) provides patients with healthcare services for their recuperation and rehabilitation after an illness or injury. Medicare designates four settings as PAC:

- Skilled nursing facilities (SNFs)
- Long-term care hospitals (LTCHs)
- Inpatient rehabilitation facilities (IRFs)
- Home health agencies (HHAs) (Medicare Payment Advisory Commission [MedPAC] 2014a, 169)

PAC allows patients to safely continue their recovery in settings less intensive and more appropriate than acute-care inpatient hospitals. Medicare has the same goal for its beneficiaries in PAC as it has for its beneficiaries across the continuum of care.

Medicare's Overarching Goal

Ensure that beneficiaries receive appropriate, high-quality care in the least costly setting appropriate for their clinical condition.

Source: MedPAC. 2014a (March). *Report to the Congress: Medicare payment policy.* (p. xvii). http://medpac.gov.

For each PAC setting, Medicare has implemented a prospective payment system (PPS). After the implementation of the inpatient PPS in October 1983, Medicare expenditures in PAC grew at a "tremendous" rate (Cotterill and Gage 2002, 1). Therefore, Congress took action to slow this tremendous growth in expenditures. Between 1998 and 2002, a series of federal laws established PPSs in the four PAC settings. Although Medicare payments still continue to increase in PAC, the rate is slower than in the past (MedPAC 2014b, 112). Currently, the increase in expenditures is mainly in payments to SNFs and HHAs (MedPAC 2014b, 112).

The PPSs in the four types of PAC have similar components. First, the PPSs require data collection on specialized instruments. Second, the PPSs are based on various types of **case-mix groups (CMGs)**. Case-mix groups classify together patients or residents with similar conditions and characteristics who use similar levels of resources. Case-mix groups have relative weights, with higher weights generally being associated with patients who are sicker and who use more resources. Third, the

base rate converts the weights to dollars. Fourth, there is an adjustment for varying costs of labor in terms of wage indexes across the nation. Finally, there are adjustments for patients with atypical characteristics and for facilities with special situations.

The Centers for Medicare and Medicaid Services (CMS) publishes the updates for these PPSs in the *Federal Register* (discussion in chapter 6). In addition, CMS has a website for each of these PPSs with data files for some of the data, such as the relative weights of the CMGs and the wage indexes.

Skilled Nursing Facility Prospective Payment System

Nursing homes are healthcare facilities that are licensed by a state to offer, on a 24-hour basis, both skilled nursing care and personal care services (see figure 8.1).

Figure 8.1. Basic concepts

Activities of daily living: Basic personal activities that include bathing, eating, dressing, mobility, transferring from bed to chair, and using the toilet. Activities of daily living are used to measure how dependent a person may be on requiring assistance in performing any or all of these activities.

Nursing home: Facility licensed by the state to offer residents personal care as well as skilled nursing care 24 hours a day. Provides nursing care, personal care, room and board, supervision, medication, therapies, and rehabilitation. Shared rooms and communal dining are common. (Licensed as nursing homes, county homes, or nursing homes/residential care facilities.)

Personal care services: Assistance with activities of daily living, self-administration of medications, and preparation of special diets. Personal care services may be expanded to include light housekeeping furnished to an individual who is not an inpatient or a resident of a group home, assisted living facility, or long-term facility such as a hospital, nursing facility, intermediate-care facility for the mentally retarded, or institution for mental disease. Personal care (also called custodial care) services are those that individuals would typically accomplish themselves if they did not have a disability.

Rehabilitation services: Services designed to improve or restore a person's functioning; include physical therapy, occupational therapy, or speech therapy or some combination of these.

Skilled care: Level of care, such as injections, catheterizations, and dressing changes, provided by trained medical professionals, such as physicians, nurses, and physical therapists.

Skilled nursing care: Daily nursing and rehabilitative care that can be performed only by or under the supervision of skilled medical personnel.

Skilled nursing facility: Facility that is certified by Medicare to provide 24-hour skilled nursing care and rehabilitation services in addition to other medical services.

Source: Assistant Secretary for Planning and Evaluation (ASPE), Office of Disability, Aging, and Long-Term Care Policy. 2011. Glossary of terms. http://aspe.hhs.gov/daltcp/diction.shtml.

Health services in nursing homes are offered as *long-stay* and chronic-care (Grabowski 2010, 2). A type of nursing home is a **skilled nursing facility (SNF)**. On an inpatient basis, SNFs provide *short-term* skilled nursing care and rehabilitation services to Medicare beneficiaries after an acute-care inpatient hospitalization.

SNFs can be freestanding facilities, hospital-based units, or swing beds in acute-care hospitals. In acute-care hospitals, swing beds are beds that may be used for both acute inpatient care and skilled nursing care. Typically, these acute-care hospitals are small, rural hospitals or critical access hospitals. CMS must approve the dual use of the beds (MedPAC 2014c, 1). About 90 percent of SNF admissions are in freestanding facilities (MedPAC 2014b, 113).

Background

Medicare Part A covers the cost of SNF services for Medicare beneficiaries. Medicare beneficiaries are eligible for SNF services immediately after an acute-care inpatient hospitalization of at least three days. They may receive up to 100 days of SNF-covered services per benefit period (see chapter 4). As described in chapter 4, Medicare beneficiaries pay cost sharing for their SNF services. SNFs are the most commonly used post-acute-care setting (MedPAC 2014c, 1).

The skilled nursing facility prospective payment system (SNF PPS) was mandated by Section 4432 of the Balanced Budget Act of 1997 and was effective in 1998. The SNF PPS pays a daily rate for each day of care (per diem). The SNF PPS covers the costs of skilled nursing care, rehabilitation services, ancillary services, capital costs, and other goods and services (MedPAC 2014c, 1). The costs included in the daily rate are for services that would be expected for a SNF to efficiently deliver routine services. High-cost, low-probability services are excluded from the daily rate and are paid separately (MedPAC 2014c, 1).

In addition, the SNF PPS mandates **consolidated billing (CB)** for SNFs. CB requires the SNF to pay for outpatient services that a resident may receive from outside vendors. Outside vendors who provide services to SNF residents with Part A benefits submit their bills to the SNF, *not* to Medicare. Examples of outside vendors under consolidated billing are laboratories, x-ray services, and pharmacies. Emergency services, inpatient services, and other extensive procedures (such as radiation therapy) are not consolidated. Operational costs associated with defined, approved educational activities are also excluded from the base rate and consolidated billing.

Data Collection and Reporting

Since the late 1980s, CMS has required SNFs to prepare the **Minimum Data Set (MDS)**. The MDS represents clinical documentation of the resident's care. Therefore, the MDS is an extensive database of clinical data. The MDS is part of the resident's health record. CMS currently requires that SNFs submit data on MDS 3.0.

The clinical data on the MDS 3.0 include comprehensive assessments. Assessments must be completed within prescribed timeframes (table 8.1) (CMS 2011a, 26389). The standard assessments represent admissions or readmissions.

There are also schedules of assessments for:

- Start of therapy (SOT)
- Change of therapy (COT)
- End of therapy (EOT)
- Significant change in status assessment (SCSA)

Reporting of these assessments may be combined.

Treatment plans are also part of the clinical data on the MDS. In the PPS, treatment plans are integral because services outside the scope of the treatment

Table 8.1.   Schedule of standard assessments

Medicare MDS Assessment Type	Assessment Reference Date (ARD) Window	Assessment Reference Date Grace Days	Applicable Medicare Payment Days
5 day	Days 1–5	6–8	1–14
14 day	Days 13–14	15–18	15–30
30 day	Days 27–29	30–33	31–60
60 day	Days 57–59	60–63	61–90
90 day	Days 87–89	90–93	91–100

Source: Adapted from Centers for Medicare and Medicaid Services. 2011a. Medicare Program; prospective payment system and consolidated billing for skilled nursing facilities; disclosures of ownership and additional disclosable parties information; Proposed Rules. *Federal Register* 76(88):26389.

plans may be excluded from payment. The PPS also requires SNFs to use ICD and HCPCS coding. Finally, timeframes also exist for transmission of required MDS data to CMS's Quality Improvement Evaluation System (QIES) Assessment Submission and Processing (ASAP) system. Generally, the transmission may be no later than 14 days from the assessment reference date (ARD) (CMS 2014a, 5-2).

Structure of Payment

There are three components in the structure of payment under the SNF PPS: the base rate, the SNF case-mix group, and adjustments (figure 8.2). Figure 8.2 shows the basic foundation of a SNF PPS payment. There are three steps based on the base rate, adjustments, and the actual payment for the number of days of the resident's hospitalization.

Base Rate (Per Diem)

The SNF PPS payment begins with a per diem (daily) rate for each day of care. This daily rate is known as the federal base rate (and also as the federal per diem). The federal base rate is calculated using allowable costs from previous SNF **cost reports**. Cost reports are reports that providers are required to submit to Medicare. To calculate the base rate, CMS typically uses the most recent year for which it has complete and available data. The year becomes the **base year**.

Adjustments to Base Rate

Several adjustments are applied to the base rate. These adjustments include

- Geographic factors and inflation

Figure 8.2.   Foundation of skilled nursing facility prospective payment system

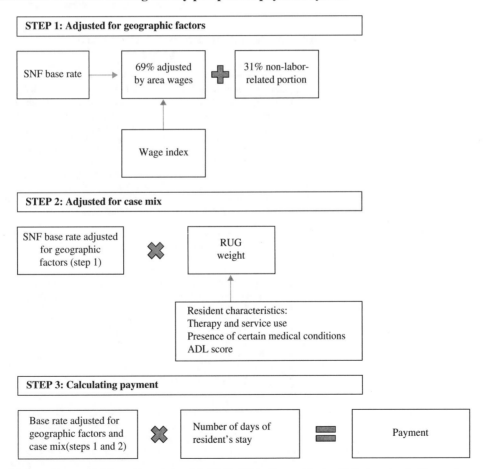

Source: Adapted from Medicare Payment Advisory Commission (MedPAC). 2014c. Payment basics: Skilled nursing facility services payment system. Pg. 2. http://www.medpac.gov.

- Other adjustments mandated by statute or regulation

- Patient **case mix** (complexity and resource intensity of residents' conditions)

The base rate is annually adjusted for differences in local markets (figure 8.3). In different geographic areas (local markets) in the United States, costs (prices) are different. These differences affect the costs that providers, such as SNFs, must expend in order to render services to residents, patients, and clients. Therefore, CMS adjusts payment rates to match local prices.

The **market basket** is a tool to make this adjustment. A market basket is a mix of goods and services. The **market basket (price) index** is a relative measure that averages the costs of an appropriate mix of goods and services for the site of care in the continuum of care. The market basket includes items related to labor and nonlabor. In its calculations, CMS

also determines the proportion of the market basket related to labor costs and the proportion of the market basket related to nonlabor costs. Wages also differ across the nation. CMS uses **wage indexes** to adjust the labor-related portion of the payment rates for these wage differences. The data are aggregated nationally by urban and rural areas so that CMS can establish separate base rates for urban and rural areas. Data gathered for the market basket also are used to adjust for inflation.

Over the years, various adjustments have been mandated by statute or regulation. Currently, three adjustments of this type are in effect in the SNF PPS:

- Multifactor productivity adjustment. The Affordable Care Act mandated that the market basket adjustment be reduced by the multifactor productivity adjustment. The multifactor productivity adjustment helps

Figure 8.3.   Common terms in payment adjustments for different costs in local markets

Term	Definition
Labor-related portion (share)	Portion of the cost of the goods and services needed to run a facility that are related to labor costs. Labor costs include wages and salaries, employee benefits, professional fees, and labor-related portion of capital costs. The labor-related portion is based on the market basket for the site of care. The market basket associated with the type of care is used to determine how much of the site's costs are related to labor. Each year, the federal government calculates the ratio of the labor-related portion because it varies slightly from year to year. The ratio is published annually in the proposed rule and in the final rule. The labor-related portion is standard across the United States.
Market basket	Mix of goods and services and their respective costs. In healthcare reimbursement, it is an appropriate mix of goods and services for the site of care in the continuum of care. Market baskets vary among sites in the continuum of care. There are market baskets for skilled nursing facilities (SNFs); rehabilitation, psychiatric, and long-term care (RPL) facilities; physicians; acute inpatient hospitals; PPS-exempt hospitals; and home health agencies (HHAs).
Market basket index (price index)	Relative measure that averages the costs of an appropriate mix of goods and services for the site of care in the continuum of care.
Non–labor-related portion (share)	Portion of the cost of the goods and services needed to run a facility that are *not* related to labor costs. Nonlabor costs include overhead (electricity, fuel, water and sewer, utilities), pharmaceuticals (prescription drugs), food and food contractor fees, medical instruments and equipment, medical materials and supplies, malpractice (liability) insurance, chemicals, nonmedical professional fees, photographic supplies, and rubber and plastic products. The non–labor-related portion is based on the market basket for the site of care. The market basket associated with the type of care is used to determine how much of the sites' costs are related to nonlabor items. Each year, the federal government calculates the ratio of the non–labor-related portion, because it varies slightly from year to year. The ratio is published annually in the proposed rule and in the final rule. The non–labor-related portion is standard across the United States. The non–labor-related portion can also be calculated: non–labor-related portion = 1.0 – labor-related portion
Wage index	Relative measure of the average of the hourly wages of health personnel within a **core-based statistical area (CBSA)**. A CBSA is a geographic area designated by the Office of Management and Budget. There is a wage index specific to each CBSA. Wages and thus the wage indexes vary annually among CBSAs. Each year, the federal government calculates, adjusts, and publishes, at the end of the final rule, the wage indexes for all CBSAs. Wage indexes can range between 0.90 and 1.2. Wage indexes also vary from year to year for a specific CBSA. For example, the wage index for Greenville, North Carolina (CBSA 24780), has ranged between 0.9098 and 0.9448.

ensure that the market basket update not only accounts for changes in the costs of goods and services used to provide patient care but also reflects increases in provider productivity that could reduce the actual cost of providing services (such as new technologies) (HHS 2014a, 45631).

- Temporary payment adjustment. The Medicare Prescription Drug, Improvement, and Modernization Act of 2003 (MMA) (P.L. 108–173) initiated an additional temporary payment adjustment. This additional temporary payment is a type of add-on. The MMA provided a temporary increase of 128 percent for SNF residents with acquired immunodeficiency syndrome (AIDS). The act identifies no particular **resource utilization group (RUG)**. The act is in effect until the Secretary of Health and Human Services certifies that the case-mix system takes into account the costs of AIDS patients. The secretary has not made this certification, so the adjustment is still in effect (HHS 2014a, 45633).

- **Budget neutrality**. In most instances, changes in federal reimbursement methods must be implemented in ways that maintain budget neutrality. In budget neutrality, federal expenditures remain essentially the same under the "old" method and the new method. To maintain budget neutrality, CMS applied a parity adjustment that recalibrated each component of the per diem rate (see figure 8.4) (HHS 2014a, 45639).

The SNF PPS base rate is adjusted for patient case mix. Case mix takes into account the differences among residents. These differences result in different uses of resources. For example, some residents require total help with their **activities of daily living (ADLs)**. These residents require the SNF to use more resources. Other residents have complex nursing care needs or require less help with their ADLs. Case mix represents the complexity and the resource intensity of the residents' conditions.

The SNF case-mix group is the RUG. Classifying a resident's care into a RUG adjusts for case mix. Residents within a group are similar (homogeneous) in terms of their health characteristics and use of

resources (services). Residents in the same RUG have similar requirements in terms of skilled nursing care and therapy. The three components of the payment rate for each RUG include

- **Nursing component**, the intensity of nursing care that resident is expected to need

- **Therapy component**, the occupational, physical, or speech therapies that residents in Rehabilitation plus Extensive Services RUGs or Rehabilitation RUGs, are expected to need

- **Non-case-mix-adjusted component**, the room and board, linens, and administrative and capital-related services (and **non-case-mix therapy component**, the standard flat amount) for residents in RUGS without rehabilitation (figure 8.4)

The current version of the RUG case-mix classification system that CMS is using is RUG-IV.

Figure 8.4.   Components of case-mix-adjusted per diem rates of SNF PPS

Nursing component	**Nursing per diem amount** is the standard that which includes direct nursing care and the cost of nontherapy ancillary services.
	Nursing index is the ratio based on the amount of staff time, weighted by salary levels, associated with each RUG; applying this ratio to the nursing per diem is the case-mix adjustment.
Therapy component	**Therapy per diem amount** is a standard amount that includes physical, occupational, and speech-language therapy services provided to beneficiaries in a Part A stay.
	Therapy index is the ratio based on the amount of staff time, weighted by salary levels, associated with each RUG; applying this ratio to the therapy per diem is the case-mix adjustment.
Non-case-mix-adjusted component	**Non-case-mix therapy component** is the standard amount to cover the cost of therapy assessments of residents who were determined not to need continued therapy services; this amount is the therapy component for nonrehabilitation groups.
	Non-case-mix component is the standard amount added to the rate for each RUG to cover administrative and capital-related costs; this standard amount is added to all groups.

Source: Centers for Medicare and Medicaid Services (CMS). 2011c. CMS Manual System, Pub 100-04. Medicare claims processing manual: Chapter 6—SNF inpatient Part A billing and SNF consolidated billing. Section 30.6.2. https://www.cms.gov/manuals/downloads/clm104c06.pdf.

RUG-IV has 66 RUGs. MDS data on health characteristics and resource utilization are used to classify a resident into a RUG.

Key data include the following:

- Therapy, such as occupational, physical, or speech therapy, and certain other services, such as respiratory therapy or feeding
  - Mode (**individual therapy**, **concurrent therapy**, or **group therapy** (see figure 8.5)
  - Number of minutes and distinct therapy days during which at least 15 minutes of therapy were provided

- Presence of certain conditions (pneumonia and sometimes depression)

- **ADL** index (standardized measure of dependency, ranging from 0 to 16) based on the resident's ability to perform four ADLs: eating, toileting, bed mobility, and transferring (the higher the ADL score, the more dependent the resident and thus the more resource-intensive)

RUG-IV schema has eight hierarchical categories from most resource-intensive to least resource-intensive (see figure 8.6). Divided among the eight categories are the 66 RUGs. The most resource-intensive RUGs are called the upper groups. The least resource-intensive RUGs are called the lower groups.

The 52 upper groups are as follow:

- 9 RUGs ranging from ultra-high to low in Rehabilitation Plus Extensive. Example: resident who is receiving rehabilitation services, is also receiving complex clinical care involving a tracheostomy, and has a qualifying ADL score.

- 14 RUGs ranging from ultra-high to low in Rehabilitation. Example: resident who is receiving rehabilitation services.

- 3 RUGs in Extensive Services. Example: resident who is receiving complex clinical care involving a tracheostomy and who has a qualifying ADL score.

Figure 8.5.   Reporting and grouping of individual, concurrent, and group therapy in MDS 3.0 and RUG-IV

Individual	Concurrent	Group
One-on-one individualized physical, occupational, or speech therapy time. All minutes are reported. All minutes used in RUG-IV classification.	Concurrent therapy is the practice of one professional therapist treating multiple patients at the same time while the patients are performing different therapeutic activities. Residents cannot benefit from observing other residents in the group, because everyone is performing different activities. CMS considers concurrent therapy an adjunct to individual therapy. Medicare Part A coverage requires that concurrent therapy consist of two residents (regardless of payer source), both of whom must be in line of sight of the treating therapist (or assistant). Medicare Part B does not cover concurrent therapy. SNF records all the minutes (unallocated). RUG grouper allocates (divides) the minutes in half.	Group therapy is the practice of one therapist providing the same therapeutic services to everyone in the group. Residents may benefit by observing other residents in the group performing the same activity. Medicare Part A coverage requires that group therapy consist of four residents (regardless of payer source), who are performing similar activities and are supervised by a therapist (or assistant) who is not supervising any other residents outside the group. Medicare Part B covers therapy of two residents (or more) at the same time (regardless of payer source) as group therapy. SNF records the total (unallocated) group therapy minutes on each MDS for each of the four residents. RUG grouper allocates (divides by 4) the total recorded minutes among the four group therapy participants. The allocated minutes are used to determine the RUG of the resident's care. The grouper applies the rule that the group minutes cannot exceed 25 percent of the total minutes. Participants' unexpected absences do *not* affect the four-part allocation.

Source: Centers for Medicare and Medicaid Services (CMS). 2011b. Medicare program; Prospective payment system and consolidated billing for skilled nursing facilities for FY 2012; Final rule. *Federal Register* 76(152):48486–48562.

Figure 8.6.   RUG-IV categories and activity of daily living indexes

RUG Category	Rehab Level	ADL Levels				
		0–1	2–5	6–10	11–14	15–16
Rehabilitation Plus Extensive	Ultra high		RUL		RUX	
	Very high		RVL		RVX	
	High		RHL		RHX	
	Medium		RML		RMX	
	Low		RLX			
Rehabilitation	Ultra high	RUA		RUB	RUC	
	Very high	RVA	RVB		RVC	
	High	RHA	RHB		RHC	
	Medium	RMA	RMB		RMC	
	Low		RLA		RLB	
Extensive Services			ES1, ES2, ES3			
Special Care High			HB2	HC2	HD2	HE2
			HB1	HC1	HD1	HE1
Special Care Low			LB2	LC2	LD2	LE2
			LB1	LC1	LD1	LE1
Clinically Complex		CA2	CB2	CC2	CD2	CE2
		CA1	CB1	CC1	CD1	CE1
Behavioral Symptoms and Cognitive Performance		BA2	BB2			
		BA1	BB1			
Reduced Physical Function		PA2	PB2	PC2	PD2	PE2
		PA1	PB1	PC1	PD1	PE1

Source: Adapted from Department of Health and Human Services. 2009. Medicare Program; Prospective Payment System and Consolidated Billing for Skilled Nursing Facilities for FY 2010; Minimum Data Set, Version 3.0 for Skilled Nursing Facilities and Medicaid Nursing Facilities; Proposed Rule. *Federal Register* 74(90):22227.

- 8 RUGs in Special Care High. Example: resident who has septicemia and a qualifying ADL score.

- 8 RUGs in Special Care Low. Example: resident who is receiving dialysis and who has a qualifying ADL score.

- 10 RUGs Clinically Complex. Example: resident who has pneumonia (CMS 2014a, 6-3 to 6-4).

Residents in the upper groups receive at least 45 minutes of therapy per week.

The 14 lower groups are

- 4 RUGs in Behavioral Symptoms and Cognitive Performance

- 10 RUGs in Reduced Physical Function

Residents in these groups do *not* receive at least 45 minutes of therapy per week.

Medicare will cover services to residents *correctly* classified by MDS data into the upper 52 RUGs. CMS presumes that these admissions are justified. This "presumption of coverage" begins when the beneficiary is admitted (or readmitted) directly after a qualifying acute-care hospitalization. By definition, these residents require skilled care. However, CMS states that the SNF still has the responsibility to document medical necessity. The lower 14 RUGS involve impaired cognition and reduced physical function. Typically, residents classified into these lower RUGs do not need skilled care (MedPAC 2014c, 2). Medicare coverage of the services to residents classified into the lower RUGs is determined on an individual basis (HHS 2014a, 45640).

Payment

The resident's RUG is derived from the MDS data. Each RUG has its own associated nursing and therapy weights that are applied to the base rate. The federal payment to a SNF for a resident's care is the base rate and the resident's RUG (see figure 8.2 and table 8.2). The base rate is adjusted for local geographic variations in wages. To adjust the base rate, its labor portion is multiplied by the local wage index, which varies from year to year. The nonlabor portion is added to the adjusted labor rate to derive the wage-adjusted federal rate. Finally, to calculate the payment, the wage-adjusted total federal rate is multiplied by the number of covered Medicare days.

The pricer is the software program that has the logic to calculate payments for SNF PPS claims (pricers exist for other federal payment systems as well). The pricer's logic contains the following data items on rates and weights:

- Components of the federal rate for rural and urban areas, including a table of the nursing and therapy indexes for each RUG
- Applicable wage index
- Changes, if applicable, to the labor and nonlabor portions (table 8.2)

CMS updates these data items periodically, usually annually and in October. However, updates may also occur at other times in the year, as required by legislation.

Other Applications

State Medicaid programs use PPSs to pay for nursing home services. Nationwide, there are about 17,000 nursing facilities (homes) that are Medicaid-certified. Of these nursing facilities, about 85 percent are also Medicare-certified (Grabowski 2010, 2).

State Medicaid payment methods vary greatly across the states. Moreover, most states have changed their payment methods multiple times since 1965 (see chapter 4) (Grabowski 2010, 2). Most states use PPSs. A few states use hybrid systems that mix aspects of prospective and retrospective payment methods (Grabowski 2010, 2). Typically, the payment is based on a per diem rate that the state Medicaid program sets prospectively. The per diem rate is calculated based on costs of direct resident care, indirect support services (such as the Business Office or Health Information Services), administration, and capital (Grabowski 2010, 2).

Table 8.2.   Sample payment calculation: RUG-IV SNF XYZ: Located in Cedar Rapids, IA[1,2,3]

RUG-IV Group	Labor	Wage Index	Adjusted Labor	Nonlabor	Adjusted Rate	Medicare Days	Payment
RVX	$478.32	0.8850	$423.31	$213.10	$636.41	14	$8,909.74
ES2	$384.06	0.8850	$339.89	$171.10	$510.99	30	$15,329.70
RHA	$241.31	0.8850	$213.56	$107.50	$321.06	16	$5,136.96
BA2	$153.36	0.8850	$135.72	$68.32	$204.04	30	$6,121.20

[1] Cedar Rapids, IA, is in an urban Core-Based Statistical Area (CBSA: 16300).
[2] The wage index for the CBSA is 0.8850.
[3] No patients have AIDS, so no 128 percent adjustment.

Source: Adapted from Department of Health and Human Services (HHS). 2014a. Medicare program; Prospective payment system and consolidated billing for skilled nursing facilities for FY 2015; Final rule. *Federal Register* 7(150):45640.

State Medicaid PPSs also vary from the federal PPS. For example, not all state Medicaid programs use the MDS for their case-mix payment systems (CMS 2014a, 6-2). Specifically, more than half of the state Medicaid programs also use the MDS for these systems. Plus, the federal system uses RUG-IV; state Medicaid programs have the option to use RUG-III (CMS 2014a, 6-2). Moreover, CMS has provided states with alternative forms of RUG-III, with 34, 44, or 53 groups, and alternative forms of RUG-IV, with 48, 57, or 66 groups. CMS gives state Medicaid programs these alternative forms so that the Medicaid programs can select the number of groups that best suits their Medicaid long-term care population (CMS 2014a, 6-2). Thus, state Medicaid programs can develop nursing home payment systems that best meet their goals (CMS 2014a, 6-2).

Long-Term Care Hospital Prospective Payment System

Patients with multiple acute and chronic diseases may require medically complex care. **Long-term care hospitals (LTCHs)** are able to provide inpatient care to these patients for extended periods.

Background

Medicare beneficiaries' long-term care hospitalizations are covered under Part A Medicare. Beneficiaries have up to 90 days of hospital services within the benefit period (see chapter 4). Admissions to both acute-care hospitals and LTCHs are counted in the benefit period. As described in chapter 4, beneficiaries pay cost-sharing for their LTCH services. One inpatient deductible is required for each 90-day benefit period. For the days 61 through 90, a daily coinsurance payment is also required. The 60 lifetime reserve days may also be used after the 90th day.

The Medicare, Medicaid, and SCHIP Balanced Budget Refinement Act (BBRA) of 1999 (P.L. 106–113), as amended by the Benefits Improvement and Protection Act of 2000 (P.L. 106–554), mandated that a PPS be implemented for LTCHs. In October 2002, CMS implemented the long-term care hospital prospective payment system (LTCH PPS).

LTCHs treat groups of patients who have longer-than-average **lengths of stay (LOS)** (days as inpatient). In general, the patients are medically complex and

need specialized care. Some patients have chronic diseases, such as tuberculosis and respiratory ailments. Other patients have acute diseases requiring long-term therapy, such as cancer and head trauma. LTCHs can provide both general acute-care and specialized services, such as comprehensive rehabilitation and ventilator-dependent therapy.

A facility can meet the CMS's definition of an LTCH in two ways:

- Its **average length of stay (ALOS)** (mean of patients' lengths of stays) is 25 days or more. The calculation is based only on the LOS of Medicare patients, and it includes both covered and noncovered days. In addition, the calculation must be based on data from the past six months.

- It was excluded from the inpatient prospective payment system on or after August 5, 1997, and has an ALOS of 20 days or more for both Medicare and non-Medicare patients. In addition, 80 percent of the hospital's annual inpatient Medicare discharges in the fiscal year (FY) had principal diagnoses of neoplastic diseases, such as cancer. These LTCHs are also known as "subclause II" or "subsection II" LTCHs (HHS 2014b, 50166).

Approximately 420 LTCHs meet these qualifying circumstances (MedPAC 2014d, 1). LTCHs can be freestanding, satellites of other larger facilities, or colocated units within acute care hospitals, inpatient rehabilitation facilities, or skilled nursing facilities. When they are colocated within larger medical facilities, they are sometimes known as **hospitals within hospitals** (HwH) (MedPAC 2014d, 1). Types of hospitals excluded from the LTCH PPS are

- Department of Veterans Affairs (VA) hospitals

- Hospitals reimbursed under state cost-control systems or authorized demonstration projects

- Nonparticipating hospitals furnishing emergency services to Medicare beneficiaries

Beginning in October 2016, under provisions of the Pathway for SGR Reform Act of 2013, only certain types of discharges from LTCHs will qualify for the LTCH PPS payment. Nonqualifying discharges will be paid under the IPPS for acute care hospitals (chapter 6). Either of two circumstances qualifies an LTCH discharge for payment under the LTCH PPS:

- An immediately preceding acute care hospital stay that included at least three days of intensive care services

- Principle diagnosis indicating the receipt of at least 96 hours of mechanical ventilation

Nonqualifying discharges are paid under the IPPS in what are called site-neutral payments. The site neutral payments are the *lesser* of the IPPS amount or 100 percent of the discharge's costs (MedPAC 2014d, 4).

Data Collection and Reporting

LTCHs are responsible to complete, submit, and maintain patient assessments using the **LTCH**

Figure 8.7.   Foundation of long-term care hospital prospective payment system

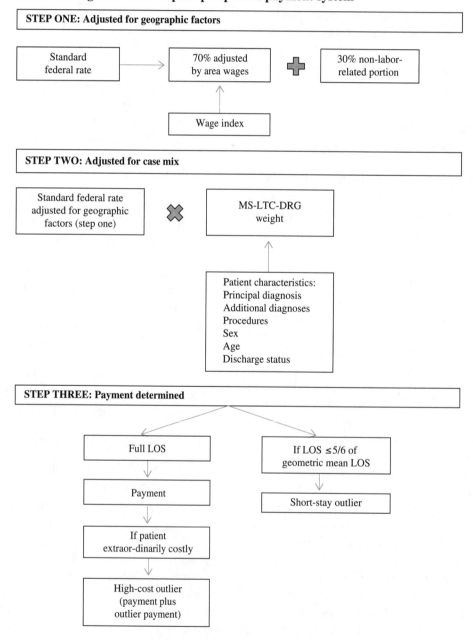

Source: Adapted from Medicare Payment Advisory Commission (MedPAC). 2014d. Payment basics: Long-term care hospitals payment system. Pg. 2. http://www.medpac.gov.

Continuity Assessment Record and Evaluation (CARE) Data Set. Similar to the MDS, the LTCH CARE Data Set has specific dates by which assessments must be completed. Moreover, data collection using the LTCH CARE Data set is applicable to all patients regardless of the patient's age, diagnosis, length of stay, or payer. Also included in the LTCH-CARE Data Set are quality measures (HHS 2014b, 50286-50308). The ACA requires LTCHs to submit data on these quality measures (see chapter 10).

Structure of Payment

The LTCH PPS is based on categorizing patients into case-mix groups with similar clinical characteristics. There are three components in the structure of payment under the LTCH PPS: the standard federal rate, the LTCH case-mix group, and adjustments (figure 8.7). Figure 8.7 shows the basic foundation of an LTCH PPS payment. There are three steps based on these components: adjustment for geographic factors, adjustment for case mix, and payment determination.

The LTCH PPS payment includes reimbursement for all the following costs related to providing covered services:

- Operating
- Capital-related
- Routine (regular room, dietary and nursing services, minor medical and surgical supplies, and equipment for which a separate charge is not usually made)
- Ancillary

Excluded from the PPS are the following costs (although the LTCH can bill them separately to CMS):

- Bad debts
- Approved educational activities
- Blood-clotting factors
- Anesthesia
- Photocopying costs for records sent to federal contractors

Standard Federal Rate (Base Rate)

The **standard federal rate** converts the LTCH case-mix group weight into a payment. The LTCH PPS payment begins with the standard federal rate for each discharge. This per discharge rate is known as the base

rate. The standard federal rate is a standardized payment amount based on average costs. The standard federal rate is calculated using data from the LTCHs' previous cost reports. These reports provide data on operating and capital costs. Into the calculation, CMS also inputs data from the prices of the market basket of goods and services (see SNF section). Thus, the standard federal rate is based on operating costs and capital costs adjusted by the data from the market basket (HHS 2014d, 50176). It is updated annually. Table 8.3 shows standard federal rates for selected years.

Adjustments to Standard Federal Rate

The standard federal rate is adjusted for geographic differences in wages and prices and for patient case mix.

Geographic Adjustments

There are two adjustments based on geography and location:

- Labor portion adjusted for area's local wage index. In different geographic areas (local markets) wages are different. A large part of the standard federal rate is based on labor (part of operating costs) (see figure 8.3 in the SNF section). The LTCH PPS uses the local wage index to factor in the effects of the area's wages (see table 8.4). The labor portion varies each year from approximately 62 percent to 71 percent (figure 8.7 and table 8.4).

- Cost-of-living adjustment (COLA) for LTCHs in Alaska and Hawaii (HHS 2014b, 50439).

Adjustments for Patient Case-Mix

The LTCH case-mix group is the **Medicare-severity long-term care diagnosis-related groups (MS-LTC-DRGs)**. MS-LTC-DRGs are a type of case-mix group. MS-LTC-DRGs account for variations in the use of resources to care for patients in LTCHs. Based on coding, patients' discharges are grouped into MS-LTC-DRGs.

The MS-LTC-DRGs are structurally identical to the acute-care MS-DRGs (HHS 2014b, 50168). Thus,

Table 8.3. Over time: select standard federal rates and fixed-loss amounts

	2011	2013	2015
Standard Federal Rate	$39,600	$40,398	$41,044
Fixed-Loss Amount	$18,785	$15,408	$14,972

Table 8.4.   Examples of calculation of adjusted LTCH PPS payments

	A	B	C	D	E	F	G	H	I	J	K
1	Rate Year	Standard federal rate	Labor-related portion	Local wage index	Nonlabor-related portion	Adj labor-related portion (unadj federal rate × labor-related portion × local wage index)	Adj nonlabor-related portion (unadj federal rate × nonlabor-related portion)	Adjusted federal rate (adj labor portion + nonlabor-related portion)	Case-mix adjustment	Weight	Adjusted payment (adj federal rate × weight)
2						B × C × D	B × E	F + G	MS-LTC-DRG		H × J
3	2010	$39,897	69%	0.9401	31%	$25,805	$12,448	$38,253	004	3.1040	$118,737
4	2015	$41,044	62%	0.9371	38%	$23,847	$15,597	$39,443	004	2.8875	$113,893
5	2010	$39,897	69%	0.9401	31%	$25,805	$12,448	$38,253	081	0.4766	$18,231
6	2015	$41,044	62%	0.9371	38%	$23,847	$15,597	$39,443	081	0.4959	$19,560

*Local wage index for CBSA 24780 (Greenville, NC)

the MS-LTC-DRGs are organized into major diagnostic categories and are divided into surgical and medical partitions. This duplication extends to their numeric titles and word titles (see table 8.5).

A computer software program called a grouper classifies patient discharges into MS-LTC-DRGs. Groupers have internal logic or an algorithm that determines the patients' groups. The grouper uses the following data to determine the patient's MS-LTC-DRG (same as MS-DRGs):

- Principal diagnosis

- Additional diagnoses (up to 24)

- Procedures (up to 25)

- Sex

- Age

- Discharge status

Primarily, the principal diagnosis determines the MS-LTC-DRG. Additional (secondary) diagnoses and certain procedure codes also affect the assignment of the MS-LTC-DRG. Additional diagnoses represent complications and comorbidities (CCs):

- Complications are conditions that occurred subsequent to the admission (during the hospitalization).

- Comorbidities were present at the time of the admission.

See chapter 6 for a detailed explanation of grouping. MS-LTC-DRGs in this chapter follow the same process as MS-DRGs in chapter 6. Both CCs affect the grouping of a patient's discharge to an MS-LTC-DRG.

MS-LTC-DRGs have assigned relative weights (table 8.5). These weights reflect the resources necessary to treat LTCH patients who require medically complex care. Patients who consume more resources are grouped to MS-LTC-DRGs that have higher relative weights.

MS-LTC-DRGs *do* differ from the MS-DRGs in terms of their relative weights and their distribution. First, the relative weights of MS-LTC-DRGs differ from the relative weights of MS-DRGs because the mix of patients in LTCHs differs from the mix of patients in acute-care inpatient hospitals. Patients in LTCHs are characterized by the complexity of their multiple medical problems. Thus, the use of resources differs between LTCHs and acute-care inpatient hospitals. The relative weights account for this difference in the use of resources.

Second, the distribution of MS-LTC-DRGs differs from the distribution of MS-DRGs. This difference results because LTCHs do not typically treat the full range of diagnoses as acute inpatient hospitals do. Therefore, some MS-LTC-DRGs have very few or no cases. CMS manages this situation by creating two subsets of MS-LTC-DRGs:

- Low-volume MS-LTC-DRGs have fewer than 25 cases (patient discharges). They are divided

Table 8.5. Comparison of relative weights for selected Medicare-severity long-term care diagnosis-related groups (MS-LTC-DRGs) and Medicare-severity diagnosis related groups (MS-DRGs)

No.	Title	MS-LTC-DRG Weight	MS-DRG Weight
052	Spinal disorders and injuries with CC/MCC*	1.2901	1.5813
056	Degenerative nervous system disorders with MCC	0.8300	1.7615
058	Multiple sclerosis and cerebellar ataxia with MCC	0.7881	1.6336
067	Nonspecific CVA and precerebral occlusion without infarct with MCC	0.4959	1.4527
189	Pulmonary edema and respiratory failure	0.9098	1.2136
190	Chronic obstructive pulmonary disease with MCC	0.7493	1.1743
191	Chronic obstructive pulmonary disease with CC	0.5967	0.9370
192	Chronic obstructive pulmonary disease without CC/MCC	0.4958	0.7190
207	Respiratory system diagnosis with ventilator support 96+ hours	1.9279	5.3425
535	Fractures of hip and pelvis with MCC	0.6214	1.2410

among five **quintiles** (one-fifth of cases in a distribution) based on average *charges* per discharge. Each quintile has a relative weight.

- No-volume MS-LTC-DRGs have no cases. CMS assigns no-volume MS-LTC-DRGs relative weights and average length of stays. To assign these relative weights and average lengths of stay, CMS crosswalks the no-volume group to another MS-LTC-DRG with clinical similarity and relative costliness. CMS assigns these relative weights and lengths of stay to prepare for the upcoming fiscal year because LTCHs *could* have patient discharges in these groups in the upcoming

year. CMS also includes MS-LTC-DRGs with relative weights of 0.0000 in the count of no-volume MS-LTC-DRGs. These MS-LTC-DRGs are the MS-LTC-DRGs for organ transplants (organ transplants should not occur at an LTCH) and the MS-LTC-DRGs for administrative errors (998, Principal Diagnosis is invalid and 999, Ungroupable).

Thus, most MS-LTC-DRGs have unique relative weights. However, low-volume MS-LTC-DRGs share the relative weight of their quintile.

The healthcare system is dynamic. CMS annually adjusts the groups and weighting factors to reflect changes in

- Treatment patterns
- Technology
- Number of discharges
- Other factors affecting the relative use of LTCH resources

These changes in the delivery of healthcare affect the use and consumption of resources. By adjusting the groups and weights, CMS accounts for these changes in use and consumption. For example, the number of MS-LTC-DRGs varies from year to year (table 8.6).

In addition, the types of patients in the LTCH vary from year to year. The numbers of low-volume and no-volume MS-LTC-DRGs representing these patients' discharges also vary from year to year (table 8.6). Finally, CMS also adjusts relative weights to reflect current use of resources. Changes in treatment patterns or technology can result in increases in relative weights or in decreases in relative weights. For example, between two fiscal years, the relative weight

Table 8.6. Variation over time in numbers of Medicare-severity long-term care diagnosis-related groups, low-volume groups, and no-volume groups

	2004	2008	2012
All Groups	518	745	751
Low-Volume Groups	173	303	277
No-Volume Groups (Including Transplants and Administrative)	167	185	236

Table 8.7. Example of refinements in weights accounting for variation in use of resources

	2008	2012
Relative Weight: MS-LTC-DRG 004 Trach w MV 96+ hrs or PDX exc face, mouth & neck w/o maj O.R.	3.0249	3.0467
Relative Weight: MS-LTC-DRG 081 Nontraumatic stupor & coma w/o MCC	0.5618	0.4607

of MS-LTC-DRG 004 *increased* while the relative weight of MS-LTC-DRG 081 *decreased* (table 8.7).

Adjustments for Individual Discharges
Case-level adjustments reflect unique aspects of patients' individual hospital stays. There are four case-level adjustments:

- A **short-stay outlier** is defined as an LTCH admission shorter than the average length of stay. There are two types: a very short-stay outlier and a short-stay outlier. A very short-stay outlier is a case with a length of stay that is less than or equal to the inpatient prospective payment system (IPPS) comparable threshold. The IPPS comparable threshold is the average length of stay for that same case-mix group in the inpatient acute care setting (MS-DRG matches the MS-LTC-DRG) plus one standard deviation. Short-stay outliers are five-sixths of the geometric average length of stay. (Tables in the LTCH PPS's proposed rules and final rules include the geometric average lengths of stay and the short-stay outlier threshold.) Short-stay outliers are paid the *least* of the following four amounts: (1) 100 percent of the cost of the case; (2) 120 percent of the MS-LTC-DRG per diem amount; (3) full MS-LTC-DRG payment; or (4) blend of an IPPS amount and 120 percent of the MS-LTC-DRG per diem amount (MedPAC 2014d, 2-3).

- An **interrupted stay** is when a patient is (1) admitted to an LTCH; (2) then discharged to home, an acute-care inpatient hospital, IRF, or SNF; and (3) readmitted to the LTCH within a fixed period of days (home, three days; acute-care inpatient hospital, nine days; IRF, 27 days; SNF,

45 days) (MedPAC 2014d, 3). An interrupted stay becomes one discharge and one payment. Admissions and discharges from colocated facilities come under this adjustment. Discharges and readmissions among colocated facilities may not exceed five percent without penalty.

- A **high-cost outlier** is a discharge with extraordinarily high costs that exceed the typical costs of its MS-LTC-DRG. To identify high-cost outliers, CMS uses a threshold. The threshold is based on the adjusted federal payment plus the fixed-loss amount (MedPAC 2014d, 3). Each year, CMS publishes the fixed-loss amount (calculated from the latest available data on LTCH cost reports). Table 8.3 shows fixed-loss amounts for selected years.

- The 50-percent rule (formerly 25-percent rule) reduces payments for HWH LTCHs and satellite LTCHs that exceed the 50-percent threshold for patients admitted from their "host" acute care hospitals during a cost reporting period. The purposes of the rule are to ensure that LTCHs do not function as units of acute care hospitals and to ensure that decisions about admission, treatment, and discharge are made for clinical rather than financial reasons (MedPAC 2014d, 3). After the threshold is exceeded, the LTCH is paid the *lesser* of the LTCH PPS rate or an amount equivalent to the IPPS rate for patients discharged from the host acute care hospital (MedPAC 2014d, 3).

Discharges can be classified into multiple case-level adjustments. For example, an interrupted stay may also be a high-cost outlier.

Payment
Under the LTCH PPS, payment for a Medicare patient is made at a predetermined, per discharge amount for each MS-LTC-DRG. A software program known as a pricer calculates the LTCH payment. The unit of payment is the discharge. To determine the federal payment rate for each patient discharge, the pricer's internal logic uses the components in figure 8.7 and table 8.4. Here are the processes illustrated in table 8.4:

- Standard federal rate is adjusted for differences in geographic areas' wages:
  ◦ Unadjusted standard federal rate is multiplied by the local wage index to adjust

for local labor costs (columns B, C, D, and F in table 8.4).

- ° Nonlabor-related portion of the standard federal rate is calculated by multiplying the unadjusted standard federal rate by the nonlabor-related portion (columns B, E, and G in table 8.4)
- ° Adjusted federal rate is calculated by adding together the two adjusted portions, the adjusted labor-related portion and the adjusted nonlabor-related portion (columns F, G, and H in table 8.4).

- Geographic adjusted standard federal rate is adjusted for case-mix by multiplying the adjusted standard federal rate by the MS-LTC-DRG relative weight (columns H, J, and K in table 8.4).

- Column K, the payment, is adjusted for short-stay outlier and high-cost outlier as necessary.

Finally, CMS reduces payments to LTCHs that do not submit quality data (see previous section LTCH CARE Data Set and chapter 10). LTCHs that fail to submit the quality data are subject to a two percent reduction in the next year's percentage increase in the market basket (HHS 2014b, 50311).

Implementation

The importance of accurate coding for the LTCH PPS cannot be overstated. By establishing the MS-LTC-DRG, correct ICD coding drives Medicare's payment of the claim. CMS emphasizes that LTCHs must follow the official coding guidelines as described in chapter 2.

Coders must be careful to record the code that occasioned the admission to the LTCH. They must be careful *not* to record the code that occasioned the admission to the acute-care hospital. For the case depicted in figure 8.8, correct LTCH coding results in MS-LTC-DRG 057. *Incorrectly* using the acute-care codes would have resulted in MS-LTC-DRG 068 (because MS-LTC-DRGs match acute MS-DRGs).

The relative weights of the two MS-LTC-DRGs differ by a small amount (cell J5 on table 8.8). However, this small amount, when multiplied by the standard federal rate, becomes sizeable (cell K5 in table 8.8). In this case, if the coder had recorded the incorrect diagnosis code (the acute-care hospital code), the LTCH would have been underpaid.

Figure 8.8.   Case study to calculate long-term care prospective payment system reimbursement

Acute Care Hospital
Patient suffers a stroke and is admitted to an acute care hospital.

The inpatient MS-DRG is 068, Nonspecific CVA and Precerebral Occlusion without infarct without MCC.

Long-term Care Hospital
Patient is discharged and then admitted to an LTCH for further treatment of left-sided hemiparesis (late effects of cerebrovascular disease, hemiplegia affecting nondominant side) and dysphasia (late effects of cerebrovascular disease, dysphasia).

The MS-LTC-DRG is 057, Disease and Disorders of the Nervous System without MCC.

Coding additional diagnoses is also critical. Additional diagnoses may represent CCs and MCCs. CCs and MCCs group patients' discharges to MS-LTC-DRGs with relative higher weights than MS-LTC-DRGs without CCs and MCCs. Higher relative weights result in higher payments. As always, the goal is accuracy to garner correct reimbursement—and always, the goal is accurate coding to garner correct payments.

Check Your Understanding 8.1

1. What tool does CMS require that SNFs use to collect and report clinical data about residents?

2. What tool does the SNF PPS use annually to adjust payment rates?

3. What cost sharing applies to beneficiaries residing in an LTCH for 90 days?

4. True or false? Even though MS-LTC-DRGs are based on the same general factors as the acute-care MS-DRGs for the IPPS, MS-LTC-DRGs differ from acute-care MS-DRGs because MS-LTC-DRGs have different relative weights and use quintiles for low volumes.

5. What converts the MS-LTC-DRG into an unadjusted payment amount?

Inpatient Rehabilitation Facility Prospective Payment System

Inpatient rehabilitation facilities (IRFs) provide intense multidisciplinary services to inpatients. The purpose of these services is to restore or enhance patients' function after injury or illness. Members of the multidisciplinary team that provides these services are physicians, nurses, physical therapists, occupational

Table 8.8. Impact of coding on grouping and payment

	A	B	C	D	E	F	G	H	I	J	K
1	Coding Quality	Standard federal rate	Labor-related portion	Local wage index*	Nonlabor-related portion	Adj labor-related portion (unadj federal rate × labor-related portion × local wage index)	Adj nonlabor-related portion (unadj federal rate × nonlabor-related portion)	Adjusted federal rate (adj labor portion + nonlabor-related portion)	MS-LTC-DRG	Weight	Adjusted payment (adj federal rate × weight)
2						B × C × D	B × E	F + G			H × J
3	Correct	$41,044	62%	0.9371	38.0%	$23,847	$15,597	$39,443	057	0.6192	$24,423
4	Incorrect	$41,044	62%	0.9371	38.0%	$23,847	$15,597	$39,443	068	0.4949	$19,521
5	Difference									-0.1243	-$4,903

*Local wage index for CBSA 24780 (Greenville, NC)

therapists, and speech therapists. The services are (1) medically necessary, (2) based on an assessment, and (3) individualized to each patient's needs.

IRFs must be licensed under applicable state laws to provide skilled nursing care to inpatients 24 hours per day. These facilities may be

- Freestanding hospitals
- Distinct specialized rehabilitation units in acute-care hospitals

The following healthcare organizations are excluded from the IRF PPS:

- Department of Veterans Affairs (VA) hospitals
- Hospitals reimbursed under state cost-control systems or authorized demonstration projects
- Nonparticipating hospitals furnishing emergency services to Medicare beneficiaries

Medicare accounts for approximately 60 percent of IRF cases. About 1,170 IRFs are Medicare-certified (MedPAC 2014d, 1).

To be classified as an IRF under the IRF PPS, a facility must meet a **compliance percentage**. The compliance percentage is the minimum percentage of

an IRF's inpatients requiring intensive rehabilitation services in one of the qualifying conditions, including comorbidities (figure 8.9). Per the Medicare, Medicaid, and SCHIP Extension Act (MMSEA) of 2007, the compliance percentage is 60 percent. This criterion is known as the "60 percent rule." The 60 percent rule must be met in order for the IRF to receive payment under the IRF PPS (MedPAC 2014d, 3).

Background

The Balanced Budget Act of 1997 authorized the development of the inpatient rehabilitation facility prospective payment system (IRF PPS). The development of the IRF PPS was also affected by amendments in the Balanced Budget Refinement Act of 1999 and the Medicare, Medicaid, and SCHIP Benefits Improvement and Protection Act of 2000. In January 2002, CMS implemented the IRF PPS.

Medicare beneficiaries' inpatient rehabilitation hospitalizations are covered under Part A Medicare. Preadmission screening establishes a Medicare beneficiary's eligibility for inpatient rehabilitation. To be eligible for treatment in an IRF, a beneficiary must be able to tolerate and benefit from three hours of therapy per day or 15 hours per week (seven consecutive days). Medicare beneficiaries admitted directly from an acute-care inpatient hospital do *not*

Figure 8.9. Thirteen conditions qualifying for designation as inpatient rehabilitation facility

Stroke
Spinal cord injury
Congenital deformity
Amputation
Major multiple trauma
Fracture of the femur (hip fracture)
Brain injury
Neurological disorders
Burns
Active, polyarticular rheumatoid arthritis, psoriatic arthritis, and seronegative arthropathies
Systemic vasculitides with joint inflammation (unresponsive to aggressive, sustained, and appropriate outpatient treatment)
Severe or advanced osteoarthritis involving two or more major weight-bearing joints
Knee or hip replacement with bilateral replacement, extreme obesity, or age 85 or older

pay a second inpatient deductible (IRF admission is part of the benefit period; see chapter 4). However, Medicare beneficiaries who are admitted from the community are beginning their benefit period and, thus, must pay the inpatient deductible.

Data Collection and Reporting

CMS requires that inpatient rehabilitation services be reasonable and medically necessary for each Medicare beneficiary. These requirements, called coverage criteria, include documentation of preadmission screening, close medical supervision, a director of rehabilitation, the plan of care, and a coordinated multidisciplinary team approach (figure 8.10). The time frames in the coverage criteria do not affect the time frames for the **inpatient rehabilitation facility patient assessment instrument (IRF PAI)**. The coverage criteria must be met for payment under the IRF PPS.

The IRF PPS features a rehabilitation-specific tool. This tool is the IRF PAI. The IRF PAI collects the information that drives payment. The IRF PAI must be completed on both Medicare Part A fee-for-service inpatients and on Medicare Advantage (Part C) inpatients. The IRF PAI must be completed for each Medicare patient twice: once upon admission and again at discharge.

Types of Patient Information

The IRF PAI consists of the following types of patient information:

- Identification information, including admission information
- Payer information
- Medical information
- Function modifiers
- Functional independence assessment information
- Discharge information
- Therapy information
- Quality indicators with admission and discharge assessments (for example, pressure ulcers or patient falls)
- Certification of information's accuracy (for example, signatures and dates)

Assignment of Codes

By the fourth day of the inpatient admission, the IRF PPS requires the assignment of codes. These codes reflect

- The reason for admission to the rehabilitation facility (using impairment group codes)
- The etiology of the impairment (using ICD codes)
- Comorbidities and complications (using ICD codes)
- The reason for interruption, transfer, or death (using an ICD code)

The functional abilities of the patient must be assigned using the functional independence assessment tool. This standardized tool, measuring patients' need for assistance, is discussed in detail in the subsequent subsection entitled "Functional Independence Assessment."

Figure 8.10.   Criteria establishing reasonableness and necessity of inpatient rehabilitation services

Criterion	Specifications
Requirements for the preadmission screening	Comprehensive preadmission screening, for all patients, serving as the basis for the initial determination of whether or not the patient meets the requirements for an IRF admission to be considered reasonable and necessary
	Includes a detailed and comprehensive review of the patient's condition and medical history, which indicates the patient's prior level of function, expected level of improvement, the expected length of time necessary to achieve that level of improvement, risk of clinical complications, conditions needing rehabilitation, therapies needed, expected frequency and duration of therapies, anticipated discharge destination, anticipated postdischarge treatment, and other relevant information
	Conducted by a licensed or certified clinician(s) designated by a rehabilitation physician
	Conducted within the 48 hours immediately preceding the admission or conducted more than 48 hours immediately preceding the admission but updated in person within the 48 hours immediately preceding the admission
	Includes informing a rehabilitation physician who reviews and documents his or her concurrence with the findings and results of the preadmission screening
	Retained in the patient's medical record
Requirement for a postadmission physician evaluation	Completed by a rehabilitation physician within 24 hours of the patient's admission
	Documents the patient's status on admission, includes a comparison with the information noted in the preadmission screening documentation, and serves as the basis for the development of the overall individualized plan of care (the history and physical does not suffice)
	Retained in the patient's medical record
Requirement for an individualized overall plan of care	Comprehensive plan
	Developed for each admission by a rehabilitation physician within 96 hours of the patient's admission with input from the interdisciplinary team as available
	Retained in the patient's medical record
Requirements for evaluating the appropriateness of an admission	Requires active and ongoing therapeutic intervention of multiple therapy disciplines, one of which must be physical or occupational therapy
	Generally requires and can reasonably be expected to actively participate in, and benefit from, an intensive rehabilitation therapy program of at least three hours of therapy per day five days per week or at least 15 hours of therapy within seven consecutive days, beginning with the date of admission
Requirement for the interdisciplinary team meetings	Uses a coordinated interdisciplinary team approach
	Approach documented by periodic clinical entries made in the medical record
	Documentation notes the patient's status in goal attainment
	Team conferences are held at least once per week to determine the appropriateness of treatment; first meeting must be within a week of the patient's admission
	Interdisciplinary team includes, at a minimum, a rehabilitation physician, registered nurse with specialized training or experience in rehabilitation, social worker or case manager (or both), and licensed or certified therapist representing each discipline providing therapy to the patient
	Team must be led by a rehabilitation physician
Requirement for physician supervision	Face-to-face visits with the patient at least three days per week throughout the patient's stay in the IRF
Requirement regarding initiation of therapy services	Therapy must begin within 36 hours from midnight of the day of admission
Provision of group therapies in IRFs	Group therapies do not substitute for one-on-one therapy services; group therapies are used primarily as an adjunct to one-on-one therapy services
Director of rehabilitation	Have a director of rehabilitation who meets the criteria

The codes on the IRF PAI are used for research, for grouping patients into CMGs, and for determining the payment tier. It must be emphasized that the codes on the IRF PAI do not follow the UHDDS and the UB-04 guidelines.

Impairment Group Code

The reason for admission is coded using an **impairment group code (IGC)** (table 8.9). CMS provides these codes in the manual. There are 85 IGCs organized into 17 impairment groups. The IGC structure consists of a

Table 8.9.   Inpatient rehabilitation facility prospective payment system's impairment groups and impairment group codes (IGCs)

Impairment group	No. of IGCs	ICG	Description of selected examples of IGCs in impairment groups
Stroke	5	01.1	Left body involvement (right brain)
		01.2	Right body involvement (left brain)
		01.3	Bilateral involvement
		01.4	No paresis
		01.9	Other stroke
Brain dysfunction	4	02.21	Traumatic, open injury
		02.22	Traumatic, closed injury
Neurologic conditions	7	03.1	Multiple sclerosis
		03.2	Parkinsonism
Spinal cord dysfunction, non-traumatic and traumatic	18	04.130	Other non-traumatic spinal cord dysfunction
		04.210	Traumatic paraplegia, unspecified
		04.211	Traumatic paraplegia, incomplete
		04.212	Traumatic paraplegia, complete
		04.220	Traumatic quadriplegia, unspecified
		04.2211	Traumatic quadriplegia, incomplete C1-4
		04.2212	Traumatic quadriplegia, incomplete C5-8
		04.2221	Traumatic quadriplegia, complete C1-4
		04.222	Traumatic quadriplegia, complete C5-8
Amputation	8	05.1	Unilateral upper limb above the elbow (AE)
Arthritis	3	06.1	Rheumatoid arthritis
		06.2	Osteoarthritis
Pain syndromes	4	07.1	Neck pain
Orthopedic disorders	12	08.11	Status post unilateral hip fracture
		08.72	Status post knee and hip replacements (different sides)
Cardiac	1	09	Cardiac
Pulmonary disorders	2	10.1	Chronic obstructive pulmonary disease
Burns	1	11	Burns
Congenital deformities	2	12.1	Spina bifida
Other disabling impairments	1	13	Other disabling impairments
Major multiple trauma	4	14.1	Brain + spinal cord injury
		14.3	Spinal cord + multiple fracture/amputation
Developmental disability	1	15	Developmental disability
Debility	1	16	Debility (non-cardiac, non-pulmonary)
Medically complex	11	17.2	Neoplasms
		17.32	Nutrition without intubation/parenteral nutrition
		17.4	Circulatory disorders
		17.51	Respiratory disorders – ventilator dependent
		17.8	Medical/surgical complications

Source: Centers for Medicare and Medicaid Services. 2014b (October). IRF Patient Assessment Instrument. Updated IRF PAI Training Manual, October 2014. http://www.cms.gov/Medicare/Medicare-Fee-for-Service-Payment/InpatientRehabFacPPS/IRFPAI.html.

two-digit ID number, a decimal point, and one to four digits representing the subgroups. The IGC describes the primary reason that the patient is being admitted to the rehabilitation program. The IGCs are subsequently classified into a **rehabilitation impairment category (RIC)** by CMS's grouper software. The RICS are the highest level of classification for the IRF payment categories. The RICs are *not* recorded on the IRF-PAI, but are assigned by the software based on the admission IGCs (see the later section "Adjustments for Case Mix").

Etiologic Diagnosis

The IRF PAI also reports the code for the etiology of the problem that led to the condition requiring the inpatient rehabilitation admission. The **etiologic diagnosis** is an ICD code. Thus, a principal diagnosis, as defined by the UHDDS, is not reported on the IRF PAI.

Comorbidities and Complications

A comorbidity is a specific condition that the patient had at admission to the IRF. Complications are comorbidities that occur after admission to the IRF (Trela 2007, 70). Some comorbidities (and complications) affect patients' care in addition to their etiologic diagnoses and their impairments. For these comorbidities (and complications), the IRFs must use additional resources (costs) to treat these patients.

To account for these additional costs, ICD coding of comorbid conditions and complications is critical (Trela 2007, 70). Complications are reported as comorbidities to be taken into account in the payment system. Codes identified the day before discharge or the day of discharge are not recorded (Trela 2007, 70). Up to 10 ICD codes for comorbid conditions (and complications) may be reported on the PAI.

About 900 comorbid conditions affect the IRF PPS payment. These comorbid conditions are divided into tiers by associated costs (table 8.10). CMS has linked the ICD codes to their respective tiers. Tier 1 is high cost, tier 2 is medium cost, and tier 3 is low cost (and a fourth tier for no cost). Conditions that are inherent to a specific RIC are excluded from the list of relevant comorbidities for that RIC. Excluded comorbidities do not affect the relative weight and, thus, do not increase the payment for that RIC.

Other Reporting

No procedures codes are reported on the IRF PAI (Trela 2007, 70). Finally, the reason for transfer or death is reported by ICD code on the IRF PAI.

Table 8.10.   Excerpt from list of comorbidities and tiers in inpatient rehabilitation facility prospective payment system

Comorbidity	Tier 1, 2, or 3	Excluded RIC
Tuberculosis of lung, infiltrative, bacteriological or histological examination unknown	3	15
Syphilitic endocarditis of valve, unspecified	3	14
Candidiasis of lung	3	15
Acute lymphoid leukemia, without mention of having achieved remission	3	–
Hemiplegia, unspecified, affecting nondominant side	3	01
Unilateral paralysis of vocal cords or larynx, partial	1	15
Dysphasia, not otherwise specified	2	01
Tracheostomy status	1	–

Source: Centers for Medicare and Medicaid Services. 2014b (October). IRF Patient Assessment Instrument. Updated IRF PAI Training Manual, October 2014. http://www.cms.gov/Medicare/Medicare-Fee-for-Service-Payment/InpatientRehabFacPPS/IRFPAI.html.

Functional Independence Assessment

Another major element of the IRF PAI is the **functional independence assessment tool** (table 8.11). This tool is an 18-item, rehabilitation-specific instrument that reflects the characteristics of patients. It captures patients' functional statuses. **Functional status** is a patient's ability to perform activities of daily living. CMS has organized this assessment by **motor** functioning (muscular activities, such as walking and eating) and **cognitive** functioning (mental abilities, such as talking and problem solving).

The functional independence measure tool was developed in the 1980s. This standardized instrument is widely used and accepted as a way to measure the severity of patients' impairments (Chumney et al. 2010, 17). The 18 items are measured on a seven-level scale that classifies patients according to their ability to perform certain activities. A score of 7 indicates complete independence. Conversely, a score of 1 indicates complete dependence. The IRF PAI added an eighth level, 0, for not assessed. Therefore, a higher score means that the patient has more functional abilities; a lower score means that the patient has fewer

Table 8.11.   Functional independence measure (FIM) and inpatient rehabilitation facility prospective payment system

CMS Motor Items		Min = 0, Max = 84
No.	Description	Score (0, 1 to 7)*
1.	Eating	
2.	Grooming	
3.	Bathing	
4.	Dressing—upper	
5.	Dressing—lower	
6.	Toileting	
7.	Bladder control	
8.	Bowel control	
9.	Bed, chair, wheelchair transfer	
10.	Toilet transfer	
11.	Tub, shower transfer (CMS excludes)	
12.	Walk/wheelchair locomotion	
13.	Stairs locomotion	
CMS Cognitive Items		**Min = 0, Max = 35**
14.	Comprehension	
15.	Expression	
16.	Social interaction	
17.	Problem solving	
18.	Memory	

*1 = complete dependence, 7 = complete independence, 0 = not assessed (0 score is unique to PAI).

Source: Adapted from Department of Health and Human Services. 2001. Medicare Program; Prospective Payment System for Inpatient Rehabilitation Facilities; Final Rule. *Federal Register* 66(152):41333, 41349.

functional abilities. Patients with fewer functional abilities (lower scores) need more assistance from facilities' personnel and thus require more resources.

All the patient's scores for the motor items are totaled and all the patient's scores for the cognitive items are totaled. These totals for the motor items and the cognitive items with the patient's diagnosis and age are data used to determine the exact case-mix group.

Time Frames and Electronic Submission

IRF staff members must complete PAIs upon admission and again at discharge. The PAI must be completed within specific timeframes. However, if entries are incorrect, facilities may update data any time before transmission of the IRF PAI.

Facilities must submit the IRF PAI to CMS electronically. The data must be encoded using CMS's free program, the **Inpatient Rehabilitation Validation and Entry (IRVEN)** software. There are strict timeframes for submission (table 8.12). Failure to follow timeframes results in a 25 percent reduction of the payment. Moreover, CMS penalizes IRFs that fail to submit IRF PAIs on all their Medicare Advantage (Part C) patients to CMS's data system per established timelines. These IRFs forfeit the use of any of the data on their Medicare Advantage (Part C) patients in the calculation of the compliance percentage.

Structure of Payment

The IRF PPS is based on classifying patients into case-mix groups with similar characteristics. There are three components in the structure of payment under the IRF PPS: the standard payment (base rate), the IRF case-mix group, and adjustments (figure 8.11). Figure 8.11 shows the basic foundation of an IRF PPS payment. There are four steps based on the standard payment conversion factor.

Standard Payment Conversion Factor

A **standard payment** conversion factor (base rate) converts the CMG weight into a payment (figure 8.11, table 8.13). The standard payment conversion factor

Table 8.12.   Inpatient rehabilitation facility prospective payment system timeframes for completion of the IRF PAI

Event	Admission	Discharge
Observation period	Days 1–3	Date of discharge or end of Medicare Part A fee-for-service coverage
Assessment reference date	Day 3	Date of discharge or discontinuation of covered services
Completion date	Day 4	Day 5 following discharge or discontinuation of covered services
Encoded date	Day 10	Day 7 following completion date (count completion date as day 1)
Transmission date	With discharge assessment	Day 7 following the encoded date

Source: Trela P. 2002. Inpatient rehabilitation PPS presents new challenges, opportunities. *Journal of AHIMA* 73(1):48A–48D.

Figure 8.11.   Foundation of inpatient rehabilitation facility prospective payment system

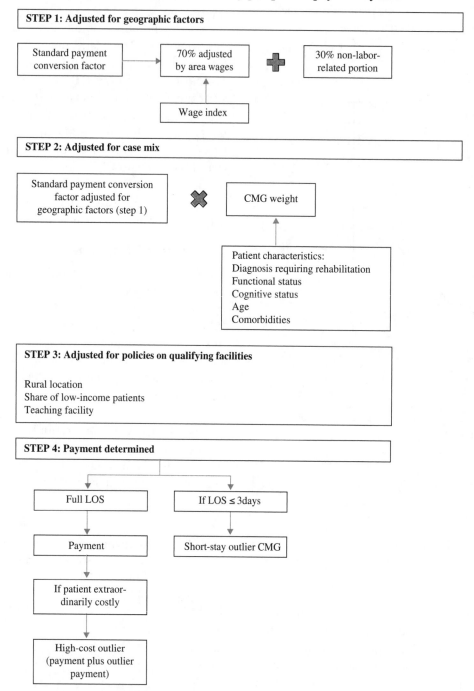

Source: Adapted from Medicare Payment Advisory Commission (MedPAC). 2014e. Payment basics: Inpatient rehabilitation facilities payment system. p. 2. www.medpac.gov.

covers all operating and capital costs that an IRF would be expected to incur to efficiently provide intensive

rehabilitation services. Excluded from the PPS are costs of bad debts and educational activities. Each year the standard payment conversion factor is updated to reflect the market basket (see SNF section). Across the years, the standard payment conversion factor has ranged between $11,838 and $15,198.

Adjustments to the Standard Payment Conversion Factor

The IRF PPS takes into account geographic factors through adjustments for local wages (figure 8.11). The case-mix adjustment accounts for the use of resources related to the patients' differing conditions and statuses (figure 8.11).

Geographic Adjustments

On figure 8.11, the adjustments for wages (labor-related portion) and the non-labor-related portion represent geographic adjustments. There are two wage-related adjustments (figure 8.3 in SNF section, figure 8.11 and table 8.13). The first is the labor-related portion (labor ratio and, correspondingly, the non-labor-related portion and non-labor ratio) and the second is the wage index. Each year, the ratios of the labor-related portion and the non-labor-related portion vary slightly. Across the years, the labor-related portions have ranged between 69 percent and 76 percent. As previously discussed in relation to SNFs, wage indexes vary annually among geographic areas, known as **core-based statistical areas (CBSAs)**. The annual differences in the labor-related portion and the wage index are small. However, to accurately estimate healthcare revenues, health personnel must identify these wage adjustments in the final rule and update their systems.

Adjustments for Case Mix

A special case-mix classification was developed unique to inpatient rehabilitation services. This special case-mix classification was specifically developed so that the IRF PPS could be implemented. This classification accounts for variations in the use of resources to care for and provide therapy to patients in rehabilitation facilities.

This special case-mix classification is called case-mix groups (CMGs). CMGs are classes of patient discharges from IRFs. These groups represent similar functional-related patient discharges based on impairment, functional capability of the patient, age, and comorbidities. There are 100 CMGs. Of the CMGs, 95 are clinical and 5 are administrative. CMGs are four-digit codes, such as 0101 and 5104. CMGs are derived from

- The rehabilitation impairment category (RIC)

- Total of the scores from the motor (M) items from the functional independence assessment tool

- Total of the scores from the cognitive (C) items from the functional independence assessment tool (used only with selected diagnoses related to stroke and traumatic brain injury)

Table 8.13.   Sample calculations of payments under inpatient rehabilitation facility prospective payment system showing effects of different wage indexes

	A	B	C	D	E	F	G	H	I	J	K
1	Standard pymt CF	Labor-related portion	Nonlabor-related portion	Local wage index*	Adj labor-related portion (unadj. pymt CF × labor-related portion × local wage index)	Nonlabor-related portion (unadj. pymt CF × nonlabor-related portion)	Labor adjusted standard pymt CF (adj. labor-related portion + adj. nonlabor-related portion)	HIPPS Code	CWG and Tier	Case-mix weight	Payment (labor adj rate × case-mix weight)
2					A × B × D	A × C	E + F				G × J
3	$15,198	69%	31%	0.7165	$7,514	$4,711	$12,225	B0109	0109 Tier 1	2.0570	$25,147
4	$15,198	69%	31%	1.0045	$10,534	$4,711	$15,245	B0109	0109 Tier 1	2.0570	$31,359
5	$15,198	69%	31%	1.6679	$17,491	$4,711	$22,202	B0109	0109 Tier 1	2.0570	$45,670

*CBSAs: 19460, Decatur, AL, 0.7165; 15380, Buffalo-Niagara Falls, NY, 1.0045; 42220, Santa Rosa-Petaluma, CA, 1.6679.

Table 8.14.   Rehabilitation impairment categories (RICs) and associated impairment group codes (IGCs)

RIC	Description	IGC	Description
01	Stroke (Stroke)	01.1	Left-body involvement (right brain)
		01.2	Right-body involvement (left brain)
		01.3	Bilateral involvement
		01.4	No paresis
		01.9	Other stroke
02	Traumatic brain injury (TBI)	02.21	Open injury
		02.22	Closed injury
04	Traumatic spinal cord injury (TSCI)	04.210	Paraplegia, unspecified
		04.211	Paraplegia, incomplete
		04.212	Paraplegia, complete
		04.220	Quadriplegia, unspecified
		04.2211	Quadriplegia, incomplete C1–4
		04.2212	Quadriplegia, incomplete C5–8
		04.2221	Quadriplegia, complete C1–4
		04.2222	Quadriplegia, complete C5–8

Source: Department of Health and Human Services. 2001. Medicare Program; Prospective Payment System for Inpatient Rehabilitation Facilities; Final Rule. *Federal Register* 66(152):41342–41344.

Table 8.15.   Rehabilitation impairment categories (RICs)

RIC	Description
01	Stroke (Stroke)
02	Traumatic brain injury (TBI)
03	Nontraumatic brain injury (NTBI)
04	Traumatic spinal cord injury (TSCI)
05	Nontraumatic spinal cord injury (NTSCI)
06	Neurological (Neuro)
07	Fracture of lower extremity (FracLE)
08	Replacement of lower extremity joint (Rep1LE)
09	Other orthopedic (Ortho)
10	Amputation, lower extremity (AMPLE)
11	Amputation, other (AMP–NLE)
12	Osteoarthritis (OsteoA)
13	Rheumatoid, other arthritis (RheumA)
14	Cardiac (Cardiac)
15	Pulmonary (Pulmonary)
16	Pain syndrome (Pain)
17	Major multiple trauma, no brain injury or spinal cord injury (MMT–NBSCI)
18	Major multiple trauma, with brain injury or spinal cord injury (MMT–BSCI)
19	Guillain Barre (GB)
20	Miscellaneous (Misc)
21	Burns (Burns)

Source: Based on Department of Health and Human Services. 2001. Medicare Program; Prospective Payment System for Inpatient Rehabilitation Facilities; Final Rule. *Federal Register* 66(152):41342–41344.

- Age (A; used only with selected diagnoses related to stroke, traumatic spinal cord injury, and joint replacement)

- Comorbid conditions

As previously noted, the IRF PAI is completed twice—once with admission data and a second time with discharge data. The admission assessment assigns patients to a CMG. The discharge assessment determines the weighting factors associated with comorbidities (if they are present and applicable).

In the admission assessment, patients are assigned to one of the 95 clinical CMGs. Patients are classified into CMGs based on admission data, clinical characteristics, and the expected improvement of the patient's functional status as reflected by the functional independence assessment tool. IRFs must complete admission assessments, which are the basis for CMG assignment, according to a specific timetable (Trela 2002, 48C).

The CMS software that assigns patients to CMGs is called the grouper. The grouper uses the impairment group codes (IGCs) on the PAI to classify patients into one of 21 RICs (tables 8.14 and 8.15). RICs are clusters of similar impairments and diagnoses. It should be noted that staff members at IRFs enter the IGC on the PAI; they do not enter the RIC. The grouper calculates the RIC from the IGC. RICs, in turn, assign patients to CMGs (table 8.16).

To summarize: IGC → RIC → CMG

Table 8.16.   Selected, representative excerpts from case-mix groups with item scores, relative weights, and tiers

CMG	CMG Description; (M = Motor, C = Cognitive, A = Age)	Tier 1	Tier 2	Tier 3	None
0101	Stroke M>51.05	0.7853	0.7150	0.6512	0.6248
0102	Stroke M>44.45 and M<51.05 and C>18.5	0.9836	0.8955	0.8155	0.7826
0109	Stroke M>22.35 and M<26.l5 and A<84.5	2.0570	1.8728	1.7055	1.6366
0110	Stroke M<22.35 and A<84.5	2.6928	2.4518	2.2328	2.1425
0202	Traumatic brain injury M>44.25 and M<53.35 and C>23.5	1.0591	0.8629	0.7741	0.7385
0204	Traumatic brain injury M>40.65 and M<44.25	1.3397	1.0915	.9793	0.9342
0404	Traumatic spinal cord injury M<16.05 and A>63.25	4.0832	3.4967	3.2348	2.8845
0405	Traumatic spinal cord injury M<16.05 and A<63.5	3.3355	2.8564	2.6425	2.3563
0501	Nontraumatic spinal cord injury M>51.35	0.8418	0.6804	0.6237	0.5643
0506	Nontraumatic spinal cord injury M<23.75	2.7066	2.1875	2.0052	1.8144
0803	Replacement of lower extremity joint M>28.65 and M<37.05 and A>83.5	1.3744	1.0963	1.0133	0.9345
0805	Replacement of lower extremity joint M>22.05 and M<28.65	1.4702	1.2503	1.1140	1.0274
5001	Short-stay cases, length of stay is 3 days or fewer				0.1549
5101	Expired, orthopedic length of stay is 13 days or fewer				0.6791
5102	Expired, orthopedic length of stay is 14 days or more				1.5539
5103	Expired, not orthopedic, length of stay is 15 days or fewer				0.7274
5104	Expired, orthopedic length of stay is 16 days or more				1.9477

Adapted source: Department of Health and Human Services. 2014c. Medicare Program; Inpatient Rehabilitation Facility Prospective Payment System for Federal Fiscal Year 2015; Final Rule. *Federal Register* 79(151):45878–45881.

Table 8.17.   Comorbidity codes

A	Without comorbidities
B	Comorbidity in tier 1
C	Comorbidity in tier 2
D	Comorbidity in tier 3

The CMGs are assigned relative weights to account for the comparative difference in resource use. Each of the 95 clinical CMGs has four relative weights (MedPAC 2014e, 1). Comorbid conditions increase the relative weight. There is one rate for cases without a comorbid condition and three rates for cases with comorbid conditions (table 8.17). The three rates with comorbid conditions correspond to the three tiers that reflect extra costs. The five administrative CMGs do not have tiers for comorbid conditions. The grouper selects the condition that assigns the case to the tier with the highest payment.

There are also special arrangements.

- The five administrative (special) CMGs are for case-level adjustments. There is one CMG for short-stay cases. Short stays comprise three days or less (including patient expirations) and do not meet the definition of a transfer. There are four CMGs for expired patients. These four CMGs are determined by the condition (orthopedic or nonorthopedic) and by the lengths of stay.

- Special payment arrangements are made for interrupted stays and transfer cases. In interrupted stays, the patient is discharged from the IRF and returns within three calendar days. Only one payment based on the CMG from the initial assessment is made. Transfer cases are paid per diem. This per diem is the facility-adjusted federal prospective payment (weight × CF) divided by the average length of stay for the tier (table 8.18).

The relative weights of the CMGs are calculated using the most current and complete Medicare claims and cost report data, in a budget-neutral manner. Similar to the SNF PPS and LTCH PPS, CMS periodically adjusts the CMGs and weighting factors to reflect changes in treatment patterns, technology, and other factors.

Table 8.18. Excerpt from average length of stay in days for case-mix groups and tiers

CMG	CMG Description; (M = Motor, C = Cognitive, A = Age)	Tier 1	Tier 2	Tier 3	None
0101	Stroke M>51.05	9	10	8	8
0102	Stroke M>44.45 and M<51.05 and C>18.5	11	11	10	10
0805	Replacement of lower extremity joint M>22.05 and M<28.65	14	14	13	12

Adapted source: Department of Health and Human Services. 2014c (August 6). Medicare Program; Inpatient Rehabilitation Facility Prospective Payment System for Federal Fiscal Year 2015; Final Rule. *Federal Register* 79(151):45878–45880.

CMS must maintain budget neutrality so that changes in federal payment systems do not result in significant differences in expenditures. To maintain budget neutrality, CMS analysts, using various mechanisms, adjust CMG weights so that total expenditures are equal to specific past periods (figure 8.12). Often aspects of the mechanisms to maintain budget neutrality are mandated under federal acts and regulations. Budget neutrality is frequently discussed in federal payment systems. Healthcare personnel and reimbursement analysts should monitor the processes by which it is maintained.

Adjustments for Policies on Qualifying Facilities

CMS has policies that increase payments by "facility-level adjustment factors." There are three facility-level adjustment factors:

- Rural location. Rural IRFs' payments are increased because they tend to have fewer

Figure 8.12. CMS's two-step process to maintain budget neutrality

Step 1 at micro-level: **Normalization** is at the micro-level of the relative weight. In normalization, CMS isolates the impact of the recalibration of relative weights of prospective payment systems. The average of all proposed relative weights is compared against the average of existing relative weights. The resulting ratio is used to reduce all proposed relative weights proportionally so that the new average equals the existing average.

Step 2 at macro-level: CMS analysts estimate aggregate payments for all facilities without and with changes in relative weights. They compare the two estimated amounts deriving a ratio. This ratio becomes the **budget neutrality factor**. Thus CMS maintains the same total of estimated aggregate payments for facilities. The budget neutrality factor serves to offset any estimated *decrease* or *increase* in aggregate IRF payments as a result of changes in relative weight.

cases, longer lengths of stay, and higher average costs per case than urban IRFs. CMS defines rural as being located outside a CBSA. To increase payments to rural IRFs, their payments are multiplied by a rural adjustment. CMS periodically recalculates the rural adjustment. Rural adjustments have ranged between 14 percent and 22 percent.

- Share of low-income patients. CMS increases payments to IRFs that treat a high percentage of low-income patients (LIP). The calculation of the LIP adjustment for an IRF with a disproportionate share of low-income patients is based on
  ° Disproportionate share hospital (DSH) patient percentage as a ratio (5 percent equals 0.05)
  ° Periodically determined power (such as squared or cubed; in the IRF PPS it is a proportion of 1.0)
  ° CMS periodical determination the of appropriate power to apply; power for the LIP adjustment has ranged from 0.4613 to 0.6229 (see table 8.19 for the calculation of the LIP adjustment)

- Teaching hospital adjustment. Teaching IRFs receive an adjustment for the additional indirect costs of providing graduate medical education. This upward adjustment is based on the ratio of full-time medical residents training in the IRF to the IRF's average daily census.

Potential Adjustments for Outliers

Two outlier calculations may be applied, if valid:

- High-cost outliers are cases in which the costs exceed an adjusted outlier threshold

Table 8.19. Calculation of low-income patient (LIP) adjustment for disproportionate share hospital (DSH) under IRF PPS

	Hosp. A	Hosp. B	Hosp. C
DSH percentage	25.97%	5%	15%
1 + DSH percentage	1.2597	1.0500	1.1500
Raised to periodically determined power (0.4838 in this example) equals LIP adjustment	1.1547	1.0309	1.0910

amount. The outlier payment is 80 percent of the difference between the estimated cost of the case and the fixed-loss threshold. The adjusted threshold includes the IRF's wage adjustment, LIP adjustment, and rural adjustment, as applicable. CMS calculates the adjusted outlier threshold periodically. Adjusted outlier thresholds have ranged between $8,848 and $10,660.

- Short-stay outliers are for patients with hospitalizations three days or less. IRFs payments are reduced for short-stay outliers. Payments for short-stay outliers are pre-established amounts that have ranged from about $1,900 to $2,300. This amount is adjusted by the local wage index.

Payment

In the IRF PPS, the unit of measure of the system is the discharge. CMS reimburses IRFs for each discharge, with all costs of covered inpatient services included (Trela 2002, 48A). CMS's pricer software calculates the payment.

Health Insurance Prospective Payment System (HIPPS) Code

IRFs report the **Health Insurance Prospective Payment System (HIPPS) code** on the claim. HIPPS codes are specialized codes created by CMS for some of its PPSs, such as the IRF PPS and the home health agency PPS (next section of this chapter) (CMS 2010, 1). The HIPPS code is a five-character alphanumeric code. The exact structure and meaning of each character varies by PPS (CMS 2010, 1).

For the IRF PPS, the HIPPS code collapses the information about the case-mix group and comorbidity into one code. The first character is the letter designation of the comorbidity tier (A to D). The last four characters are the four-digit CMG (table 8.16). Thus, the HIPPS code for a patient with a tier 1 comorbidity and a CMG of 0109 is B0109. Only one HIPPS code is allowed per claim.

Calculation

To calculate the federal payment for each patient discharge, the pricer's internal logic uses the components in figure 8.11 and table 8.13. Following are the processes illustrated in table 8.13:

- The standard payment conversion factor begins the calculation.

- Area wage adjustments are applied to the labor-related portion of the unadjusted standard payment conversion factor. The application of the wage-related adjustments on the calculations of the IRF payment is demonstrated in columns A, B, D, and E in table 8.13.

- The non-labor-related portion is calculated (columns A, C, and F in table 8.13).

- The adjusted labor-related portion and the non-labor-related portion are added together to obtain the labor-adjusted standard payment conversion factor (column G in table 8.13).
  ° If the local wage index is less than 1.0, the adjusted standard payment conversion factor is *less* than the standard payment conversion factor (most CBSAs; see row 3 of table 8.13).
  ° If the local wage index is approximately 1.0, the adjusted standard payment conversion factor almost equals the standard payment conversion factor (row 4 of table 8.13).
  ° If the local wage index is greater than 1.0, the adjusted standard payment conversion factor is *greater* than the standard payment conversion factor (such as affluent CBSAs, Alaska, and Hawaii; see row 5 of table 8.13).

- The labor-adjusted standard payment conversion factor is adjusted for case mix. The labor-adjusted standard payment conversion factor and the relative weight of the HIPPS code (CMG and tier) are multiplied together (columns G, J, and K in table 8.13). This product is the labor and case-mix adjusted federal payment.

- As necessary, outlier adjustments are applied to the case-mix adjusted federal payment.

Implementation

Comprehensiveness and accuracy in coding and reporting the items of the IRF PAI are essential to generate correct Medicare payments. Documentation in the patient record should support the IGC and the ICD codes. The guidelines for reporting codes on the IRF PAI need careful review.

The IRF and its agents must ensure the confidentiality of the information collected in accordance with the Conditions of Participation and HIPAA requirements. Patients must be informed of their rights regarding the collection of patient assessment data and the release of patient-identifiable information.

An IRF must maintain all patient assessment data sets completed on Medicare Part A fee-for-service patients within the previous five years and on Medicare Part C (Medicare Advantage) patients within the previous 10 years. The IRF may maintain these sets either in a paper format in the patient's clinical record or in an electronic computer file format that the IRF can easily obtain.

Home Health Prospective Payment System

Home health agencies (HHAs) provide skilled care to people in their homes, typically people who are homebound. Health professionals may provide these services on either a part-time basis or an intermittent basis. HHAs may be freestanding or based in hospitals or other healthcare organizations. HHAs must be licensed per state or local law. In addition, Medicare-certified HHAs must meet Medicare's Conditions of Participation (CoP) and comply with its requirements for the collection and transmission of data. There are more than 12,000 HHAs. Medicare payments for HHA services total about $18 billion (MedPAC 2014f, 1).

Background

The home health prospective payment system (HHPPS) went into effect on October 1, 2000. The HHPPS was authorized by the Balanced Budget Act of 1997, as amended by the Omnibus Consolidated and Emergency Supplemental Appropriations Act (OCESAA) of 1999.

Benefit

Home health services are covered under both Medicare Part A and Medicare Part B. Beneficiaries can receive an *unlimited* number of episodes (60-day periods of care) so long as they continue to meet the coverage (eligibility) criteria (see next section). Medicare beneficiaries have *no* cost sharing for

home health services, except for a 20 percent coinsurance for **durable medical equipment (DME)** (see chapter 4). Durable medical equipment is equipment designed for long-term use in the home, such as specialized beds, walkers, wheelchairs, and other supplies.

Eligibility Criteria

The coverage (eligibility) criteria for home health services are delineated in the specifications for **certification**. Under both Part A and Part B Medicare, home health services must be certified. Certification may be made by the home health physician, a nonphysician practitioner (NPP) working in collaboration with the certifying physician, or, after an acute or postacute hospitalization, a physician who cared for the patient in the acute-care or post-acute-care facility. The "certification" (documentation of continued eligibility) must state that

- A face-to-face encounter occurred within the 90 days prior to the start of home health care or within the 30 days after the start of care.

- The home health services are needed because the individual is confined to the home (figure 8.13) and needs intermittent skilled nursing care, physical therapy, speech-language pathology services, or a combination of services or continues to need occupational therapy.

- A plan for furnishing such services to the individual has been established and is periodically reviewed by a physician.

- The services are or were furnished while the individual was under the care of a physician (Medicare Learning Network 2014, 2–3).

Certifications must be obtained when the plan of care is established or as soon thereafter as possible. For continuing services, the physician must recertify the services at intervals of at least once every 60 days. In the recertification, the physician recertifies that a continuing need exists for the services and estimates how long services will continue to be needed. The recertification should be obtained when the plan of care is reviewed because the same interval (at least

Figure 8.13.   Definition of "confined to the home" from the Centers for Medicare and Medicaid Services

An individual shall be considered "**confined to the home**" (homebound) if the following two criteria are met:

Criterion-One:

The patient must either:
Because of illness or injury, need the aid of supportive devices such as crutches, canes, wheelchairs, and walkers; the use of special transportation; or the assistance of another person in order to leave their place of residence

OR

Have a condition such that leaving his or her home is medically contraindicated.
If the patient meets one of the Criterion-One conditions, then the patient must ALSO meet two additional requirements defined in Criterion-Two below.

Criterion-Two:

There must exist a normal inability to leave home;

AND
Leaving home must require a considerable and taxing effort.

Source: Medicare Learning Network 2013 (November). MLN Matters MM8444, Home Health-Clarification to Benefit Policy Manual Language on "Confined to the Home" Definition. http://www.cms.gov/Outreach-and-Education/Medicare-Learning-Network-MLN/MLNMattersArticles/Downloads/MM8444.pdf.

once every 60 days) is required for the review of the plan.

Consolidated Payment

The unit of payment is the **episode of care**. The episode of care is all the home health care services delivered to a patient during a 60-day period. Claims for episodes of care usually include more than one date of service. As previously stated, beneficiaries may have multiple 60-day episodes. The per episode payment consolidates, into one payment, reimbursement for

- All physical, occupational, and speech-language therapies

- Skilled nursing care

- Home health aide services

- Medical social work services

- All medical supplies, including **nonroutine medical supplies (NRS)**, such as supplies specifically ordered by the physician and particular to a condition

The services must be ordered by a physician. Excluded from the HHPPS are DME and osteoporosis drugs. The HHA, however, may bill these items separately to CMS (Medicare Learning Network 2014, 5).

Data Collection and Reporting

The goals of the data collection and reporting are to document the delivery of appropriate and quality care and to support accurate claims for reimbursement. This section covers the data collection instrument for home health, special issues related to coding, and electronic collection and transmission of data.

Outcome Assessment Information Set

In HHAs, data are collected on an instrument called the **Outcome Assessment Information Set (OASIS)**. The version that is currently used is OASIS-C1. HHA personnel use the OASIS data in the comprehensive assessment that underlies the patient's care plan. OASIS collects data in six major domains:

1. Sociodemographic

2. Environment

3. Support system

4. Health status

5. Functional status

6. Behavioral status

CMS requires specific timeframes for the collection of OASIS data and the completion of comprehensive assessments. OASIS data are collected at the following times:

- Start of care (SOC)

- Significant change in condition (SCIC), such as unexpected decline or improvement

- Transfer to inpatient facility

- Resumption of care (ROC) after inpatient hospitalization situation occurs

- Discharge from care of HHA

- Death at home

For all these events, OASIS data must be collected within 48 hours (Gaboury 2008, 6–7). For patients whose care is continuing, the HHA must recertify their medical eligibility within five days of the end the 60-day episode of care (days 56 through 60). The OASIS data set does not substitute for the comprehensive assessment and care plan. The comprehensive assessment is a Medicare Condition of Participation.

Coding for Home Health

OASIS uses ICD codes to represent the health status of patients. CMS requires that coding on the OASIS be based on official guidelines (see chapter 2).

CMS requires that HHAs list in the OASIS all diagnoses for which the patient is receiving home care (Columns 1 and 2 in table 8.20). The sequencing of the diagnoses should reflect the seriousness of each condition and should support the disciplines (skilled nursing, HH aide, physical therapy, speech-language pathology, occupational therapy, and medical social services) rendering care and the services being provided. The primary (principal) diagnosis for the HHPPS is the diagnosis most related to the current plan of care. The diagnosis may or may not be related to the patient's most recent hospital stay but must relate to the services rendered by the HHA. Other (secondary) diagnoses are conditions that exist when the plan of care is established, subsequently develop, or affect the treatment or care. Examples of conditions or diagnoses that may affect treatment or care are those that affect patients' responsiveness to treatment or their

rehabilitative prognosis. Symptom control ratings are entered for all diagnoses (Column 2 in table 8.21).

In infrequent instances, following official coding guidelines results in codes in OASIS that are not **case-mix diagnoses** that drive (affect) payment (figure 8.14 and table 8.20). In those instances, HHAs may provide additional information in OASIS (columns 3 and 4 in table 8.20).

Other Data Collection

CMS requires that HHAs collect and report data on quality measures. CMS publicly posts these quality data to the CMS website. Consumers may use these results to compare the quality of HHAs. Submission of data on quality measures affects payment (discussed in later section on payment).

Home health claims must record and report all home health services provided to the beneficiary within each 60-day episode. Each service must be reported in line item detail. Healthcare Common Procedure Coding System (HCPCS) G codes are recorded to reflect details of skilled nursing and therapy services. HCPCS G codes are used to report the following:

- Skilled nursing services provided by a licensed nurse directly to a patient

- Nursing visits for management and evaluation, observation and assessment, and training and education.

Table 8.20. OASIS diagnoses, symptom control, and payment diagnoses

Column 1	Column 2	Column 3	Column 4
Descriptions	Codes	Optional Payment (Case-Mix) Diagnosis	Optional Payment (Case-Mix) Diagnosis
Descriptions of all diagnoses for which patient is receiving home care sequenced in order of the seriousness of the condition and support the disciplines and services provided.	ICD codes for each condition and symptom control rating (0 to 4). Codes for "Factors Influencing Health Status and Contact with Health Services" and "External Causes" are allowed. Order may differ from Column 1.	Complete using case-mix diagnosis if codes for "Factors Influencing Health Status and Contact with Health Services" are assigned in Column 2. Codes for "Factors Influencing Health Status and Contact with Health Services" and "External Causes" are *not* allowed.	Complete using case-mix diagnosis *only* if codes for "Factors Influencing Health Status and Contact with Health Services" *and* multiple codes for manifestations are assigned in Column 2. Codes for "Factors Influencing Health Status and Contact with Health Services" and "External Causes" are *not* allowed.
Primary diagnosis	Primary diagnosis code with rating	Description of primary diagnosis and code	Description of primary diagnosis and code
Other diagnoses	Other diagnoses codes with rating	Description of other diagnoses and codes	Description of other diagnoses and codes

Source: Centers for Medicare and Medicaid Services. 2015a (January). Final OASIS-C1/ICD-9 Version Item Set. http://www.cms.gov/Medicare/Quality-Initiatives-Patient-Assessment-Instruments/HomeHealthQualityInits/Downloads/Final-OASIS-C1-ICD-9-Version-Item-Set-effective-01-01-2015.pdf.

Table 8.21. Symptom control rating scale for primary and secondary diagnoses in OASIS

Rating	Description
0	Asymptomatic; no treatment needed at this time
1	Symptoms well controlled with current therapy
2	Symptoms controlled with difficulty, affecting daily functioning; patient needs ongoing monitoring
3	Symptoms poorly controlled; patient needs frequent adjustment in treatment and dose monitoring
4	Symptoms poorly controlled; history of rehospitalizations

Source: Centers for Medicare and Medicaid Services. 2015a (January). Final OASIS-C1/ICD-9 Version Item Set. http://www.cms.gov/Medicare/Quality-Initiatives-Patient-Assessment-Instruments/HomeHealthQualityInits/Downloads/Final-OASIS-C1-ICD-9-Version-Item-Set-effective-01-01-2015.pdf.

Figure 8.14. Diagnostic categories of case-mix diagnoses

Blindness and low vision	Ortho 1 (leg disorders)
Blood disorders	Ortho 2 (other orthopedic disorders)
Cancer and selected benign neoplasms	Psych 1 (affective and other psychoses, depression)
Diabetes	
Dysphagia	Psych 2 (degenerative and other organic psychiatric disorders)
Gait abnormality	Pulmonary disorders
Gastrointestinal disorders	Skin 1 (traumatic wounds, burns, and postoperative complications)
Heart disease	
Hypertension	Skin 2 (ulcers and other skin conditions)
Neuro 1 (brain disorders and paralysis)	Tracheostomy care
Neuro 2 (peripheral neurological disorders)	Urostomy or cystostomy care
Neuro 3 (stroke)	
Neuro 4 (multiple sclerosis)	

Source: Department of Health and Human Services. 2007. Medicare Program; Home Health Prospective Payment System Refinement and Rate Update for Calendar Year 2008; Final Rule. Federal Register 72(167):49787–49817.

- Services and therapy maintenance programs provided by a qualified physical or occupational therapist or a speech-language pathologist. Visits by qualified therapy assistants are separately coded. CMS uses these codes to differentiate services delivered by therapists from services delivered by assistants (Medicare Learning Network 2011, 2–5).

Appropriate HCPCS codes may also be recorded to report nonroutine supplies for CMS's tracking purposes.

The number of therapy hours that the patient has received in the 60-day episode also requires documentation. The documentation should focus on functional, measurable, and objective goals in the treatment plan and progress being made toward those goals. Specifically, Medicare requires documentation of

- Initial assessment by a qualified therapist (not an assistant) from *each* discipline providing services to the patient. For example, a physical therapist would assess the patient's need for physical therapy, an occupational therapist would assess the patient's need for occupational therapy, and so forth.

- Subsequent provision of needed therapy services and assessments at least once every 30 days by the pertinent qualified therapist or therapists (not assistants) to confirm the continued need for therapy (HHS 2014d, 66104).

Electronic Collection and Transmission

HHAs use a special software, the Java-based **home assistance validation and entry (jHAVEN)** system, to electronically collect and transmit the OASIS data. jHAVEN is replacing HAVEN as the software tool for the collection and submission of data. It is made publicly available by CMS. Through HAVEN, OASIS data are entered, formatted, and locked for electronic transmission to state agencies. HAVEN also includes a grouper (CMS 2015b).

Structure of Payment

The HHPPS is based on a predetermined rate for a 60-day episode of home health care. Figure 8.15 shows the basic foundation of an HHPPS payment. OASIS data are essential to HHAs' reimbursement under the HHPPS. OASIS data drive the determination of the case-based adjustment (figure 8.15). There are three components in the structure of payment under the HHPPS: the national standardized episode rate, the HHA case-mix group, and adjustments.

Figure 8.15.   Foundation of home health prospective payment system

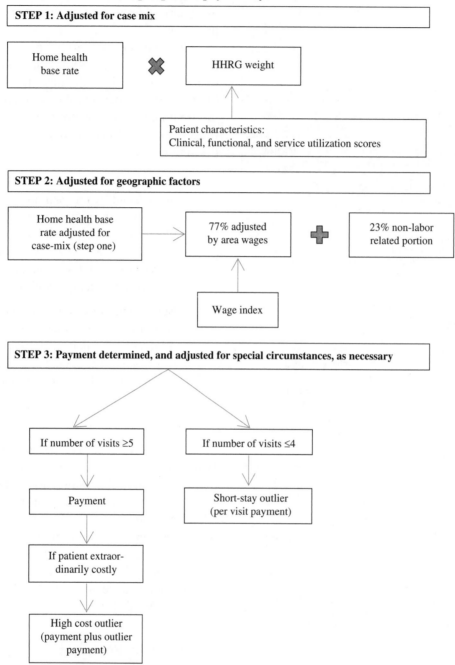

Source: Medicare Payment Advisory Commission (MedPAC). 2014f (October). Payment basics: Home health care services payment system. http://www. medpac.gov.

National Standardized Episode Rate

The **national standardized episode rate** is a predetermined base rate for the calculation of the home health payment (table 8.22). This base rate is derived from data from the most recent audited cost reports on all covered home health services. The national standardized episode rate converts the CMG into a payment (figure 8.15). The national standardized episode rate is recalibrated annually for changes in the home health market basket (mix of goods and services appropriate to home health services).

Table 8.22. National standardized episode rates, selected years

	2009	2012	2015
Amount with submission of quality data	$2,271.92	$2,138.52	$2,961.38
Amount without submission of quality data	$2,227.75	$2,096.34	$2,903.37

Adjustments to the National Standardized Episode Rate

In the HHPPS, the case-mix adjustment accounts for differing use of resources related to patients' conditions and need for therapies (figure 8.15). The HHPPS takes into account geographic factors through the adjustments for local wages (figure 8.15).

Adjustments for Case Mix

HHAs enter data from their patients' OASIS assessments, including the ICD codes, into HAVEN. The grouper in HAVEN uses these data to classify patients into a **home health resource group (HHRG)**. An HHRG is a CMG that includes patients with similar conditions and resource utilization (figure 8.16). HHRGs exist for a wide spectrum of patients, from relatively uncomplicated patients to severely ill, functionally limited patients requiring extensive therapy. There are 153 HHRGS. Each HHRG has a case weight (HHS 2014d, 66035).

The grouper uses three dimensions to calculate an HHRG code:

- Clinical severity (C): The clinical severity is the patient's characteristics and health status. The grouper adds scores for certain wound and skin conditions, such as infected wounds, abscesses, chronic ulcers, and gangrene; for specific diagnosis groups, such as pulmonary, cardiac, and cancer; and for certain secondary diagnoses (table 8.23). Scores in multiple groupings are added. These scores are factored into the case weight.

- Functional status (F): Limitations.

- Service utilization (S). Service utilization represents the patient's consumption of therapy resources. Service utilization is defined as the number of therapy visits by physical therapy, speech-language pathology, or occupational

therapy. High is 14 or more, and low is 13 or fewer therapy visits. There are also three thresholds of therapy visits (6, 14, and 20 visits) with graduated steps of one to four visits per grouping (HHS 2007, 49776). See tables 8.24, 8.25, and 8.26.

These dimensions and their severity are represented in the HHRG codes' six alphanumeric characters. An example of an HHRG code is C1F1S1.

- Clinical severity is the first position; its severity is in the second position.

- Functional status (F) is the third position; its severity is in the fourth position.

- Service utilization (S) is the fifth position; its severity is in the sixth position.

C1F1S1 represents a patient with the lowest severity in the clinical, functional, and service dimensions (tables 8.24 and 8.25). HHRGs with lower severity levels are associated with lower weights (table 8.26).

In the HHPPS, the HHRG *contributes* to the calculation of the case weight; the HHRG is *not* the sole determinant of the case weight. The timing of the episode and its sequence are also taken into account. The grouper uses complex statistical procedures based on **regression analyses** to combine the dimensions (HHRG) and the episodes' timing (table 8.24). CMS calls these calculations the four-equation model. This combination divides the 153 HHRGs into five categories based on the amount of therapy provided and the episode's timing in the sequence (MedPAC 2014f, 1).

The four-equation model also adjusts for the costs of nonroutine medical supplies (NRS). Examples of NRS include catheter bags, urinary and stool collection pouches, irrigation trays, and appliance cleaners. These supplies are not bundled into typical (routine) medical care (such as swabs, bandages, and sterile gloves). Often physicians specifically order NRS. CMS found that use of NRS varies greatly among patients with different clinical characteristics. To account for these costs, CMS developed six severity groups based on points assigned to the clinical characteristics (table 8.27). Classification into one of the six severity groups is based on points. CMS believes that the six groups of NRS severity reflect the variations in costs across patients with different conditions.

Figure 8.16.   Home health resource group from OASIS data on clinical, functional, and service dimensions

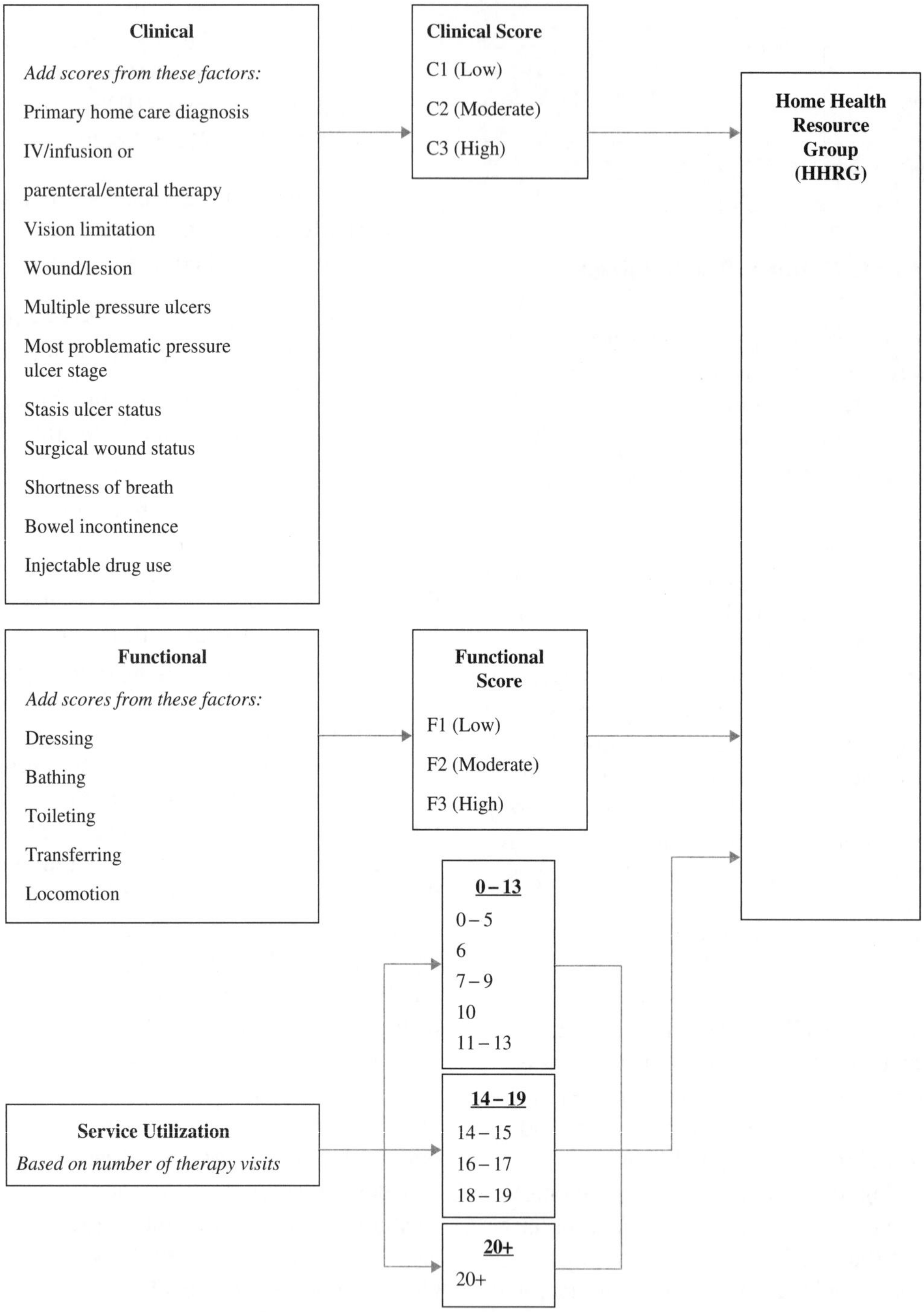

Source: Medicare Payment Advisory Commission (MedPAC). 2014f (October). Payment basics: Home health care services payment system. http://www .medpac.gov.

Geographic Adjustments

There are two geographic adjustments to the national standardized episode rate (see previous detailed discussion in section on SNFs). First are the percentages for the labor-related portion and the non-labor-related portion. These two percentages are usually 77 percent for the labor-related portion and 23 percent for the non-labor-related portion (MedPAC 2014f, 3). Second is

Table 8.23. Case-mix adjustment variables and scores

		1 or 2	1 or 2	3+	3+
	Episode number within sequence of adjacent episodes				
	Therapy visits	0 to 13	14+	0 to 13	14+
	EQUATION:	1	2	3	4
CLINICAL DIMENSION					
2	Primary or Other Diagnosis = Blood disorders Vision		6		3
6	Primary or Other Diagnosis = Dysphagia *AND* Primary or Other Diagnosis = Neuro 3 – Stroke	2	16	1	9
17	Primary or Other Diagnosis = Neuro 3 – Stroke *AND* M1860* (Ambulation) = 4 or more				
FUNCTIONAL DIMENSION					
49	M1840* (Transferring) = 2 or more	3	4	2	1

*Data item numbers in OASIS-C1

Source: Excerpts from Department of Health and Human Services. 2014d. Medicare and Medicaid Programs; CY 2015 Home Health Prospective Payment System Rate Update; Home Health Quality Reporting Requirements; and Survey and Enforcement Requirements for Home Health Agencies; Final Rule. *Federal Register* 79(215):66056–66059.

the adjustment for the differing wage indexes among CBSAs (figure 8.15). The wage index is based on the site of the service to the beneficiary and *not* on the site of the HHA.

Potential Adjustments for Special Circumstances

Other adjustments may be applied to HHA payments for special circumstances. These potential payment adjustments include **low-utilization payment adjustments (LUPAs)**, partial episode payment (PEP) adjustments, and high-cost outlier payments (figure 8.15).

- Low-utilization payment adjustment (LUPA): LUPA is the term used in the HH PPS for short-stay outliers. LUPAs are applied when an HHA provides four or fewer visits in an episode. Under the LUPA, the HHA is reimbursed for each visit rather than for the 60-day episode (table 8.30). For the initial or only visit, a special calculation is made rather than using the amounts published in

the pertinent Final Rule (see table 8.28). Effective in 2014, for the initial or only visit, the rate for skilled nursing, physical therapy, or speech-language pathology is multiplied by a LUPA factor (see table 8.28). Skilled nursing, physical therapy, and speech-language pathology are the only three disciplines allowed to conduct the initial assessment visit, per the Medicare Conditions of Participation (HHS 2013, 72305).

- Partial episode payment (PEP) adjustment: Intervening events, such as a patient's elective transfer or a patient's discharge and then return to care, may initiate the PEP adjustment. The PEP adjustment is based on the span of days of the shortened episode. The proportion of the 60-day episode that the span of days represents is calculated. For example, a 45-day span equals 75 percent of a 60-day episode. The original, potential payment, had the patient not left before the end of the 60-day episode, is multiplied by this proportion, 75 percent (HHS 2014d, 66107).

- High-cost outlier: For cases incurring excessive costs, an outlier payment is made. The outlier payment is in addition to the 60-day episode payment. HHAs receive outlier payments when costs exceed the fixed-loss threshold. CMS established thresholds for each CMG by estimating costs per visit and including a fixed-loss amount (HHS 2014d, 66092).

Payment

For an episode of care, HHAs usually receive payment in the form of two partial payments. These two partial payments are the initial payment and the final payment. These two payments are known as percentage payments or as split percentage payments. For special circumstances, other potential payment adjustments exist.

Percentage Payments

Payment begins when the HHA submit a **Request for Anticipated Payment (RAP)** to the Medicare Administrative Contractor (MAC). A RAP is the first of two transactions submitted for a HHPPS

Table 8.24. Clinical and functional thresholds in home health resource groups

Dimension	Severity Level	1st and 2nd episodes		3rd+episodes		All episodes
		0–13 therapy visits	14–19 therapy visits	0–13 therapy visits	14–19 therapy visits	20+ therapy visits
Grouping step:		1	2	3	4	5
Equation(s):		1	2	3	4	(2&4)
Clinical	C1 (low)	0–1	0–1	0	0–5	0–3
	C2 (medium)	2–3	2–7	1	6–12	4–16
	C3 (high)	4+	8+	2+	13+	17+
Functional	F1 (low)	0–14	0–3	0–9	0	0–2
	F2 (medium)	15	4–13	10	1–7	3–5
	F3 (high)	16+	14+	11+	8+	6+

Source: Adapted from Department of Health and Human Services. 2014d. Medicare and Medicaid Programs; CY 2015 Home Health Prospective Payment System Rate Update; Home Health Quality Reporting Requirements; and Survey and Enforcement Requirements for Home Health Agencies; Final Rule. *Federal Register* 79(215):66060–66066.

Table 8.25. Therapy thresholds for service utilization in home health resource groups

Dimension	Severity Level	1st and 2nd episodes		3rd+episodes		All episodes
		0–13 therapy visits	14–19 therapy visits	0–13 therapy visits	14–19 therapy visits	20+ therapy visits
Grouping step:		1	2	3	4	5
Equation(s):		1	2	3	4	(2, 4)
Service utilization (number of therapy visits)	S1 (minimum)	0–5	14–15	0–5	14–15	20+
	S2 (low)	6	16–17	6	16–17	
	S3 (moderate)	7–9	18–19	7–9	18–19	
	S4 (high)	10		10		
	S5 (maximum)	11–13		11–13		

Source: Adapted from Department of Health and Human Services. 2007 Medicare Program; Home Health Prospective Payment System Refinement and Rate Update for Calendar Year 2008; Final Rule. *Federal Register* 72(167):49825. Department of Health and Human Services. 2014d. Medicare and Medicaid Programs; CY 2015 Home Health Prospective Payment System Rate Update; Home Health Quality Reporting Requirements; and Survey and Enforcement Requirements for Home Health Agencies; Final Rule. *Federal Register* 79(215):66062–66066.

episode. Based on the RAP, the HHA receives the first split percentage payment for that episode. A RAP may be submitted when the following four following conditions are met:

- OASIS assessment is complete, locked, or export-ready.

- Physician's verbal orders for home care have been received and documented.

- Plan of care has been established and sent to the physician.

- First service visit under that plan has been delivered.

Table 8.26. Home health resource groups and case-mix weights

HHRG	Step (Episode and or Therapy Visit Ranges)	Case Mix Weight
C1F1S1	1st and 2nd Episodes, 0 to 5 Therapy Visits	0.5985
C1F1S1	1st and 2nd Episodes, 14 to 15 Therapy Visits	1.2270
C1F1S1	3rd+ Episodes, 0 to 5 Therapy Visits	0.4942
C1F1S1	3rd+ Episodes, 14 to 15 Therapy Visits	1.2407
C1F1S1	All Episodes, 20+ Therapy Visits	1.8122
C1F1S5	1st and 2nd Episodes, 11 to 13 Therapy Visits	1.1013
C1F3S2	1st and 2nd Episodes, 6 Therapy Visits	0.9056
C3F3S3	1st and 2nd Episodes, 18 to 19 Therapy Visits	2.0718
C3F3S3	3rd+ Episodes, 18 to 19 Therapy Visits	2.0901
C3F2S1	All Episodes, 20+ Therapy Visits	2.2135
C3F3S1	All Episodes, 20+ Therapy Visits	2.2950

Source: Department of Health and Human Services. 2014d (November 6). Medicare and Medicaid Programs; CY 2015 Home Health Prospective Payment System Rate Update; Home Health Quality Reporting Requirements; and Survey and Enforcement Requirements for Home Health Agencies; Final Rule. *Federal Register* 79(215):66062–66066.

Table 8.27. Severity groups for nonroutine medical supplies (NRS)

Severity Level	Points (Scoring)
1	0
2	1 to 14
3	15 to 27
4	28 to 48
5	49 to 98
6	99+

Source: Adapted from Department of Health and Human Services. 2014d (November 6). Medicare and Medicaid Programs; CY 2015 Home Health Prospective Payment System Rate Update; Home Health Quality Reporting Requirements; and Survey and Enforcement Requirements for Home Health Agencies; Final Rule. *Federal Register* 79(215):66062–66066.

The pricer software is used to process all HHPPS claims and is integrated into the Medicare claims processing systems. The pricer makes all reimbursement calculations applicable under the HHPPS. The MAC uses the pricer to calculate

- Percentage payments on RAPs
- Claim payments for full episodes of care
- Potential payment adjustments for special circumstances

HHAs may download the pricer software from the CMS website. For the HHAs, the pricer is a tool to estimate HHPPS payments. The CMS official payment may differ slightly from the HHA's estimated payment because the public pricer may not contain the most up-to-date data from HHA cost reports. The MAC pricer contains these updated cost data.

The MAC makes the second (final) split percentage payment in response to a claim from the HHA. HHAs may submit claims at the end of the 60-day episode or after the patient is discharged, whichever is earlier. HHAs may *not* submit the claim until *after* all services are provided for the episode *and* the physician has signed the plan of care and any subsequent verbal order. Signed orders are required every time a claim is submitted.

Added together, the initial and final payment equal 100 percent of the permissible payment for the episode. For all initial episodes, the percentage split for the two payments is 60 percent in response to the RAP and 40 percent in response to the claim. For all subsequent episodes in periods of continuous care, each of the two percentage payments is 50 percent of the estimated case-mix-adjusted episode payment.

Health Insurance Prospective Payment System (HIPPS) Code

Payment in the HHPPS is based on the HIPPS codes (see IRF section for definition). HIPPS codes are derived from the HHRG codes. HIPPS codes are five-character alphanumeric codes (table 8.28). The codes are "intelligent" because the number or letter in each position provides information:

- First position: payment grouping step for episode; 1, 2, 3, 4, or 5 (numeric characters only)
- Second position: clinical dimension; C1, C2, or C3 converted to A, B, or C (alphabetic characters only)
- Third position: functional dimension; F1, F2, or F3 converted to F, G, or H (alphabetic characters only)
- Fourth position: service dimension; S1, S2, S3, S4, or S5 converted to K, L, M, N, or P (alphabetic characters only)
- Fifth position: severity group of nonroutine medical supplies (NRS severity) for supplies provided, S, T, U, V, W, or X, and for supplies not provided, 1, 2, 3, 4, 5, or 6

Table 8.28. HHA standard payment rates

	2009		2012		2015	
	With Submission of Quality Data	Without Submission of Quality Data	With Submission of Quality Data	Without Submission of Quality Data	With Submission of Quality Data	Without Submission of Quality Data
National standard episode amount	$2,271.92	$2,227.75	$2,138.52	$2,096.34	$2,961.38	$2,903.37
Low-utilization payment adjustment (LUPA) by home health discipline						
Home health aide	$48.89	$47.94	$51.13	$50.12	$57.89	$56.75
Medical social services	$173.05	$169.68	$180.96	$177.39	$204.91	$200.89
Occupational therapy	$118.83	$116.52	$124.26	$121.80	$140.70	$137.95
Physical therapy	$118.04	$115.74	$123.43	$121.39	$139.75	$137.02
Skilled nursing	$107.95	$105.85	$112.88	$110.65	$127.83	$125.33
Speech-language pathology	$128.26	$125.77	$134.12	$131.48	$151.88	$148.90
*Low-utilization payment adjustment (LUPA) for initial or only visit	$90.48	$88.72	$94.62	$92.75	Differential LUPA factor applied to rate of discipline making visit; nursing(1.8451), physical therapy (1.67), or speech-language pathology (1.6266)	
Nonroutine medical supplies (NRS) by severity rating						
Severity level 1 (0 points, relative weight 0.2698)	$14.13	$13.86	$14.37	$14.09	$14.36	$14.08
Severity level 2 (1–14 points, relative weight 0.9742)	$51.04	$50.04	$51.91	$50.87	$51.86	$50.84
Severity level 3 (15–27 points, relative weight 2.6712)	$139.94	$137.22	$142.32	$139.49	$142.19	$139.51
Severity level 4 (28–48 points, relative weight 3.9686)	$207.91	$203.86	$211.45	$207.24	$211.25	$207.12
Severity level 5 (49–98 points, relative weight 6.1198)	$320.62	$314.37	$326.06	$319.58	$325.76	$319.39
Severity level 6 (99+ points, relative weight 10.5254)	$551.43	$540.67	$560.79	$549.64	$560.27	$549.32

*LUPA calculation changed in 2014 to factor from amount.

Source: Department of Health and Human Services. 2014d. Medicare and Medicaid Programs; CY 2015 Home Health Prospective Payment System Rate Update; Home Health Quality Reporting Requirements; and Survey and Enforcement Requirements for Home Health Agencies; Final Rule. *Federal Register* 79(215):66088–66090.

The 153 HHRGs are represented by the first four positions of the HIPPS code (see table 8.29). The 1,836 HIPPS codes are the combination of the 153 HHRGs with the 12 NRS severity levels (two, provided or not provided, per each of the six NRS severity levels) (153 × 12). Each HIPPS code represents a distinct payment amount, without any duplication of payment weights across codes (CMS 2010, 7).

Using table 8.29, a HIPPS code can be "decoded" to determine the data that will drive payment in table 8.29. See the Examples 1 and 2.

Example 1:

First episode, 10 therapy visits, with lowest scores in the clinical, functional, and service dimensions and lowest supply severity level and NRS were not provided:

- First episode, 10 therapy visits is 1 (cell B3)

- Lowest scores in clinical, functional, and service dimensions are A, F, K (cells C3, D3, E3)

- NRS not provided is 1 (cell G3)

- HIPPS code is 1AFK1

Example 2:

Third episode, 22 therapy visits; clinical dimension score is low; functional dimension score is moderate; service dimension score is minimum; and supply severity level 6:

- Third episode, 22 therapy visits is 5 (cell B7)

- Clinical dimension low, functional dimension moderate; service dimension minimum are B, H, K (cells C4, D5, E3)

- Supply severity level 6 is X (cell F8)

- HIPPS is 5BHKX

As "intelligent" codes, the HIPPS codes represent patients' characteristics and other key data that determine payment.

Table 8.29. Creation of health insurance prospective payment system (HIPPS) codes for HHPPS

	A	B	C	D	E	F	G	H
1		Position #1	Position #2	Position #3	Position #4	Position #5		
2		Grouping step	Clinical domain	Functional domain	Service domain	NRS provided	NRS not provided	Domain levels
3	Early episodes (1st and 2nd)	1 (0–13 visits)	A (HHRG:C1)	F (HHRG:F1)	K (HHRG:S1)	S (Severity level: 1)	1 (Severity level: 1)	= minimum
4		2 (14–19 visits)	B (HHRG:C2)	G (HHRG:F2)	L (HHRG:S2)	T (Severity level: 2)	2 (Severity level: 2)	= low
5	Late episodes (3rd and later)	3 (0–13 visits)	C (HHRG:C3)	H (HHRG:F3)	M (HHRG:S3)	U (Severity level: 3)	3 (Severity level: 3)	= moderate
6		4 (14–19 visits)			N (HHRG:S4)	V (Severity level: 4)	4 (Severity level: 4)	= high
7	Early or late episodes	5 (20+ visits)			P (HHRG:S5)	W (Severity level: 5)	5 (Severity level: 5)	= maximum
8						X (Severity level: 6)	6 (Severity level: 6)	
9		6 thru 0	D thru E	I thru J	Q thru R	Y thru Z	7 thru 0	Expansion values for future use

Source: Centers for Medicare and Medicaid Services (CMS). 2010. Definition and uses of health insurance prospective payment system codes, version 5. http://www.cms.hhs.gov/ProspMedicareFeeSvcPmtGen/downloads/hippsusesv4.pdf.

Calculation

To calculate the episode payment, the pricer's internal logic uses in the components in figure 8.15 and data from tables 8.22, 8.28, and 8.30.

To make these calculations, the pricer contains

- National standardized episode rate tables
- Pricing of the HIPPS codes for HHRGs
- Labor-related portion
- Non-labor-related portion
- Wage indexes for all CBSAs and rural areas
- Rules for calculating adjustments

Here is the process shown in figure 8.15 and table 8.31:

- National standardized episode rate begins the calculation (cell A3 in table 8.31).
- The national standardized episode rate and the HIPPS relative weight of the applicable HIPPS code are multiplied together (cells A3 and C3 in table 8.31). This product is the case-mix adjusted rate (cell D3 in table 8.31).
- The labor adjustment to the case-mix adjusted national standardized episode rate is calculated by applying the labor-related portion and the local wage index (cells D3, E3, G3, and H3 in table 8.31).
- The non-labor-related portion is calculated by multiplying the case-mix adjusted national episode rate by the non-labor-related portion (cells D3, F3, and I3 in table 8.31).
- The labor-related adjusted portion and the non-labor-related adjusted portion are added together to obtain the case-mix, wage-adjusted episode payment (cells H3, I3, and J3 in table 8.31).
- To the case-mix, wage-adjusted episode rate is added the appropriate adjustment for NRS (cells J3 and K3 in table 8.31), resulting in the total payment (cell L3 in table 8.31).

Finally, CMS reduces payments to HHAs that do not submit data on the quality measures. The quality measures are included in the OASIS data set (see previous discussion in OASIS and table 8.28). HHAs

Table 8.30. Excerpted selected representative HIPPS weights

HIPPS Code	Description	Case-Mix Weight (Positions 1–4)	Supply Amount (Position 5)
1AFKS	Early Episode, 0–13 therapies, Clinical Severity Level 1, Functional Severity Level 1, Service Severity Level 1, Supply Severity Level 1, supplies provided	0.5985	$14.36
1AFMX	Early Episode, 0–13 therapies, Clinical Severity Level 1, Functional Severity Level 1, Service Severity Level 3, Supply Severity Level 6, supplies provided	0.8499	$560.27
2CHLT	Early Episode, 14–19 therapies, Clinical Severity Level 3, Functional Severity Level 3, Service Severity Level 2, Supply Severity Level 2, supplies provided	1.8487	$51.86
3AFLS	Late Episode, 0–13 therapies, Clinical Severity Level 1, Functional Severity Level 1, Service Severity Level 2, Supply Severity Level 1, supplies provided	0.6435	$14.36
4CHMV	Late Episode, 14–19 therapies, Clinical Severity Level 3, Functional Severity Level 3, Service Severity Level 3, Supply Severity Level 4, supplies provided	2.0718	$211.25
5BHKX	Early or Late Episode, 20+ therapies, Clinical Severity Level 2, Functional Severity Level 3, Service Severity Level 1, Supply Severity Level 6, supplies provided	2.0532	$560.27
5CHKX	Early or Late Episode, 20+ therapies, Clinical Severity Level 3, Functional Severity Level 3, Service Severity Level 1, Supply Severity Level 6, supplies provided	2.2950	$560.27

Source: Centers for Medicare and Medicaid Services. Home Health PPS, Coding and Billing Information. HH PPS HIPPS Code Weight Table. http://www.cms.gov/Medicare/Medicare-Fee-for-Service-Payment/HomeHealthPPS/coding_billing.html.

Department of Health and Human Services. 2014d (November 6). Medicare and Medicaid Programs; CY 2015 Home Health Prospective Payment System Rate Update; Home Health Quality Reporting Requirements; and Survey and Enforcement Requirements for Home Health Agencies; Final Rule. *Federal Register* 79(215):66089.

Table 8.31. Calculation of home health payment with submission of quality data

	A	B	C	D	E	F	G	H	I	J	K	L
1	Nat'l 60-day episode rate with qual data (CY 20**)	HIPPS Code or Case-Mix Severity	Weight (Positions 1-4)	Case-mix adjusted rate (nat'l episode rate × HIPPS weight)	Labor-related portion	Nonlabor-related portion	Local wage index*	Labor-related portion of rate (case-mix adj. rate × labor-related portion × local wage index)	Nonlabor-related portion of rate (case-mix adj. rate × nonlabor-related portion)	Adjusted rate (adj. labor-related portion + adj. nonlabor-related portion)	Supply Add-on (Position 5, NRS)	Payment
2				A × C				D × E × G	D × F	H + I		J + K
3	$2,961.38	1AFK1	0.5985	$1,772.39	77%	23%	0.9343	$1,275.07	$407.65	$1,682.72	0	$1,682.72

*CBSA 24780, Greenville, NC.

that do not submit the quality data are subject to a two percent reduction in the next year's percentage increase in the home health market basket (HHS 2014d, 66035). Table 8.28 shows the effect of the two percent reduction.

Implementation

The home health sector is dynamic and under intense scrutiny. Healthcare policy analysts find that Medicare payments to HHAs substantially exceed their costs (MedPAC 2014a, 214). Moreover, a US Senate Finance Committee report concluded that among the major for-profit home health providers, more therapy was often provided than clinically needed in an attempt to maximize Medicare reimbursement. The result has been waste of taxpayer dollars and the delivery of what could be medically unnecessary patient care to increase companies' profits (US Senate Committee on Finance 2011, 2). The US Senate Committee concluded that home health agencies' practices "at best represent abuses of the Medicare home health program. At worst, they may be examples of for-profit companies defrauding the Medicare home health program at the expense of taxpayers" (US Senate Committee on Finance 2011, 2).

To operate in this environment and to provide quality care to home health patients, implementation of HHPPS demands the management of details such as

- Processing with attention to timeframes, flow of information, and quality

- Coding and reporting following official guidelines (chapter 2)

- Data entry into OASIS and HAVEN and using updated instructions

- Identification of current payment rates for national standardized episode rates, labor-related portions, wage indexes, and other adjustments

To collect and report accurate data, ongoing training of HHA personnel is important. Training should focus on consistently applying CMS guidelines. Consistency supports accurate data collection, coding, and reimbursement (Niewenhous 2009, 378). Training should also include information on changes in the HHPPS. The CMS Manual, OASIS, the HAVEN, the grouper, and the pricer are often updated. Key personnel for training include clinicians, administrators, middle managers, and reimbursement specialists. Given the close scrutiny under which the HHA sector is currently operating, leaders and personnel should monitor the environment and its changes.

Check Your Understanding 8.2

1. What tool is used to collect the information about Medicare patients that drives payment in the IRF PPS?

2. True or false? IRF staff members record RICS on patients' PAIs to classify their impairment categories.

3. What home health care services are consolidated into a single payment to HHAs?

4. When is a LUPA used, and how does it affect reimbursement?

5. Name the three dimensions of case mix measured using data elements from OASIS for the HHPPS.

Trends in Postacute Care

Healthcare policy makers recognize that the multiple data collection instruments used in the PAC sector contribute to its complexity. SNFs must use the MDS, LTCHs, the LTCH Continuity Assessment and Record Evaluation (LTCH-CARE) Data Set, IRFs, the IRF-PAI, and HHAs the OASIS. As a result, Congress passed the Improving Medicare Post-Acute Care Transformation Act (IMPACT) of 2014, which requires the following:

*   PAC providers must report standardized patient assessment data.

*   PAC providers must report standardized quality measures and resource-use measures.

*   HHS must modify the existing PAC assessment instruments to allow for (1) submission of standardized patient assessment data and (2) comparison of such data across all PAC providers.

The standardized data are used to assess patients, to improve the quality of care, and to support reimbursement. Finally, the submission of standardized patient data, quality measures, and resource-use measures allows CMS and other health policy analysts to make comparisons across the PAC settings.

The use of PAC services will continue to increase; greater integration of services across the continuum of care is needed. People are living longer with multiple chronic conditions. However, it is difficult to match the patient with the appropriate setting. This difficulty occurs for the following reasons:

*   Medicare per capita spending (adjusted for prices and health status) on PAC varies more than on most other covered services.

*   Services overlap among PAC settings (and with inpatient acute care). Patients after a joint replacement may be discharged to home

health, to outpatient therapy, to a SNF, or to an IRF, or may remain in the acute-care inpatient hospital because of complications. These settings have very different costs.

*   PAC services are poorly defined. SNFs vary greatly in the range of complex cases they will admit; LTCHs are not located in some geographic areas. SNFs and acute-care inpatient hospitals may substitute for LTCHs.

Thus, to begin to resolve these problems, MedPAC recommends that CMS consider an integrated approach to acute care and postacute care (MedPAC 2014a, 172). The implementation of the site-neutral payments for LTCHs under the Pathway for SRG Reform Act of 2013 is one example of this integrated approach (see previous section in LTCH). In the future, integration could also be achieved through readmission policies and bundled payments. Readmission policies could align payment incentives so that providers across acute care and PAC have a common interest in preventing, and responsibility to prevent, premature discharges and inappropriate readmissions. In addition, bundled payments for services across acute and postacute settings are seen as a way to reduce fragmentation. MedPAC envisions that one payment would be made for the acute inpatient admission, outpatient services, and postacute services (MedPAC 2014a, 172). CMS's responses to these recommendations bear monitoring by healthcare analysts and personnel.

Chapter 8 Review Quiz

1. What services are included in the consolidated billing of the SNF PPS? What services are excluded from the consolidated billing of the SNF PPS?

2. How are per diem rates for SNF PPS patients determined for various cases?

3. For CMS to define a facility as an LTCH, how many days must its Medicare patients' average length of stay be?

4. How are MS-LTC-DRGs determined?

5. On the IRF PAI, the patient's ability to perform activities of daily living, or _____, is recorded on the _____.

6. True or false? For inpatient rehabilitation facility patients, codes on the IRF PAI should follow the UHDDS and the UB-04 guidelines.

7. True or false? Facilities transmit IRF PAIs to the Centers for Medicare and Medicaid Services using CMS's free IRVEN software.

8. In the HHPPS, the _____ software is used to collect and submit OASIS data.

9. How is durable medical equipment (DME) reimbursed in the HHPPS?

10. Why is the home health HIPPS code called an "intelligent" code?

References

Assistant Secretary for Planning and Evaluation (ASPE), Office of Disability, Aging, and Long-Term Care Policy. 2011. Glossary of terms. http://aspe.hhs.gov/daltcp/diction.shtml.

Centers for Medicare and Medicaid Services (CMS). 2010. Definition and uses of health insurance prospective payment system codes, version 5. http://www.cms.hhs.gov/prospmedicarefeesvcpmtgen/downloads/hippsusesv4.pdf.

Centers for Medicare and Medicaid Services (CMS). 2011a. Medicare Program; prospective payment system and consolidated billing for skilled nursing facilities; disclosures of ownership and additional disclosable parties information; Proposed Rules. *Federal Register* 76(88):26364–26429.

Centers for Medicare and Medicaid Services (CMS). 2011b. Medicare program; Prospective payment system and consolidated billing for skilled nursing facilities for FY 2012; Final rule. *Federal Register* 76(152):48486–48562.

Centers for Medicare and Medicaid Services (CMS). 2011c. CMS Manual System, Pub 100-04. Medicare claims processing manual: Chapter 6—SNF inpatient Part A billing and SNF consolidated billing. Section 30.6.2. https://www.cms.gov/manuals/downloads/clm104c06.pdf.

Centers for Medicare and Medicaid Services (CMS). 2014a (October). MDS 3.0 RAI Manual v1.12R and Change Tables. *Long-Term Care Facility Resident Assessment Instrument User's Manual*, version 3.0. Chapters 5 and 6. http://www.cms.gov/Medicare/Quality-Initiatives-Patient-Assessment-Instruments/NursingHomeQualityInits/MDS30RAIManual.html.

Centers for Medicare and Medicaid Services (CMS). 2014b (October). IRF Patient Assessment Instrument. Updated IRF PAI Training Manual, October 2014. http://www.cms.gov/Medicare/Medicare-Fee-for-Service-Payment/InpatientRehabFacPPS/IRFPAI.html.

Centers for Medicare and Medicaid Services. 2015a (January). Final OASIS-C1/ICD-9 Version Item Set. http://www.cms.gov/Medicare/Quality-Initiatives-Patient-Assessment-Instruments/HomeHealthQualityInits/Downloads/Final-OASIS-C1-ICD-9-Version-Item-Set-effective-01-01-2015.pdf.

Centers for Medicare and Medicaid Services. 2015b (February). jHAVEN/HAVEN. http://www.cms.gov/Medicare/Quality-Initiatives-Patient-Assessment-Instruments/OASIS/HAVEN.html.

Chumney, D., K. Nollinger, K. Shesko, K. Skop, M. Spencer, and R.A. Newton. 2010. Ability of Functional Independence Measure to accurately predict functional outcome of stroke-specific population: Systematic review. *Journal of Rehabilitation Research and Development* 47(1):17–29.

Cotterill, P.G., and B.J. Gage. 2002. Overview: Medicare post-acute care since the Balanced Budget Act of 1997. *Health Care Financing Review* 24(2):1–6.

Department of Health and Human Services. 2001. Medicare program; Prospective payment system for inpatient rehabilitation facilities; Final rule. *Federal Register* 66(152):41316–41427.

Department of Health and Human Services. 2007. Medicare program; Home health prospective payment system refinement and rate update for calendar year 2008; Final rule. *Federal Register* 72(167):49762–49945.

Department of Health and Human Services. 2009. Medicare program; Prospective payment system and consolidated billing for skilled nursing facilities for FY 2010; Minimum Data Set, version 3.0 for skilled nursing facilities and Medicaid nursing facilities; Proposed rule. *Federal Register* 74(90):22208–22316.

Department of Health and Human Services. 2013. Medicare and Medicaid Programs; Home Health Prospective Payment System Rate Update for CY 2014, Home Health Quality Reporting Requirements, and Cost Allocation of Home Health Survey Expenses; Final Rule. *Federal Register* 78(231):72255–72320.

Department of Health and Human Services. 2014a. Medicare Program; Prospective Payment System and Consolidated Billing for Skilled Nursing Facilities for FY 2015; Final Rule. *Federal Register* 79(150):45627–45659.

Department of Health and Human Services. 2014b (August 22). Medicare Program; Hospital Inpatient Prospective Payment Systems for Acute Care Hospitals and the Long-Term Care Hospital Prospective Payment System and Fiscal Year 2015 Rates; Quality Reporting Requirements for Specific Providers; Reasonable Compensation Equivalents for Physician Services in Excluded Hospitals and Certain Teaching Hospitals; Provider Administrative Appeals and Judicial Review; Enforcement Provisions for Organ Transplant Centers; and Electronic Health Record (EHR) Incentive Program; Final Rule. *Federal Register*, book 2 of 2 books, 79 Part II(13):49853–50536.

Department of Health and Human Services. 2014c (August 6). Medicare Program; Inpatient Rehabilitation Facility Prospective Payment System for Federal Fiscal Year 2015; Final Rule. *Federal Register* 79(151):45871–45936.

Department of Health and Human Services. 2014d (November 6). Medicare and Medicaid Programs; CY 2015 Home Health Prospective Payment System Rate Update; Home Health

Quality Reporting Requirements; and Survey and Enforcement Requirements for Home Health Agencies; Final Rule. *Federal Register* 79(215):66031–66118.

Gaboury, M.A. 2008. *Home Health Pocket Guide to OASIS*, 2nd ed. Marblehead, MA: HCPro.

Grabowski, D.C. 2010. Postacute and long-term care: A primer on services, expenditures and payment methods. Prepared for Office of Disability, Aging and Long-Term Care Policy, Office of the Assistant Secretary for Planning and Evaluation. http://aspe.hhs.gov/daltcp/reports/2010/paltc.htm.

Medicare Learning Network. 2011. MLN Matters Number MM7182. New home health claims reporting requirements for G codes related to therapy and skilled nursing services. https://www.cms.gov/MLNMattersArticles/downloads/MM7182.pdf.

Medicare Learning Network. 2013 (November). MLN Matters MM8444, Home Health-Clarification to Benefit Policy Manual Language on "Confined to the Home" Definition. http://www.cms.gov/Outreach-and-Education/Medicare-Learning-Network-MLN/MLNMattersArticles/Downloads/MM8444.pdf.

Medicare Learning Network. 2014 (January). Quick Reference Information: Home Health Services, ICN908504. https://www.cms.gov/Outreach-and-Education/Medicare-Learning-Network-MLN/MLNProducts/Downloads/Quick_Reference_Home_Health_Services_Educational_Tool_ICN908504.pdf.

Medicare Payment Advisory Commission (MedPAC). 2014a (March). Report to the Congress: Medicare Payment Policy. http://medpac.gov.

Medicare Payment Advisory Commission (MedPAC). 2014b (June). A data book: Health care spending and the Medicare program. http://medpac.gov.

Medicare Payment Advisory Commission (MedPAC). 2014c (October). Payment basics: Skilled nursing facility services payment system. http://www.medpac.gov.

Medicare Payment Advisory Commission (MedPAC). 2014d (October). Payment basics: Long-term care hospitals payment system. http://www.medpac.gov.

Medicare Payment Advisory Commission (MedPAC). 2014e (October). Payment basics: Inpatient rehabilitation facilities payment system. http://www.medpac.gov.

Medicare Payment Advisory Commission (MedPAC). 2014f (October). Payment basics: Home health care services payment system. http://www.medpac.gov.

Niewenhous, S.S. 2009. April 2009 OASIS questions and answers. *Home Health Care Management and Practice* 21(5):378–383.

Trela, P. 2002. Inpatient rehabilitation PPS presents new challenges, opportunities. *Journal of AHIMA* 73(1):48A–48D.

Trela, P. 2007 (May). IRF PPS coding challenges. *Journal of AHIMA* 78(5):70–71.

U.S. Senate Committee on Finance. 2011 (September). Staff Report on Home Health and the Medicare Therapy Threshold. http://permanent.access.gpo.gov/gpo14737/Home_Health_Report_Final.pdf.

Chapter 9
Revenue Cycle Management

Objectives

- To recall and describe the components of the revenue cycle

- To define revenue cycle management

- To describe the importance of effective revenue cycle management for a provider's fiscal stability

Key Terms

Accounts receivable (AR)
Charge capture
Charge description master (CDM)
Claim processing activities
Claims reconciliation and collection
Explanation of benefits (EOB)
Hard coding
Integrated revenue cycle
Key performance indicator (KPI)

Medicare Administrative Contractor (MAC)
Medicare Summary Notice (MSN)
Outpatient service-mix index (SMI)
Preclaims submission activities
Remittance advice (RA)
Revenue cycle (RC)
Revenue cycle management (RCM)
Scrubber

Portions of this chapter are adapted from the AHIMA Press publication The Charge Description Master Handbook, *by Anne B. Casto, RHIA, CCS.*

Introduction to Revenue Cycle Management

Prospective payment systems have been implemented in virtually every service area in the healthcare arena. To maintain profitability under the prospective payment systems, healthcare facilities are incentivized to constantly examine and implement methods to either increase reimbursement or decrease costs. Managers of many facilities understand the importance of decreasing payment delays and lost revenue through **revenue cycle management (RCM)**. RCM is the supervision of all administrative and clinical functions that contribute to the capture, management, and collection of patient service revenue. This text discusses a standard **revenue cycle**, or the regular set of tasks and activities producing revenue for the facility or practice, and the management of that cycle in an acute care setting. Though many of the components are similar across various healthcare settings, there may be differences in the revenue cycle flow and management dependent upon institution size, approach to charge capture, and availability of coding professionals.

Multidisciplinary Approach

In the past, RCM used a silo approach in which each clinical department was responsible for its own functions and contributions to the revenue cycle. However, this linear approach was often reactive in nature, and rather than promoting communication between departments, it tended to foster hostility and division. The twenty-first-century approach to RCM in healthcare facilities is based on a multidisciplinary model. This dynamic management style promotes cooperation among various clinical departments by creating an RCM team composed of representatives from all revenue cycle areas. An emphasis on education encourages all team members to be updated on changing market forces such as payer trends, government and regulatory modifications, and organization strategy. As a result of each member of the team better understanding other members' contributions and their importance to the revenue cycle, this modern management approach has influenced the team as a whole to take a proactive stance in regard to reimbursement issues.

Components of the Revenue Cycle

Each section of the revenue cycle is vital to creating efficient and compliant reimbursement processes. The basic components of the revenue cycle are similar at each facility or physician practice even though there is varying nomenclature used between facility, practices, and healthcare systems. One difference between the revenue cycles at many facilities and physician practices is the size. At a facility, the revenue cycle is typically comprised of numerous units and service areas (registration, laboratory, coding, and such). At a physician practice, there may be one service area and one business office in which the majority of revenue cycle tasks and functions are completed. Although each unit in a facility setting is responsible for its own functions and tasks, cooperation from outside departments and clinical areas is often critical for timely and accurate completion and submission of healthcare claims. Likewise, in the physician practice setting, each team member of the business office may be responsible for a set of tasks; however, all team members must work together to create a successful revenue cycle. The major components of the revenue cycle are

- Preclaims submission activities
- Claims processing activities
- Accounts receivable
- Claims reconciliation and collections

Preclaims Submission Activities

Preclaims submission activities comprise tasks and functions from the patient registration and case management areas. Specifically, this portion of the revenue cycle is responsible for collecting the patient's and responsible parties' information completely and accurately for determining the appropriate financial class, for educating the patient about his or her ultimate financial responsibility for services rendered, for collecting waivers when appropriate, and for verifying data prior to procedures or services being performed and submitted for payment. For example, when a Medicare patient arrives for admission into the cardiology unit for a coronary artery stent placement, the admitting representative is responsible for collecting the patient demographic data, including the individual's Medicare healthcare identification claim number (HICN). Additionally, the Medicare patient may need to be educated about any annual deductible amount or copayment responsibilities if the inpatient stay should last longer than 60 days.

Claims Processing Activities

Claims processing activities include the capture of all billable services, claim generation, and claim corrections. **Charge capture** is a vital component of the revenue cycle. All clinical areas that provide services to a patient must report charges for the services that they have performed. Failure to report charges for these services will result in lost reimbursement for the healthcare facility. Charge capture can be accomplished in a variety of ways depending on the technological capabilities of the healthcare facility.

Order Entry

Electronic order entry systems have been implemented at hospitals to help capture the charge at the point of service delivery. With an electronic order entry system, the charge for the service or supply is automatically transferred to the patient accounting system and posted to the patient's claim. Facilities without electronic systems and most physician practices use paper-based processes such as charge tickets, superbills, and encounter forms to assist in charge collection. With a paper-based process, the paper forms are collected and then entered into the patient accounting system, where the charge is then transferred to the claim. The paper system leaves more room for error because charges can be posted to the wrong patient's account, digits can be transposed during data entry, and backlogs can occur when data entry clerks are absent or pulled off task.

Charge Description Master

Coding is a major portion of charge capture. Claims submission regulations require ICD and/or HCPCS codes to be reported on a patient's claim. Several types of visits, such as clinic visits, or services, such as laboratory or radiology, are designed to have procedure codes posted to the claim via the **charge description master (CDM)**. During order entry, electronic or paper-based, a unique identifier for each service is entered. This unique identifier triggers a charge from the CDM to be posted to the patient's account. This process is known as **hard coding**.

Different facilities use different terminology for the CDM. Some more common synonyms include chargemaster, charge compendium, service master, price list, service item master, and charge list (Schraffenberger and Kuehn 2011, 222). The CDM is a large database maintained by the facility that houses the price list and

required claim data elements for all services provided to patients. The primary function of the CDM is to produce hospital claims. It is used to translate services rendered to the patient into the data elements required for reporting services on the hospital claim. Without the CDM, a clerk would have to manually enter data elements into the claim form for each claim. With use of the CDM, the data elements can be transferred to the claim form electronically and with speed and consistency that manual data entry cannot ensure.

Each time a unit of service is transferred to a patient claim, the CDM tracks the usage of that service. Thus, at any given time, the number of services performed or the number of units of rendered services can be calculated. This is very helpful for utilization management. For example, the Radiology department may want to track how many chest x-rays are performed per month. Further, the department manager wants to confirm that every chest x-ray procedure was billed. The department will most likely have internal records of the number of x-rays performed by month, but comparing that volume with the units of service billed according to the CDM will allow the Radiology department to identify whether there is a charge capture issue.

Like utilization management, the resource consumption level can be monitored in a consistent and communicable manner with the help of the CDM. The CDM, by using standardized code sets, allows a facility to track the type of services utilized by a specific patient population. For example, the cardiac catheterization unit wants to know what drugs were given to patients who underwent catheterization in May. By using the charge identifier for cardiac catheterization procedures, the department can pull line item level detail from the facility's data warehouse. The department can then analyze the data to determine which types of resources are most often consumed by patients. The department may be particularly interested in recovery room time. Because recovery room time is reported on claims, the service has a unique charge identifier. Therefore, the analysis would be able to determine the average length of time that patients spend in the recovery room post procedure. This is important not only for cost determination, but also for staffing and patient scheduling considerations. With the use of CDM data elements, this review can be performed by a data analyst very easily. This is in contrast to requiring a data abstraction professional to review medical records, which can be very time-consuming.

Traditionally, the CDM is housed in the finance department. However, many clinical and ancillary areas share in the maintenance responsibility. Nonetheless, the CDM coordinator typically reports to a finance management team member. Of course, there are different models available for use. Some facilities have moved the responsibility to the HIM department because of the strong coding background of many HIM professionals.

The size of the CDM unit or team will vary from facility to facility. The number of full-time equivalents (FTEs) in the unit depends on the size of the CDM as well as how many facility satellite areas require CDM line item management. Typically, there is a CDM coordinator position that manages the CDM unit. CDM coordinator position requirements vary from facility to facility based on the philosophy and complexity of CDM management of the facility or practice. In general, CDM coordinators should possess

• Considerable knowledge of the revenue cycle

• Good communication skills, both verbal and written

• Understanding of coding and reimbursement systems

• Management experience

The CDM coordinator position is one of great importance. Even though it is a very detail-oriented position, the coordinator must also be able to engage others in the maintenance process. Individuals interested in this position must be able to strike a balance between control and delegation—not always an easy task.

Though the CDM function has been, and continues to be, housed primarily in the finance department at many facilities, HIM professionals have an important role in the maintenance of the CDM. The coding and reimbursement experience of CDM coordinators varies from hospital to hospital. Thus, the coding and reimbursement expertise of HIM professionals is often sought after by the CDM team. The HIM professional may help the CDM team understand the intent of a CPT/HCPCS code, may help the CDM team understand new coding guidelines released for a CPT code, may help the CDM team understand how new CMS regulations affect the CDM, and may help the CDM team communicate coding rules and regulations to various clinical or ancillary department managers.

Additionally, it is valuable for the HIM department and CDM team to have a good working relationship. By exploring each professional's roles and responsibilities,

they will see that they may have more in common than they thought. When these two units work together, they can significantly affect key performance indicators established for the revenue cycle, improving the efficiency of providing quality service for all patients.

Coding by HIM

Other types of visits, such as inpatient or complex ambulatory surgery, require that diagnoses and operating room procedures be coded by health information management (HIM) professionals. During the coding process, medical records are viewed and read by the coding staff. All diagnoses and procedures are identified, coded, and then abstracted into the HIM coding system. This system then transfers the diagnoses and procedure codes to the patient accounting system, where they are posted to the patient's claim prior to submission for payment.

Auditing and Review

After all data have been posted to a patient's account, the claim can be reviewed for accuracy and completeness. Many facilities have internal auditing systems, known as scrubbers. The auditing system runs each claim through a set of edits specifically designed for that third-party payer. The auditing system identifies data that has failed edits and flags the claim for correction. Examples of errors that cause claim rejections or denials if not caught by the scrubber are

• Incompatible dates of service

• Nonspecific or inaccurate diagnosis and procedure codes

• Lack of medical necessity

• Inaccurate revenue code assignment

The auditing process prevents facilities from sending incomplete or inaccurate claims to the payer. Facilities that do not have an editing system may perform a hand audit of a sample of claims. HIM and reimbursement specialists review claims with the medical record to determine whether all services, diagnoses, and procedures were accurately reported. If errors are found, they can be corrected before claim submission.

Submission of Claims

After being reviewed and corrected, the claim can be submitted to the third-party payer for payment.

The Health Insurance Portability and Accountability Act of 1996 (HIPAA) added a new part to the Social Security Act, titled Administrative Simplification. The purpose of this section is to improve the efficiency and effectiveness of the healthcare delivery system. Through this section, Medicare has established standards and requirements for the electronic exchange of certain health information (HHS 2003a, 8381). The final rule on Standards for Electronic Transactions and Code Sets, also known as the Transactions Rule, identified eight electronic transactions and six code sets (tables 9.1 and 9.2). This rule ensures that all providers, third-party payers, claims clearinghouses, and so forth use the same sets of codes to communicate coded health information, ensuring standardization for systems and applications across the healthcare continuum. Not only does this support standardization, but it also supports administrative simplification. Providers can now maintain a select number of code sets at their current version, rather than maintaining different versions (current and old) of many code sets based on payer specification, as required in the past.

Healthcare claims, healthcare payment and remittance advice, and coordination of benefits are included in the electronic transactions. Since October 16, 2003, all healthcare facilities have been required to electronically submit and receive healthcare claims, remittance advices, and coordination of benefits. Thus, today, facilities submit claims via the 837I electronic format, which replaces the UB-04 or CMS-1450 billing form. Physicians submit claims via the 837P electronic format, which takes the place of the CMS-1500 billing form.

Table 9.1. HIPAA electronic transactions

Healthcare claims or equivalent encounter information
Eligibility for a health plan
Referral certification and authorization
Healthcare claim status
Enrollment and disenrollment in a health plan
Healthcare payment and remittance advice
Health plan premium payments
Coordination of benefits

Source: Department of Health and Human Services. 2003. Health insurance reform. Security standards; Final rule. *Federal Register* 68(34):8382.

Table 9.2. HIPAA code sets

International Classification of Diseases, 9th Revision, Clinical Modification, vols. 1 and *2; replacement by 10th revision expected 10/1/2015*
International Classification of Diseases, 9th Revision, Clinical Modification, vol. 3; replacement by Procedure Coding System (PCS) expected 10/1/2015
National Drug Codes
Code on Dental Procedures and Nomenclature
Health Care Financing Administration Common Procedure Coding System
Current Procedural Terminology, 4th ed.

Source: Department of Health and Human Services. 2003. Health insurance reform. Security standards; Final rule. *Federal Register* 68(34):8382.

Centers for Medicare and Medicare Services. 2014. Press Release: "Deadline for ICD-10 allows health care industry ample time to prepare for change."

Accounts Receivable

The accounts receivable department manages the amounts owed to a facility by customers who received services but whose payments will be made at a later date by the patients or their third-party payers. After the claim is submitted to a third-party payer for reimbursement, the accounts receivable clock begins to tick. Typical performance statistics maintained by the accounts receivable department include days in accounts receivable and aging of accounts. Days in accounts receivable is calculated by dividing the ending accounts receivable balance for a given period by the average revenue per day. Facilities typically set performance goals for this standard. Aging of accounts is maintained in 30-day increments (0–30 days, 31–60 days, and so forth). Facilities monitor the number of accounts and the total dollar value in each increment. The older the account or the longer the account remains unpaid, the less of a chance that the facility will receive reimbursement for the encounter.

Insurance Processing

Once a claim is received by the third-party payer (TPP), the insurance processing of the claim begins. Medicare claims for Part A services and hospital-based Medicare Part B services are submitted to a designated A/B **Medicare Administrative Contractor (MAC)**. MACs contract with Medicare to process claims for a specific area or region. The MAC determines costs and reimbursement amounts, conducts reviews and audits, and makes payments to providers for covered services on behalf of Medicare. Figure 9.1 shows the A/B MAC jurisdictions.

Benefits Statements

In addition to processing the claim for payment, TPPs prepare an **explanation of benefits (EOB)** that is delivered to the patient. The EOB is a statement that describes services rendered, payment covered, and benefits limits and denials. Specifically for Medicare patients, claims payment contractors prepare **Medicare Summary Notices (MSNs)**. The MSN details amounts billed by the provider, amounts approved by Medicare, how much Medicare reimbursed the provider, and what the patient must pay the provider by way of deductible and copayments. EOBs and MSNs are part of the Transactions Rule and are provided to the facility via electronic data interchange (EDI) and are sent to the patient via postal mail.

Remittance Advice

After the claim is processed by the TPP, a **remittance advice** (RA) is electronically returned to the provider via the 835A or 835B electronic format. The RA is sent to the provide by third-party payers and outlines claim rejections, denials, and payments to the facility. Payments are typically made in batches, with the RA sent to the facility and payments electronically transferred to the provider's bank.

Claims Reconciliation and Collection

The last component of the revenue cycle is reconciliation and collections. The healthcare facility uses the EOB, MSN, and RA to reconcile accounts. EOBs and MSNs identify the amount owed by the patient to the facility.

Figure 9.1.   A/B MAC jurisdictions

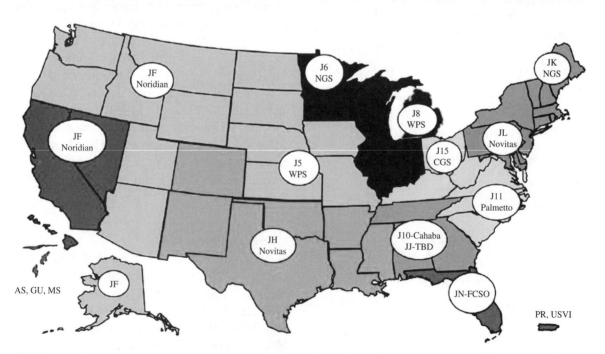

Source: CMS 2015. http://www.cms.gov/Medicare/Medicare-Contracting/Medicare-Administrative-Contractors/Downloads/AB-Jurisdiction-Map-Feb-2014.pdf.

Collections can contact the patient to collect outstanding deductibles and copayments. RAs indicate rejected or denied line items or claims. Facilities can review the RAs and determine whether the claim error can be corrected and resubmitted for additional payment. If a correction is not warranted, reconciliation can be made via a write-off or adjustment to the patient's account. After the account has been settled, the revenue cycle is completed. Figure 9.2 provides a flow chart of the revenue cycle.

CDM Structure, Maintenance, and Compliance

The CDM is a vital component of claims processing activities as the majority of outpatient and several inpatient supplies and services are placed on the claim via the CDM. The accuracy of the data elements are critical to ensure that claims are accurate and complete. The governance of the data elements in a year-round endeavor requiring a multidisciplinary team.

CDM Structure

Although each CDM is unique to a hospital or hospital system, standard data elements are included in each

CDM. It is important that HIM professionals be familiar with each of the CDM data elements and that they understand the elements' importance to the claim production process. Table 9.3 displays sample line items from a CDM.

Charge Code

The charge code, also known as the service code, charge description number, or charge identifier, is a hospital-specific internally assigned code used to identify an item or service. The code is typically numeric, but that is dependent upon a hospital's CDM strategy or structure.

Charge code numbers are assigned or distributed by a designated person, the IT department, or the CDM coordinator. The methodology for distribution depends on the facility. Similar to typical medical record number schemes, the charge code number may be distributed in straight numerical order, or a facility may reserve numerical sections by ancillary service. For example, charge code number set 100000–199999 is reserved for radiology.

Regardless of the distribution methodology, each charge code number must be unique, so the CDM unit

Figure 9.2.   Flowchart of the revenue cycle

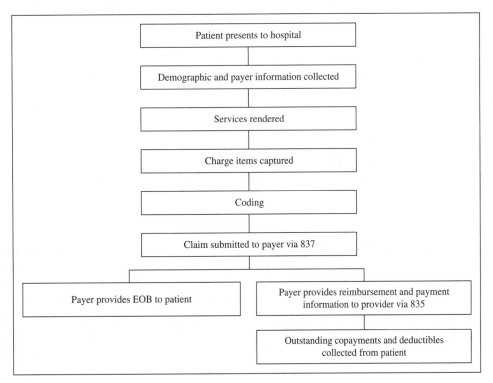

Table 9.3.   Sample charge description master

Department Code	Charge Code*	Code Description	Revenue Code	HCPCS Code**	Charge***	Active/Inactive Status
700	7008989	Dermagraft (Synth skin graft)	252	Q4106	$1,525.00	Active
700	7005202	Minor surgery—½ hour	360		$1,203.00	Active
700	7005203	Regular OR—1st hour	360		$4,687.00	Active
700	7005205	Regular OR—½ hour	360		$1,682.00	Active
715	7157059	Open heart—1st hour	360		$5,589.00	Active
715	7157060	Open heart—½ hour	360		$2,782.00	Active
760	7605161	OB/GYN surgery	360		$1,975.00	Active
800	8004557	Rabies vaccine-IM use	450	90675	$632.00	Active
822	8224210	Albumin 5% saline	250	P9045	$265.00	Active
367	3675839	Speech screening	440	V5362	$298.00	Active
367	3675840	Language screening	440	V5363	$298.00	Active
367	3675841	Dysphagia screening	440	V5364	$298.00	Active
200	2578961	Venipuncture	300	G0001	$18.00	Inactive
200	2578989	Venipuncture	300	36415	$18.00	Active
110	1478951	MRI upper extremity without dye	610	73218	$817.00	Active
110	1478952	MRI upper extremity with dye	610	73219	$857.00	Active
110	1478953	MRI upper extremity without and with dye	610	73220	$897.00	Active

* Also called item number, charge number, item code, service code, and service number.

** When blank, Healthcare Common Procedure Coding System (HCPCS) code is determined via coding in health information management (HIM) department for certain revenue codes.

*** Charge is fictitious and should not be used for rate setting.

must ensure that there are not duplicate charge codes in the CDM. The CDM coordinator should schedule and complete duplicate charge code audits throughout the year.

Department Code

Department code is a hospital-specific number that is assigned to each clinical or ancillary department that provides services to patients and has at least one charge item in the CDM. Alternative terminology for this data element may be general ledger number. This code is used to identify the area within the healthcare facility that is providing the service. The codes usually correspond with an ancillary or clinical service such

as speech therapy or by physical area, such as the emergency department.

Some facilities accomplish having multiple charge items for the same service that are performed in different areas by combining the department number and a service code to create the unique charge code. For example, venipunctures are often performed in various areas for the healthcare facility and are prime candidates for this type of structure. Table 9.4 provides an illustration of this methodology. By using this methodology, charge entry users within the healthcare facility can look at the unique charge code and know that the venipuncture (12345) was performed in the emergency department (123) when the charge code 12312345 appears on the claim.

Table 9.4.   Combination of department code and service code to create unique charge code

Department Code	Venipuncture Service Code	Unique Charge Code
123—Emergency department	12345	12312345
124—Clinic	12345	12412345
125—Pre-operative holding	12345	12512345

Revenue Code

A revenue code is a four-digit numeric code required for billing on the UB-04 claim form or the 8371 ETS. Revenue codes are maintained by the National Uniform Billing Committee, so revenue codes are standard, with the same code set used by all facilities. What vary from facility to facility are the services or CPT/HCPCS codes assigned to a revenue code or code group. However, revenue code assignment is usually driven by the ancillary department or location where the service was rendered. Revenue code reporting requirements for Medicare are detailed in the *Medicare Claims Processing Manual*, chapter 25, section 75.4 (CMS 2005a). At each facility, the revenue code reported on individual claims is used at the end-of-year cost reporting process.

Although the revenue code list is standardized, the combination of CPT/HCPCS code and revenue code can be somewhat facility-specific. However, Medicare and other third-party payers issue transmittals and bulletins that provide revenue code instruction for use with specific CPT/HCPCS codes. Additionally, the Medicare Code Editor (MCE) and the Integrated Outpatient Code Editor (OCE) used by the Medicare Administrative Contractors (MACs) contain revenue code and CPT/HCPCS code edits to ensure that appropriate combinations are reported on a claim when required.

In addition to identifying the service area or type of service performed, revenue codes are used by third-party payers to identify payment methodologies for specific services in their contracts. Therefore, the use of revenue codes for services must be reviewed very closely by the hospital contract management team. For example, consider the following contract language for three payers at a facility. Payer one indicates in the contract that he or she will pay 60 percent of billed charges for MRI services identified by revenue code 0610. The second payer, Medicare, specifies that the most specific revenue code be used for MRI services and that facilities report the applicable code in range 0610–0614. The third payer

specifies that he or she will reimburse MRI services based on the CPT code regardless of the revenue code used. The CDM unit must work closely with hospital contract managers to ensure that the CDM is meeting the reporting needs for all three of these payers, not just major payers such as Medicare.

CPT/HCPCS Code

CPT/HCPCS codes are the current code set assigned by the American Medical Association (AMA) and CMS to be reported for individual services, procedures, and supplies rendered to the patient. Code use requirements may be payer-specific—Medicare, Medicaid, Blue Cross, and the like. It is important to remember that CPT/HCPCS codes are not provided for all line items. Several services or supplies billed to the patient do not have associated CPT/HCPCS codes (room rates, general supplies), so this data element will be blank for these line items.

The CPT/HCPCS code delineates several data pieces within the charge item. The CPT/HCPCS code sets were established by the Health Insurance Portability and Accountability Act of 1996 (HIPAA) as the designated code set to be used on certain electronic transactions by all healthcare facilities and insurers for the services, procedures, and supplies rendered in the outpatient settings. Thus, the use of CPT/HCPCS codes is mandatory when codes are available for reporting.

There are instances in which Medicare and other third-party payers may require different codes to report a service. Medicare maintains the HCPCS Level II system that in part contains temporary codes developed for use in various Medicare Prospective Payment Systems (PPS). In such instances, the facility must make accommodations in the CDM for both codes for that specific service. Currently, CMS requires different codes for some (but not all) coronary artery stent placement services. CMS has created C-codes for hospital outpatient departments to use for Medicare patients as outlined in table 9.5. Other third-party payers may not follow Medicare reporting guidance and may require the CPT codes rather than the HCPCS C-codes. Thus, facilities serving both a Medicare and a commercial patient population must be able to report the correct code for services based on the patient's financial class. Some facilities accomplish this by creating different charge items based on financial class. (See table 9.6.) Other facilities may add a column in the CDM for "Medicare CPT/HCPCS code," as

Table 9.5.   Coronary artery stent placement services CPT/HCPCS codes

Code	Description
92928	Percutaneous transcatheter placement of intracoronary stent(s), with coronary angioplasty when performed; single major coronary artery or branch
92929	Percutaneous transcatheter placement of intracoronary stent(s), with coronary angioplasty when performed; each additional branch of a major coronary artery
C9600	Percutaneous transcatheter placement of drug-eluting intracoronary stent(s), with coronary angioplasty when performed; single major coronary artery or branch
C9601	Percutaneous transcatheter placement of drug-eluting intracoronary stent(s), with coronary angioplasty when performed; each additional branch of a major coronary artery

Source: AMA 2014; CMS 2014.

shown in table 9.7. Either way, the facility must have a procedure in place to ensure that the required code is placed on the claim in order to prevent rejections and denials issued by the payer as well as to receive proper reimbursement.

Charge Description

Charge description is an explanatory phrase that has been assigned to describe a procedure, service, or supply. The charge description is usually based on the official CPT/HCPCS description when applicable, but the field is often limited by the character length allowed by the financial system, so shorter descriptions are used.

The AMA and CMS provide an official long description for each code. Additionally, a short description is provided for use in space-limited fields

within hospital systems. The CDM team must decide whether the short description of the code should be used as the hospital description or whether a modified description would better suit the facility. Likewise, a list of commonly used abbreviations should be maintained to provide consistency through the CDM. The dilemma lies in that most practitioners are not familiar with the official CPT/HCPCS code description; rather, they use working lay titles for the procedures and services they perform or provide. Therefore, using the official short descriptions in the computerized or manual order entry system or CDM may be confusing for the service providers. On the flip side, consumers of healthcare may better understand the official short or long description than the lay term used by practitioners. As hospitals work to improve customer service with their patients, they are striving to produce a patient bill that the patient can easily comprehend.

To illustrate this point, compare a few lay descriptions to some official short descriptions that are located in table 9.8. In examples A and B, would the average patient be able identify the service they received from the charge description? If someone did not know coding, would they know what "SLP treatment" represents? It is likely that only ancillary therapists might understand the hospital lay description for these therapy services. Likewise, in examples C and D, perhaps only radiology technicians, radiologists, physicians, and coders might understand the hospital lay descriptions for these services. Do you think that the average patient would be able to connect "SP Arterio Renal Bilateral" to the catheterization that they received? What description would be even more patient-friendly for examples B and D?

Table 9.6.   Coronary stent placement, drug-eluting stent, by payer example 1

Charge Code	Department Number	Revenue Code	HCPCS Code	Description	Charge*
12345	301	0481	C9600	Coronary stent placement, drug-eluting stent—Medicare	$12,375.00
12346	301	0481	92928	Coronary stent placement, drug-eluting stent—non-Medicare	$12,375.00

*Charge is fictitious and should not be used for rate setting.

Table 9.7.   Coronary stent placement, drug eluting stent, by payer example 2

Charge Code	Department Number	Revenue Code	HCPCS Code	HCPCS Code CMS	Description	Charge*
12345	301	0481	92928	C9600	Coronary stent placement, drug-eluting stent—Medicare	$12,375.00

*Charge is fictitious and should not be used for rate setting.

Table 9.8.   Sample charge descriptions (lay descriptions) versus short descriptions

Example	Charge Description	Code	Short Description
A	SLP treatment	92507	Speech/hearing therapy
B	CPM setup	97001	PT evaluation
C	Treatment aids—interm	77333	Radiation treatment aid(s); intermediate
D	SP arterio renal bilateral	36246	Place catheter in artery; initial second order

Source: AMA 2014; CMS 2015a.

There are no hard and fast rules regarding the description that must be used in the CDM charge description field. Each facility must determine which methodology works best for their facility. The Healthcare Financial Management Association (HFMA) published significant work in the area of patient-friendly billing. HFMA has launched the Patient Friendly Billing Project (HFMA 2015a) to encourage facilities to improve billing for patients. The philosophy of the project is based on the following ideals:

- The needs of patients and family members should be paramount when designing administrative processes and communications.

- Information gathering should be coordinated with other providers and insurers, and this collection process should be done efficiently, privately, and with as little duplication as possible.

- When possible, communication of financial information should not occur during the medical encounter.

- The average reader should easily understand the language and format of financial communications.

- Continuous improvement of the billing process should be made by implementing better practices and incorporating feedback from patients and consumers (HFMA 2014a).

Though many revenue cycle areas are impacted by this project, it is clear that there is emphasis on the charge descriptions used by facilities on the patient bill.

Charge (Price)

The charge, or price, is the dollar amount that the hospital is charging for the item or service rendered to the patient. Though the charge itself is a data element within the CDM, the finance department within the healthcare facility typically manages this data element. Statistics gathered from the CDM may be useful in analyzing charge structure. Likewise, oddities that are identified should be investigated by the revenue cycle team, but the actual setting of rates is typically not performed by the CDM team.

Modifier

Modifiers are codes used by providers and facilities to identify or flag a service that has been modified in some way or to provide more specific information about the procedure or service. There are two sources of modifiers. The first source of modifiers includes those that are part of the CPT code set. The second source of modifiers includes those that are part of the HCPCS Level II code set.

Because the use of a modifier can alter the meaning of the code, it is important that modifiers only be applied to CPT and HCPCS codes when documentation in the medical record supports the application of the modifier. Thus, hard-coding of modifiers in the CDM is rare, but some facilities do use this practice. CDM units should pay close attention to modifier reporting guidelines if they choose to hard-code a modifier into the CDM. CDM units should consider all compliance implications that could arise as a result of the hard-coded modifier appearing with the associated CPT/HCPCS code every time the charge code is activated by the order entry process.

Charge Status (Active or Inactive)

Charge status is an identifier used to indicate whether a line item charge is currently being used by the facility to report a service or supply. Hospitals may or may not maintain an active indicator status in the CDM. Most facilities will not delete charge items from their CD to preserve historic practices and thus use a charge status indicator instead. This allows the facility to maintain the integrity of charge items that have been used in the past and that may be reviewed at later dates by Medicare and other third-party payers. It is also a way to identify whether new charge items are needed. In the charge item addition process, the requested charge item can be compared to inactive charge items. If there is a match, the appropriate discussions can then take place about why the charge item was moved to inactive status and to determine whether the new charge is necessary.

Payer Identifier

Payer identifier codes are used to differentiate among payers that may have specific or special billing protocol in place. Illustration of this practice was described in the CPT/HCPCS code section. It is important for the CDM team to review the payer identifier assignment on a regular basis. Each time a payer contract is revised, the CDM team must work with the contract management unit to determine whether changes in payer identifier assignment are warranted.

For example, a facility's largest payer (Super Payer) is adopting the CMS Outpatient Prospective Payment System (OPPS) methodology. Previously, Super Payer paid a percent of charge and did not require facilities to use HCPCS Level II codes. However, with the movement to OPPS, now they will require HCPCS Level II codes, and the Super Payer is adopting the same reporting requirements as Medicare. The payer identifier assignment for Super Payer may need to be revisited before the switch in their methodology, as displayed in table 9.9.

CDM Maintenance

CDM maintenance is an ongoing process at any healthcare facility, physician office, hospital, imaging center, or freestanding laboratory facility. Numerous events throughout the year provide cause for CDM maintenance. CPT/HCPCS codes are updated regularly throughout the year, as is billing and coding guidance.

Likewise, payer contracts are usually negotiated based on the facility's fiscal year, which may or may not correspond with Medicare's various payment system updates. Understanding the hospital's financial calendar is an important part of planning for ongoing maintenance to the CDM.

Each year, the CDM coordinator should ensure that the proper resources are acquired for CDM maintenance. Updated codebooks as well as national, uniform billing data set information are required. Additionally, payer instructions such as the *Medicare Claims Processing Manual* should be available so that crucial instructions can be easily located and reviewed. Any publications specific to the state in which the facility operates should be present as well (Dietz 2005, 3). Many resources, such as the *Medicare Claims Processing Manual*, are available online, but your CDM team may consider having a shared location to house the links to these documents to ensure that all team members are able to access the necessary documents without having to spend time searching online.

Although facilities may use different management structures, the CDM unit or team, CDM committee, or revenue cycle team will need to oversee the CDM maintenance process. The oversight should not be a single individual's responsibility, as varying perspectives and expertise are required to create a comprehensive plan. One of the major responsibilities of the team is to develop policies and procedures for the CDM review plan (Bielby, et al. 2010). As the CDM team is developing policies and procedures for the CDM maintenance process, they should consider the following questions:

Table 9.9.   Example of effect on payer identifier by payer reimbursement methodology change

Super Payer—Reimbursement Methodology Is Percent of Billed Charges						
Charge Code	Department Number	Revenue Code	HCPCS Code	HCPCS Code CMS	Description	Charge*
12345	301	0481	92928	C9600	Coronary stent placement, drug eluting sent—Medicare	$12,375.00
Super Payer—Reimbursement Methodology Is OPPS						
Charge Code	Department Number	Revenue Code	HCPCS Code	HCPCS Code CMS and Super Payer	Description	Charge*
12345	301	0481	92928	C9600	Coronary stent placement, drug eluting sent—Medicare	$12,375.00

- Do our policies cover how coding and billing regulations are communicated within the organization? Do we expect a response?

- Do our policies address resources and instructions for code updates?

- Do our policies require coders and billers to document any advice received from the Medicare Administrative Contractor?

- Are we addressing CDM risk areas in our policies and procedures?

- Do our policies define how consultants may be used in CDM maintenance? Should they? (Acumentra Health 2005, 11–12)

After the policies and procedures are in place, the team can start to build their maintenance plan.

Maintenance Plan

CDM maintenance is a very detailed process and must be approached very methodically. Thus, the maintenance plan should consist of several organized and structured processes, and CDM coordinators might want to consider a project plan approach to CDM maintenance. A CDM maintenance plan will allow all individuals and departments that are included in the maintenance process to understand how their components fit into the larger maintenance plan. Likewise, each participant will understand his or her duties and be fully aware of the expected timeline for completion. Not only does this help individuals stay on task, but it can be very beneficial to new employees who may not be familiar with the facility's internal process.

Working with Hospital Departments

Ancillary and other clinical areas play a large role in CDM maintenance. Their clinical expertise combined with the coding knowledge of the CDM coordinator or HIM representative will allow a facility to have a current, accurate, and complete CDM. It is important to remember that the primary focus of clinical and ancillary areas is patient care, so the CDM coordinator must engage the departments in the CDM maintenance process.

Understanding Services

Having a good working relationship with clinical and ancillary areas is important for the maintenance process.

Who better to explain services, service components, and service delivery techniques than health professionals themselves? Understanding the service is the key to assigning the appropriate CPT or HCPCS code for the charge item. For example, interventional radiology is a very challenging service area for many coders and CDM professionals. This service area requires code selection from both the surgical and radiology sections. Understanding which codes are used together for which procedures is critical, so having a clinician from the interventional radiology department explain which procedures are performed by the facility and how the components work together is paramount. This type of valuable interaction will provide clinical insight to help ensure that these complex cases are accurately and completely reported by the facility.

Understanding the CDM

As important as it is for clinical and ancillary areas to share their expertise with the CDM coordinator, it is equally important for the CDM coordinator to explain the compliance or billing implications with the clinical areas. It is much easier to get buy-in from healthcare professionals when they understand the reasoning behind a set process or protocol. Providing an example with significant financial implications is an effective way to help ancillary and clinical professionals understand why proper code selection is vital in the CDM maintenance process. For example, suppose a CDM team member is updating the charge ticket for the neurology clinic. The team member identifies three charge codes with the same description: autonomic nerve function test. The neurology manager may not understand the issue, as the clinical professionals in the clinic understand the difference between tests one, two, and three. However, what if the charge entry staff do not? Further review of the utilization report for this clinic reveals that the first listed charge code is reported 98 percent of the time. Is that the actual utilization? A sample of medical records are reviewed, and it is determined that the wrong charge code was activated 65 percent of the time. To make matters worse, because the wrong charge code was activated, the wrong CPT code (95921 rather than 95922 or 95923) was reported on the claim for several encounters. Because of the charging error, the facility was overpaid by Medicare for several claims and must now resubmit the claims with the corrected CPT code and pay back the overpayment amount. How can this be prevented in the future? The CDM team must take the time to work with the neurology clinic manager and revise the charge descriptions so that they better differentiate among the three tests. Although similar descriptions may not be an issue for the clinicians, clearly they can be for other hospital staff members. Appreciating the complexities of each other's roles and responsibilities will strengthen the relationship between the CDM team and the clinical and ancillary areas.

Components of a CDM Maintenance Plan

The CDM team will engage in numerous maintenance activities throughout the year. To be able to understand and effectively communicate the intent of the maintenance activities, the CDM team should establish a scope of review for each review. By defining the scope, each participant will understand the intent and extent of the review. The CDM coordinator will be able to communicate what is included and what is not included in each review activity to the finance team and the revenue cycle team.

Although each facility is different, the following technical activities should be included in the CDM maintenance plan for each review:

- Review of current statistics
- CPT/HCPCS code review
- Revenue code review
- Modifier review (Dietz 2005, 3)

Each of these line item components should be addressed in the review. However, it is not enough to just review each component individually to ensure that it is a valid code. Rather, the whole line item should be reviewed to ensure that the components fit together properly. This is where CDM maintenance can become very complex. The reviewer must ensure that the line item components meet the requirements for each payer as well as meet the requirements established under compliance guidance.

There is much to remember, research, and verify during the CDM maintenance process, so having a thorough review plan is critical. Mapping out each task in the plan will force the reviewer to complete all planned activities. Likewise, it is during this process that the CDM review policies and procedures must be adhered to.

The responsibility of charge or price setting varies from hospital to hospital. Most often this activity is the responsibility of the finance department, so charge or price review may or may not be performed by the CDM team. However, the CDM team can assist the finance department by identifying charges that appear to be outside normal limits. For example, the CDM team could identify all line items that are missing charges or prices. Likewise, it could identify line items that have charges or prices lower than the Medicare reimbursement rate under the current OPPS.

Ongoing Maintenance

The CDM team must regularly complete ongoing maintenance activities. There will always be issues that arise and that must be addressed immediately. However, the majority of maintenance can be scheduled, so staffing of the CDM team for these activities can be projected.

CPT Updates

The CPT Editorial Research and Development department supports the modification process for the CPT code set. The CPT Editorial Panel meets three times per year to consider proposals for changes to CPT (AMA 2010). The Editorial Panel is supported by the CPT Advisory Committee, which comprises representatives of more than 90 medical specialty societies and other healthcare professional organizations. To stay current with new technologies and pioneering procedures, CPT is revised each year, with changes effective the following January 1.

The updated code set is released before January 1, so the CDM maintenance plan should include steps for the acquisition of the new code set as well as adequate time for additions, deletions, and modifications to be reviewed and incorporated into the CDM as warranted. This makes December a very busy time of year for the CDM team. The CDM coordinator should give special attention to time-off requests for the CDM team members to ensure that line items will be ready for use by January 1. Additionally, the CDM coordinator needs to schedule the annual maintenance with IT and other revenue cycle team representatives. Not only do the CDM line items need to be up to date, but the team must ensure that adequate time is provided for IT to update computerized order entry and to ensure that CDM to finance system interfaces remain intact. If charge tickets are used, the ancillary or clinical units must have adequate time to ensure that the tickets are up to date and staff is properly educated on charge entry changes.

HCPCS Level II Updates

Permanent HCPCS Level II codes are maintained by the CMS HCPCS workgroup. Permanent national codes are updated annually every January 1. Temporary codes can be added, changed, or deleted quarterly.

Like the CPT code updates, the HCPCS Level II code updates must be planned for as well. But in addition to the yearly updates, CDM coordinators must plan for quarterly updates to the temporary HCPCS Level II codes as well. HCPCS Level II code updates require coordination with a variety of areas in the healthcare facility. Not only does the code set contain procedure or service codes, but also included are drug codes, supply codes, durable medical equipment (DME) codes, and implantable device codes. The CDM team must work closely with materials management and the pharmacy department to ensure that the CDM line items properly represent the drugs, biologicals, and devices used by the facility.

New drug, device, and supply codes should be closely reviewed during the HCPCS Level II update. Just because the HCPCS Level II code is new does not mean that the drug, device, or supply is a recently created item that is new to the marketplace. Perhaps, the drug has been manufactured and administered for several years but has just now been assigned a HCPCS Level II code. Remember, numerous drugs are reported under revenue code 025x without a HCPCS Level II code.

Prospective Payment System Updates

The Centers for Medicare and Medicaid (CMS) update their prospective payment systems on a regular schedule throughout the year. For example, the CMS Inpatient Prospective Payment System (IPPS) is updated on the federal fiscal year, with an effective date of October 1. However, the Outpatient Prospective Payment System (OPPS) is updated on the calendar year, with an effective date of January 1. Depending on the type of facility or facilities included under the healthcare entity, the CDM coordinator will need to plan for the review of PPS rules and the incorporation of rule changes into the CDM. For example, a CDM coordinator that manages the CDM for the acute care facility as well as the psychiatric unit and the rehabilitation unit will need to be aware of the IPPS, OPPS, Inpatient Rehabilitation Facilities (IRF PPS), and Inpatient Psychiatric Facilities (IPF PPS) rules to ensure a complete and accurate

CDM. CMS proposed and final rules are posted on the CMS website. Choose the desired payment system area under the Medicare Fee-for-Service Payment section at http://www.cms.hhs.gov/home/medicare.asp.

Policy Alerts

Throughout a payer contract effective period, the payer may send out policy alerts. The policy alerts may contain billing and coding requirements specific to that payer. It is important that the payer contract unit at the facility provide a copy or summary of the policy alerts to the revenue cycle team or CDM unit. Not only may the policy alert require modification to the CDM, but it may also warrant changes to order entry, as well as education for clinical or ancillary areas.

Payer Updates

Although hospitals and other healthcare facilities may prefer to have payer contracts in alignment with their fiscal year, there may be payers that have a set effective period that differs from the facility's fiscal year. Thus, a schedule of payer contract updates should be considered in the CDM maintenance plan. The CDM coordinator and payer contract unit must work together to ensure that the CDM reflects billing and coding protocol outlined in the payer contracts.

Other Maintenance

Even with policies, procedures, and maintenance plans in place, issues will always arise that need immediate attention. When issues come to the surface, the CDM coordinator must be ready to execute a CDM review to help identify the root cause of the issue at hand. It is important to address the issue quickly. Not only is reimbursement for rendered services at stake, but the internal cost of claim correct and resubmission can be significant.

Monitoring Rejections and Denials

The CDM coordinator should have constant communication with the claims reconciliation unit. The claims reconciliation unit reviews payer documents to identify whether the expected reimbursement matches the actual reimbursement for claims. During data analysis, the reconciliation area may uncover billing, coding, or CDM issues. It is important for the reconciliation, CDM, and coding units to work together to resolve systematic issues.

Human Errors

A common adage is "to err is human," meaning that mistakes are inevitable. Thus, it is important to make corrections and provide education when human errors are identified. For example, numeric digits may be transposed when entered by hand into the CDM, as indicated in table 9.10. The internal scrubber may not catch the code transposition error because code 11442 is a valid code. But for the charge item with charge code 8756214, it is the wrong CPT code. Thus, a CDM review should be conducted so that the charge item can be corrected. Not only do the two charge items in question have different charges, they also have very different Medicare reimbursement rates. The date of the data entry error should be pinpointed and all claims with charge code 8756214 should be located and corrected. Resubmission of claims may be warranted so that the correct code and charge are reported for the service provided to the patient and so that accurate reimbursement can be received.

System Errors in Bill Production or Bill Transmission

Not only may the reconciliation unit uncover human errors, but the unit may also uncover system errors in claim production and claim transmission. No matter how much system testing the information technology unit provides, there may still be claim production or claim transmission errors. It is important for the CDM coordinator to be aware of and participate in system testing when the CDM is involved. The CDM coordinator may be called upon to communicate the expected outcome for required CDM data elements. For example, it is common for individuals to leave off the leading zero for revenue codes when verbally discussing or informally writing revenue codes. Many say revenue code 360 not 0360. But if the leading zero for revenue codes is left off in data transmission, there can be a significant issue. At the payer end, revenue code 360 may be accepted as 3600 instead of 0360. The result is that the line item on the claim is rejected because of the invalid revenue code. Not only will the system issue need to be corrected, but again, all claims containing a 0360 revenue code will need reviewing, and those where the line item was rejected will need to be adjusted with the payer, as the line item denial or rejection most likely affected the reimbursement level.

Automation of Chargemaster Maintenance

Not only is CDM maintenance very detail-oriented and complicated, but it is time-consuming. To assist facilities with CDM maintenance, many companies have begun to sell CDM maintenance software packages. Although each maintenance program will have unique and proprietary features, most provide software that will identify revenue codes, CPT/HCPCS codes, and compliance issues for the facility. For example, the

Table 9.10.   Example of digit transposition

Charge Code	Revenue Code	HCPCS Code	Description	Charge*	OPPS Rate 2015
Charge Code 8756214 with Incorrect CPT Code						
8756214	0360	*11442*	Excision benign lesion, scalp, neck, hands, feet, genitalia, 3.1 to 4.0 cm	$2,000.00	$826.58
8756849	0360	11442	Excision benign lesion, face, ears, eyelids, nose, lips, mucous membrane, 3.1 to 4.0 cm	$1,500.00	$826.58
Charge Code 8756214 with Correct CPT Code						
8756214	0360	*11424*	Excision benign lesion, scalp, neck, hands, feet, genitalia, 3.1 to 4.0 cm	$2,000.00	$1,341.41
8756849	0360	11442	Excision benign lesion, face, ears, eyelids, nose, lips, mucous membrane, 3.1 to 4.0 cm	$1,500.00	$826.58

*Charge is fictitious and should not be used for rate setting.

Source: CMS 2015a.

program will identify all codes in the client CDM that have been deleted according to the CPT annual update and will provide the facility with replacement choices.

Some of the maintenance programs are installed at the facility and some are provided online. It is important to remember that many of these packages are based on Medicare guidelines, though some also provide state-level Medicaid regulations. Individual payer regulations are typically not included in these packages, so specific coding and billing guidance by private payers must be considered and monitored by the facility.

Failure to effectively maintain the CDM puts a facility at risk for compliance violations and lost reimbursement, as outlined in table 9.11. With the implementation of PPS in various healthcare settings, it is vital that the correct information be reported to third-party payers. Because key information used to determine payment is transmitted to the claim via the CDM, it is critical that the CDM always be precise. Whereas the focus of the CDM may have been simply the charge value in the past, it is clearly now the accuracy of the entire line item.

Compliance

In today's healthcare environment, every facility has a compliance plan. It is important for the CDM unit's policies and procedures to be in alignment with the facility's compliance plan. Because coding and billing affect reimbursement, this is a highly regulated area (Bowman 2008, 115). The CDM unit must pay close attention and develop protocol to ensure compliance with the laws, regulations, and requirements for all payers, both government and private. It is definitely a challenge to stay up to date with all the compliance guidance. Making compliance guidance a part of

Table 9.11. Charge description master maintenance issues

Issue	Possible Result	Risk Area
Undercharging for services	Underpayment	Lost revenue
Overcharging for services	Overpayment	Compliance
Incorrect HCPCS or diagnosis code	Claims rejection/denial	Lost revenue
Incorrect revenue code	Claims rejection/denial	Lost revenue

regular activities in the CDM maintenance plan will help ensure that the CDM team stays focused on compliance. Likewise, a good working relationship with the facility's compliance department will help the CDM team address and resolve difficult compliance issues.

Compliance Guidance
Numerous publications and policy documents must be reviewed and assessed throughout the year to keep the CDM compliant with coding and billing regulations. This section provides an overview of many publications that affect CDM (and revenue cycle) maintenance. Though many of these documents pertain to Medicare, private payer regulations should not be forgotten. Although numerous private payers have adopted compliance guidelines similar to Medicare, the specifics for each payer should be closely examined and incorporated into the facility's CDM.

Medicare Claims Processing Manual
The CMS *Claims Processing Manual* (Publication 100-04) is one of the many manuals included in the CMS Internet-Only Manuals System. The Internet-Only Manuals System is used by CMS program components, partners, contracts, and other agencies to administer CMS programs. Day-to-day operating instructions, policies and procedures based on statutes, regulations, guidelines, models, and directives are included in the manuals (CMS 2010a). Though three manuals are still provided in hard copy, the majority of manuals were converted to an online, user-friendly system in 2003, now at http://www.cms.hhs.gov/Manuals/IOM/list.asp.

The *Medicare Claims Processing Manual* currently has 38 chapters and provides guidance for producing claims for all healthcare settings (inpatient, outpatient rehabilitation, and the like). General billing requirements as well as service area-specific requirements are provided. A CDM coordinator may need to be familiar with many of the chapters, and he or she may study more closely the requirements outlined for the service areas included in their hospital's own book of business. For example, the CDM coordinator may have a cursory understanding of Ambulatory Surgical Center regulations but may have a detailed understanding of hospital inpatient requirements.

Updates to the *Medicare Claims Processing Manual* are made throughout the year based on changes made to the unique prospective payment systems. For example, changes brought about by the final IPPS rule in August would be incorporated in the *Medicare Claims Processing Manual* by October 1. However, the modifications from the final OPPS rule in November would be incorporated by January 1. One great feature is that CMS displays changes to the Claims Processing Manual in red, allowing the CDM coordinator can browse the individual chapter and easily locate recent changes.

CMS Program Transmittals

Program transmittals are used by CMS to communicate policies and procedures for the specific prospective payment systems' program manuals. Current and historic transmittals dating back to 2000 can be found at www.cmshhs.gov/transmittals/01_overview.asp (CMS 2005b).

CDM professionals should stay up to date with program transmittals released for Part A and Part B Medicare payment systems. The transmittals should be read carefully and the information communicated effectively to the compliance department, revenue cycle team, and CDM team. Any issues related to the CDM should be incorporated into the facility's active CDM as warranted. The CDM coordinator should keep an audit trail of changes made to the CDM based on program transmittal guidance.

National and Local Coverage Determinations

National Coverage Determinations (NCDs) describe the circumstances under which specific medical supplies, services, or procedures are covered nationwide by Medicare under title XVIII of the Social Security Act and other medical regulations and rulings. After the NCD has been published, it is binding for all Medicare contractors (Medicare Administrative Contracts [MACs], Durable Medical Equipment Regional Contractors [DMERCS], Quality Improvement Organizations [QIOs], and so on) (CMS 2008). Additionally, contractors are responsible for notifying the provider community of an NCD release. Contractors do not have the authority to deviate from an NCD when absolute words such as "never" or "only if" are used in the policy. When reviewing coverage issues, the contractors may cover services at their own discretion based on a local coverage determination if an NCD is not established (CMS 2008).

Local Coverage Determinations (LCDs), formerly Local Medical Review Policies or LMRPs, provide facilities and physicians with the circumstances under which a service, procedure, or supply is considered medically necessary. An LCD is used to determine coverage on a Medicare Administrative Contractor–wide, intermediary-wide, or carrier-wide basis (rather than nationwide, as with an NCD). There are regional differences in medical necessity, and thus differences in coverage, for Medicare supplies, services, and procedures (CMS 2008). LCDs are educational materials intended to assist facilities and providers with correct billing and claim processing. Within the LCD is a listing of ICD-9-CM codes that indicate what is covered and what is not covered. Additionally, there may be a listing of the HCPCS codes for which the LCD applies.

It is important to understand the difference between coverage and medical necessity. For example, chest x-rays are covered by Medicare. However, the service is only reimbursed by Medicare when it is deemed medically necessary. This means that the physician has to provide sufficient medical documentation, through ICD diagnosis coding, to substantiate that the service is warranted for diagnostic or therapeutic treatment of the patient. Medicare does not pay for services that are not medically necessary.

The *Medicare National Coverage Determinations Manual* (NCD) is an Internet-Only Manual (IOM) published by CMS. This manual provides a listing of all topics included in the numerous active NCDs. The publication number for the NCD manual is 100-03.

The NCD manual consists of two chapters: (1) Coverage Determinations and (2) HCPCS Codes for Services Described in *National Coverage Determinations Manual*. However, only chapter 1, Coverage Determinations, parts 1–4, is ready for use by providers. Chapter 1 lists all NCDs currently in effect.

To gain a clear understanding of coverage issues, let us examine NCD 140.2, shown in Figure 9.3. From the information provided in this NCD, it is clear that Medicare program payment will not be made for breast reconstruction for cosmetic reasons. Cosmetic surgery is excluded from coverage under §1862(a)(10) of the Act. However, breast reconstruction following the removal of a breast for any medical reason is a covered procedure. This coverage determination applies to both the affected and the contralateral unaffected breast (CMS 2010b).

Additional information regarding LCDs can be located in the *Medicare Program Integrity Manual* (Publication 100-08), chapter 13, Local Coverage

Figure 9.3.   NCD 140.2—Breast Reconstruction Following Mastectomy

> **140.2 - Breast reconstruction following mastectomy**
>
> **(Rev. 1, 10-03-03)**
>
> **CIM 35-47**
>
> During recent years, there has been a considerable change in the treatment of diseases of the breast such as fibrocystic disease and cancer. While extirpation of the disease remains of primary importance, the quality of life following initial treatment is increasingly recognized as of great concern. The increased use of breast reconstruction procedures is due to several factors:
>
> - A change in epidemiology of breast cancer, including an apparent increase in incidence;
> - Improved surgical skills and techniques;
> - The continuing development of better prostheses; and
> - Increasing awareness by physicians of the importance of postsurgical psychological adjustment.
>
> Reconstruction of the affected and the contralateral unaffected breast following a medically necessary mastectomy is considered a relatively safe and effective non-cosmetic procedure. Accordingly, program payment may be made for breast reconstruction surgery following removal of a breast for any medical reason.

Source: CMS 2010b

Determinations. Chapter 13 outlines Medicare policy regarding NCDs and LCDs and then provides the regulations for LCD creation, modification, distribution, execution, and appeals.

When examining LCDs, it is important to understand the difference between policies and articles. An LCD policy contains only the reasonable and necessary provision regarding a supply, procedure, or service. For example, a list of codes describing which conditions provide for medical necessity and which conditions do not warrant medical necessity may be provided in a LCD policy.

An article is used by the Medicare Administrative Contractor (MAC) to provide guidelines about the benefit category, statutory exclusions, and coding provisions. For example, coding guidelines relating to diagnosis codes in the medical necessity code list would be provided in an article, not in the LCD policy itself. Thus, to fully understand an LCD and effectively implement it, a CDM professional must read the policy as well as any associated articles.

To find NCDs and LCDs for a specific geographical area, CDM professionals can access the Medicare Coverage Database at http://www.cms.gov/medicare-coverage-database/overview-and-quick-search.aspx. This search engine allows the user to search documents of national coverage or local coverage. Additionally, the user can search articles and policies by geographic area or MAC. It also allows the user to enter search criteria, such as CPT/HCPCS code, keywords, ICD codes, coverage topics, and date criteria.

National Correct Coding Initiative

National Correct Coding Initiative (NCCI) edits have been in place for outpatient claim editing since January 1, 1996. There are two sets of NCCI edits, one for the physician setting and one for the hospital outpatient setting. The hospital outpatient setting edits are embedded in the Integrated Outpatient Code Editor (OCE) used by Medicare Administrative Contractors (MACs) to process claims under OPPS.

The purpose of the NCCI edits is to ensure proper CPT and HCPCS coding for Medicare Part B services. This set of edits are not medical necessity denial edits, rather they are in place to ensure correct coding and payment. The edits are designed to audit CPT codes based on the CPT coding conventions, national and local policies and edits, coding guidelines developed by national societies, analysis of standard medical and surgical practices, and a review of current coding practices (CMS 2010c).

Within the set of edits, there are two types: comprehensive code edits and mutually exclusive code edits. The comprehensive code edits are designed to identify instances in which the most comprehensive code was not reported, but rather components of that service were reported, or when a comprehensive code and a component code are reported together, also known as unbundling of services. Reporting component codes rather than a comprehensive code is against coding guidelines and could lead to overpayment. This set of edits ensures that only the comprehensive code will receive payment. Additionally, the NCCI contains mutually exclusive edits. These code combinations consist of codes that would not reasonably be reported together or that should not be reported together. All edits (comprehensive and mutually exclusive) are released quarterly on the CMS website. Figure 9.4 provides an example of a NCCI edit.

Claims violating NCCI edits will receive a rejection or denial message on the Medicare correspondence. Remember that the Medicare Summary Notice is provided to the patient and the remittance notice is issued to the facility.

Figure 9.4. NCCI edit

CPT code 80061 (lipid panel) includes the following tests:
CPT code 82465—Cholesterol, serum or whole blood, total
CPT code 83718—Lipoprotein, direct; HDL cholesterol
CPT code 84478—Triglycerides
When all tests are performed, the panel test, CPT code 80061, should be reported in place of the individual tests.

Source: CMS 2015b.

CMS publishes the *National Correct Coding Initiative Policy Manual for Medicare Services*, available on the CMS website. Additionally, the Medicare Claims Processing Manual contains information regarding the NCCI edits in chapter 23, section 20.9. Chapter 23, section 20.9.1, Correct Coding Modifier Indicators and HCPCS Codes Modifiers, discusses the NCCI edits that allow providers to use modifiers to indicate special circumstances when the code edit should be bypassed based on the patient's specific course of treatment (CMS 2009). Several modifiers have specific usage guidelines to prevent fraud and abuse situations.

Integrated Outpatient Code Editor

The Medicare Integrated Outpatient Code Editor (OCE) is a software program designed to process data for OPPS pricing and to audit facility claims data. The processing function prepares submitted claims data for the Medicare pricer by

- Assigning appropriate Ambulatory Payment Classifications (APCs)
- Assigning CMS-designated status indicators
- Computing applicable discounts
- Determining a claim disposition based on generated edits
- Determining whether packaging is applicable
- Determining applicable payment adjustments (3M 2010, 1.6)

The editing function audits claims for coding and data entry errors. The extensive edits in the OCE are applied to claims, individual diagnoses and procedures, and code sets. Table 9.12 provides a sample of edits included in the OCE. When activated, OCE edits have an associated line or claim disposition attached to them. Table 9.13 provides a listing of the edit dispositions and their definitions.

Depending on the claim disposition, providers or facilities may correct the claim or process write-offs based on facility policy. It is critical for facilities to monitor and analyze claim disposition composition. Possible reasons for claim errors should be investigated, with corrective action taken when applicable. Most revenue cycle teams have an ongoing quality monitoring process in place so that resolutions to claim errors can be incorporated into the process.

For example, in January the reconciliation unit at Hospital A begins to see Medicare bills with rejections for IOC edit #48, revenue center requires HCPCS. Upon investigation, it is found that a line item for a newly added CPT code is missing the CPT code in the CDM, so when the charge identifier is sent to the patient's account, the revenue code is sent, but the CPT code is not. Perhaps during the annual update, the line item was created, but the CPT code was not entered into the line item. Though this is a somewhat simple fix to the CDM—the CPT code is added to the line item— it is a wake-up call to the CDM unit that quality review of the CDM annual update may need to be revisited and the process improved.

The edits are updated quarterly and posted at http://www.cms.gov/Medicare/Medicare-Fee-for-Service-Payment/HospitalOutpatientPPS/index.html. CDM professionals should review the edits annually to ensure that all devices used by the facility have line item charges with the correct HCPCS Level II supply code included in the CDM. CDM professionals must also confirm that the line item charge is also included in the order entry system and, in addition, provide education to charge entry staff.

Payer-Specific Edits

Payer-specific edits must also be taken into consideration by the compliance department and the CDM team. For example, state workers compensation (WC) provisions may not cover preventive immunizations. However, they may cover tetanus shots post-injury and have advised facilities to report these charges in revenue code 0450 via a policy alert. The claims processing system at the WC contains an edit to deny claim line items reported with revenue codes 0770–0779, preventive care services. Thus, when a tetanus administration is provided to a WC patient in the emergency department, the code would need to be reported with revenue code 0450, rather than 0771, for that specific payer.

Table 9.12.   Sample of the edits included in the OCE

Edit	Generated when....
1. Invalid diagnosis code	The principal diagnosis field is blank, there are no diagnoses entered on the claim, or the entered diagnosis code is not valid for the selected version of the program.
2. Diagnosis and age conflict	The diagnosis code includes an age range, and the age is outside that range.
8. Procedure and sex conflict	The procedure code includes sex designation, and the sex does not match.
19. Mutually exclusive procedure that is not allowed by NCCI even if appropriate modifier is present	The procedure is one of a pair of mutually exclusive procedures in the NCCI table coded on the same day, where the use of a modifier is not appropriate. Only the code in column 2 of a mutually exclusive pair is rejected; the column 1 code of the pair is not marked as an edit.
20. Code 2 of a code pair that is not allowed by NCCI even if appropriate modifier is present	The procedure is identified as part of another procedure on the claim coded on the same day, where the use of a modifier is not appropriate. Only the code in column 2 of a code pair is rejected; the column 1 code of the pair is not marked as an edit.
28. Code not recognized by Medicare; alternate code for same service may be available	The procedure code has a "Not recognized by Medicare" indicator.
41. Invalid revenue code	The revenue code is not in the list of valid revenue code entries.
43. Transfusion or blood product exchange without specification of blood product	A blood transfusion or exchange is coded but no blood product is coded.
71. Claim lacks required device code	The code for a device designated as necessary for an outpatient procedure coded on the claim is missing. This edit is bypassed when the modifier is 52, 73, or 74.

Source: CMS 2015a

Table 9.13.   Listing of the edit dispositions and their definitions

Disposition	Definition
Claim rejection	The provider can correct and resubmit the claim but cannot appeal the rejection
	Currently not assigned to edits
Claim denial	The provider cannot resubmit the claim but can appeal the denial
	Example: Edit 27 – Only incidental services reported (all line items are bundled services under HOPPS)
Claim return to provider (RTP)	The provider can resubmit the claim once the problems are corrected
	Example: Edit 1 – Invalid diagnosis code
Claim suspension	The claim is not returned to the provider, but it is not processed for payment until the fiscal intermediary (FI) makes a determination or obtains further information
	Example: Edit 12 – Questionable covered service
Line Item rejection	The claim can be processed for payment with some line items rejected for payment (that is, the line item can be corrected and resubmitted but cannot be appealed)
	Example: Edit 19 – Mutually exclusive procedure that is not allowed by NCCI even if appropriate modifier is present
Line item denial	There are one or more edits that cause one or more individual line items to be denied. The claim can be processed for payment with some line items denied for payment (that is, the line item cannot be resubmitted but can be appealed)
	Example: Edit 9 – Non-covered for reasons other than statute

Source: CMS 2015a

1. What is the first component in the revenue cycle?

2. How are charges for healthcare at all of the points of services collected and reported to the appropriate patient account for entry onto the provider's claim?

3. What is the function of scrubbers in the claims processing component of the revenue cycle?

4. List the basic data elements of a CDM, identifying which data elements are hospital-specific and which are nationally recognized.

5. Discuss how NCDs are different from LCDs.

Revenue Cycle Management Team

The purpose of a revenue cycle management (RCM) team is to improve the efficiency and effectiveness of the revenue cycle process. Each team will develop different goals and objectives to guide their focus and discussions. Some sample objectives follow:

- To identify issues to improve accounts receivable

- To communicate issues with appropriate areas

- To develop educational materials, such as a revenue cycle manual

- To create a map or blueprint for how to bring up new services

- To review denials and actively discuss the appeal process and successes

- To discuss key performance indicators (KPI) and measures

After an RCM team establishes goals and objectives, team members must define optimal performance for their facility or practice. Many teams define optimal performance by establishing **key performance indicators** and by setting a standard for each indicator. Key performance indicators are a performance measurement tool that should represent areas that need improvement. The facility or practice should design indicators so that they can be measured to gauge performance improvement. The Healthcare Financial Managers Association (HFMA) created a task force to develop national standard key performance indicators both for facility-based revenue cycle management and for physician practice management. The key performance indicators are called MAP Keys. The task force reviewed numerous key performance indicators used throughout the United States and evaluated the indicators for completeness, validity, relevancy, ability to support performance conclusions and value (HFMA, http://www.hfma.org). Many facilities have adopted the use of the MAP Keys and are able to benchmark performance across institutions and peer groups. Table 9.14 provides the MAP Keys for Revenue Cycle Excellence. Table 9.15 provides the MAP Keys for Physician Practice Management. Individual facilities and physician practices may choose to adopt all MAP Keys or may adopt a portion of them to be incorporated into their RCM plan. By reviewing the MAP Keys, it is clear that there are some similarities and some differences between facility and physician practice RCM. Healthcare systems that are comprised of both facilities and physician practices must utilize both sets of key performance indicators in order to effectively manage both revenue cycles.

Current levels for each key indicator should be determined and compared to a standard. For example, if the standard for key performance indicator "dollar value of discharged, not final billed, encounters" is $2 million and the current value is $10 million, the facility is exceeding the standard by $8 million, so significant focus should be placed on reducing that total. Perhaps the facility is experiencing a coder shortage or there is a backlog in the prepping and scanning area, so the coders are unable to review the records online. The HIM management team must investigate the issues and practice performance improvement techniques to improve coding and record processing procedures so that the standard can be met. Key indicators should be continuously monitored until their related standard is consistently met, after which facilities typically review the indicator quarterly or semiannually to ensure continued optimal performance.

With the publication of the Accountable Care Organizations final rule (discussed in detail in chapter 10 of this text), more emphasis has been placed on healthcare systems purchasing physician practices. As physician practices are integrated into the revenue cycle and business practices of healthcare systems, close attention must be given to some of the nuances

Table 9.14.   HFMA's MAP Keys for Revenue Cycle Excellence

MAP Category	Measure	Purpose	Value	Equation
Patient Access	Point-of-Service (POS) Cash Collections	Trending indicator of POS collection efforts	Indicates potential exposure to bad debt, accelerates cash collections, and can reduce collection costs	N: POS payments D: Total patient cash collected
Patient Access	Charity Care	Trending indicator of local ability to pay	Indicates services provided to patients deemed unable to pay	N: Charity care write-off D: Gross patient service revenue
Patient Access	Preregistration Rate	Trending indicator that patient access processes are timely, accurate, and efficient	Indicates revenue cycle efficiency and effectiveness	N: Number of patient encounters preregistered D: Number of scheduled patient encounters
Patient Access	Insurance Verification Rate	Trending indicator that patient access functions are timely, accurate, and efficient	Indicates revenue cycle process efficiency and effectiveness	N: Total number of verified encounters D: Total number of registered encounters
Patient Access	Service Authorization Rate	Trending indicator that patient access functions are timely, accurate, and efficient	Indicates revenue cycle process efficiency and effectiveness	N: Number of encounters authorized D: Number of encounters requiring authorization
Patient Access	Conversion Rate of Uninsured Inpatient to Payer Source	Trending indicator of qualifying uninsured inpatients for a funding source	Indicates organization's ability to successfully secure funding for uninsured inpatients and improve customer satisfaction	N: Total inpatient cases approved D: Total uninsured inpatient discharges
Revenue Integrity	Days in Total Discharged Not Final Billed (DNFB)	Trending indicator of claims generation process	Indicates revenue cycle performance and can identify performance issues that affect cash flow	N: Gross dollars in accounts receivable (A/R) (not final billed) D: Average daily gross revenue
Revenue Integrity	Days in Total Discharged Not Submitted to Payer (DNSP)	Trending indicator of total claims generation and submission process	Indicates revenue cycle performance and can identify performance issues that affect cash flow	N: Gross dollars in DNFB + gross dollars in final billed not submitted to payer (FBNS) D: Average daily gross revenue
Revenue Integrity	Late Charges as % of Total Charges	Measure of revenue capture efficiency	Identify opportunities to improve revenue capture, reduce unnecessary cost, enhance compliance, and accelerate cash flow	N: Charges with post date greater than three days from last service date D: Total gross charges
Revenue Integrity	Net Days Revenue in Credit Balance	Trending indicator to accurately report account values, ensure compliance with regulatory requirements, and monitor overall payment system effectiveness	Indicates whether credit balances are being managed to appropriate levers and are compliant to regulatory requirements	N: Dollars in credit balance D: Average daily net patient services revenue

(Continued on next page)

Table 9.14.   (Continued)

MAP Category	Measure	Purpose	Value	Equation
Revenue Integrity	Denial Write-Offs as a Percent of Net Revenue	Trending indicator of final disposition of lost reimbursement, where all efforts of appeal have been exhausted or provider chooses to write off expected payment amount	Indicates provider's ability to comply with payer requirement and payer's ability to accurately pay the claim	N: Net dollars written off as denials D: Net patient services revenue
Claims Adjudication	Aged A/R as a % of Billed A/R by Payer Group	Trending indicator of receivable collectability by payer group	Indicates revenue cycle's ability to liquidate A/R by payer group	N: Billed payer group by aging (>30, >60, >90, >120 days) D: Total billed A/R by payer group
Claims Adjudication	Days in FBNS	Trending indicator of claims affected by payer/regulatory edits within claims processing system	Track the impact of internal/external requirements to clean claim production, which affects positive cash flow	N: Gross dollars in FBNS D: Average daily gross revenue
Claims Adjudication	Initial Denial Rate-Zero Pay	Trending indicator of % claims not paid	Indicates provider's ability to comply with payer requirements and payer's ability to accurately pay the claim	N: Number of zero paid claims denied D: Number of total claims remitted
Claims Adjudication	Initial Denial Rate-Partial Pay	Trending indicator of % claims partially paid	Indicates provider's ability to comply with payer requirements and payer's ability to accurately pay the claim	N: Number of partially paid claims denied D: Number of total claims remitted
Claims Adjudication	Denials Overturned by Appeal	Trending indicator of hospital's success in managing the appeal process	Indicates opportunities for payer and provider process improvement and improves cash flow	N: Number of appeal claims paid D: Total number of claims appealed and finalized or closed
Claims Adjudication	UB04 (8371) Clean Claim Rate	Trending indicator of claims data as it affects revenue cycle performance	Indicates quality of data collected and reported	N: Number of claims that pass edits requiring no manual intervention D: Total claims accepted into claims scrubber tool for editing prior to submission
Management	Aged A/R as a Percentage of Billed A/R	Trending indicator of receivable collectability	Indicates revenue cycle's ability to liquidate A/R	N: >30, >60, >90, >120 days D: Total billed A/R
Management	Net Days in A/R	Trending indicator of overall A/R performance	Indicates revenue cycle efficiency	N: Net A/R D: Average Daily Net Patient Service Revenue
Management	Cost to Collect	Trending indicator of operational performance	Indicates the efficiency and productivity of revenue cycle (RC) process	N: Total RC Cost D: Total cash collected

Table 9.14.   (Continued)

MAP Category	Measure	Purpose	Value	Equation
Management	Cash Collection as a Percentage of Adjusted Net Patient Services Revenue	Trending indicator of revenue cycle to convert net patient services revenue to cash	Indicates fiscal integrity/financial health of the organization	N: Total cash collected / D: Average monthly net revenue
Management	Bad Debt	Trending indicator of the effectiveness of self-pay collection efforts and financial counseling	Indicates organization's ability to collect self-pay accounts and identify payer sources for those who cannot meet financial obligations	N: Bad debt write-off / D: Gross patient service revenue
Management	Charity as a Percent of Uncompensated Care	Trending indicator that monitors charity care versus bad debt	Reflection of charity care (provided to the community)	N: Charity care / D: Total uncompensated care (bad debt + charity care)
Management	Case-Mix Index	Trending indicator of patient acuity, clinical documentation, and coding	Supports appropriate reimbursement for services performed and accurate clinical reporting	N: CMI (average RW/patient) = Sum of relative weights for all Patients (exclusions: healthy newborns and medicare-exempt units) / D: Number of patients in the month (exclusions: healthy newborns and medicare-exempt units)
Management	Cost to Collect by Functional Area	Trending indicator of operational performance by functional area as reported in KI Cost to Collect	Indicates the efficiency and productivity of revenue cycle process by functional area	N: Total x (x = the cost of each functional area) cost, which Should equal total cost of KPI *Cost to Collect* / D: Total cash collected

Source: Healthcare Financial Management Association. http://www.hfma.org.

of the physician practice structure that can affect RCM, such as

- Organization structure
- Payment methodology
- Payer classifications
- Systems
- Metrics and monitoring system
- Denial management
- Point-of-service patient collection opportunities (Sorrentino and Sanderson 2011, 88–92)

Probably the most significant difference between facility-based and physician-based revenue cycles is the payment systems (Sorrentino and Sanderson 2011, 89). Most facility-based payment systems utilize a case-based payment (MS-DRGs, LTCH DRGs, and OPPS). Physician practices are reimbursed via RBRVS, a transaction-based payment system (see chapter 7 of this text for more about the structure of RBRVS). Though facilities may be familiar with negotiating case rates with their payer population, physician practice contracts require more negotiation and a clear understanding of the types of services, or book of business, for the physician practice that has been acquired (Sorrentino and Sanderson 2011, 89). Incorporating the existing expertise from the physician practice would provide significant benefits to healthcare.

Many systems are moving toward an **integrated revenue cycle** (IRC) approach. Integrated IRC means different things to different systems, but at a basic level, an IRC is the coordination of revenue cycle activities under a single leadership and team structure (Colton and Davis 2015, 56). Systems can have a lower level of integration at which the oversight is united but there are separate physician and hospital divisions all the way to a fully integrated system in which oversight, as well as function managers, monitor both facility

Table 9.15.   HFMA's MAP Keys for Physician Practice Management

Measure	Purpose	Equation
Practice Operating Margin	Measures financial performance of a physician entity on an accrual basis	N: Net income from operations / D: Operating revenue
Practice Net Days in Accounts Receivable	Calculates the average number of days it takes to collect payment on services rendered and measures revenue cycle effectiveness and efficiency	N: Average monthly net patient service accounts receivable / D: Average daily net patient service revenue
Practice Cash Collection Percentage	Measures revenue cycle efficiency and supports valuation of current accounts receivable and predicts income	N: Actual patient service cash collections / D: Net patient service revenue
Total Physician Compensation as a Percentage of Net Revenue	Demonstrates ability to afford physician compensation in relation to revenue of the physician enterprise	N: Total physician salary / D: Net patient service revenue
Professional Services Denial Percentage	Tracks payer denials and effect on cash flow, and trends payment and process improvement opportunity	N: ΣCPT (units of service) codes denied / D: ΣCPT codes billed
Point-of-Service (POS) Collection Rate	Provides opportunity to decrease collection costs, accelerate cash flow, and increase collections	N: Total point of service collections / D: Total patient cash collected
Total Charge Lag Days	Measures charge capture workflow efficiency and identifies delays in cash	N: Σdays from revenue recognition date less date of service date (by CPT code) / D: ΣCPT codes billed
Percentage of Patient Schedule Occupied	Identifies opportunity to maximize slot utilization and improve practice productivity	N: Number of patient hours occupied (average weekly) / D: Number of patient hours available (average weekly)

Source: Healthcare Financial Management Association. http://www.hfma.org.

and physician revenue cycle activities. There are three primary benefits a system can experience from an IRC (Colton and Davis 2015, 57):

- Reduced cost to collect—combine strategic and operational elements including resources, management, overhead, vendors, IT platforms, and business intelligence

- Performance consistency—combine job codes and pay rates, clearly define roles and responsibilities, and strive for consistent production and quality rates through improved information sharing

- Coordinated strategic goals—develop a shared focus on strategic goals and to promote improved coordination between financial and nonfinancial units

Not all systems may move directly to a fully IRC; many may face resistance from physician practices arising from a fear that lower-dollar encounters will not receive the attention that high-dollar inpatient admissions receive. However, many systems will move to a form of IRC that fits the needs and environment of the individual system.

Revenue Cycle Analysis

Establishing good focus areas for revenue cycle analysis takes a considerable amount of research by the revenue cycle team. Team members must stay up to date on compliance issues published and discussed in various government and other third-party payer documents. For example, the OIG Workplan should be reviewed each year. This document provides insight into the directions the OIG is taking and highlights hot areas of compliance. In addition, the CERT and National Recovery Audit programs issue summaries of improper Medicare fee-for-service payments throughout the year. These reports provide insight into payment errors identified across the nation and can be downloaded from www.cms.gov. The following case studies show how a manager can use auditing results with internal and external benchmarking to monitor compliance.

Case-Mix Index Analysis

Analyzing the growth or decline of a facility's CMI is the beginning phase for assessing the quality of its coding and billing practices for hospital acute care encounters (IPPS). Managers begin by comparing the CMI of the facility to that of its peers and the state or nation for the past three years. Questions posed include the following:

- Is the CMI steady?

- Does it increase steadily, or drastically?

- Is there a sharp or sudden decline?

To explore the analysis issues, consider data for a medium-sized (250–400-bed) not-for-profit facility (hospital A), its peer facilities, and the nation. Peer facilities included in this example are local hospitals with which this facility competes for market share. Figure 9.5 displays CMI trend over a three-year study period.

Clearly, this facility's CMI has increased at a much greater rate than the national average or that of its peers. In addition, figure 9.6 shows that hospital

Figure 9.5.   CMI—Three-year study period

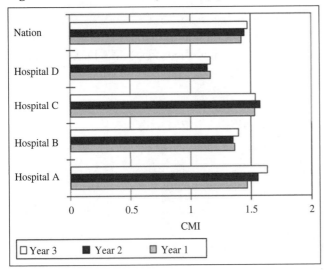

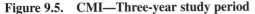

Figure 9.6.   CMI percent change—from year 1 to year 3

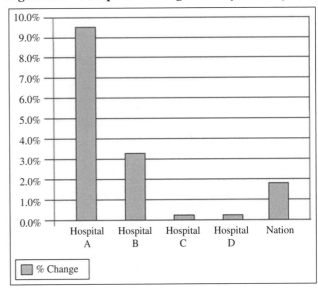

A's CMI is greater than that of the nation and its peers. So not only has its CMI increased at a fast pace, but it is also the highest in this data set. What has caused this major shift? The facility can now drill down to the major diagnostic category (MDC) level to pinpoint noteworthy changes at the service area level.

Figure 9.7 shows that the CMI for MDC 05, Diseases of the Circulatory System, increased greatly during the three-year study period (15.7 percent). One cannot tell from the data alone what has caused this increase. However, by performing a thorough investigation, the issue(s) can be identified. Several areas to consider include

- Coding and billing errors

- Changes in MS-DRG assignments

- Equipment purchases

- New or expanded service areas

- Acquisition of new facilities

- Changes in physician personnel

Regardless of the root cause of the data deviations, compliance with established rules and regulations must be verified. If coding practices are questionable, a medical record review should

Figure 9.7.   MDC 05 CMI trend—three-year study period

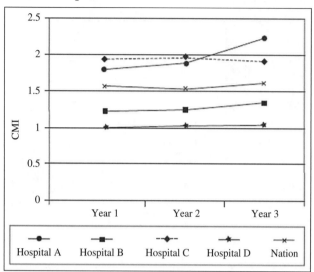

be completed to identify whether a compliance infraction has occurred. Managers should follow established procedures for correcting and reporting a compliance lapse. This exercise can also be completed for the facility's **outpatient service-mix index (SMI)**, the sum of the weights of ambulatory payment classification groups for patients treated during a given period divided by the total volume of patients treated.

MS-DRG Relationships Reporting

Within the MS-DRG system, there are MS-DRGs that have a relationship or similar grouping methodology to other MS-DRGs. For example, MS-DRG sets exist where the listings of diagnoses used to drive the grouping are the same, but the presence or absence of a complication or comorbidity (CC) diagnosis or major complication or comorbidity (MCC) diagnosis assigns the case to a higher or lower MS-DRG. MS-DRG sets may contain two MS-DRGs or three MS-DRGs. These MS-DRG relationships and sets pose a compliance concern because the medical record documentation used to support the coding of the principal diagnosis, complications, and comorbidities may not always be clear or used appropriately by the coder. Thus, inaccurate coding can lead to incorrect MS-DRG assignment and thereby inappropriate reimbursement.

Example:

Included in many Medicare and third-party payer audits is the comparison of the reporting rates of simple pneumonia with complication(s) or comorbidity(ies) versus simple pneumonia without complication(s) or comorbidity(ies). MS-DRG 193, Simple Pneumonia and Pleurisy with MCC, has a higher relative weight than the other MS-DRGs in this relationship and should be closely monitored (table 9.16). Hospital reporting of MCCs is closely monitored to ensure that all coding rules and regulations have been followed. Furthermore, the medical record documentation is scrutinized to ensure its adequacy for coding purposes. Reporting MS-DRG 193 at a higher rate than warranted will cause the facility to receive reimbursement of which it is not entitled, creating noncompliance.

Again, hospital A is a medium-sized, not-for-profit facility, and the peer facilities are local hospitals. Figure 9.8 compares hospital A's reporting rate for the MS-DRG 193 relationship group to its peers and state for the study period. Hospital A's reporting rate, 31 percent, is much higher than the state average and that of all of its peers. It is clear that a medical record review is warranted to determine whether inaccurate coding practices (upcoding) are the root cause of the reporting differences. Medical records assigned to MS-DRG 193 should be reviewed to determine whether the assignment of this MS-DRG is supported through documentation in the medical record. Again, established procedures for compliance issues should be followed.

Poor documentation identified during the intensive medical record review should be addressed with the medical staff, and incorrect code assignments should be immediately discussed with the coding staff.

Site of Service: Inpatient versus Outpatient

The following example illustrates the concept of a site-of-service review focused on MS-DRGs prone to compliance problems.

Table 9.16.   MS-DRG 193 family

MS-DRG Number	DRG Title	FY 2015 Relative Weight
193	Simple Pneumonia and Pleurisy with MCC	1.4491
194	Simple Pneumonia and Pleurisy with CC	0.9688
195	Simple Pneumonia and Pleurisy without MCC/CC	0.7044

Example:

Several MS-DRGs are under a site-of-service review by improper payment review entities such as the MACs and RACs. Documentation and admission criteria are reviewed to determine whether the inpatient setting is the most efficient and effective treatment area for patients. One focus area is diabetes: MS-DRGs 637, Diabetes with MCC, 638, Diabetes with CC; and 639, Diabetes without MCC or CC.

Compliance investigators examine the reporting rates for MS-DRG 637 at one facility. Hospital A is a medium-sized not-for-profit facility. Analysis of figure 9.9 shows the reporting rate for MS-DRG 637 or the percent of MS-DRG 637 cases to total discharges for the facility in the study period. Hospital A reported MS-DRG 637 at a much higher rate than its peers and the nation.

Compliance investigators next examine whether this is a trend or a new risk area. Figure 9.10 displays the reporting rate for MS-DRG 637 for a three-year period for hospital A. The data show that diabetes encounters have been reported at a significantly high level for the past three years, peaking in year 2 of the study period.

Because this MS-DRG family is under close review owing to site-of-service questions, the coding manager should also review the length of stay (LOS) for these MS-DRGs. Do the majority of cases follow the average length of stay (ALOS) for this MS-DRG, or is there a much lower LOS? A lower LOS could indicate that the patients could have been treated as outpatients rather than as inpatients. The ALOS for MS-DRG 637 at hospital A in year 3 of the study period was 4.73. The national ALOS for MS-DRG 637 is 4.1. The data show that hospital A's LOS is consistent with what is expected for patients grouping to this MS-DRG.

However, examiners look more deeply and examine the frequency of LOS values for MS-DRG 637. Figure 9.11 displays the LOS distribution for MS-DRG 637 in the study period. Again, the data show that the LOS reporting for this MS-DRG is consistent with the national expected ALOS. Investigators review encounters in the one-day stay category to verify that admission criteria and medical necessity were met. After drill-down analysis, it appears that this MS-DRG is being appropriately reported at this facility. However, if other MS-DRGs show deviation, they should be investigated by a Utilization Review Committee consisting of representatives from HIM, Quality, Utilization, and Medical Staff. Together, this interdisciplinary team can determine whether the site or service was appropriate for the encounters under review.

Figure 9.8.   Percent assigned to MS-DRG 193

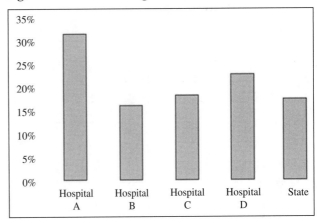

Figure 9.9.   MS-DRG 637 reporting rate

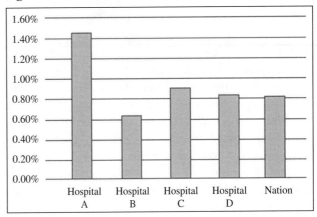

Figure 9.10.   Hospital A reporting trend MS-DRG 637

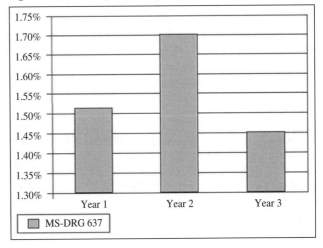

Figure 9.11.   Hospital ALOS distribution for MS-DRG 552

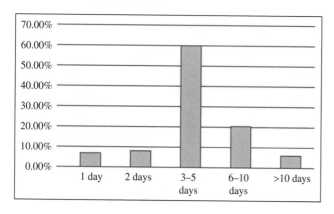

codes 99284 and 99285 (high-level emergency department visits) at a much higher percentage than hospital C and the nation. CMS has suggested that emergency department APC distribution should follow somewhat of a bell-curved shape. Clearly, hospital A deviates far from this configuration.

Again, it is important to examine the trend for hospital A. Figure 9.13 displays a trending graph for the past four years. The data show that hospital A's reporting of higher-level E/M codes has increased from 25 percent of the total cases in year 1 to 80 percent of total cases in year 4. This drastic increase in the reporting of levels 4 and 5 E/M codes should be addressed by this facility. A medical record audit should be performed to verify that medical record documentation supports the assignment of these higher-level CPT codes.

Evaluation and Management Facility Coding in the Emergency Department

The implementation of the Hospital Outpatient Prospective Payment System (OPPS) has brought about new compliance challenges for hospitals. One area under review is evaluation and management (E/M) coding. Because the CPT code reported on a Medicare outpatient claim drives the ambulatory payment classification (APC) assignment and hence the level of reimbursement, the code assignment should be closely monitored. Currently each facility determines its hospital-specific criteria for level of service determination for emergency department visits. Thus, auditing is necessary to validate that the levels are correctly assigned based on the established criteria and that the criteria are reflective of resource consumption experienced at that facility for the services rendered (table 9.17).

Outpatient Code Editor Edit Review for Hospital Outpatient Services

The following examples illustrates how ongoing analysis of OCE results can improve a facility's revenue cycle performance. Facility A submitted one month of Medicare outpatient claims for auditing by the Medicare Outpatient Code Editor (OCE). The data set contained 2,530 claims, 17,710 line items, and $5,457,513 in charges. The results of an OCE audit are displayed in table 9.18.

Several edits were evoked during the audit. To improve the revenue cycle process, the RCM team investigates each edit to uncover its root problems.

OCE Edit 41

OCE edit 41 (invalid revenue code) has been evoked, which usually arises when the revenue code reported on the claim is not in the list of valid revenue codes for OPPS. When this edit is activated, the claim is returned to the provider for correction. Therefore, this error is delaying payment of several claims and is also costing the facility staff time in rework. Each claim must be corrected and resubmitted to the MAC for payment.

Example:

Code distribution may be compared among a medium-sized not-for-profit hospital, two peer facilities, and the nation. Figure 9.12 shows the E/M code distribution during the study period. The data show that hospital A reported

Table 9.17.   E/M emergency department CPT codes and APC groupings (CY 2015)

	99281	99282	99283	99284	99285
APC Group	0609—Level 1 Emergency Visit	0613—Level 2 Emergency Visit	0614—Level 3 Emergency Visit	0615—Level 4 Emergency Visit	0616—Level 5 Emergency Visit
APC Relative Weight	0.8155	1.5206	2.6747	4.5003	6.6424
APC Payment (unadjusted)	$60.49	$112.79	$198.39	$333.80	$492.69

Figure 9.12.   E/M code distribution

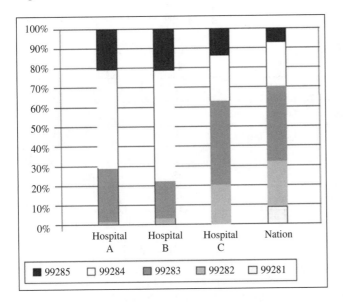

Figure 9.13.   Hospital A E/M distribution trend—four-year study period

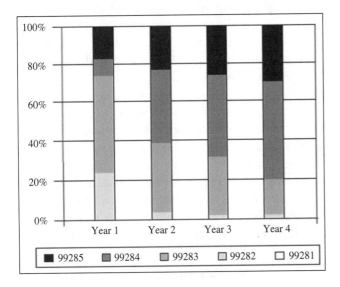

Clearly, this situation raises revenue code issues. Revenue codes are stored in the charge description master (CDM) and are placed on the claim via charge/order entry. A CDM review is thus warranted because several line items obviously are stored with incorrect revenue codes. Perhaps a program transmittal was incorrectly interpreted, or a typing mistake was made during data entry in the CDM.

A review of the 65 error claims shows that two line items in the ancillary section of physical therapy have incorrect information. The two line items represent physical therapy evaluation services, which should be reported using revenue code 0424. However, these line items had been assigned revenue code 0425—not a valid revenue code. This was a simple data entry mistake, but it resulted in delayed payment for several claims. This error is easy to correct, but it reveals the need for the CDM update process to be reviewed to identify risk areas for typing errors. Facility A subsequently implements a review component as part of its CDM update process.

OCE Edit 48

OCE edit 48 (Revenue center requires HCPCS code) is triggered when a HCPCS code is not reported with a revenue code on the claim, and the revenue center status indicator is not bundled. This edit is not applicable for revenue codes 100x, 210x, 310x, 099x, 0905–0907, 0500, 0509, 0583, 0660–0663, 0669, 0931–0932, 0521–0522, 0524–0525, 0527–0528, 0637, or 0948. Because this edit is activated, claims are being returned to the facility for correction. Like OCE edit 41, this error is also delaying the payment of several claims and is costing facility A staff time for rework.

Review of these 29 claims reveals they all included the line item number 3268916, used to report lithotripsy. Facility A had recently hard-coded the lithotripsy services in the CDM, so the RCM team could not understand why the HCPCS code was not appearing on the claim. Furthermore, the lithotripsy unit was contacted, and its staff confirmed that they performed 35 procedures last month, so why did only 29 claims evoke this edit? What happened to the other six claims? The RCM team asked the CDM coordinator to review all line items for lithotripsy services.

The CDM review revealed that there were duplicate line items for this service. Apparently the previous line item for this service was not marked as inactive when the hard-coding update occurred; thus the CDM contained two active line items for the same service. However, the RCM team was still puzzled, thinking they had thoroughly educated the charge entry staff about the line item changes. After further investigation, the RCM team discovered that one charge entry staff member had been vacationing during the training, and upon returning to work, she was not informed about the line item changes. She had thus continued to use the previous line item number.

Two fixes were implemented. First, line item number 3268916 was marked inactive. Second, the

Table 9.18.   Hospital A OCE Audit Results

OCE Edit	Edit Description	Violations	Claims Processing Area
01	Invalid diagnosis code	23	Coding
06	Invalid procedure code	21	Coding/CDM
27	Only incidental services reported	16	Order entry/coding/CDM
28	Code not recognized by Medicare; alternate code for same service may be available	54	Coding/CDM
38	Inconsistency between implanted device or administered substance and implantation or associated procedure	47	Order entry/CDM
41	Invalid revenue code	65	CDM
43	Transfusion or blood product exchange without specification of blood product	15	Order entry/CDM
44	Observation revenue code on line item with nonobservation HCPCS code	49	Order entry/CDM
48	Revenue center requires HCPCS code	29	CDM
61	Service can only be billed to the DMERC	14	Order entry/CDM
68	Service provided before date of National Coverage Determination (NCD) approval	32	Coding/CDM
71	Claim lacks required device code	28	Order entry/CDM

charge entry staff member was scheduled for training immediately. Additionally, the RCM team and coding manager learned two lessons. An additional component was needed in the hard-coding conversion plan to review all previous line items for inactive status, and a sign-in sheet was needed for use during training sessions and following up on missing attendees to ensure the education of all staff members in the future.

OCE Edit 38

OCE edit 38 (Inconsistency between implanted device and implantation procedure) is triggered when an HCPCS code with APC payment status indicator H (pass-through device) or APC 0987–0997 (implant) is present on the claim, but no APC with a payment status indicator of S (significant), T (surgical), or X (ancillary—nonimplant) is reported. This edit causes the claim to be returned to the provider for correction.

To determine whether this situation resulted from a CDM error or a flaw in the order entry process, facility A required a claim analysis. Claim review showed that the 47 cases evoking OCE edit 38 were all cardiac pacemaker claims. Further investigation of the cardiac encounters revealed that the order entry process included reporting the device code via the CDM, but the facility's chart flow process was bypassing the HIM department. Thus, the code for the pacemaker

insertion procedure was not being coded or reported on the claim.

Not only did facility A require rework and resubmission for these 47 claims, but the HIM and cardiac departments and the RCM team had to work together to change claims-processing flow.

This case study shows that each claim that evokes an edit from an internal or external auditing system or process should be investigated and corrected, if warranted. Facilities should resubmit all possible claims in order to achieve optimal reimbursement. Failure to review and rework error claims will result in significant lost payment. A facility's RCM team should facilitate this process so that efforts can be coordinated and streamlined.

Check Your Understanding 9.2

1. Healthcare facilities should design key performance indicators so that they _____.

2. Identify one MAP KPI and identify the revenue cycle component it represents.

3. What are three benefits of an integrated revenue cycle?

4. What system is typically used to audit outpatient Medicare claims?

5. In MS-DRG relationships reporting, MS-DRG families are examined for _____.

Chapter 9 Review Quiz

1. Which provider order entry system is usually more reliable, paper-based or electronic? Why?

2. What are two sources of new charge description master codes?

3. What risk areas are concerns when the charge description master is not properly maintained and revised?

4. How has HIPAA changed claims processing?

5. What are two roles of EDI in claims processing?

6. List ways that discrepancies between submitted charges and paid charges are reconciled by the provider.

7. How do providers decide what optimal performance is for units of their facility?

8. Facility B just completed an analysis of its alarmingly high balance of unpaid claim amounts. What are some key performance indicators a provider's RCM team could use to learn the reason(s) for the surge in unpaid balances?

9. Describe at least three sources of errors that cause claim denials.

10. True or false? Use of the charge description master has made manual coding by HIM coders obsolete.

References

3M Health Information System. 2010 (January). *Outpatient Code Editor with Ambulatory Payment Classification Software; Installation and User's Manual*. 3M: Wallingford, CT.

Acumentra Health. 2005 (December). Hospital Payment Monitoring Program (HPMP) Compliance Workbook. Prepared under contract with CMS. http://www.acumentra.org.

American Medical Association. 2010. CPT™ Process—How a Code Becomes a Code. http://www.ama-assn.org/ama/no-index/physician-resources/3882.shtml.

Bielby, Judy A., et al. Care and maintenance of charge masters. *Journal of AHIMA* (Updated March 2010). http://library.ahima.org/xpedio/groups/public/document/ahima/bok1_047258.hcsp?dDocName=bok1_04728.

Bowman, S. 2008. *Health Information Management Compliance: Guidelines for Preventing Fraud and Abuse*, 4th ed. Chicago: AHIMA.

Casto, A. 2011. *The Charge Description Master Handbook*. Chicago: AHIMA.

Centers for Medicare and Medicaid Services. 2005a. Overview. http://www.cms.gov/Manuals/01_Overview.asp.

Centers for Medicare and Medicaid Services. 2005b. Program Transmittals Overview. http://www.cms.hhs.gov/transmittals/01_overview.asp.

Centers for Medicare and Medicaid Services. 2008 (rev. April 25). *Medicare Program Integrity Manual*: Chapter 13—Local Coverage Determinations. http://www.cms.gov/manuals/downloads/pim83c13.pdf.

Centers for Medicare and Medicaid Services. 2009 (rev. Nov. 13). *Medicare Claims Processing Manual*. Chapter 23, Section 20.9. http://www.cms.gov/manuals/downloads/clm104c23.pdf.

Centers for Medicare and Medicaid Services. 2010a. Internet-Only Manuals (IOMs). http://www.cms.hhs.gov/Manuals/IOM/list.asp.

Centers for Medicare and Medicaid Services. 2010b (rev. May 28). *Medicare National Coverage Determinations Manual*: Chapter 1, Part 2 (Sections 90–160.26)—Coverage Determinations. http://www.cms.gov/manuals/downloads/ncd103c1_Part2.pdf.

Centers for Medicare and Medicaid Services. 2010c. *National Correct Coding Initiative Policy Manual for Medicare Services*, Version 15.3, Chapter 10, page X-5. http://www.cms.hhs.gov/NationalCorrect CodInitEd/.

Centers for Medicare and Medicaid Services. 2014. Healthcare Procedure Coding System (HCPCS) Level II.

Centers for Medicare and Medicaid Services. 2015a. Outpatient Code Editor. http://www.cms.gov/Medicare/Coding/OutpatientCodeEdit/.

Centers for Medicare and Medicaid Services. 2015b. Addendum B—OPPS Payment by HCPCS Code for CY 2015. http://www.cms.gov/Medicare/Medicare-Fee-for-Service-Payment/HospitalOutpatientPPS/Addendum-A-and-Addendum-B-Updates.html.

Centers for Medicare and Medicaid Services. 2015c. NCCI Coding Edits. http://www.cms.gov/Medicare/Coding/NationalCorrectCodInitEd/NCCI-Coding-Edits.html.

Colton, B., and A. Davis. 2015. Integrating the Revenue Cycle for Improved Health System Performance. *Healthcare Financial Management* 65:12, 56–61

Department of Health and Human Services. 2003a (February 20). Health insurance reform: Security standards; Final rule. *Federal Register* 68(34):8333–8399.

Department of Health and Human Services. 2003b (February 20). Health insurance reform: Modifications to electronic data transaction standards and code sets. *Federal Register* 68(34):8381–8399.

Dietz, M. S. 2005 (October). Ensure equitable reimbursement through an accurate charge description master. *Proceedings from AHIMA's 77th National Convention and Exhibit*. Chicago: AHIMA.

Healthcare Financial Management Association. 2015a. Patient Friendly Billing Project. http://www.hfma.org/Content.aspx?id=1033.

Healthcare Financial Management Association. 2015b. Map Keys. http://www.hfma.org/Content.aspx?id=13116.

Schraffenberger, L.A., and L. Kuehn. 2011. *Effective Management of Coding Services*. Chicago: American Health Information Management Association.

Sorrentino, P.A., and B. Sanderson. 2011. Managing the physician revenue cycle. *Healthcare Financial Management* 69:1, 88–94.

Additional Resources

AHIMA. 1999. Practice brief: The care and maintenance of charge masters. *Journal of American Health Information Management Association* 70(7):80A–B.

Berkey, T. 1998. Reducing accounts receivable through benchmarking and best practices identification. *Journal of American Health Information Management Association* 69:10, 30–34.

Bohley, M., and B. Kost. 2005. Beyond APCs: New challenges with outpatient coding, compliance, and reimbursement. Do you know where you stand? *Proceedings of AHIMA's 77th National Convention and Exhibit*. Chicago: AHIMA.

Centers for Medicare and Medicaid Services. July 31, 2014. Press Release: Deadline for ICD-10 allows health care industry ample time to prepare for change. http://www.cms.gov/Newsroom/MediaReleaseDatabse/Pressreleases/2014-Press-releases-items/2014-07-31/html.

Cummins, R., and J. Waddell. 2005 (July–August). Coding connections in revenue cycle management. *Journal of AHIMA* 76(7):72–74.

Drach, M., A. Davis, and C. Sagrati. 2001. Ten steps to successful chargemaster reviews. *Journal of AHIMA* 72(1):42–48

Grzybowski, D., and L. Schraffenberger. 2006. Double duty: Where HIM and chargemaster coding intersect. *Proceedings of AHIMA's 78th National Convention and Exhibit Proceedings.* Chicago: AHIMA.

Healthcare Financial Management Association. Summer 2003 Patient Friendly Billing Report. http://www.hfma.org/HFMA-Initiatives/Patient-Friendly-Billing/Patient-Friendly-Billing-Project-Reports/.

Hirschl, N., and P. Belton. 2005 (October) Revenue integrity and coding compliance: The sharp experience. *Proceedings from AHIMA's 77th National Convention and Exhibit*. Chicago: AHIMA.

Kuehn, L., and L. Schraffenberger. 2009. *Effective Management of Coding Services*, 4th ed. Chicago: AHIMA.

Leeds, E. 2001 (October). When good chargemasters go bad. *Proceedings from AHIMA's 73rd National Convention and Exhibit*. Chicago: AHIMA.

National Uniform Billing Committee. 2010. www.nubc.org.

Richey, J. 2001. A new approach to chargemaster management. *Journal of AHIMA* 72(1):51–55.

VHA. 2002. Revenue cycle management: The paradigm shift to success. VHA, Inc. http://www.vha.com.

Work, M. 2005. Best practices in revenue cycle management. *Journal of American Health Information Management Association* 76:7, 31.

Youmans, Karen. 2004. An HIM spin on the revenue cycle. *Journal of American Health Information Management Association* 75:3, 32–36.

Chapter 10
Value-Based Purchasing

Objectives

- To describe the origins and evolution of value-based purchasing and pay-for-performance

- To describe models of value-based purchasing and pay-for-performance

- To explain models of value-based purchasing implemented by the Centers for Medicare and

Medicaid Services for various healthcare settings and payment systems

- To describe how compliance with the Centers for Medicare and Medicaid Services value-based purchasing programs affects healthcare reimbursement for a facility, entity, or professional

Key Terms

Accountability
Accountable care organization (ACO)
Attribution
Hospital Quality Alliance (Hospital) Consumer Assessment of Healthcare Providers and Systems (HCAHPS)
Measure (indicator)
Measurement
Patient-centered medical home (PCMH)
Pay-for-performance (P4P)

Pay-for-reporting
Purchaser
STEEEP (safe, timely, effective, efficient, equitable, and patient-centered)
Target
Transparency
Triple aim
Value
Value-based purchasing (VBP)

Introduction to Value-Based Purchasing and Pay-for-Performance Systems

Value-based purchasing (VBP) and pay-for-performance (P4P) systems reflect a widespread movement in the healthcare industry toward improving the quality, safety, efficiency, and the overall value of healthcare. The rising costs of healthcare have motivated payers to establish VBP/P4P systems. Underpinning this decision is payers' perception that quality and safety have not concomitantly improved with healthcare's increasing costs.

VBP/P4P systems link quality, performance, and payment. These payment systems are growing in their influence and prevalence. In the private sector, VBP/P4P systems are endorsed by large private employers and coalitions that seek to increase the quality and safety of healthcare. In the public sector, this movement has become known as VBP and is an element of federal and state healthcare reimbursement systems.

The first half of this chapter provides a general overview of these systems' origins and some common models. The second half of this chapter details the history and features of the VBP programs used in the payment systems of the Centers for Medicare and Medicaid Services (CMS).

Definitions

The fundamental characteristics that VBP/P4P systems share are **measurement**, **transparency**, and **accountability** (figure 10.1). This order is important. Measurement comes first because stakeholders, such as patients, consumers, payers, and other decision makers must have facts. Transparency is essential because stakeholders need information about the cost and quality

Figure 10.1.   Fundamental characteristics of value-based purchasing and pay-for-performance systems

Measurement: Systematic process of data collection, repeated over time or at a single point in time (CMS 2006, n.p.).

Transparency: Act of making available to the public, in a reliable and understandable manner, information regarding a healthcare organization's quality, efficiency, and consumer experience with care, which includes price and quality data, so as to influence the behavior of patients, providers, payers, and others to achieve better outcomes (Committee on Quality 2001, 8).

Accountability: Obligation of individuals or organizations to provide information about, to be answerable for, and to justify their actions to other actors, along with the imposition of sanctions for failure to comply, to engage in appropriate action, or both (Brinkerhoff 2004, 372).

of healthcare so that they can make informed choices. Finally, accountability holds individuals and organizations responsible for their actions (O'Kane 2007, S3).

Pay-for-performance (P4P) may be defined as any type of payment arrangement to reimburse providers that is performance-based and that includes incentives (Pope 2011, 33). P4P systems align payment incentives with contractually-specified performance **targets**. Targets are specific, measurable objectives against which performance can be judged. Examples of performance targets include maintaining or improving the quality of care or meeting benchmarks on profitability or efficiency. Quality is often assessed by conformance with quantifiable and evidence-based standards, known as measures. Process measures reflect compliance with guidelines or standards of care, such as the number of smoker patients to whom physicians provide advice on smoking cessation. A target for increased profitability could be lowering costs for referrals to specialists (Dudley and Rosenthal 2006, 1). Incentives are broadly defined. Incentives may be rewards, such as bonuses, or may be penalties, such as reduced payments.

Value-based purchasing (VBP) is defined as a system in which **purchasers** hold providers of healthcare accountable for both the costs of healthcare and its quality (Meyer et al. 1997, 1). Purchasers are "public and private sector entities that subsidize, arrange and contract for—and in many cases bear the risk for—the cost of health care services received by a group" (Agency for Healthcare Research and Quality [AHRQ] 2002, n.p.). These entities include employers, federal and state governments, health plans, and other payers. In VBP, **value** is "usually defined as *focusing on both quality and cost at the same time in purchasing and delivering health care*" (Thomas and Caldis 2007, 1; Trisolini 2011, 11). Value is a "function of quality, efficiency, safety, and cost" (Keckley et al. 2011, 1). Value includes the delivery of timely, effective, appropriate, and high-quality services that result in the best possible outcomes (Medicaid and CHIP Payment and Access Commission [MACPAC] 2012, 10).

VBP does the following (Meyer et al. 1997, 1):

- Integrates information on healthcare quality with cost data

- Focuses on managing the use of the healthcare system to reduce inappropriate care

- Identifies and rewards the best-performing providers

Although some healthcare experts use the terms *VBP* and *P4P* interchangeably, others make distinctions. Common distinctions are made on cost, setting, and duration:

- Cost
  - VBP is improved quality for the same cost to the purchaser (Tompkins et al. 2009, w252).
  - P4P is additional payments for high or increasing quality (Briesacher et al. 2009, 1; Tompkins et al. 2009, w252).

- Setting
  - P4P is common in the private sector, such as health plans and employer–payer coalitions.
  - VBP is the current term of the public sector, such as Medicare's payment systems.

- Duration
  - P4P is associated with systems that have been established since approximately 2004.
  - Common use of VBP dates to its use in the Deficit Reduction Act (DRA) of 2005, although analysts and researchers used the term as early as 1997 (Meyer et al. 1997, 1).

Other terms for VBP/P4P systems include value-oriented payment, value-based care, quality compensation programs, quality-based purchasing, performance-based contracting, and shared savings/risks programs. The use of many terms reflects the dynamic nature of these payment systems.

Goals

The visions and missions of healthcare organizations differ. As a result, their goals for VBP/P4P systems differ. However, organizations typically list some of or all the following goals:

- Reward the provision of quality care

- Improve the quality of care

- Control costs by reducing errors, waste, inappropriate utilization, and expensive inpatient admissions

Generally, organizations merge these goals into achieving (1) higher quality care for the same cost, (2) the same quality care for lower cost, or (3) higher quality care for lower cost (Trisolini 2011, 11). These goals are broad and all-inclusive. Some healthcare organizations may have additional subgoals, such as achieving a competitive edge through a focus on cost-effective quality or improving coordination of care among providers.

Background

On a limited basis, forms of P4P have existed since the early 1970s. At that time, the "Buy Right" program was aimed at corporate purchasers of healthcare. It combined quality improvement, incentives, and efficiency measures (Millenson 2004, 324). In the late 1990s and early 2000s, both the public and private sectors within the healthcare industry began VBP/P4P initiatives.

By the mid-2000s, more than 100 organizations had initiated VBP/P4P systems (Rowe 2006, 695). These organizations included health plans, employer–payer coalitions, and Medicare and Medicaid programs. During the period, P4P systems targeted individual physicians and HMOs (Rose 2008, 27; Rosenthal and Frank 2006, 152). The P4P system's incentives were based on the measures in the Healthcare Effectiveness Data and Information Set (HEDIS) of the National Committee for Quality Assurance (NCQA) (see chapter 5 and next section on Drivers) and on clinical practice guidelines published by medical specialty societies (Rose 2008, 27).

Over the past decade, the VBP/P4P systems have continued to progress by

- Expanding to more types of providers, such as preferred provider organizations, medical specialists, and hospitals

- Extending beyond payers and providers to consumers, such as dissemination of performance results in public reports and involvement in consumer-directed care (see chapter 3)

- Developing more performance measures, such as adoption of health information technologies, specific population measures, clinical practice guidelines (evidence-based process measures), cost savings, and return on investment

- Advancing incentives to tiered fee schedules (Keckley et al. 2011, 5–8)

The Affordable Care Act of 2010 expanded the use of VBP and P4P in Medicare. Today, VBP/P4P systems are widespread. For example, approximately 66 percent of members of commercial insurance plans and 35 percent of Medicare beneficiaries receiving care from providers under P4P systems (Long et al. 2014, 883; Wouters and McGee 2014, e285). VBP/P4P systems are continuing to emerge and evolve.

Drivers

Drivers in the development of VBP/P4P systems are reports on the US healthcare system, private-sector coalitions and associations, and the federal government.

In the late 1990s and into the 2000s, drivers of the VBP/P4P initiatives were a series of reports calling into question the quality, safety, and cost of US healthcare and recommending new designs of payment systems:

- *To Err Is Human: Building a Safer Health System*. This report from the Committee on Quality of Health Care in America of the Institute of Medicine (IOM) stated that a large number of hospital deaths, possibly as many as 98,000 per year, were caused by medical errors. The size of the problem in other healthcare settings was unknown but was suspected to be as great (Kohn et al. 1999, 1–2).

- *Crossing the Quality Chasm: A New Health System for the 21st Century*. This IOM report stated that the US healthcare delivery system needed fundamental change as "quality problems are everywhere, affecting many patients" (Committee on Quality 2001, 1). The report's authors called for the redesign of the US healthcare system to support the delivery of quality healthcare. One characteristic of that redesign was the alignment of payment incentives and quality, such as in P4P systems (Committee on Quality 2001, 4–5).

- *Rewarding Provider Performance: Aligning Incentives in Medicare*. The authors of this IOM report also stated that poor quality was a problem in the US healthcare delivery system. The poor quality of healthcare, that had been described in *Crossing the Quality Chasm, still existed (Committee on Redesigning 2007, 1). Moreover, the report's authors* specifically recommended that "new payment incentives must be created to encourage the redesign of structures and processes of care to promote higher *value* and to encourage progress toward significant *quality improvement*" (emphases added; Committee on Redesigning 2007, 1–2).

Recent information shows continued problems with quality, safety, and cost in the US health system. In its most recent report on quality, the Agency for Healthcare Research and Quality (AHRQ) graded the quality of healthcare in the United States only as "fair." On average, Americans receive 70 percent of the healthcare services that they need to treat or prevent particular medical conditions and fail to receive 30 percent of the healthcare services that they needed. The authors of the report concluded that the gap between best possible care and what is routinely delivered remains substantial across the entire country (AHRQ 2014, 2). The US healthcare system's safety is similarly disappointing. Recent research shows that the US healthcare system's safety has not significantly improved since the release of *To Err Is Human* in 1999. Each year, between 210,000 and 440,000 hospital patients suffer preventable harms that contribute to their deaths. These deaths are roughly one-sixth of all deaths in the United States (James 2013, 127).

The increasing costs of healthcare have been discussed previously in chapters 1 and 3. Moreover, fee-for-service (FFS) payment systems have perverse incentives that reward overutilization without regard for quality and cost. In FFS payment systems, providers are paid based on the volume of services rather than on the quality of services. Proponents of VBP/P4P contend that these systems can contain costs.

Private-sector associations and coalitions have been influential in the development of VBP/P4P systems since the 1990s. Major players in the private sector include the following:

- Leapfrog Group. The Leapfrog Group, established in November 2000, includes large employers. These large employers represent 26 million covered lives and $45 billion in healthcare expenditures (Moran and Scanlon 2013, 27). The goal of the Leapfrog Group is to positively affect the quality and affordability of healthcare by "leaping" forward improvements in hospitals' quality and safety through rewards. For example, Leapfrog Group promoted the use of computerized drug order entry in hospitals to automate prescription drug ordering and thus reduce medication errors. The Group also promoted staffing hospital intensive care units with intensivists, physicians specially trained in critical care medicine (Moran and Scanlon 2013, 27).

- Health Care Incentives Improvement Institute (HCI3). HCI3 is a nonprofit multi-stakeholder organization that develops and disseminates programs and resources to help payers and providers design innovative incentive systems. It was created when Bridges to Excellence® (BTE) merged with PROMETHEUS Payment®, an approach to bundled payments. Established in 2002, BTE is a family of programs to recognize and reward physicians, nurse practitioners, and physician assistants for reengineering and improving their practices' systems, for adopting health information technology, and for delivering quality outcomes to their patients (de Brantes and D'Andrea 2009, 305). BTE's programs are organized by diseases, such as asthma and diabetes. BTE's programs emphasize all characteristics described as key to the Institute of Medicine's redesigned healthcare system: safe, timely, effective, efficient, equitable, and patient-centered (**STEEEP**).

- Integrated Healthcare Association (IHA) of California. This nonprofit multi-stakeholder group was established in 2003. IHA is statewide coving seven health plans, 225 physician organizations (35,000 physicians), purchasers, consumer-advocate groups, and 6.2 million enrollees (Damberg et al. 2009, 518). The IHA applies one common, uniform set of performance measures to all of its participating physician organizations. The performance measures are similar to the HEDIS of the NCQA. Annually, the IHA produces performance scores, based on these measures, for the physician organizations. The IHA is an example of a model in which quality and efficiency are successfully integrated (Harbaugh 2009, 1004).

- National Business Coalition on Health (NBCH). Established in 1992, the NBCH is an umbrella organization at the national level for employer-based health coalitions (Webber 2012, 30). The purpose of the NBCH and its member coalitions is to improve the value of healthcare provided through employer-sponsored health plans. The NBCH and its members achieve this purpose through the collective action of public and private purchasers. NBCH seeks

to accelerate the nation's progress toward safe, efficient, high-quality health care and to improve the health status of the US population. NBCH provides expertise, resources, and a voice to its member coalitions. Examples of member coalitions include the Colorado Business Group on Health, the Florida Health Care Coalition, and the Memphis Business Group on Health. In total, there are 55 member coalitions. The NBCH represents over 4,000 employers and about 35 million employees and their dependents.

- National Committee for Quality Assurance (NCQA). The NCQA is a nonprofit organization aiming to improve the quality of health care and to transform healthcare quality through measurement, transparency, and accountability. The NCQA was formed in 1979 by the managed care industry and the Group Health Association of America (now known as America's Health Insurance Plans, AHIP) (Ohldin and Mims 2002, 344–345). Between 1979 and 1990, the NCQA grew with the support of large employers, consumers, labor unions, quality experts, and policy experts. In 1990, aided by a grant from the Robert Wood Johnson Foundation, the NCQA was established as an independent organization. The NCQA provides standards with which healthcare entities can measure their performance. Its HEDIS indicators are used by 90 percent of health plans to measure their performance (Harbaugh 2009, 1003). NCQA has multiple accreditation, certification, and recognition programs addressing many aspects of performance (NCQA 2012, n.p.). Moreover, NCQA certification is a prerequisite to participation in the BTE program (Harbaugh 2009, 1003). The widespread adoption of its performance indicators and programs makes NCQA an influential organization in healthcare quality.

Federal and state governments have gradually introduced VBP/P4P into public sector healthcare payment programs. Over the past 10 years, Medicare has established VBP/P4P programs for almost all its major provider types (Medicare Payment Advisory Commission [MedPAC] 2014, 41). These provider types include inpatient hospitals, post-acute care providers, physicians and professionals, dialysis facilities, and federally qualified health centers. VBP/P4P, called the shared-savings program, is a central component of Medicare's payment policy for accountable care organizations (ACOs) (see section on accountable care organizations later in the chapter). Many state Medicaid and Children's Health Insurance Program (CHIP) programs attempt to align their payments with value (MACPAC 2012, 10). For example, to enhance the quality of care, 34 states' Medicaid programs added or enhanced their pay-for-performance arrangements to enhance the quality of care (Smith et al. 2014, 2). By aligning payments to value, federal and state payers are striving to provide access to appropriate services while ensuring quality, economy, and efficiency.

Finally, many policymakers in the private and public sectors believe that VBP/P4P systems offer potential countermeasures to failures in quality, safety, and costs of the US healthcare system. VBP/P4P systems attempt to address the system's shortcomings by rewarding quality, performance, and efficiency. In VBP/P4P systems, incentives are directly linked to quality, to performance measures, and to financial targets. Therefore, VBP/P4P systems work to motivate providers, through incentives, to deliver high-quality care in a cost-effective and cost-efficient manner.

International Movement

VBP/P4P is an international movement. P4P systems have been implemented in many countries, from developing to industrialized. These countries include Australia, Austria, Belize, Burundi, Canada, China, the Democratic Republic of the Congo, Estonia, France, Germany, Iran, Italy, Kenya, the Netherlands, the Philippines, Rwanda, Tanzania, Uganda, United Kingdom, Vietnam, and others (Aryankhesal et al. 2013, 207; Bowser et al. 2013, 1064; Menya et al., 2013, n.p.; Merilind et al. 2014, 110; Tsiachristas et al. 2013, 296; Wilson 2013, 2; Witter et al. 2013, n.p.). The P4P systems vary. Some focus on one provider, such as general practitioners or hospitals. Others are specific programs that focus on improving outcomes for certain conditions, such as diabetes or on improving the delivery of care, such as integrating chronic care. Selected representative examples of international P4P systems and programs follow:

- The United Kingdom (UK) introduced a P4P program for general practitioners in 2004. The UK's program is called the Quality and Outcomes Framework (QOF). The QOF is an incentive-based, quality-improvement program (Greene and Nash 2009, 140). The QOF is one of the world's largest P4P systems (Langdown and Peckham 2014, 251). A recent literature review found that the QOF improved outcomes for certain conditions, such as diabetes, and had mixed results for others, such as chronic heart disease. Generally, though, in the QOF, improvements initially occurred in outcomes for conditions, but as time went on, the improvements plateaued. Researchers concluded that the plateau in improvements was related to the QOF's focus on process measures rather than on outcome measures (Langdown and Peckham 2014, 251, 255).

- In Canada, two provinces have instituted P4P programs. Ontario implemented P4P for physician payments in 2004. Since then Ontario has established the program, Paying-for-Results, to reduce nonurgent patients' waiting times in emergency departments (Wilson 2013, 32). British Columbia, in fiscal year 2007–2008, also established a P4P pilot program to reduce wait times in the emergency departments of the province's hospitals. In this pilot program, only selected hospitals, usually urban hospitals with long wait times, participate (Cheng and Sutherland 2013, 87).

- Australia began to implement P4P in 1997 (Wilson 2013, 3). Two early programs were the General Practice Immunization Incentives Scheme and the Practice Incentives Program. Australia's Veteran's Affairs Department also implemented a P4P system for inpatient hospital services (Wilson 2013, 3). In addition, in 2008, Queensland province introduced a P4P system for its hospital prospective payment system. This P4P system is known as the Clinical Practice Improvement Payment (CPIP). The CPIP uses financial incentives to reward clinical practices that have a direct, positive effect on patient outcomes (Duckett et al. 2008, 174).

- In Italy, much like in Canada, adoption of P4P systems has been at the province level. Italian provinces in the central and north-central regions have initiated P4P. For example, the Emilia Romagna region ties general practitioners' compensation to achievement of diabetes care goals (Wilson 2013, 4). In Tuscany, bonuses are paid to chief executive officers when their organizations meet performance targets (Wilson 2013, 7). The Lazio region implemented a P4P program to reduce time-to-surgery for elderly patients with hip fractures (Colais et al. 2013, n.p.).

The general effect of P4P systems internationally is still unknown. Some research has shown gains in quality for specific targets. Other research shows little or no effect. The quality of the research itself is questionable with small samples and weak designs. Internationally, the ability of financial incentives to improve performance is still uncertain (Wilson 2013, 12).

Research on Impact

There is little evidence to support the use of VBP/P4P systems despite their proliferation (Werner et al. 2013, 1394). Recently conducted comprehensive and systematic reviews of the research literature on the effects of VBP/P4P systems generally found that the evidence was inconclusive or that the results were only modestly positive.

- A study by the RAND Corporation reported on 129 different VBP/P4P arrangements. The analysts examined peer-reviewed articles published between 2000 and 2013. Generally, the analysts reported that the effect of VBP/P4P was inconclusive. Some studies showed modest improvements in cost and quality, while other studies showed no substantial improvements. The methodologically strong research studies tended to show no substantial improvements (Damberg et al. 2014, 8, 18–23).

- An overview of systematic literature reviews was performed to examine the effectiveness of financial incentives to change health professionals' behavior and patients' outcomes. The time period was the inception of the literary databases through 2010. Only four reviews met the criteria of the researchers. These four reviews reported on 32 research studies. The authors of the overview reported that financial incentives may be effective in changing health professionals' behavior. No review reported evidence on the effect of financial incentives on patients' outcomes (Flodgren et al. 2011, n.p.).

- An overview of systematic literature reviews was performed to examine the effects of P4P in healthcare. The review was similar to the previous review by Flodgren and colleagues. This review, however, was conducted for an additional 18 months and was able to include two more systematic reviews. The authors of this review also broadened their inclusion criteria. Therefore, these authors examined 22 reviews. These authors found that P4P had the potential to be cost-effective, but that the evidence was unconvincing. The research studies were of low quality and failed to disentangle the effects of the P4P initiative from other simultaneous improvement initiatives (Eijkenaar et al. 2013, 115).

- A systematic review of the literature was conducted to determine the efficiency of P4P systems based on economic evaluations. Efficiency is achieving improved quality of care with equal or lower costs or is achieving the same quality of care with lower costs. During 2000–2010, the researchers found nine studies that met their criteria. Based on their analysis of these nine studies, the researchers concluded that evidence of P4P efficiency was scarce and was not shown (Emmert et al. 2012, 755).

- A systematic review of the literature was performed to obtain insights into the effects of P4P programs aimed at improving the delivery of health services for chronic care through disease management (see chapter 5). During 2000–2010, the researchers identified eight articles describing research on this type of program, with six programs based in the United States. Most studies showed positive effects on healthcare quality, but no study evaluated the effects of the P4P program on costs. The researchers concluded that hardly any information is available about the effects of P4P disease management programs on quality and cost (de Bruin et al. 2011, n.p.).

In sum, research has provided little evidence upon which leaders can base decisions about healthcare policy. These thorough reviews suggest that little is known about factors associated with successful VBP/P4P systems. Many questions still remain about how to design and implement VBP/P4P systems to achieve their stated goals. Answering these questions through well-conducted research will help leaders as they determine healthcare policy.

Advantages and Disadvantages

Both advantages and disadvantages can accrue to healthcare organizations that implement VBP/P4P systems.

The advantages include the following (Bell and Levinson 2007, 1718):

- Demonstrated commitment to providing quality care

- Establishment of infrastructure for reporting on quality

- Rewards for providing quality healthcare

- Transparent process of rewards

- Ability to focus on underserved or high-risk groups

The disadvantages include the following (Bell and Levinson 2007, 1718):

- Implementation of intervention that is not evidence-based (paucity of literature on VBP/P4P)

- Potential for unintended consequences, such as poor quality in unmeasured processes or inappropriate reduction of needed services

- Lack of accepted model with each system uniquely tailored for a specific healthcare entity

- Difficulty in measuring processes and outcomes in populations of patients or clients with complex diseases and conditions

- Difficulty in assessing measures that involve patients' or clients' compliance, such as smoking cessation

- Potential that costs of implementation could be better spent on other efforts

- Better documentation of care rather than actual better quality of care

Thus, despite having significant disadvantages, VBP/P4P systems are firmly entrenched in public and private healthcare payment systems.

Models

Models of VBP/P4P systems are evolving. Additionally, the models are diverse, having developed in both the private and public sectors. The ACA also encouraged experimentation in the design of these initiatives (James 2012, 1). Moreover, models differ because the missions and goals of healthcare organizations differ. Thus, the models vary from payer to payer, plan to plan, and program to program.

This section first describes design considerations for VBP/P4P models. Then, the section describes two current models, patient-centered medical homes and ACOs, that are generating much discussion in the healthcare sector.

Design Considerations

Two key considerations in the design of existing models of VBP/P4P systems are

- Recipient of reward or penalty (individual or group)

- Mechanism of payment

Based on these two key considerations, the current models fit two major categories (Bell and Levinson 2007, 1717):

- Reward-based
  - Individual, group, hospital, or region
  - Rewards (compensation) when targets are met or exceeded
  - Higher fee schedule for superior performance
  - Increased payment rates for superior providers

- Penalty-based
  - Individual, group, hospital, or region
  - Compensation withheld when targets are not met or performance is not improved
  - Lower fee schedule for inferior performance

VBP/P4P systems are more likely to use reward-based incentives than penalty-based incentives (Trisolini 2011, 23). The few penalty-based VBP/P4P systems include state Medicaid payment systems and some aspects of the CMS's VBP initiatives (see the second half of this chapter).

Patient-Centered Medical Home (PCMH)

A **patient-centered medical home (PCMH)** is a model of primary care "that seeks to meet the health care needs of patients and to improve patient and staff experiences, outcomes, safety, and system efficiency" (Jackson et al. 2013, 169). Many other definitions exist. Varying widely, operational definitions of PCMH are often specific to the site and organization (Jackson et al. 2013, 176).

The concept of PCMHs is not new. The American Academy of Pediatrics first used the term "medical home" in 1967 (Iglehart 2008, 1200). At that time, a "medical home" was described as a central source of a child's health records, particularly a child with a chronic disease or disabling condition (Sia et al. 2004, 1473). Since 1967, the concept has expanded "across multiple patient populations, disease states, geographies, and payers" (Fields et al. 2010, 819). PCMH initiatives are often organized by health plans, states, payers, providers, or multistakeholder groups. The number of initiatives is increasing, with 26 in 2009 and 114 in 2013 (Edwards et al. 2014, 1823). Fueled by the support of state Medicaid programs and the federal Medicare program, it is expected that this trend will continue (Edwards et al. 2014, 1824–1825).

The PCMH model combines the core functions of primary care with the innovations of 21st-century practice. Therefore, the PCMH model integrates the following features of primary care:

- Continuous and long-term
- Comprehensive including prevention and wellness, acute care, and chronic care
- Coordinated across the continuum of care, including specialty care, hospitals, home health care, and community services and supports
- Patient-centered being focused on the needs and preferences of patients and being relationship-based with (1) an orientation toward the whole person, (2) informed engagement of the patient and family, and (3) recognition of each patient's unique needs

with the use of the following:

- Multidisciplinary team
- Electronic information systems and on-line patient portals
- Chronic disease registries
- Population-based management of chronic disease
- Continuous quality improvement (Edwards et al. 2014, 1823; Jackson et al. 2013, 169; Rittenhouse et al. 2009, 2301).

In current PCMHs, the most common payment method is fee-for-service that is increased with per-member-per-month payments and P4P bonuses (Edwards et al. 2014, 1829).

Research on the effect of PCMHs on cost and quality has had mixed results. A comprehensive review of the research literature was conducted to summarize PCMHs' effects on patient and staff experiences, process of care, and clinical and economic outcomes. During the period from the inception of the literary databases through 2012, the researchers found 19 studies that met their criteria. The researchers found that PCMHs had a small positive effect on patients' experience of care and a small to moderate positive effect on staffs' experiences. However, generally, based on their analysis of these 19 studies, the researchers concluded that evidence on the PCMH model's effect was scarce and was insufficient to determine the model's effects on clinical and economic outcomes. Finally, there was no evidence for overall costs savings (Jackson et al. 2013, 169).

As a specific example, recent research evaluated a large PCMH initiative over a three-year period. The PCMH included 32 physician practices providing care to over 64,000 patients. The participant-practices were recognized by the NCQA as meeting its standards for PCMHs. The PCMH initiative's results were compared to 29 similar physician practices providing care to over 55,000 patients. The initiative did not reduce total costs or utilization of emergency, hospital, or ambulatory services. There was improvement in only one of 11 quality measures of chronic disease management (Friedberg et al. 2014, 815).

A related concept is the medical neighborhood. In a medical neighborhood, interactions between practices, such as a general practice and a specialty practice, are integrated and coordinated (Laine 2011, 60). In this way, specialists are incorporated into the care of patients. Thus, a medical neighborhood promotes the provision of efficient, high-quality health services (Laine 2011, 60).

Accountable Care Organization (ACO)

An **accountable care organization (ACO)** is a model for healthcare delivery and payment. Around 2005, researchers at Dartmouth first coined the term *accountable care organization* (MacKinney et al. 2011, 132). An ACO is a set of "providers who are jointly held accountable for achieving measured quality improvements and reductions in the rate of spending growth" (McClellan et al. 2010, 982). The purposes of ACOs are to improve the quality of care and curb its costs by reducing fragmentation and increasing coordination of healthcare services (Fisher et al. 2007, w44). An ACO is accountable for all the healthcare costs of its designated population. The concept of ACOs has been adopted by commercial payers, state Medicaid programs, and Medicare (Shortell et al. 2014, 1883).

There are three essential characteristics of ACOs (Devers and Berenson 2009, 2):

- Ability to manage patients across the continuum of care, including acute, ambulatory, and postacute health services

- Capability to prospectively plan budgets and resources needs

- Sufficient size to support comprehensive, valid, and reliable measurement of performance

Some analysts liken ACOs to managed care (Diamond 2009, 15; Knickman 2011, 58).

Local healthcare providers in a city or region are integrated in an ACO. The integrated providers may include primary care physicians, specialists, hospitals, healthcare insurance plans, suppliers of durable medical equipment or other services and items, and other stakeholders. The exact makeup of the ACO depends on its sponsoring healthcare organization. Experts describe three categories of ACOs based on size, scope of services, governance, ability to manage patients with complex chronic diseases, and other characteristics:

- Larger, integrated systems that offer a broad scope of services and frequently include one or more postacute care facilities

- Smaller, physician-led practices, centered in primary care

- Moderately sized, joint hospital-physician and coalition-led groups that offer a moderately broad scope of services with some involvement of postacute care facilities (Shortell et al. 2014, 1883).

ACOs are present in most healthcare markets. Recent publications show that there are more than 600 ACOs and that their numbers are rapidly increasing (Shortell et al. 2014, 1884; Petersen et al. 2014, n.p.).

The Affordable Care Act (ACA; Section 3022) required that the CMS promote the development of ACOs by establishing a Shared Savings Program. The Shared Savings Program has a **triple aim**: (1) better quality of care for individuals, (2) greater health for populations, and (3) lower growth in healthcare costs (CMS 2011a, 67803–67804). The general concept of shared savings programs is that providers are rewarded with a portion of the savings if they reduce the total healthcare spending for their patients below the level that the payer expected. The overarching result is that payer spends less money that it expected and the provider receives more revenue than it expected.

CMS has refined and further delineated the general definition of ACOs. Per CMS, an ACO is a legal entity recognized under state law. It is composed of a group of ACO participants (providers of services and suppliers) that have established a mechanism for shared governance. Under a three-year agreement with the CMS, the ACO participants coordinate the care of traditional Medicare fee-for-services beneficiaries. The ACO is accountable for the quality, cost, and overall care of all the beneficiaries assigned to it (CMS 2011a, 67974). Expanding on the specific components of this definition yields the following:

- A legal entity that is recognized and authorized under applicable state, federal, or tribal law

- Identified by a taxpayer identification number (TIN)

- Is formed by one or more the following ACO participants (providers or suppliers) or others:
  ○ Group practice of ACO professionals (physicians, physician assistants, nurse practitioners, clinical nurse specialists, or a combination)
  ○ Network of individual practices
  ○ Partnership or joint venture arrangements between hospitals and ACO professionals
  ○ Hospital employing ACO professionals
  ○ Critical access hospitals that bill outpatient services under the optional method for outpatient services with the cost based on the facility services plus a 115-percent fee schedule payment for professional services (Method II)
  ○ Rural health clinic
  ○ Federally qualified health center
- ACO participants working together to manage and coordinate care for Medicare fee-for-service beneficiaries
- Accountable for the quality, cost, and overall care for Medicare fee-for-service beneficiaries assigned to the ACO
- Operating under a risk model
  ○ One-sided model (Track 1) (available to ACOs only for their *initial* agreement period): ACOs share savings with the Medicare program, if they meet the requirements, but the ACOs do *not* share losses
  ○ Two-sided model (Track 2): ACOs share savings with the Medicare program, if they meet the requirements, and the ACOs share losses with the Medicare program
- Maintaining shared governance through an identifiable, authoritative governing body (at least one Medicare beneficiary and 75 percent ACO participants) with transparent processes that promote evidence-based medicine and patient engagement, that report on quality and cost measures, and that coordinate care
- A leadership and management structure that includes clinical and administrative systems supportive of the triple aim, executive officer, senior-level medical director, and other ACO participants must demonstrate meaningful commitment to the ACO's mission

- Providing primary care (outpatient, home, and wellness visits) to at least 5,000 assigned Medicare beneficiaries with at least a sufficient number of primary care ACO professionals for at least three years (term of agreement)
- Required explicitly to
  ○ Promote evidence-based medicine
  ○ Promote beneficiary engagement adopting patient-centeredness
  ○ Report on quality and cost metrics
  ○ Coordinate care across providers

Operating under this model, ACOs that meet the quality performance standards and generate savings will share a percentage of the savings with the CMS (CMS 2011a, 67974–67977).

Looking into future trends for ACOs, healthcare professionals should be aware of recent recommendations of the MedPAC. The MedPAC analyzed the functioning of ACOs under the Medicare program based on three years of experiences. Five issues emerged that must resolved for ACOs and the Shared Saving Program to be successful. In the short term, attribution of patients to providers must be improved and quality measurement and evaluation simplified. In the long term, the program should shift to the two-sided model; waive some regulations meant as constraints on overutilization, such as the skilled nursing facility three-day rule (required inpatient stay of at least three days prior to admission); and lower beneficiaries' cost sharing and allow additional engagement (Hackbarth 2014, 1–2). Finally, though, "ACOs represent an opportunity to transform the delivery system, but realizing that opportunity will require providers to change their practices and take a risk on a novel payment system, and CMS to be flexible and responsive as the program evolves" (Hackbarth 2014, 18).

Operations

In the operation of VBP/P4P systems, leaders face several considerations. Six important considerations are allocation and reward of incentives, types of incentives, method of implementation, performance dimensions and targets, performance measures, and information systems.

Allocation and Reward of Incentives

VBP/P4P systems are incentive-based. In the operation of VBP/P4P systems, the allocation and reward of incentives must be fair. In fairness, the provider or providers who rendered the care should receive the incentive. In addition, the allocation and reward of incentives must be transparent. The methods of allocation and reward of incentives should be clear and known to all involved providers.

Determining who rendered care is termed **attribution**. Another term for attribution and used by Medicare is *assignment*. Attribution is important because it allows the costs of a patient's care and the outcomes of that care to be specified to a provider. Subsequently, attribution determines which provider receives the incentive.

Attribution is not straightforward when multiple providers are involved. For example, some patients, including Medicare patients, have multiple, complex diseases that require multiple providers of care. One research study of Medicare claims found that Medicare beneficiaries saw a median of two primary care physicians and five specialists working in four different physician groups (Pham et al. 2007, 1132–1133). Moreover, for a third of Medicare beneficiaries, their assigned physicians were changed from one year to the next, with 97 percent being changed to different physician groups (Pham et al. 2007, 1134). To address this issue, healthcare analysts have created attribution algorithms.

Many attribution algorithms exist. Attribution algorithms that can be applied to individual providers are known as single attribution. Attribution algorithms that can be applied to multiple providers are known as multiple attribution. Algorithms select providers based on rules. Following are examples of some of the rules (Sorbero et al. 2006, 41):

- Gatekeeper or primary care provider for HMOs and other health plans that assign enrollees to providers (physicians)

- Highest volume of Evaluation and Management (E&M) visits (see chapter 2, CPT codes)

- Greatest share of overall, allowable patient costs

- Greatest share of E&M services costs

- Highest volume of preventive care

- All providers who cared for the patient

Under methods based on these rules, no more than half of the Medicare beneficiaries' visits could be attributed (Pham et al. 2007, 1131–1132, 1136).

Subsequently, CMS tested six approaches to attributing episodes of care to providers (MedPAC 2009, 65). These six approaches were variations on some of the algorithm rules previously listed (Sorbero et al. 2006, 41). The MedPAC analyzed the approaches of the CMS. In its analyses, MedPAC focused on four variations of CMS's methods of attributing episodes of care (MedPAC 2009, 72–73):

- Single attribution
  - Identifying physician billing most E&M costs (dollars)
  - Identifying physician billing most total costs (dollars)

- Multiple attribution
  - Identifying physicians billing most E&M costs (dollars)
  - Identifying physicians billing most total costs (dollars)

MedPAC reported that all four attribution methods gave similar results. Thus, MedPAC stated that the ultimate choice of method depended on Medicare's goals (MedPAC 2009, 74). Finally, MedPAC concluded that CMS could decide to use more than one method of attribution.

Types of Incentives

VBP/P4P systems link incentives and performance. Incentives may be positive in the form of rewards or negative in the form of penalties. Incentives can be financial or nonfinancial. Positive financial incentives include bonuses or higher fee structures. Positive nonfinancial incentives include public recognition, altruism, and alignment with professionalism (Dudley et al. 2004, 2). Negative financial incentives include penalties such as lowered bonuses or reduced payments. Negative nonfinancial incentives include poor public report cards.

The use of rewards, penalties, or both depends upon the individual program. The amount of incentives in VBP/P4P systems may vary by type of measure achieved. Weighting in payment formulae is a way to emphasize quality indicators over administrative indicators. For example, clinical measures (indicators) may be weighted more heavily than measures of patient satisfaction or cost efficiency (Sorbero et al. 2006, 41). Clinical measures are those that affect the care of patients, such as the number of patients with diabetes and who have undergone a key laboratory test (Hb A1c) within the past 12 months. Finally, the amount of bonuses should be tied to the costs associated with adherence or nonadherence to guidelines (Rosenthal and Dudley 2007, 741).

The level of the incentive must be sufficient to induce a change in behavior. It is difficult to determine exactly what this level must be, for the amount sufficient to induce change varies by the setting and situation. In one study, set in 1984, $2.00 was sufficient to have an effect (Hickson et al. 1987, 346–347). Yet, in another study, $10,000 was insufficient to have an effect (Roski et al. 2003, 294, 297). A comprehensive review of the literature on financial incentives and their link to quality in primary care found only a few research studies (Scott et al. 2011, 9–10). These authors reported a range of levels of incentives:

- Forty-nine clinics in a health system were eligible for a $5,000 bonus for referring 50 smokers to a telephone smoking counseling service during a nine-month period. After reaching the 50-smoker threshold, the clinic was eligible for $25 per smoker referral.

- Physician group practices were eligible for a quarterly bonus based on meeting or exceeding thresholds on five clinical measures. The bonus was $0.6795 per member per quarter per measure met or exceeded. The maximum annual bonus for a group with 2,000 eligible members was $27,180.

- A health plan was eligible for a quarterly bonus based on meeting or exceeding three performance measures. The bonus was $0.23 per member per month per performance measure met or exceeded. A health plan with 10,000 members and perfect performance could earn up to $270,000.

- Clinics were eligible for an annual bonus based on meeting or exceeding thresholds for documentation, in patients' health records, of patients' smoking status and providers' provision of advice to quit smoking. Clinics with one to seven providers could earn a maximum bonus of $5,000; clinics with more than eight providers could earn a maximum bonus of $10,000.

- Individual general practitioners were eligible for an approximately $130 bonus per smoker patient who was confirmed, by blood test, as having been abstinent at 12 months (Scott et al. 2011, 9–10).

The review authors noted that important details were absent. For example, there was a lack of information about how payments were distributed and used within the physician groups. Also, only two studies reported the financial incentive "in terms of the percentage of annual revenue delivered by the incentive scheme. This is important information to report about in this type of intervention, as incentives that are a larger proportion of revenue are expected to have a larger effect" (Scott et al. 2011, 12). Based on the evidence, the authors concluded that leaders should carefully design incentive schemes and proceed cautiously when implementing them.

As a rough guide, Rosenthal and colleagues observe that bonuses should be 5 percent or more of payments because this rate is prevalent among private payers (Rosenthal et al. 2005, 1902). Goldfield and colleagues suggest that, to be effective, the incentives must be large enough to make providers take notice (Goldfield et al. 2005, 32–33). They recommend that 20 percent is an amount substantial enough to make providers "relentlessly" pursue quality (Goldfield et al. 2005, 33). Moreover, they recommend that this 20 percent be carved out of current payments rather than bonuses on top of current payments (Goldfield et al. 2005, 33). They take this controversial stance because they believe that dramatic changes need to be made to the current healthcare delivery system—and that VBP/P4P systems that put providers at significant financial risk are the means to achieve these changes and quality improvement (Goldfield et al. 2005, 32–33).

Method of Implementation

Most healthcare entities implement VBP/P4P systems incrementally. They begin small and expand operations over time. Following are key advantages to incremental implementation (Dudley and Rosenthal 2006, 12):

- Measures are tested before full-scale use.
- Providers have time to prepare.
- Sponsors can evaluate policies, procedures, and results before full-scale use.

Incremental implementations can be pilot projects that focus on the following (Dudley and Rosenthal 2006, 12):

- Specific providers, patient populations, or geographic areas
- National measures
- Existing administrative or billing data
- Volunteers
- Specific processes, such as data collection, reporting, or benchmarking

CMS uses an incremental implementation. CMS withheld 0.4 percent of the payment update from hospitals that did not participate in the public reporting of a set of quality measures (Dudley and Rosenthal 2006, 12). A comprehensive description of this incremental approach is provided in the second half of the chapter.

Performance Dimensions and Targets

Determining the dimensions of performance to reward is critical. Dimensions of performance are broad functional areas. VBP/P4P systems may focus on a single performance dimension or may combine multiple dimensions (table 10.1). The choice of dimension or dimensions depends upon and link to the goals of the organizations. Dimensions are sometimes called domains.

Table 10.1.   Selected performance dimensions and examples

Performance Dimension	Example
Clinical outcomes	Monitoring mortality rates and other results of medical care or health services
Clinical process quality	Measuring the number of screening examinations, administration of vaccinations, and other activities related to quality outcomes
Patient safety	Reductions in medication errors and other preventable adverse events
Access to and availability of care	Patients' ability to schedule visits with the provider of their choice when they choose, regardless of the reason for their visit.
Service quality	Friendliness and competence of the office staff, along with other nonclinical factors
Patient experience or satisfaction	Patients' assessments of changes in their health status or other reports of their observations or participation in their healthcare
Patient engagement	Patient portals that facilitate patients' access to their own health record and other actions taken by patients, families, and healthcare providers to help patients
Cost efficiency or cost of care	Comparisons of the relative costs of inpatient hospital admissions for conditions
Cost effectiveness	Comparisons of the relative costs of inpatient hospital admissions for conditions with and without complications and other ways of incorporating quality considerations into efficiency measures
Adherence to evidence-based medical practice	Percentage of heart attack patients who received aspirin at admission and discharge per recommended guidelines and the percentages of patients who received care and treatment per other valid standards of care and service
Utilization	Overuse or underuse of emergency care and other health services
Productivity	Total relative value units divided by clinical work hours and other measures dividing output by input
Administrative efficiency and compliance	Medical loss ratio (MLR), the portion of premium income that insurers pay out in the form of healthcare claims and other indicators of administrative efficiency
Adoption of information technology	Implementation of computerized drug order entry and using other information and communication technologies
Reporting of performance indicators	Pay-for-reporting and other incentives for reporting quality data (see detailed discussion in second half of the chapter)
Participation in performance-enhancing activities	Pay-for-participation and other forms of incentives for participating in quality improvement initiatives

Sources: Chung and Shauver 2009, 77; Cowing 2009, 75; McGlynn 2008, 18; Pope 2011, 34–37; Waldman and Bailit 2014, 4; Woodcock 2013, 317–318.

After determining the dimension or dimensions to reward, leaders must choose specific targets of performance improvement. Researchers at the AHRQ recommend that VBP/P4P systems focus on the following performance targets (Dudley and Rosenthal 2006, 6):

- Most significant problems in terms of quality or cost

- Proportion of population covered by the service or provider

- Availability of valid and reliable performance measures

Success of operations also depends on other factors, such as the characteristics of the incentives, the organizational infrastructure, the culture of quality, and effective leadership (table 10.2).

Analysis of organizational data may reveal problems in delivery of services in terms of quality and cost. Sources of these data include quality and utilization reports, claims data, lawsuits, and patients' or clients' complaints. The literature may also suggest problems prevalent in many healthcare entities that could become the basis of the VBP/P4P program.

VBP/P4P systems should focus on services or providers that affect many patients or enrollees. Although services or providers that affect only a few enrollees are important to those few patients or enrollees, the overall effect of changing behaviors will be small. Moreover, there may be little, if any, return on investment. Thus, experts recommend focusing on services or providers that affect a large proportion of the healthcare entities' populations (Dudley and Rosenthal 2006, 6). In addition to these considerations, other experts recommended that the problems be important to patients or clients (Damberg et al. 2005, 68).

Performance Measures

Measures (indicators) are quantitative tools that provide an indication of an individual's or organization's performance in relation to specified processes or outcomes via the measurement of actions, processes, or outcomes of care or services (Health Level Seven 2014, n.p.). Measures (indicators) may be called performance measures, quality measures, clinical measures, structure measures, process measures, or outcomes measures, depending on the specific activity they are measuring.

Table 10.2. Additional factors in success of value-based purchasing and pay-for-performance systems

Factors	Features
Characteristics of the incentive	• Magnitude affected by overarching payment system, such as fee-for-service or capitation, or other requirements, such as accreditation • Provision of additional funds directly, in the form of revenue, or indirectly, through reduced costs • Ability to determine, using organizational health information technology, the proportion of providers' patients to which the incentive applies • Return on investment as affected by risk, complexity, and socioeconomic factors • Individual, group, hospital, or region (incentives beyond individual involve sophisticated data collection and algorithms)
Infrastructure of health information technologies	• Ability to collect data for measures • Ability to manipulate data for reporting • Capability to provide timely and reliable feedback • Capability to calculate incentives, especially for group recipients of incentives
Shared culture of quality	• Buy-in obtained of all stakeholders • Collaborative focus among healthcare personnel, including physicians, nurses, allied health providers, administrators, and technical and clerical staff on quality and quality improvement • Collective actions among all healthcare personnel • Shared accountability
Effective leadership	• Communication • Clear goals • Effectual teams • Efficient management

Sources: Campbell et al. 2005; Damberg et al. 2005; Dudley 2005.

Common types of performance measures are structure, process, and outcome:

- Structure measures: Characteristics of the healthcare organization, such as the existence of health information technology and its degree of implementation.

- Process measures: Compliance with treatment guidelines or standards of care. Many VBP/P4P measures are focused on activities, such as prescribing appropriate medications for patients.

- Outcome measures: End result of activities or process, such as mortality rates.

In 2009, the NQF endorsed composite measures (NFQ 2009, 2). Composite measures are a combination of two or more individual quality measures in a single measure that results in a single score (NQF 2009, v). These new composite measures address mortality for selected conditions, patient safety for selected indicators, and pediatric patient safety for selected indicators (NQF 2009, vi).

Using good measures is essential. VBP/P4P systems based on poor or weak measures are a waste of time and resources, lack credibility, and do not inspire providers' support and commitment (O'Kane 2007, S4). Good measures have several characteristics:

- Validity: Clinical relevance, scientific soundness, and evidence-based foundation. Valid measures measure what they are intended to measure.

- Reliability: Consistency over time, site, and data collectors.

- Attributability: Being within the control of providers, such as ordering appropriate laboratory tests or prescribing correct medications, rather than measures dependent on patients' or clients' compliance (Damberg et al. 2005, 68).

- Acceptability: Recognition as valid and reliable by the providers whose performance is being assessed (Lester and Campbell 2010, 107).

- Feasibility: Based on data that are available and collectable. Experts recommend that both administrative data and clinical data be used, because administrative data cannot represent all processes of care (Lester and Campbell 2010, 107; Damberg et al. 2005, 77).

- Sensitivity: Capacity for being adjusted for risk and socioeconomic status, for detecting changes, and for discerning differences (Casalino et al. 2007, 495; Tabak et al. 2007, 790; Lester and Campbell 2010, 107).

- Relevance: The area in which a gap in performance affects outcomes and is meaningful to providers, patients, policymakers, and other stakeholders (Lester and Campbell 2010, 107).

Adoption of poor or weak performance measures may have unintended and undesirable consequences and contrary results (Casalino et al. 2007, 495). The accuracy and fairness of a VBP/P4P system is based upon the soundness of its measures.

Sources of good performance measures include the following:

- Joint Commission (Core Measures and ORYX Noncore Measures)

- National Quality Measures Clearinghouse

- National Quality Forum (NQF; endorsed measures)

- NCQA (HEDIS)

- Hospital Quality Alliance (Hospital Consumer Assessment of Healthcare Providers and Systems [HCAHPS])

- AQA Alliance (formerly Ambulatory Care Quality Alliance)

- AHRQ (Consumer Assessment of Healthcare Providers and Systems [CAHPS])

- Leapfrog measures

- CMS (core sets and measures, Medicare Advantage Stars Program measures, Hospital Compare, Nursing Home Compare, and others)

In addition, specialty medical organizations, such as the American College of Rheumatology; American Diabetes Association; National Heart, Lung, and Blood Institute; and National Osteoporosis Foundation provide disease-specific guidelines that some organizations adopt as measures.

Analysts have explored the functioning of VBP/P4P systems for physicians who care for patients with multiple chronic diseases (Boyd et al. 2005, 717). Many medical specialty groups have disseminated clinical practice guidelines for each of these chronic diseases. The VBP/P4P systems have adopted many of the clinical practice guidelines, or standards derived from them, as evidence of the provision of quality of care (superior performance). Thus, these systems reward physicians for providing the elements of the guidelines. Unfortunately, the guidelines are single-disease guidelines; they were developed for each single disease in isolation, not for complex combinations of these chronic diseases. The analysts targeted guidelines for combinations of the following: hypertension, chronic heart failure, stable angina, atrial fibrillation, hypercholesterolemia, diabetes mellitus, osteoarthritis, chronic obstructive pulmonary disease, and osteoporosis (Boyd et al. 2005, 717). The analysts found that single-disease clinical practice guidelines "do not provide an appropriate, evidence-based foundation for assessing quality of care in older adults with several chronic diseases" (Boyd et al. 2005, 720). Moreover, using these clinical practice guidelines to assess the care of these complex cases could lead to inaccurate judgments about the quality of care provided, erroneous calculations of rewards, and potentially, creation of disincentives to treating these patients (Boyd et al. 2005, 722).

Information Systems

Operations of VBP/P4P systems depend on reliable and timely information (Bell and Levinson 2007, 1718). To make this information available to organizational leaders, internal systems of data collection need to be in place. These internal systems include clinical data capture, administrative databases, provider surveys, patient surveys, and longitudinal claims data. These internal systems also must be able to report to the external entities that require the performance and quality data.

This measurement will be greatly enhanced by an infrastructure of health information technology, such as electronic health records and data warehouses. The NQF, Health Level 7, American Health Information Management Association, and several other organizations are beginning to build this infrastructure for performance and quality reporting. These organizations have worked together to develop the Health Quality Measures Format (HQMF) and the Quality Reporting Document Architecture (QRDA). The HQMF is a standard for communicating and incorporating representative measures in electronic health records (and other electronic documents). The QRDA is a standard for collecting and reporting data that documents compliance with performance or quality measures. The QRDA allows the creation and submission of reports in interoperable formats across vendors and disparate health information technology systems (Alschuler et al. 2007, 9). Together, the HQMFs and QRDAs will be able to import, calculate, and export scores on measures in a quality report (Rosenthal 2009, n.p.). These standards advance the automation of performance measurement.

Operations of successful VBP/P4P systems depend on fair methods of allocating rewards, meaningful incentives, effective implementations, significant targets, and suitable performance measures. Success

of operations also depends on other factors, such as the characteristics of the incentives, the organizational infrastructure, the culture of quality, and the effectiveness of leadership (table 10.2).

Check Your Understanding 10.1

1. What three components do value-based purchasing (VBP) systems and pay-for-performance (P4P) systems typically link?

2. What three reports provided the impetus for VBP/P4P systems?

3. True or false? VBP/P4P systems only include financial rewards.

4. True or false? VBP/P4P systems have been slow in getting established since 2004.

5. What are the two major categories of VBP/P4P models?

6. What targets should be the focus of VBP/P4P systems?

Centers for Medicare and Medicaid Services—Linking Quality to Reimbursement

The CMS has articulated its vision for healthcare quality—the right care for every person, every time (CMS 2007a, 3). From this vision and with the support of various laws, CMS has made significant strides to link quality to reimbursement. The Medicare Prescription Drug, Improvement, and Modernization Act of 2003 (MMA) established the framework for CMS to meld together quality and reimbursement. The MMA established the Reporting of Hospital Quality Data for Annual Payment Update (RHQDAPU) program. The move to a P4P component within the inpatient prospective payment system (IPPS) and other medical settings was further strengthened by the DRA when a call for a VBP program was signed into law.

Value-Based Purchasing

Several pieces of legislation, including the MMA and the DRA, set in motion the requirement and need for CMS to develop a VBP program. The DRA, in fact, required CMS to develop a plan for implementation of a VBP program. As established by Congress, the plan had to consider the following issues (CMS 2007a, 2):

- The ongoing development, selection, and modification process for measures of quality and efficiency in hospital inpatient settings
- The reporting, collection, and validation of quality data
- The structure of payment adjustments, including the determination of thresholds of improvements in quality that would substantiate a payment adjustment, the size of such payments, and the sources of funding for the payments
- The disclosure of information on hospital performance

CMS created the Hospital Pay-for-Performance Workgroup to prepare plan options, create a draft plan, and finalize the CMS VBP plan. As stated in the *Medicare Hospital Value-Based Purchasing Plan Issues Paper*, it was expected that CMS would adhere to the following guiding principles in establishing the Medicare Hospital Value-Based Purchasing program (CMS 2007a, 4–6):

- The VBP program will be budget-neutral.
- The VBP program will build on the existing Medicare performance measurement and reporting infrastructure—specifically, the components for the RHQDAPU.
- The VBP performance measures will apply to a broad range of care delivered in the acute-care setting and will address clinical quality, patient-centered care, and efficiency.
- CMS will continue to work collaboratively with the Hospital Quality Alliance, NQF, and Joint Commission.
- The design of the VBP program will avoid creating additional disparities in healthcare and reduce existing disparities.
- CMS will develop and implement ongoing evaluation process to assess effects, examine the utility of the measures, and monitor unintended consequences of the program.

On November 21, 2007, the CMS Hospital Value-Based Purchasing Workgroup presented its Report to Congress: Plan to Implement a Medicare Hospital Value-Based Purchasing Program (CMS 2007a). Furthermore, CMS has published a *Roadmap for Implementing Value Driven Healthcare in the Traditional Medicare Fee-for-Service Program* (CMS 2009). This document provided CMS's vision, goals, key initiatives, demonstration projects, and timeline for its VBP program. Before discussing key initiatives and demonstration projects, it is important to review the vision and goals for VBP. CMS's Vision for America is patient-centered, high-quality care delivered efficiently (CMS 2009, 1–3) with the following goals:

- Financial viability—where the financial viability of the traditional Medicare fee-for-service program is protected for beneficiaries and taxpayers
- Payment incentives—where Medicare payments are linked to the value (quality and efficiency) of care provided
- Joint accountability—where physicians and providers have joint clinical and financial accountability for healthcare in their communities
- Effectiveness—where care is evidence-based and outcomes-driven to better manage diseases and prevent complications from them
- Ensuring access—where a restructured Medicare fee-for-service payment system provides equal access to high-quality, affordable care
- Safety and transparency—where a value-based payment system gives beneficiaries information on the quality, cost, and safety of their healthcare
- Smooth transitions—where payment systems support well-coordinated care across different providers and settings
- Electronic health records—where value-driven healthcare supports the use of information technology to give providers the ability to deliver high-quality, efficient, well-coordinated care

CMS definitely has a transformative effect on the American healthcare system. There is no doubt that VBP will transform healthcare to an environment where clinical and financial outcomes are tied together. The ACA of 2010 mandated the establishment of additional VBP programs in a variety of service areas. Not only did the ACA increase the number of pay-for-reporting programs, but the law also created additional P4P programs for hospital inpatient services, physician services, and the end-stage renal disease benefit under CMS.

Pay-for-Reporting

The development of quality measures is the first step in the establishment of a VBP program. Thus, CMS has established pay-for-reporting programs in several service areas. That is, CMS allows a facility to maintain the full payment for services when it successfully participates in a quality-measure reporting program. In this type of program, quality is not measured per se; rather, the action of reporting data in proper format in the given timeframe is what allows facilities to receive full payment. To monitor the development and implementation of high-caliber quality measures, CMS has created the Measures Management System, which comprises various processes and decision criteria used across service area quality programs. The Measures Management System has been developed in collaboration with the NQF, the AHRQ, the Joint Commission, the NCQA, the American Medical Association Physician Consortium for Performance Improvement, and other measure stakeholders. (More information about the Measures Management System, along with numerous downloads, can be found at http://www.cms.gov/MMS/.) The following text further discusses the hospital inpatient, hospital outpatient, ambulatory surgical center (ASC), long-term healthcare hospital, inpatient rehabilitation, hospice, and physician pay-for-reporting programs.

Hospital Inpatient Quality Reporting

Formerly named the RHQDAPU and the National Voluntary Hospital Reporting Initiative (NVHRI), the Hospital Inpatient Quality Reporting (Hospital IQR) is a quality-based, pay-for-reporting program of CMS. Introduced in section 501(b) of the MMA, this program requires that hospitals report quality information for established quality measures.

Although the MMA created the requirement for hospitals to report quality information, the DRA expanded it. DRA changed the penalty for noncompliance from 0.4 percent reduction to the payment update to 2 percent from FY 2007 on. The standardized amount reduction applies only with respect to the FY involved and will not be taken into account for computing the applicable

percentage increase for a subsequent FY. The DRA also requires that CMS establish procedures for making quality data available to the public after ensuring that a hospital has the opportunity to review, in advance, its data. It also requires that quality measures of process, structure, outcome, and patients' perspectives on care, efficiency, and costs of care are reported on the CMS website. In addition, the DRA required that the quality reporting measures be expanded beginning in 2007. The DRA provides the secretary with the discretion to retire and add quality measures. CMS has modified the measures list each year since 2007 during the IPPS rulemaking process. The measures applicable for data reporting during each payment year are discussed in full detail in the final rule for the IPPS, published in the *Federal Register*.

In 2008, in addition to expanding the quality measures, CMS implemented the **Hospital Quality Alliance (Hospital) Consumer Assessment of Healthcare Providers and Systems (HCAHPS)** patient survey for adoption in FY 2007 (October 1, 2006). HCAHPS is designed to make apples-to-apples comparisons of patients' perspectives on hospital care, including communications with doctors, communications with nurses, hospital staff responsiveness, hospital cleanliness and quietness, pain control, communication about medicines, and discharge information. HCAHPS continues to be used by CMS under Hospital IQR.

Under this program, quality data are reported for both Medicare and non-Medicare patients. Submitted data must pass the validation requirement of a minimum of 80 percent reliability. CMS uses a two-step process that includes a chart review. Facilities have been instructed to submit data through the QualityNet Exchange secure website (http://www.qnetexchange. org). Data populates the Hospital Compare website (http:// www.medicare.gov/hospitalcompare/).

Hospital Outpatient Quality Reporting

Section 109(a) and (b) of the Medicare Improvements and Extension/Tax Relief and Health Care Act of 2006 (MIEA-TRHCA) extended the financial ramification and requirement of reporting quality results to the hospital outpatient and ASC areas. This law established the Hospital Outpatient Quality Reporting (Hospital OQR) program, formerly known as the Hospital Outpatient Quality Data Reporting Program, for hospital outpatient departments.

In the 2008 Final Rule for outpatient prospective payment system (OPPS) and the ASC Payment System, seven quality measures were finalized. Outpatient facilities were required to report quality data on outpatient-specific measures beginning with services provided in April 2008. Hospitals must meet administrative requirements, data collection and submission requirements, and validation requirements under the OQR. Facilities that do not meet all requirements, or those that choose not to participate in the quality program, will receive a two percent reduction in their OPPS rate for the upcoming calendar year.

Similar to the Hospital IQR, CMS updates the outpatient quality measures each year during the OPPS rulemaking process. The measures applicable for data reporting during each payment year are discussed in full detail in the final rule for the OPPS that is published in the *Federal Register*.

Ambulatory Surgical Center Quality Reporting Program

Although section 109(b) of MIEA-TRHCA established the requirement of reporting quality data for the ASC setting, rulemaking for this area was delayed so ASCs could become familiar with the APC-based payment system. The ASC PPS final rule for 2012 released the program details for the ASC Quality Reporting Program (ASCQR). Like the hospital inpatient and outpatient programs, ASC annual update amount is reduced by two percent for facilities that do not adequately or fail to report quality data. In alignment with the other quality reporting programs, the measures applicable for data reporting during each payment year are discussed in full detail in the final rule for the ASC PPS that is published in the *Federal Register*.

Long-Term Care Hospital Quality Reporting Program

Section 3044 of the ACA directed the Secretary of the Department of Health and Human Services (HHS) to establish quality reporting requirements for long-term care hospitals (LTCHs) no later than October 1, 2012. Like the other pay-for-reporting programs, LTCH annual payment update will be reduced by two percent for facilities that do not adequately or fail to report quality data. The quality measures are discussed in detail in the LTCH PPS final rule. Proposed and final rules for each payment system are published in the *Federal Register*.

Inpatient Rehabilitation Hospital Quality Reporting Program

Section 3044 of the ACA directed the secretary of the HHS to establish quality reporting requirements for inpatient rehabilitation hospitals no later than October 1, 2012. Inpatient rehabilitation facilities (IRFs) began reporting quality data beginning October 1, 2012. The reporting or nonreporting of quality data will affect the annual update percentage by negative two percent for the applicable payment year. Discussion regarding the selection of the quality measures can be found in the IRF PPS final rule. Proposed and final rules for each payment system are published in the *Federal Register*.

Hospice Quality Reporting Program (HQRP)

Section 3044 of the ACA directs the secretary of the HHS to establish quality reporting requirements for hospice no later than October 1, 2012. Hospices will report quality information through the Hospice Item Set (HIS). Though the quality measures have the potential to be expanded or retired each year, the 2015 the HIS contains seven measures. The reporting or nonreporting of the data will negatively impact the annual payment update for hospice by two percent. The data quality measures selected for the implementation of the reporting program are as discussed in the *hospice final rule. The final rule should be reviewed each year to identify the quality measures applicable to the year under review.* Proposed and final rules for each payment system are published in the *Federal Register*.

Home Health Quality Reporting

Section 5201(c)(2) of the DRA called for the development of a pay-for-reporting program for home health agencies. The requirements call for quality assessments and Home Health Care Consumer Assessment of Healthcare Providers and Systems Survey (HH CAHPS) data. Providers must submit a minimum set of two assessments for each patient. Valid types of assessments include start of care (SOC), resumption of care (ROC), and end of care (EOC). HHAs report the required quality information through the Outcome and Assessment Information Set (OASIS). Similar to HCAHPS, the HH CAHPS takes into consideration patients' perspectives about the care they receive from a HHA. Thus, this quality program takes into consideration the quality of care provided and the consistency of that care.

CMS has implemented a tiered approach for compliance. For the 7/1/2015 through 6/30/16 reporting period, facilities must meet a 70 percent compliance standard. For the 7/1/2016 through 6/30/17 reporting period, the compliance standard increases to 80 percent. And for 7/1/2017 through 6/30/18 and beyond, providers must meet a compliance standard of 90 percent. (CMS 2015a, n.p.) Providers that fail to meet the compliance standard will receive a two percent reduction from the home health market basket.

Physician Quality Reporting System

TRHCA required that CMS establish a pay-for-reporting system for professionals. The Physician Quality Reporting System (PQRS), formerly known as the Physician Quality Reporting Initiative, inaugurated in 2007, includes an incentive payment for professionals who satisfactorily report data on included quality measures. In 2007, 74 quality measures were available under PQRS. Each year, the number of measures under this program has increased. For CY 2015, there are more than 250 measures from which professionals could select for PQRS reporting. To satisfy the PQRS requirements, providers must submit data for at least nine quality measures across three domains. Providers having at least one face-to-face encounter with a Medicare beneficiary must report one measure from the cross-cutting measure list. The one cross-cutting measure counts as one of the nine required measures. The measures available for each year can be downloaded from the Medicare PQRS webpage (http://www.cms.gov/Medicare/Quality-Initiatives-Patient-Assessment-Instruments/PQRS/index.html).

Providers may submit quality data via their Part B claims, through a Medicare qualified registry, or through a Medicare qualified electronic health record product. Beginning in 2011, group practices could choose a group practice reporting option rather than individual submission. CMS provides numerous informational manuals available to assist professional and group practices with the reporting system. These materials are available via download from the Medicare PQRS webpage.

At inception, professionals who satisfactorily reported quality measures under PQRS received incentive payments of 1.5 percent of their allowed charges for covered professional services. The Medicare Improvements for Providers and Patients Act of 2008 increased the incentive from 1.5 percent to 2.0 percent for 2009 and 2010. However, the adjustment was decreased each year from 2012 through 2014. For CY 2015, the adjustment is 0 percent. Physicians who do not satisfy the PQRS reporting requirements will encounter a PQRS penalty of two percent beginning in 2016.

Pay-for-Performance

After establishing the need to collect data on quality measures comes the need to pay for quality performance. CMS has investigated P4P through several demonstration projects, including the Premier Hospital Quality Incentive Demonstration. The success of this demonstration project was reported to Congress in 2007. In this report, CMS supports the introduction of a broad VBP payment policy for hospitals, which includes payment for quality performance (CMS 2009, 8).

Hospital Value Based Purchasing

Section 3001(a)(1) of the ACA requires CMS to implement a Hospital VBP program that rewards hospitals for the quality of care they provide (CMS 2011b, 26493). In April, 2011, CMS released final rule for a Hospital VBP Program. The Hospital VBP takes the Hospital IQR program to the next level by providing incentive payments for performance achievement and performance improvement. This is a significant VBP step for CMS because hospital payments account for the largest share of Medicare spending, with more than 12.4 million inpatient hospitalizations in 2009 (CMS, 2011c). The MS-DRG base operating payment amounts will be reduced by one percent in FY 2013, rising to two percent by FY 2017 to fund the incentive payments. One hundred percent of the reduction of MS-DRGs base amounts will be redistributed among the participating providers based on their total performance scores. Not all providers are eligible for participation in the incentive program. Providers that are excluded are providers that are

- Subject to payment reductions under Hospital IQR
- Cited for deficiencies during the performance period that pose immediate jeopardy to the health or safety of patients
- Hospitals without a minimum number of cases, measures, or surveys

It is important to note that hospitals excluded from the incentive program will not have the one percent withheld from their operating base MS-DRG amount.

The Hospital VBP will measure hospital performance using four domains: the clinical care domain, safety domain, efficiency and cost reduction domain, and patient experience of care domain. Additional measures will be added for future payment determination years. For each measure, hospitals are scored based on their performance achievement as well as their performance improvement. Performance achievement compares a facility's performance with all other facilities' performance. Performance improvement compares a facility's current performance with the facility's baseline performance. When calculating a facility's total performance score, the safety domain is weighted at 20 percent, the clinical care domain is weighted at 30 percent (outcomes 20 percent and process 15 percent), efficiency and cost reduction domain is weighted at 25 percent and the patient experience of care domain is weighted at 25 percent. These weights apply to the 2015 reporting year for 2017 payment rate determination.

The measures within each domain are scored to determine a score for the domain. The domain scores are combined (based on the above mention weights) resulting in a total performance score (TPS). A facility's TPS determines what portion of the holdback amount (total dollar reduction of base payments for the year) the facility will earn back. For every point increase in the TPS, the provider will increase payment by a portion of the holdback dollars, so in this VBP, a higher TPS score is desired.

ESRD Quality Incentive Program

The End-Stage Renal Disease Quality Incentive Program (ESRD QIP) was established in accordance with Section 153(c) of MIPPA of 2008. The ESRD QIP is a pay-for-performance program linking quality measure performance directly to payment for ESRD services. When a facility's Total Performance Score does not meet standards, the facility will receive a maximum reduction of two percent to all payments during the applicable payment year.

First, data are gathered from all dialysis facilities during a comparison period in order to establish performance standards. Then data from the actual performance period are gathered and compared to the performance standards from the comparison period. To avoid payment reductions, facilities strive to perform at least as well as they did during the comparison period.

Measures are updated each year in the ESRD PPS final rule, published in the *Federal Register*. Examples of ESRD measures include anemia management required for the administration of erythropoiesis-stimulating agents (ESAs) and hemodialysis adequacy. Facilities are provided with a performance score certificate, which must be displayed in English and Spanish in a prominent location at their facility. Scores are also displayed on the Medicare Dialysis Compare website (http://www.Medicare.gov/dialysisfacilitycompare/).

Paying for Value

To move to a mature VBP program, CMS desires to pay for value—that is, to promote efficiency in resource use while providing high-quality care. To achieve this goal, CMS was charged with developing efficiency models that inform providers about the value of their care delivery (CMS 2009, 10). As the first step, CMS established the hospital-acquired conditions provision in the acute-care inpatient setting. Recently, as required by the Affordable Care Act, CMS added the Hospital Readmission Reduction Program and the Physician Feedback Program/Value-Based Modifier adjustment.

Hospital-Acquired Condition Reduction Program

Section 5001(c) of P.L. 109-171, the DRA, required the secretary to implement the hospital-acquired conditions (HAC) provision to IPPS. This additional component of P4P used reported *International Classification of Diseases, Clinical Modification* (ICD) diagnosis codes and the present-on-admission indicator to identify quality issues. The Secretary included in the program conditions that

- Are high-cost or high-volume, or both
- Result in the assignment of a case to a DRG that has a higher payment when present as a secondary diagnosis
- Could reasonably have been prevented through the application of evidence-based guidelines

Under this program IPPS payments were adjusted when HAC conditions were reported as occurring during the hospitalization (the condition(s) was not present on admission). MS-DRG payments were made at a lower level within a MS-DRG family for the admission under review.

Section 3008 of the Affordable Care Act added section 1886(p) to the Act which modified and changed the name of the HAC provision. The HAC Reduction Program incentivizes a facility to reduce HAC conditions beginning October 1, 2014. Hospitals with HAC scores in the lowest-performing quartile will have payments for all encounters reduced by 1 percent beginning in FY 2015. Unlike the Hospital VBP program and the Hospital Readmission Reduction program, the payment reduced under the HAC program is the payment amount after the application of program adjustments such as outlier, DSH, and IME.

There are two domains included in the total HAC score. Measures included in the program are discussed each year during the rule making process. Final measures are reported in the IPPS final rule. Table 10.3 indicates the domains and measures for 2015 through 2017. For 2015, domain I is weighted at 35 percent of the total HAC score and domain II is weighted at 65 percent. For FY 2016, the weighting is modified so that domain I is 25 percent and domain II is 75 percent of the total HAC score.

Each facility receives a confidential HAC report providing the facility's measure scores, domain scores, and total HAC score. Facilities have an opportunity to review the report and to submit changes to the report prior to the data being posted for public viewing on the Hospital Compare website.

Hospital Readmission Reduction Program

Section 3025 of the Affordable Care Act amended by Section 10309 of the ACA added section 1886(q) of the Act to establish the Hospital Readmissions Reduction Program beginning October 1, 2012. Under the Hospital Readmission Reduction Program, IPPS base operating MS-DRG payment amounts are reduced by a hospital-specific adjustment factor that accounts for the hospital's excess readmissions. This program collects readmission data for all patients, not just Medicare beneficiaries. For each applicable year, CMS determines which types of admissions will be included in the readmission measurement. Table 10.4 shows the applicable conditions included in the program for 2015–2017. An encounter is counted as a readmission when the patient returns to an IPPS hospital for the focus conditions within 30 days of discharge from the original admission and the admission is not a planned readmission. CMS has established exclusions to the formula to account for planned readmissions for the focus admissions.

Base operating MS-DRG payments (payment rate prior to application of outlier, IME, DSH, etc) are reduced by the greater of the hospital-specific adjustment amount for the floor adjustment amount. For 2013, the floor adjustment amount was 0.99, in 2014 it was 0.98, and for 2015 and beyond, the floor adjustment amount is 0.97 (HHS 2014, 50025). Thus hospitals that have excess readmissions will have up to three percent of their base MS-DRG operating amount reduced for all admissions during the applicable payment year. Reduction adjustments do not carry over from year to year; rather, hospitals can improve their performance during the measurement year and in turn reduce their reduction during the applicable payment year.

Table 10.3.   HAC Domains and Measures

Domain	Measure
I	AHRQ Patient Safety Indicators (PSI) – 90 composite
II	CDC NHSN* Measures: Catheter associated urinary tract infection (CAUTI) and Central-line associated bloodstream infection (CLABSI) [2015]
	CDC NHSN* Measure: Surgical Site Infection (SSI) for colon and abdominal hysterectomy procedures [added 2016]
	CDC NHSN* Measures: Methicillin-Resistant *Staphylococcus aureus* (MRSA), Bacteremia, and *C. difficile* [added 2017]

*Centers for Disease Control (CDC) National Healthcare Safety Network (NHSN)

Source: CMS 2015 (IPPS), 50090–50091.

Table 10.4.   Hospital Readmissions Reduction Program Focus Areas

Measurement Year	Focus Readmissions	Total Number of Focus Areas
2015	Acute Myocardial Infarction	3
	Heart Failure	
	Pneumonia	
2016	Chronic Obstructive Pulmonary Disease	5
	Total Hip Arthroplasty and Total Knee Arthroplasty	
2017	Coronary Artery Bypass Graft (CABG) surgery	6

Source: CMS 2014 (IPPS), 50025–50028.

Physician Feedback Program/Value-Based Payment Modifier

As CMS moves to be an active purchaser of higher quality, more efficient healthcare through VBP programs, CMS continues to add additional programs to reward physicians whose performance is superior to their counterparts. The Physician Feedback/Value-Based Payment Program provides comparative performance information to physicians and medical practice groups. The underlying concept is that through this information sharing process, physicians will improve the quality of the care they deliver. This concept supports CMS's aim to move toward a physician reimbursement system that rewards value rather than volume.

This program, which applies to fee-for-service Medicare (not Medicare Advantage, Part C) has two primary components. First is the use of Physician Quality and Resource Use Reports (QRURs). The QRURs contain quality information (from PQRS), resource utilization, and cost data for the physician or medical practice group. The data is compared to similar physicians or medical practice groups to add perspective to the gathered information. The second component of this program is the value-based payment modifier (VM). Section 3007 of the ACA mandated that CMS begin to apply the VM to physician payments for all physicians who bill Medicare for services provided under the physician fee schedule (RBRVS). The VM combines the physician's quality level with his or her cost per beneficiary level. In 2015, CMS will apply the VM to all payments for physicians in groups of 100 or more eligible providers. In 2016, the program will be expanded to physician groups of 10 or more eligible providers. All physicians, solo practitioners, and groups will be included in the program for 2017. Physicians can add to their payments by having higher quality and lower cost than their peers. The reduction amount at risk is two percent for 2015. Table 10.5 provides the VM reduction grid for 2016. The reduction amount will increase to four percent in 2017. Interested parties should view modifications and further instructions for this program at the Medicare website, www.cms.gov.

The Future of Value-Based Purchasing

With the passage of the ACA, CMS has made great strides in implementing and successfully executing some components of a VBP program, but there are still many more programs in various patient care settings yet

Table 10.5.   Physician VM Reduction Grid for 2016

	Low Quality	Average Quality	High Quality
Low Cost	+0.0%	+1.0%*	+2.0%*
Average Cost	–1.0%	+0.0%	+1.0%*
High Cost	–2.0%	–1.0%	+0.0%

*Groups of physicians eligible for an additional +1.0%/+2.0% if reporting Physician Quality Reporting System quality measures and average beneficiary risk score is in the top 20 percent of all beneficiary risk scores.
Source: CMS 2013 (MPFS Final Rule), 74770.

to come. On September 8, 2014, Congress passed the Improving Medicare Post-Acute Care Transformation Act (IMPACT), which calls for the Secretary of Health and Human Services to develop a standardized data submission system for long-term care hospitals, skilled nursing facilities, home health agencies and inpatient rehabilitation facilities. The data submission system must be standardized and interoperable to allow for the exchange of information among post-acute care providers and other providers that will facilitate coordinated care and improve outcomes for Medicare beneficiaries. Sample domains to be included in the system include medication reconciliation, incidence of major falls, and discharge to the community.

IMPACT supports the three broad aims of the National Quality Strategy (CMS 2015b, n.p.):

- Better care: Improve the overall quality of care by making healthcare more patient-centered, reliable, accessible and safe.

- Healthy people, healthy communities: Improve the health of the US population by supporting proven interventions to address behavioral, social, and environmental determinants of health in addition to delivering higher-quality care.

- Affordable care: reduce the cost of quality healthcare for individuals, family, employers, and government.

To support the National Quality Strategy, IMPACT upholds CMS Quality Strategy goals:

- Making care safer by reducing harm caused in the delivery of care

- Ensuring that each person and family is engaged as partners in care

- Promoting effective communication and coordination of care

- Promoting the most effective prevention and treatment practices for the leading causes of mortality, starting with cardiovascular disease

- Working with communities to promote wide use of best practices to enable healthy living

- Making quality care more affordable for individuals, families, employers, and governments by developing and spreading new healthcare delivery models.

Parties interested in following the development of the PAC quality initiative can follow the progress at http://www.cms.gov/Medicare/Quality-Initiatives-Patient-Assessment-Instruments/Post-Acute-Care-Quality-Initiatives/PAC-Quality-Initiatives.html.

Several VBP programs are under way, but many stakeholders in the healthcare community continue to request that CMS consider socioeconomic status (SES) within the VBP framework. Comments during the IPPS Final Rule suggested the following regarding the current VPB programs (HHS 2014, 50026):

- Penalize hospitals serving high proportions of low-SES patients.

- Penalize conditions outside a hospital's control.

- Decrease financial resources to the hospitals most likely to treat low-SES patients, which could ultimately lead to lower quality of care.

Some commenters suggested that CMS consider adopting recommendations from the technical report from NQF's Expert Panel on Risk-Adjustment for Socioeconomic Status or Other Sociodemographic Factors. Other commenters supported efforts during the 113th Congress for two bills that supported risk adjustments: S. 2501, "The Hospital Readmissions Program Accuracy and Accountability Act," and H.R. 4188, the Establishing Beneficiary Equity in the Hospital Readmission Program Act. Both of these bills attempt to address the effect of payment penalties on hospitals treating a low-SES population (HHS 2014,

50026). CMS indicated that it will continue to monitor the work of NQF in this area and will work with stakeholders to improve and refine the VBP program.

Check Your Understanding 10.2

1. What is the ramification for hospitals that do not participate in, or do not submit sufficient data under, the Hospital IQR program?

2. How did the hospital penalty change under the revised Hospital-Acquired Conditions Reduction Program?

3. Which focus areas and conditions are included in the Hospital Readmissions Reduction Program?

4. What four domains are included in the Hospital Value-Based Purchasing Program?

5. How does the Physician Feedback Program/Value-Based Payment Modifier support the move to reimbursing physicians for quality rather than quantity?

Chapter 10 Review Quiz

1. What three fundamental characteristics do value-based purchasing (VBP) systems and pay-for-performance (P4P) systems share?

2. Why did VBP/P4P systems emerge?

3. What is attribution, and by what other term is this process known?

4. The very first P4P systems emerged in the early 1990s. True or false?

5. The Centers for Medicare and Medicaid Services (CMS) has attempted to slow the trend toward VBP/P4P systems because its experts believe the linkage of quality and rewards jeopardizes the care of patients. True or false?

6. List at least three other countries that have implemented VBP/P4P systems in their healthcare delivery systems.

7. Withholding compensation would be considered a penalty-based model of VBP/P4P. True or false?

8. What piece of legislation mandated that CMS develop a VBP program?

9. Discuss the difference between "Pay for Reporting" and "Paying for Value."

10. What type of VBP program is the Hospital-Acquired Conditions Reduction Program?

References

Agency for Healthcare Research and Quality. 2002. Evaluating the impact of value-based purchasing: A guide for purchasers. AHRQ Publication no. 02-0029. Rockville, MD: AHRQ. http://archive .ahrq.gov/professionals/quality-patient-safety/quality-resources/ value/valuebased/evalvbp2.html.

Agency for Healthcare Research and Quality (AHRQ). 2014 (August). Highlights: 2013 National Healthcare Quality and Disparities Reports. AHRQ Pub. No. 14-0005-1. Rockville, MD: Agency for Healthcare Research and Quality. http://www.ahrq .gov/research/findings/nhqrdr/nhqr13/2013highlights.pdf.

Alschuler, L., C. Bennett, C. Kallem, J. Kuhl, and F. Yu. 2007. Quality reporting document architecture: Phase I final report. http://www.alschulerassociates.com/library/documents/QRDA_ Phase_I_Public_Report.pdf.

Aryankhesal, A., T.A. Sheldon, and R. Mannion. 2013 (May). Role of pay-for-performance in a hospital performance measurement system: A multiple case study in Iran. *Health Policy and Planning* 28(2):206–214.

Bell, C.M., and W. Levinson. 2007. Pay for performance: Learning about quality. *Canadian Medical Association Journal* 176(12):1717–1719.

Bowser, D.M., R. Figueroa, L. Natiq, and A. Okunogbe. 2013. A preliminary assessment of financial stability, efficiency, health systems and health outcomes using performance-based contracts in Belize. *Global Public Health* 8(9):1063–1074.

Boyd, C.M., J. Darer, C. Boult, L.P. Fried, L. Boult, and A.W. Wu. 2005. Clinical practice guidelines and quality of care for older patients with multiple comorbid diseases. *JAMA* 294(6):716–724.

Briesacher, B.A., T.S. Field, J. Baril, and J.H. Gurwitz. 2009. Pay-for-performance in nursing homes. *Health Care Financing Review* 30(2):1–13.

Brinkerhoff, D.W. 2004. Accountability and health systems: Toward conceptual clarity and policy relevance. *Health Policy and Planning* 19(6):371–379.

Campbell, S., A. Steiner, J. Robison, D. Webb, A. Raven, S. Richards, and M. Roland. 2005. Do personal medical services contracts improve quality of care? A multi-method evaluation. *Journal of Health Services Research and Policy* 10(1):31–39.

Casalino, L.P., G.C. Alexander, L. Jin, and R.T. Konetzka. 2007. General internists' views on pay-for-performance and public reporting of quality scores: A national survey. *Health Affairs* 26(2):492–499.

Centers for Medicare and Medicaid Services (CMS). 2006 (May 14). Glossary. https://www.cms.gov/apps/glossary/default .asp?Letter=M&.

Centers for Medicare and Medicaid Services (CMS). 2007a. Report to Congress: Plan to implement a Medicare hospital value-based purchasing program. Prepared by the CMS Hospital Value-Based Purchasing Workgroup. http://www.cms.hhs.gov/ AcuteInpatientPPS/downloads/HospitalVBPPlanRTCFINAL SUBMITTED2007.pdf.

Centers for Medicare and Medicaid Services. 2009. Roadmap for implementing value driven healthcare in the traditional Medicare fee-for-service program. http://www.cms.hhs.gov/Quality InitiativesGenInfo/.

Centers for Medicare and Medicaid Services (CMS). 2011a. Medicare program; Medicare shared savings program: Accountable care organizations; Final rule. *Federal Register* 76(212):67802–67990.

Centers for Medicare and Medicaid Services (CMS). 2011b. Medicare program: Hospital inpatient value-based purchasing program; Final rule. *Federal Register* 76(88):26490–26547.

Centers for Medicare and Medicaid Services (CMS). 2011c. CMS issues final rule for first year of hospital value-based purchasing program. Press release. http://www.cms.gov/apps/media/press/ factsheet.asp?Counter=3947.

Centers for Medicare and Medicaid Services. 2015a. Home Health Quality Initiative. http://www.cms.gov/Medicare/ Quality-Initiatives-Patient-Assessment-Instruments/ HomeHealthQualityInits/index.html.

Centers for Medicare and Medicaid Services. 2015b. Improving Medicare Post-Acute Care Transformation Act. http://www.cms. gov/Medicare/Quality-Initiatives-Patient-Assessment-Instruments/ Post-Acute-Care-Quality-Initiatives/IMPACT-Act-of-2014-and- Cross-Setting-Measures.html.

Cheng, A.H., and J.M. Sutherland. 2013. British Columbia's pay-for-performance experiment: Part of the solution to reduce emergency department crowding? *Health Policy* 113(1–2):86–92.

Chung, K.C., and M.J. Shauver. 2009. Measuring quality in health care and its implications for pay-for-performance initiatives. *Hand Clinics* 25(1):71-81.

Colais, P., L. Pinnarelli, D. Fusco, M. Davoli, M. Braga, and C.A. Perucci. 2013. The impact of a pay-for-performance system on timing to hip fracture surgery: Experience from the Lazio Region (Italy). *BMC Health Services Research* 13:393: no pages.

Committee on Quality of Health Care in America of the Institute of Medicine. 2001. *Crossing the quality chasm: A new health system for the 21st century*. Washington, DC: National Academy Press.

Committee on Redesigning Health Insurance Performance Measures, Payment, and Performance Improvement Programs, Board on Health Care Services of the Institute of Medicine. 2007. *Rewarding provider performance: Aligning incentives in Medicare*. Washington, DC: National Academies Press.

Cowing, M., C.M. Davino-Ramaya, K. Ramaya, and J. Szmerekovsky. 2009. Health care delivery performance: Service, outcomes, and resource stewardship. *Permanente Journal* 13(4):72–77.

Damberg, C.L., K. Raube, T. Williams, and S.M. Shortell. 2005. Paying for performance: Implementing a statewide project in California. *Quality Management in Health Care* 14(2):66–79.

Damberg, C.L., K. Raube, S.S. Teleki, and E. de la Cruz. 2009. Taking stock of pay-for-performance: A candid assessment from the front lines. *Health Affairs* 28(2):517–525.

Damberg, C.L., M.E. Sorbero, S.L. Lovejoy, G. Martsolf, L. Raaen, and D. Mandel. 2014. *Measuring Success in Health Care Value-based Purchasing Programs. Summary and Recommendations*. Santa Monica, CA: RAND Corporation. http://www.rand.org/pubs/research_reports/RR306.html.

de Brantes, F.S., and B.G. D'Andrea. 2009. Physicians respond to pay-for-performance incentives: Larger incentives yield greater participation. *American Journal of Managed Care* 15(5):305–310.

de Bruin, S.R., C.A. Baan, and J.N. Struijs. 2011. Pay-for-performance in disease management: A systematic review of the literature. *BMC Health Services Research* 11:272: no pages.

Department of Health and Human Services (HHS). 2014. Medicare program: Prospective payment system for Acute Care Hospitals and the Long-Term Care Hospital Prospective Payment System and Fiscal Year 2015 Rates; Quality Reporting Requirements for Specific Providers; Reasonable Compensation Equivalents for Physician Services in Excluded Hospital and Certain Teaching Hospitals; Provider Administrative Appeals and Judicial Review; Enforcement Provisions for Organ Transplant Centers; and Electronic Health Record (HER) Incentive Program; Final Rule. *Federal Register* 79(163):49853–50536.

Devers, K., and R. Berenson. 2009. Timely analysis of immediate health policy issues: Can accountable care organizations improve the value of health care by solving the cost and quality quandaries? Robert Wood Johnson Foundation. http://www.rwjf.org/qualityequality/product.jsp?id=50609.

Diamond, F. 2009. Accountable care organizations give capitation surprise encore. *Managed Care* 18(9):14–15, 21–24.

Dudley, R.A., A. Frolich, D.L. Robinowitz, J.A. Talavera, P. Broadhead, and H.S. Luft. 2004. Strategies to support quality-based purchasing: A review of the evidence. Technical review summary. Technical review 10. Prepared by the Stanford-University of California San Francisco Evidence-based Practice Center under Contract No. 290-02-0017. AHRQ Publication No. 04-0057. Rockville, MD: AHRQ. http:// www.ahrq.gov/downloads/pub/evidence/pdf/qbpurch/qbpurch.pdf.

Duckett, S., S. Daniels, M. Kamp, A. Stockwell, G. Walker, and M. Ward. 2008. Pay for performance in Australia: Queensland's new clinical practice improvement payment. *Journal of Health Services Research and Policy* 13(3):174–177.

Dudley, R.A., and M.B. Rosenthal. 2006. Pay for performance: A decision guide for purchasers. AHRQ Publication No. 06-0047. Rockville, MD: AHRQ. http://archive.ahrq.gov/professionals/quality-patient-safety/quality-resources/tools/p4p/p4pguide.pdf.

Eijkenaar, F., M. Emmert, M. Scheppach, and O. Schöffski. 2013 (May). Effects of pay for performance in health care: A systematic review of systematic reviews. *Health Policy* 110(2–3):115–130.

Emmert, M., F. Eijkenaar, H. Kemter, A.S. Esslinger, and O. Schöffski. 2012. Economic evaluation of pay-for-performance in health care: A systematic review. *European Journal of Health Economics* 13(6):755–767.

Edwards, S.T., A. Bitton, J. Hong, and B.E. Landon. 2014. Patient-centered medical home initiatives expanded in 2009–13: Providers, patients, and payment incentives increased. *Health Affairs* 33(10):1823–1831.

Fields, D., E. Leshen, and K. Patel. 2010. Driving quality gains and cost savings through adoption of medical homes. *Health Affairs* 29(5):819–826.

Fisher, E.S., D.O. Staiger, J.P.W. Bynum, and D.J. Gottlieb. 2007. Creating accountable care organizations: The extended hospital medical staff. *Health Affairs Web Exclusive* 26(1):w44–w57.

Flodgren, G., M.P. Eccles, S. Shepperd, A. Scot, E. Parmelli, and F.R. Beyer. 2011. An overview of reviews evaluating the effectiveness of financial incentives in changing healthcare professional behaviours and patient outcomes. *Cochrane Database of Systematic Reviews* 7(CD009255):no pages.

Friedberg, M.W., E.C. Schneider, M.B. Rosenthal, K.G. Volpp, and R.M. Werner. 2014. Association between participation in multipayer medical home intervention and changes in quality, utilization, and costs of care. *Journal of the American Medical Association* 311(8):815–825.

Goldfield, N., R. Burford, R. Averill, B. Boissonnault, W. Kelly, T. Kravis, and N. Smithline. 2005. Pay for performance: An excellent idea that simply needs implementation. *Quality Management in Health Care* 14(1):42–44.

Greene, S.E., and D.B. Nash. 2009. Pay for performance: An overview of the literature. *American Journal of Medical Quality* 24(2):140–163.

Hackbarth, G.M. 2014 (June 16). Comment letter to CMS on accountable care organizations. http://www.medpac.gov/documents/comment-letters/comment-letter-to-cms-on-accountable-care-organizations-(june-16-2014).pdf?sfvrsn=0.

Harbaugh, N. 2009. Pay for performance: Quality-and value-based reimbursement. *Pediatric Clinics of North America* 56(4):997–1007.

Health Level Seven. 2014. HL7 Version 3 Standard: Representation of the Health Quality Measure Format (eMeasure) DSTU, Release 2. http://www.hl7.org/implement/standards/product_brief.cfm?product_id=97.

Hickson, G.B., W.A. Altemeier, and J.M. Perrin. 1987. Physician reimbursement by salary or fee-for-service: Effect on physician practice behavior in a randomized prospective study. *Pediatrics* 80(3):344–350.

Iglehart, J.K. 2008. No place like home—testing a new model of care delivery. *New England Journal of Medicine* 395(12):1200–1202.

Jackson, G.L., B.J. Powers, R. Chatterjee, J.P. Bettger, A.R. Kemper, V. Hasselblad, R.J. Dolor, R.J. Irvine, B.L. Heidenfelder, A.S. Kendrick, R. Gray, and J.W. Williams. 2013. The patient-centered medical home: A systematic review. *Annals of Internal Medicine* 158(3):169–178.

James, J. 2012 (October 11). Health policy brief: Pay-for-performance. *Health Affairs*. http://m.healthaffairs.org/healthpolicybriefs/brief.php?brief_id=78

James, J.T. 2013. A new, evidence-based estimate of patient harms associated with hospital care. *Journal of Patient Safety* 9(3):122–128.

Keckley, P.H., S. Coughlin, and S. Gupta. 2011. Value-based purchasing: A strategic overview for health care industry stakeholders. Deloitte Center for Health Solutions. http://www.orthodirectusa.com/wp-content/uploads/2013/07/US_CHS_ValueBasedPurchasing_031811.pdf.

Knickman, J.R. 2011. Health care financing. Chapter 3 in *Jonas and Kovner's health care delivery in the United States*, 10th ed. A.R. Kovner and J.R. Knickman, eds. New York: Springer Publishing.

Kohn, L.T., J.M. Corrigan, and M.S. Donaldson, eds. Committee on the Quality of Health Care in America, Institute of Medicine. 1999. *To Err Is Human: Building a Safer Health System.* Washington, DC: National Academy Press.

Laine, C. 2011. Welcome to the patient-centered medical neighborhood. *Annals of Internal Medicine* 154(1):60.

Langdown, C., and S. Peckham. 2014 (June). The use of financial incentives to help improve health outcomes: Is the quality and outcomes framework fit for purpose? A systematic review. *Journal of Public Health* 36(2):251–258.

Lester, H., and S. Campbell. 2010. Developing Quality and Outcomes Framework (QOF) indicators and the concept of 'QOFability.' *Quality in Primary Care* 18(2):103–119.

Long, G., R. Mortimer, and G. Sanzenbacher. 2014 (December). Evolving provider payment models and patient access to innovative medical technology. *Journal of Medical Economics* 17(12):883–893.

MacKinney, A.C., K.J. Mueller, and T.D. McBride. 2011. The march to accountable care organizations—how will rural fare? *Journal of Rural Health* 27(1):131–137.

McClellan, M., A.N. McKethan, J.L. Lewis, J. Roski, and E.S. Fisher. 2010. A national strategy to put accountable care into practice. *Health Affairs* 29(5):982–990.

McGlynn, E.A. 2008 (April). *Identifying, Categorizing, and Evaluating Health Care Efficiency Measures Final Report* (prepared by the Southern California Evidence-based Practice Center—RAND Corporation, under Contract No. 282-00-0005-21). AHRQ Publication No. 08-0030. Rockville, MD: Agency for Healthcare Research and Quality.

Medicaid and CHIP Payment and Access Commission (MACPAC). 2012 (June). Report to the Congress on Medicaid and CHIP. http://www.macpac.gov.

Medicare Payment Advisory Commission (MedPAC). 2009 (June). Report to the Congress: Improving incentives in the Medicare program. http://www.medpac.gov.

Medicare Payment Advisory Commission (MedPAC). 2014 (June). Report to the Congress: Medicare and the Healthcare Delivery System. http://www.medpac.gov.

Menya, D., J. Logedi, I. Manji, J. Armstrong, B. Neelon, and W.P. O'Meara. 2013. An innovative pay-for-performance (P4P) strategy for improving malaria management in rural Kenya: Protocol for a cluster randomized controlled trial. *Implementation Science* 8:48 (no pages).

Merilind, E., K. Vstra, R. Salupere, A. Kolde, and R. Kalda. 2014. The impact of pay-for-performance on the workload of family practices in Estonia. *Quality in Primary Care* 22(2):109–114.

Meyer, J., L. Rybowski, R. Eichler, and I. Fraser. 1997. Theory and reality of value-based purchasing: Lessons from the Pioneers. AHCPR Publication No. 98-0004. Rockville, MD: AHRQ. http://www.ahrq.gov/professionals/quality-patient-safety/quality-resources/tools/meyer/ and http://www.ahrq.gov/professionals/quality-patient-safety/quality-resources/tools/meyer/meyer2.html.

Millenson, M.L. 2004. Pay for performance: The best worst choice. *Quality and Safety in Health Care* 13(5):323–324.

Moran, J., and D. Scanlon. 2013. Slow progress on meeting hospital safety standards: Learning from the Leapfrog Group's efforts. *Health Affairs* 32(1):27–35.

National Committee for Quality Assurance (NCQA). 2012. About NCQA. http://www.ncqa.org/tabid/675/Default.aspx.

National Quality Forum (NQF). 2009 (August). Composite measure evaluation framework and national voluntary consensus standards for mortality and safety—composite measures: A consensus report. http://www.qualityforum.org/Publications/2009/08/Composite_Measure_Evaluation_Framework_and_National_Voluntary_Consensus_Standards_for_Mortality_and_Safety%e2%80%94Composite_Measures.aspx.

Ohldin, A., and A. Mims. 2002. The search for value in health care: A review of the National Committee for Quality Assurance Efforts. *Journal of the National Medical Association* 94(5):344–350.

O'Kane, M.E. 2007. Performance-based measures: The early results are in. *Journal of Managed Care Pharmacy* 13(2 Suppl B):S3–S6.

Petersen, M., P. Gardner, T. Tu, and D. Muhlestein. 2014 (June). Growth and Dispersion of Accountable Care Organizations: June 2014 Update. http://leavittpartners.com/aco-publications/.

Pham, H.H., D. Schrage, A.S. O'Malley, B. Wu, and P.B. Bach. 2007. Care patterns in Medicare and their implications for pay for performance. *New England Journal of Medicine* 356(11):1130–1139.

Pope, G.C. 2011. Overview of Pay for Performance Models and Issues. Chapter 2 in *Pay for Performance in Health Care: Methods and Approaches*. J. Cromwell, M.G. Trisolini, G.C. Pope, J.B. Mitchell, and L.M. Greenwald, eds. Raleigh, NC: RTI Press. http://www.rti.org/rtipress.

Rittenhouse, D.R., S.M. Shortell, and E.S. Fisher. 2009. Primary care and accountable care—Two essential elements of delivery-system reform. *New England Journal of Medicine* 316(24):2301–2303.

Rose, J. 2008. Industry influence in the creation of pay-for-performance quality measures. *Quality Management in Health Care* 17(1):27–34.

Rosenthal, D. 2009. Automating quality management. Presentation at the American Medical Informatics Association Spring Congress, Orlando, FL. http://2009springcongress.amia.org/files/congress2009/S12-Rosenthal.pdf.

Rosenthal, M.B., and R.A. Dudley. 2007. Pay-for-performance: Will the latest payment trend improve care? *JAMA* 297(7):740–744.

Rosenthal, M.B., and R.G. Frank. 2006. What is the empirical basis for paying for quality in health care? *Medical Care Research and Review* 63(2):135–157.

Rosenthal, M.B., R. G. Frank, Z. Li, and A.M. Epstein. 2005. Early experience with pay-for-performance: From concept to practice. *JAMA* 294(14):1788–1793.

Roski, J., R. Jeddeloh, L. An, H. Lando, P. Hannan, C. Hall, and S.H. Zhu. 2003. The impact of financial incentives and a patient registry on preventive care quality: Increasing provider adherence to evidence-based smoking cessation guidelines. *Preventive Medicine* 36(3):291–299.

Rowe, J.W. 2006. Pay-for-performance and accountability: Related themes in improving health care. *Annals of Internal Medicine* 145(9):695–699.

Scott, A., P. Sivey, D. Ait Ouakrim, L. Willenberg, L. Naccarella, J. Furler, and D. Young. 2011. The effect of financial incentives on the quality of health care provided by primary care physicians (Review). *Cochrane Database of Systematic Reviews* 9:CD008451.

Shortell, S.M., F.M. Wu, V.A. Lewis, C.H. Colla, and E.S Fisher. 2014. A taxonomy of accountable care organizations for policy and practice. *Health Services Research* 49(6):1883–1899.

Sia, C., T.F. Tonniges, E. Osterhus, and S. Taba. 2004. History of the medical home concept. *Pediatrics* 113(5):1473–1478.

Smith, V.K., K. Gifford, E. Ellis, R. Rudowitz, and L. Snyder. 2014 (October 14). Medicaid in an Era of Health & Delivery System Reform: Results from a 50-State Medicaid Budget Survey for State Fiscal Years 2014 and 2015. http://kff.org/

Sorbero, M.E.S., C.L. Damberg, R. Shaw, S. Teleki, S. Lovejoy, A. Decristofaro, J. Dembosky, and C. Schuster. 2006. Assessment of pay-for-performance options for Medicare physician services: Final report. RAND Health Working Paper Series. http://aspe.hhs.gov/health/reports/06/physician/report.pdf.

Tabak, Y.P., R.S. Johannes, and J.H. Silber. 2007. Using automated clinical data for risk adjustment: Development and validation of six disease-specific mortality predictive models for pay-for-performance. *Medical Care* 45(8):789–805.

Thomas, F.G., and T. Caldis. 2007. Emerging issues of pay-for-performance in health care. *Health Care Financing Review* 29(1):1–4.

Tompkins, C.P., A.R. Higgins, and G.A. Ritter. 2009. Measuring outcomes and efficiency in Medicare value-based purchasing. *Health Affairs-Web Exclusive* 28(2):W251–W261.

Trisolini, M.G. 2011. Introduction to Pay for Performance. Chapter 1 in *Pay for Performance in Health Care: Methods and Approaches*. J. Cromwell, M.G. Trisolini, G.C. Pope, J.B. Mitchell, and L.M. Greenwald, eds. Raleigh, NC: RTI Press. http://www.rti.org/rtipress.

Tsiachristas, A., C. Dikkers, M.R.S. Boland, and M.P.M.H. Rutten-van Mölken. 2013. Exploring payment schemes used to promote integrated chronic care in Europe. *Health Policy* 113(3):296–304.

Waldman, B., and M. Bailit. 2014 (September). Considerations for State Development of Performance Measure Sets. Robert Wood Johnson Foundation. http://www.rwjf.org/en/research-publications/find-rwjf-research/2014/09/considerations-for-state-development-of-performance-measure-sets.html.

Webber, A. 2012. Eyes on the prize. *Modern Healthcare* 42(46):30–31.

Werner, R.M., R.T. Konetzka, and D. Polsky. 2013. The effect of pay-for-performance in nursing homes: Evidence from state Medicaid programs. *Health Services Research* 48(4):1393–1414.

Wilson, K.J. 2013. Pay-for-performance in health care: What can we learn from international experience? *Quality Management in Health Care* 22(1):2–15.

Witter, S., A. Fretheim, F.L. Kessy, and K.A. Lindahl. 2013. Paying for performance to improve the delivery of health interventions in low- and middle-income countries. *Cochrane Database of Systematic Reviews* 5: (no pages).

Woodcock, E. 2013. Practice Benchmarking. Chapter 11 in *Physician Practice Management: Essential Operational and Financial Knowledge*, 2nd ed. L.F. Wolper, ed. Burlington, MA: Jones & Bartlett Learning.

Wouters, A.V., and N. McGee. 2014. Synchronization of coverage, benefits, and payment to drive innovation. *American Journal of Managed Care* 20(8):e285–e293.

Additional Resources

Center for Medicare and Medicaid Services. 2007. Medicare hospital value-based purchasing plan issues paper. http://www.cms.hhs.gov.

Centers for Medicare and Medicaid Services. 2007. Premier hospital quality incentive demonstration fact sheet. http://www.cms.hhs.gov.

Centers for Medicare and Medicaid Services. 2007. Premier hospital. Quality incentive demonstration project white paper, second year. http://www.premierinc.com/quality-safety.

Centers for Medicare and Medicaid Services (CMS). 2009. http://www.cms.hhs.gov/QualityInitiativesGenInfo.

Centers for Medicare and Medicaid Services. 2011. Hospital value-based purchasing proposal for FY 2014. http://www.cms.gov/apps/media/press/factsheet.asp?Counter=4008.

Centers for Medicare and Medicaid Services. 2015. Post-Acute Care Quality Initiative. http://www.cms.gov/Medicare/Quality-Initiatives-Patient-Assessment-Instruments/Post-Acute-Care-Quality-Initiatives/PAC-Quality-Initiatives.html.

Centers for Medicare and Medicaid Services. 2015. End Stage Renal Disease Quality Incentive Program. http://www.cms.gov/Medicare/Quality-Initiatives-Patient-Assessment-Instruments/ESRDQIP/index.html.

Centers for Medicare and Medicaid Services. 2015. Value-Based Payment Modifier. http://www.cms.gov/Medicare/Medicare-Fee-for-Service-Payment/PhysicianFeedbackProgram/ValueBasedPaymentModifier.html.

Centers for Medicare and Medicaid Services. 2015. ASC Quality Reporting. http://www.cms.gov/Medicare/Quality-Initiatives-Patient-Assessment-Instruments/ASC-Quality-Reporting/index.html.

Centers for Medicare and Medicaid Services. 2015. LTCH Quality Reporting. http://www.cms.gov/Medicare/Quality-Initiatives-Patient-Assessment-Instruments/LTCH-Quality-Reporting/index.html.

Centers for Medicare and Medicaid Services. 2015. Inpatient Rehabilitation Facilities Quality Reporting Program. http://www.cms.gov/Medicare/Quality-Initiatives-Patient-Assessment-Instruments/IRF-Quality-Reporting/index.html.

Centers for Medicare and Medicaid Services. 2015. Hospice Quality Reporting. http://www.cms.gov/Medicare/Quality-Initiatives-Patient-Assessment-Instruments/Hospice-Quality-Reporting/index.html.

Department of Health and Human Services. 2006. Medicare program; Revisions to Hospital Outpatient Prospective Payment System and calendar year 2007 payment rates; Final rule. *Federal Register* 71(226):67960–68401.

Department of Health and Human Services. 2007. Medicare program; Proposed changes to Hospital Outpatient Prospective Payment System and calendar year 2008 payment rates; Proposed rule. *Federal Register* 72(448):42801.

Department of Health and Human Services. 2007. Medicare program; Revisions to inpatient prospective payment system and fiscal year 2008 payment rates; Final rule. *Federal Register* 72(162):47130–48175.

Department of Health and Human Services. 2007. Medicare program; Medicare and Medicaid programs; Interim and final rule. *Federal Register* 72(227):66860–66876.

Department of Health and Human Services (HHS). 2014. Medicare program: Prospective payment system for Acute Care Hospitals and the Long-Term Care Hospital Prospective Payment System and Fiscal Year 2015 Rates; Quality Reporting Requirements for Specific Providers; Reasonable Compensation Equivalents for Physician Services in Excluded Hospital and Certain Teaching Hospitals; Provider Administrative Appeals and Judicial Review; Enforcement Provisions for Organ Transplant Centers; and Electronic Health Record (HER) Incentive Program; Final Rule. *Federal Register* 79(163):49853–50536.

Department of Health and Human Services. 2014. Medicare Program; Revisions to Payment Policies Under the Physician Fee Schedule, Clinical Laboratory Fee Schedule, Access to Identifiable Data for the Center for Medicare and Medicaid Innovation Models and Other Revisions to Part B for CY 2014; Final Rule. *Federal Register* 79(219):67547–68010.

National Business Coalition on Health. Value-based Purchasing Guide. http://www.nbch.org/VBP-Home.

National Quality Forum. 2014. Risk Adjustment for Socioeconomic Status or Other Sociodemographic Factors. www.qualityforum.org/Publications/2014/08/Risk_Adjustment_for_Socioecomic_statuss_or_othter_Sociodemogrpahic_Factors.aspx.

Stanek, M., and M. Takach. 2014 (October). The Essential Role of States in Financing, Regulating, and Creating Accountable Care Organizations. http://www.nashp.org/sites/default/files/The_Essential_Role_of_States_in_Financing_final.pdf.

Appendix A
Glossary

Abuse Unknowing or unintentional submission of an inaccurate claim for payment.

Accountability Obligation of individuals or organizations to provide information about, to be answerable for, and to justify their actions to other actors, along with the imposition of sanctions for failure to comply, to engage in appropriate action, or both.

Accountable care organization (ACO) Primary-care led physician and hospital organization that has voluntarily formed a network to provide coordinated care and to receive a share of the savings it produces while meeting quality and cost targets.

Accounts receivable One of the four components of the revenue cycle; includes the management of the amounts owed to the facility by customers who have received services but whose payment is made at a later date.

Activities of daily living (ADL) Everyday tasks that people can perform without assistance and that are used to measure their functional status and, thus, their need for institutional or assisted care. Representative basic activities of self-care include grooming, dressing the upper and lower body, bathing, transferring, ambulating, toileting, feeding, and eating.

Actual charge Amount provider actually bills a patient, which may differ from the allowable charge.

Add-on Payment adjustment in a federal system that increases reimbursement; often temporarily authorized.

Adjudication The determination of the reimbursement payment based on the member's insurance benefits.

Adjustment Amount that healthcare insurers deduct providers' payments per contracted discounts. *See also* write-off.

Adverse selection Enrollment of excessive proportion of persons with poor health status in a healthcare plan or healthcare organization.

Affordable Care Act (ACA) Brief name for Patient Protection and Affordable Care Act of 2010 (P.L. 111-148), as amended by the Health Care and Education Reconciliation Act of 2010 (P.L. 111-152). Collectively, these two acts are known as the ACA (occasionally PPACA).

AHA Coding Clinic for HCPCS Official coding guidance for Healthcare Common Procedure Coding System (HCPCS) Level II procedure, service, and supply codes.

AHA Coding Clinic for ICD-9-CM A publication issued quarterly by the American Hospital Association and approved by the Centers for Medicare and Medicaid Services (CMS) to give coding advice and direction for *International Classification of Diseases, 9th Revision, Clinical Modification* (ICD-9-CM).

AHA Coding Clinic for ICD-10-CM and ICD-10-PCS A publication issued quarterly by the American Hospital Association and approved by the Centers for Medicare and Medicaid Services (CMS) to give coding advice and direction for *International Classification of Diseases, 10th Revision, Clinical Modification and Procedure Coding System (ICD-10-CM/PCS).*

AHIMA Standards of Ethical Coding Standards developed by the Council on Coding and Classification of the American Health Information Management Association (AHIMA) to give health information coding professionals ethical guidelines for performing their coding and grouping tasks.

All-inclusive rate (AIR) Reimbursement rate for federally qualified health centers and rural health centers. The rate, based on reasonable costs as reported on the healthcare organization's cost report, is subject to annual reconciliation and to a maximum payment per visit (also known as encounter rate).

Allowable charge Average or maximum amount the third-party payer will reimburse providers for the service.

Allowable fee *See* Allowable charge.

Ambulatory payment classification (APC) Hospital Outpatient Prospective Payment System (HOPPS). The classification is a resource-based reimbursement system. The payment unit is the ambulatory payment classification group (APC group).

Ambulatory payment classification group (APC group) Basic unit of the ambulatory payment classification (APC) system. Within a group, the diagnoses and procedures are similar in terms of resources used, complexity of illness, and conditions represented. A single payment is made for the outpatient services provided. APC groups are based on HCPCS/CPT codes. A single visit can result in multiple APC groups. APC groups consist of five types of service: significant procedures, surgical services, medical visits, ancillary services, and partial hospitalization. The APC group was formerly known as ambulatory visit group (AVG) and ambulatory patient group (APG).

Ambulatory surgery center list of covered procedures (ASC list) Procedures that Medicare will cover when they are performed in the ambulatory setting.

Ambulatory surgical center (ASC) Freestanding outpatient facility in which outpatient surgeries are performed.

Ancillary services Professional healthcare services such as radiology, laboratory, or physical therapy.

Appeal Request for reconsideration of denial of coverage or rejection of claim.

Arithmetic mean length of stay (AMLOS) Sum of all lengths of stay in a set of cases divided by the number of cases. The national average number of days patients within a given diagnosis-related group (DRG) are hospitalized.

Assignment of benefits 1. Assignment of benefits is a contract between a physician and Medicare in which the physician agrees to bill Medicare directly for covered services, to bill the beneficiary only for any coinsurance or deductible that may be applicable, and to accept the Medicare payment as payment in full. Medicare usually pays 80 percent of the approved amount directly to the provider of services after the beneficiary meets the annual Part B deductible. The beneficiary pays the other 20 percent (coinsurance). 2. Contract between a health provider and a health insurer (such as Blue Cross and Blue Shield or Aetna) in which the provider directly bills the health insurer on behalf of the patient or client and the health insurer makes payment directly to the provider. The provider agrees to accept the insurer's allowance (allowable charge) as full payment for covered services, less the patient's cost sharing, such as deductibles, co-payments, and coinsurance.

Attribution Assignment of the costs of a patient's care and the outcomes of care to a specific individual provider or group of providers; allows allocation of rewards or penalties (also known as assignment in Medicare).

Average length of stay (ALOS) Average number of days patients are hospitalized. Calculated by dividing the total number of hospital bed days in a certain period by the admissions or discharges during the same period.

Bad debt Services for which healthcare organizations expected, but did not receive, payment.

Balanced Budget Act (BBA) of 1997 Legislation that affected several aspects of the healthcare industry, including the Hospital Outpatient Prospective Payment System (HOPPS), fraud and abuse, and Programs of All-Inclusive Care for the Elderly (PACE).

Base (payment) rate 1. Rate per discharge for operating and capital-related components for an acute-care hospital. 2. Prospectively set payment rate made for services that Medicare beneficiaries receive in healthcare settings. The base rate is adjusted for geographic location, inflation, case mix, and other factors.

Base year 1. Most recent 12-month period for which the Centers for Medicare and Medicaid Services (CMS) has complete and available data on which to calculate and calibrate rates and weights. 2. Cost reporting period on which a rate is based.

Benchmarking The process of comparing performance with a preestablished standard or performance of another facility or group.

Beneficiary An individual who is eligible for benefits from a health plan.

Benefit Healthcare service for which the healthcare insurance company will pay. *See* Covered service.

Benefit cap Total dollar amount that a healthcare insurance company will pay for covered healthcare services during a specified period, such as a year or lifetime.

Benefit period Length of time that a health insurance policy will pay benefits for the member, family, and dependents (if applicable) (also known as policy limit).

Block grant Fixed amount of money given or allocated for a specific purpose, such as a transfer of governmental funds to cover health services.

Budget neutrality Adjusting payment rates so that total expenditures are equal to specified past periods, often mandated under federal acts and regulations.

Budget neutrality adjustor (BN adjustor) Percentage, weight, proportion, or other mechanism that alters payment to maintain budget neutrality.

Budget neutrality factor Percentage in the Inpatient Rehabilitation Facility Prospective Payment System that alters payment to maintain budget neutrality. *See* Budget neutrality adjustor.

Bundling Combination of supply and pharmaceutical costs or medical visits with associated procedures or services for one lump sum payment.

Calendar year (CY) Twelve-month period (year) beginning January 1 and ending December 31.

Capitated payment method Method of payment for health services in which an individual or institutional provider is paid a fixed, per capita amount for each person enrolled without regard to the actual number or nature of services provided or number of persons served. *See also* capitation.

Capitation Method of payment for health services in which an individual or institutional provider is paid a fixed, per capita amount for each person enrolled without regard to the actual number or nature of services provided or number of persons served. *See also* capitated payment method.

Carrier Entity that has a contract with the Centers for Medicare and Medicaid Services (CMS) to determine and make Medicare payments for Part B benefits.

Carve-out Contracts that separate out services or populations of patients or clients to decrease risk and costs.

Case Patient, resident, or client with a given condition or disease.

Case-based payment Type of prospective payment method in which the third-party payer reimburses the provider a fixed, preestablished payment for each case.

Case management Coordination of individuals' care over time and across multiple sites and providers, especially in complex and high-cost cases. Goals include continuity of care, cost-effectiveness, quality, and appropriate utilization.

Case mix Set of categories of patients (type and volume) treated by a healthcare organization and representing the complexity of the organization's caseload.

Case-mix diagnoses Diagnoses in the home health prospective payment system that feed into the home health case-mix grouper.

Case-mix group (CMG) Class of functionally similar discharges in the inpatient rehabilitation facility prospective payment system (IRF PPS). Basis of similarity is impairment, functional capability, age, and comorbidities.

Case-mix index (CMI) Single number that compares the overall complexity of the healthcare organization's patients with the complexity of the average of all hospitals. Typically, the CMI is for a specific period and is derived from the sum of all diagnosis-related group (DRG) weights divided by the number of Medicare cases.

Catastrophic expense limit Specific amount, in a certain timeframe, such as one year, beyond which all covered healthcare services for that policyholder or dependent are paid at 100 percent by the healthcare insurance plan. *See* Maximum out-of-pocket cost *and* Stop–loss benefit.

Category I Code (CPT) A Current Procedural Terminology (CPT) code that represents a procedure or service that is consistent with contemporary medical practice and that is performed by many physicians in clinical practice in multiple locations.

Category II Code (CPT) A Current Procedural Terminology (CPT) code that represents services and/or test results contributing to positive health outcomes and high-quality patient care.

Category III Code (CPT) A Current Procedural Terminology (CPT) code that represents emerging technologies for which a Category I Code has yet to be established.

Center of excellence Healthcare organization that performs high volumes of a service with correspondingly high quality; often recognized by medical peers for its expertise, cost-effectiveness, and superior outcomes. Health insurers may negotiate discounted rates at the organization for the service. To receive full coverage for the service, insureds may be required to receive their service at the healthcare organization.

Centers for Medicare and Medicaid Services (CMS) A division of the Department of Health and Human Services (DHHS) that is responsible for administering the Medicare program and the federal portion of the Medicaid program; responsible for maintaining the procedure portion of the *International Classification of Diseases, 9th Revision, Clinical Modification* (ICD-9-CM). Before 2001, CMS was named the Health Care Financing Administration (HCFA).

Certificate holder Member of a group for which the employer or association has purchased group healthcare insurance. *See* Insured, Member, Policyholder, *and* Subscriber.

Certificate number Unique number identifying the holder (enrollee, member, or subscriber) of a healthcare insurance policy (also known as identification number, member number, policy number, and subscriber number).

Certificate of insurance Formal contract between healthcare insurance company and individuals or groups purchasing the healthcare insurance, detailing the provisions of the healthcare insurance policy (certificate of coverage, evidence of coverage, or summary plan description).

Certification 1. Approval based on inspection by state health agencies. Certified healthcare providers include home health agencies, hospitals, nursing homes, and dialysis facilities. Medicare and Medicaid cover only services rendered by Medicare-certified providers. 2. Process in which a physician verifies and documents that the health services that a patient receives are medically necessary.

Charge Price assigned to a unit of medical or health service, such as a visit to a physician or a day in a hospital. The charge for a service may be unrelated to the actual cost of providing the service. *See* Fee.

Charge capture The process of collecting all services, procedures, and supplies provided during patient care.

Charge description master (CDM) Database used by healthcare facilities to house the price list for all services provided to patients.

Charity care Services for which healthcare organizations did not expect payment because they had previously determined the patients' or clients' inability to pay.

Cherry-picking Targeting the enrollment of healthy patients to minimize healthcare costs.

Civilian Health and Medical Program: Veterans Administration (CHAMPVA) A benefits program administered by the Department of Veterans Affairs for the spouse or widow(er) and children of a veteran who meets specified criteria.

Claim Request for payment, or itemized statement of healthcare services and their costs, provided by a hospital, physician's office, or other healthcare provider. Claims are submitted for reimbursement to the healthcare insurance plan by either the policy or certificate holder or the provider. Also called bills for Medicare Part A and Part B, services billed through fiscal intermediaries, and for Part B, physician or supplier services billed through carriers.

Claim attachment Documentation of supplemental information that assists in the understanding of specific services received by an individual and in the determination of payment (such as documentation that supports medical necessity).

Claim processing activities One of the four components of the revenue cycle; includes charge capture of all billable services, claim generation, and claim corrections occurring before submission to the payer.

Claims reconciliation and collection One of the four components of the revenue cycle; includes reconciling payments, denials, and rejections via write-offs and adjustments. This component also includes the facility's attempts at collecting cost-sharing provisions still due to the facility by the patient.

Claim submission Process of transmitting claims requesting payment to payers.

Classification system 1. A system for grouping similar diseases and procedures and organizing related information for easy retrieval. 2. A system for assigning numeric or alphanumeric code numbers to represent specific diseases and/or procedures.

Clean claim Request for payment that contains only accurate information (no errors in data).

Clearinghouse Entity that acts as an intermediary between providers and payers and that converts health data in nonstandardized formats, such as paper, into standardized electronic formats for processing. May also run software-based audits to verify compliance with payers' edits (internal consistency checks) and accuracy.

Closed panel Type of health maintenance organization that provides hospitalization and physicians' services through its own staff and facilities (also known as staff model or group model).

Code range Applicable set of diagnosis or procedure codes.

Coding Clinic for ICD-10-CM/PCS Official coding guidance for the *International Classification of Diseases, 10th Revision, Clinical Modification and Procedure Coding System* (ICD-10-CM/PCS) diagnosis and procedure codes.

Coding compliance plan A component of a health information management compliance plan or a corporate compliance plan that focuses on the unique regulations and guidelines with which coding professionals must comply.

Cognitive Related to mental abilities, such as talking, memory, and problem solving.

Coinsurance Cost sharing in which the policy or certificate holder pays a preestablished percentage of eligible expenses after the deductible has been met. The percentage may vary by type or site of service.

Community rating Method of determining healthcare premium rates by geographic area (community) rather than by age, health status, or company size. This method increases the size of the risk pool. Costs are increased to younger, healthier individuals who are, in effect, subsidizing older or less healthy individuals.

Comorbidity Pre-existing condition that, because of its presence with a specific diagnosis, causes an increase in length of stay by at least one day in approximately 75 percent of the cases (as in complication and comorbidity [CC]).

Compliance Managing a coding or billing department according to the laws, regulations, and guidelines governing it.

Compliance officer Designated individual who monitors the compliance process at a healthcare facility.

Compliance Program Guidance Information provided by the Office of Inspector General (OIG) of the Department of Health and Human Services (DHHS) to assist healthcare organizations with the development of compliance plans and programs.

Compliance percentage Minimum percentage of inpatient patients receiving intensive rehabilitation services for 13 qualifying conditions to be classified as an inpatient rehabilitation facility.

Complication 1. A medical condition that arises during an inpatient hospitalization (for example, a postoperative wound infection). 2. A condition that arises during the hospital stay that prolongs the length of stay at least one day in approximately 75 percent of the cases (as in complication and comorbidity [CC]).

Comprehensive Error Rate Testing (CERT) program Measures improper payments for the Medicare fee for services payment systems as mandated by the Improper Payments Elimination and Recovery Improvement Act of 2012.

Concurrent therapy The practice of one professional therapist treating multiple patients at the same time while the patients are performing different therapeutic activities in which residents cannot benefit from observing other residents in the group because everyone is performing different activities.

Confined to the home Normal inability to leave the home in which leaving the home requires considerable and taxing effort, requires physical assistance, or is medically contraindicated.

Consolidated billing (CB) Facility submits one consolidated bill to Medicare Administrative Contractor covering the services, such as laboratory, x-ray, and pharmacy, received by the patient, client, or resident during admission to the facility, including services from outside vendors.

Consumer-directed (consumer-driven) healthcare plan (CDHP) Form of healthcare insurance characterized by influencing patients and clients to select cost-efficient healthcare through the provision of information about health benefit packages and through financial incentives.

Contracted discount rate Type of fee-for-service reimbursement in which the third-party payer has negotiated a reduced (discounted) fee for its covered insureds. *See* Discounted fee-for-service.

Conversion factor (CF) National dollar multiplier that sets the allowance for the relative values; a constant.

Coordination of benefits (COB) Method of integrating benefits payments from multiple healthcare insurers to ensure that payments do not exceed 100 percent of the covered healthcare expenses.

Copayment Cost-sharing measure in which the policy or certificate holder pays a fixed dollar amount (flat fee) per service, supply, or procedure that is owed to the healthcare facility by the patient. The fixed amount that the policyholder pays may vary by type of service, such as $20 per prescription or $15 per physician office visit.

Core-based statistical area (CBSA) Statistical geographic entity consisting of the county or counties associated with at least one core (urbanized area or urban cluster) of at least 10,000 population, plus adjacent counties having a high degree of social and economic integration with the core as measured through commuting ties with the counties containing the core. Metropolitan and micropolitan statistical areas are two components of CBSAs.

Cost-of-living adjustment (COLA) Alteration that reflects a change in the consumer price index (CPI), which measures purchasing power between time periods. The CPI is based on a market basket of goods and services that a typical consumer buys.

Cost report Report required from providers on an annual basis for the Medicare program to make a proper determination of amounts payable to providers under its provisions.

Cost sharing Provision of a healthcare insurance policy that requires policyholders to pay for a portion of their healthcare services; a cost-control mechanism.

Covered condition Health condition, illness, injury, disease, or symptom for which the healthcare insurance company will pay.

Covered service (expense) Specific service for which a healthcare insurance company will pay. *See* Benefit.

CPT Assistant Official coding guidance for Current Procedural Terminology (CPT) codes.

Critical access hospital (CAH) Small facility that gives limited outpatient and inpatient hospital services to people in rural areas.

Critical care services Evaluation and management of critically ill or critically injured patients.

Current Procedural Terminology (CPT) Coding system created and maintained by the American Medical Association that is used to report diagnostic and surgical services and procedures.

Customary, prevailing, and reasonable (CPR) Type of retrospective fee-for-service payment method in which the third-party payer pays for fees that are customary, prevailing, and reasonable.

Deductible Annual amount of money that the policyholder must incur (and pay) before the health insurance will assume liability for the remaining charges or covered expenses.

Dependent An insured's spouse, children and young adults until they reach age 26, and dependents with disabilities without an age limit. The definition of children includes natural children, legally adopted children, stepchildren, and children who are dependent during the waiting period before adoption. Children and young adults are eligible regardless of any, or a combination of any, of the following factors: financial dependency, residency with parent, student status, employment, and marital status; except for employer-based plans existing before March 23, 2010, which may state that young adults can qualify for dependent coverage only if they are not eligible for an employment-based health insurance plan. Some healthcare insurance policies also allow same-sex domestic partners to be listed as dependents.

Dependent (family) coverage Healthcare insurance benefits for spouses, children, or both of the member (enrollee, subscriber, certificate holder); coverage is dependent on relationship with member.

Diagnosis-related group (DRG) Inpatient classification that categorizes patients who are similar in terms of diagnoses and treatments, age, resources used, and lengths of stay. Under the prospective payment system (PPS), hospitals are paid a set fee for treating patients in a single DRG category, regardless of the actual cost of care for the individual.

Dirty (dingy, unclean) claim Claim that has a defect or impropriety. *See* Clean claim.

Discounted fee-for-service Type of fee-for-service reimbursement in which the third-party payer has negotiated a reduced ("discounted") fee for its covered insureds. *See* Contracted discount rate.

Discounting Reducing the payment in the Hospital Outpatient Prospective Payment System (OPPS) (payment status indicator = T). In the CMS discounting schedule, Medicare will pay 100 percent of the Medicare allowance for the principal procedure (exclusive of deductible and copayment) and 50 percent (50 percent discount) of the Medicare allowance for each additional procedure. For example, if two CT scans (APC group 0349) are performed in the same visit, the first is reimbursed at the full APC group rate and the second at 50 percent of the APC group rate.

Disease management Program focused on preventing exacerbations of chronic diseases and on promoting healthier lifestyles for patients and clients with chronic diseases.

Disproportionate share hospital (DSH) Healthcare organizations meeting governmental criteria for percentages of indigent patients. Hospital with an unequally (disproportionately) large share of low-income patients. Federal payments to these hospitals are increased to adjust for the financial burden.

Dual eligible (dual) Person who qualifies for both Medicare and Medicaid.

Durable medical equipment (DME) Equipment and supplies, such as oxygen equipment, wheelchairs, crutches, or blood testing strips for diabetics, ordered by a healthcare provider for everyday or extended use.

Edit Algorithm in computer software applications that is an internal check for consistency and accuracy.

Editor Logic (algorithms) within computer software that evaluates data for inconsistencies and other errors and is used during claim submission.

Electronic claim submission Paperless transmission of claims with health data in standardized format through a computer software system or via the Internet. *See* Claim submission.

Electronic funds transfer (EFT) Electronic exchange or transfer of money from one account to another through computer software systems.

Electronic prescribing (e-prescribing or eRx) Transmission of prescription or prescription-related information through electronic media among prescriber, dispenser, pharmacy, benefit manager, or a health plan.

Electronic Prescribing (E-prescribing) Incentive Program Initiative under Section 132 of the Medicare Improvements for Patients and Providers Act (MIPPA) of 2008 in which eligible professionals who are successful e-prescribers receive an incentive payment. *See* Eligible professional.

Electronic remittance advice (ERA) Electronic document that details the payer's determination of the payment, denial, or suspension of a provider's claim.

Eligibility Set of stipulations that qualify a person to apply for healthcare insurance, examples include percentage of the appointment or duration of employment.

Eligible professional (EP) Physician, practitioner, or therapist defined by statute who is eligible to participate in the Medicare Physician Quality Reporting Initiative and in the Medicare E-Prescribing Incentive Program. The eligible professionals' services must be paid under the Medicare physician fee schedule and not under some other fee schedule or reimbursement method.

Encounter Professional, direct personal contact between a patient and a provider who delivers services or is professionally responsible for services delivered to a patient. Face-to-face contact between a patient and a provider who has primary responsibility for assessing and treating the condition of the patient at a given contact and exercises independent judgment in the care of the patient.

Endorsement Language or statements within a healthcare insurance policy providing additional details about coverage or lack of coverage for special situations that are not usually included in standard policies. May function as a limitation or exclusion.

Enrollee Covered member or covered member's dependent of a health maintenance organization (HMO).

Enrollment Initial process in which new individuals apply and are accepted as members (subscribers, enrollees) of healthcare insurance plans.

Episode of care One or more healthcare services given by a provider during a specific period of relatively continuous care in relation to a particular health or medical problem or situation. In home health, the episode of care is all home care services and nonroutine medical supplies delivered to a patient during a 60-day period. In the home health prospective payment system (HHPPS), the episode of care is the unit of payment.

Episode-of-care reimbursement Healthcare payment method in which providers receive one lump sum for all care they provide related to a condition or disease. *See* Episode of care.

Etiologic diagnosis Underlying cause of the problem that led to the condition requiring admission to an inpatient rehabilitation facility.

Evidence-based clinical practice guideline Explicit statement that guides clinical decision making and has been systematically developed from scientific evidence and clinical expertise to answer clinical questions. Systematic use of guidelines is termed evidence-based medicine.

Exclusion Situation, instance, condition, injury, or treatment that the healthcare plan states will not be covered and for which the healthcare plan will pay no benefits (synonym is *impairment rider*).

Exclusive provider organization (EPO) Hybrid managed care organization that is sponsored by self-insured (self-funded) employers or associations and exhibits characteristics of both health maintenance organizations and preferred provider organizations.

Explanation of benefits (EOB) Report sent from a healthcare insurer to the policyholder and to the provider that describes the healthcare service, its cost, applicable cost sharing, and the amount the healthcare insurer will cover. The remainder is the policyholder's responsibility.

False Claims Act Legislation passed during the Civil War that prohibits contractors from making a false claim to a governmental program; used to reinforce healthcare against fraud and abuse.

Family coverage Healthcare insurance coverage for dependents of the policyholder, such as spouses and children.

Federal Employees' Compensation Act (FECA) of 1916 A benefit program that ensures that civilian employees of the federal government are provided medical, death, and income benefits for work-related injuries and illnesses.

Federal Register The daily publication of the US Government Printing Office that reports all regulations (rules); legal notices of federal administrative agencies, of departments of the executive branch, and of the president; and federally mandated standards, including Healthcare Common Procedure Coding System (HCPCS) and *International Classification of Diseases, 9th Revision, Clinical Modification* (ICD-9-CM) codes.

Federally qualified health center (FQHC) Nonprofit, patient-governed, and community-directed healthcare organization with the purpose of increasing access to comprehensive basic healthcare services.

Federally qualified health center prospective payment system (FQHC PPS) Medicare reimbursement system implemented in 2014 to compensate federally qualified health centers according to a prospectively established base rate for geographic locality and patients' characteristics.

Fee Price assigned to a unit of medical or health service, such as a visit to a physician or a day in a hospital. A fee for a service may be unrelated to the actual cost of providing the service. *See* Charge.

Fee schedule Third-party payer's predetermined list of maximum allowable fees for each healthcare service.

Fee-for-service (FFS) reimbursement Healthcare payment method in which providers retrospectively receive payment for each service rendered.

Final rule Regulation published by an agency, commented on by public comment, and published in its official form in the *Federal Register*. Has the force of law on its effective date.

First mover Initial innovators; other organizations follow trying to obtain success similar to first organization.

Fiscal intermediary (FI) Local payment branch of the Medicare program. Intermediaries are public or private insurance companies that contract with the Centers for Medicare and Medicaid Services (CMS) to act as agents of the federal government in dealing directly with participating providers of Medicare services. An intermediary is usually, but not necessarily, an insurance company, such as Blue Cross. FIs reimburse for inpatient or hospital services (Part A Medicare) and some Part B services.

Fiscal year (FY) Yearly accounting period; the 12-month period on which a budget is planned. The federal fiscal year is October 1 through September 30 of the next year. Some state fiscal years are July 1 through June 30 of the next year. Often, agencies and companies match their fiscal years to the state and federal governments with which they contract.

Flexible spending (savings) account (FSA) Special account, funded by employees' contributions, to pay for qualified medical care and expenses. Employees determine the pretax deduction deposited into the account, up to the limit set by the employer. Funds from one FSA plan year cannot roll forward (carry over) to the next FSA plan year.

Formulary Continually updated list of safe, effective, and cost-effective drugs, generic and brand name, that the health plan prefers that insureds use. *See also* Preferred drug list.

Fraud Intentionally making a claim for payment that one knows to be false.

Functional independent assessment tool Standardized tool to measure the severity of patients' impairments in rehabilitation settings. The tool captures characteristics that reflect the functional status of patients. Patients with lower scores on the tool have less independence and need more assistance than patients with higher scores.

Functional status Patient's ability to perform the activities of daily living.

Gatekeeper Healthcare provider or entity responsible for determining the healthcare services a patient or client may access. The gatekeeper may be a primary care provider, a utilization review or case management agency, or a managed care organization.

Geographic practice cost index (GPCI) Index based on relative difference in the cost of a market basket of goods across geographic areas. A separate GPCI exists for each element of the relative value unit (RVU), which includes physician work, practice expenses, and malpractice. GPCIs are a means to adjust the RVUs, which are national averages, to reflect local costs of service.

Geometric mean length of stay (GMLOS) Statistically adjusted value of all cases of a given diagnosis-related group (DRG), allowing for the outliers, transfer cases, and negative outlier cases that would normally skew the data. The GMLOS is used to compute hospital reimbursement for transfer cases.

Global payment method Method of payment in which the third-party payer makes one consolidated payment to cover the services of multiple providers who are treating a single episode of care.

Group number Number identifying the employer, association, or other entity that purchases healthcare insurance for the individual members of the group. Individuals in the group have the same set of healthcare benefits.

Group practice model Type of health maintenance organization (HMO) in which the HMO contracts with a medical group and reimburses the group on a fee-for-service or capitation basis. *See* Closed panel.

Group (practice) (clinic) without walls (GWW, GPWW, CWW) Type of integrated delivery system in which the individual physicians share administrative systems but maintain their separate practices and offices distributed over a geographic area. (Also known as clinic without walls [CWW].)

Group therapy The practice of one therapist providing the same therapeutic services to everyone in the group, in which residents may benefit by observing other residents in the group performing the same activity.

Grouper Computer program using specific data elements to assign patients, clients, or residents to groups, categories, or classes.

Guaranteed issue Federal requirement that a healthcare insurer allow individuals to enroll in the health plan regardless of their health, age, gender, or other factors that might predict use of health services.

Guarantor Person who is responsible for paying the bill or guarantees payment for healthcare services. Patients who are adults are often their own guarantor. Parents guarantee payments for the healthcare costs of their children.

Hard coding Use of the charge description master to code repetitive services.

Health Care and Education Reconciliation Act of 2010 (P.L. 111-152) *See* Affordable Care Act (ACA).

Health disparity Population-specific difference in the presence of disease, health outcomes, quality of healthcare, and access to healthcare services that exists across racial and ethnic groups.

Health Insurance Portability and Accountability Act (HIPAA) of 1996 Significant piece of legislation aimed at improving healthcare data transmission among providers and insurers; designated code sets to be used for electronic transmission of claims.

Health Insurance Prospective Payment System (HIPPS) code Five-character alphanumeric code used in the home health prospective payment system (HHPPS) and in the inpatient rehabilitation facility prospective payment system (IRF PPS). In the HHPPS, the HIPPS code is derived or computed from the home health resource group (HHRG). In the IRF PPS, the HIPPS code is derived from the case-mix group and comorbidity. Reimbursement weights for each HIPPS code correspond to the levels of care provided.

Health maintenance organization (HMO) Entity that combines the provision of healthcare insurance and the delivery of healthcare services. Characterized by (1) organized healthcare delivery system to a geographic area, (2) set of basic and supplemental health maintenance and treatment services, (3) voluntarily enrolled members, and (4) predetermined fixed, periodic prepayments for members' coverage. Prepayments are fixed, without regard to actual costs of healthcare services provided to members.

Health reimbursement arrangement (HRA) Combination of an employee-benefit health insurance plan and a separate arrangement to reimburse employees for all or a portion of the qualified medical expenses not paid by the health insurance policy. Though often referred to as health reimbursement accounts, no separately funded account is required.

Health savings account (HSA) Special pretax saving account into which employees, and sometimes employers, deposit money that subscribers can later withdraw to pay for qualified medical care and expenses. Unused funds can roll forward to subsequent years.

Healthcare Common Procedure Coding System (HCPCS) Coding system created and maintained by the Centers for Medicare and Medicaid Services (CMS) that provides codes for procedures, services, and supplies not represented by a Current Procedural Terminology (CPT) code.

High-cost outlier Case with extraordinarily high costs exceeding the typical costs of similar cases. *See also* Outlier.

High-cost threshold Criterion for assessing whether technologies would be inadequately paid under the inpatient prospective payment system (IPPS). The sum of the geometric mean and the lesser of 0.75 of the national adjusted operating standardized payment amount (increased to reflect the difference between costs and charges) or 0.75 of one standard deviation of mean charges by diagnosis-related group (DRG).

High deductible health plan (HDHP) Most common type of consumer-directed healthcare; insurance policy's deductibles are higher than traditional healthcare insurance plans. Combined with health savings accounts or health reimbursement arrangements, HDHPs allow subscribers to pay for qualified medical care and expenses on a pretax basis.

High-risk pool An insurance plan (often a state healthcare insurance plan) that covers unhealthy or medically uninsurable people whose healthcare costs will be higher than average and whose utilization of healthcare services will be higher than average. Also the term for the small group of unhealthy individuals who have the high probability of incurring many healthcare services at high costs.

Hold-harmless status Status in which one party does not hold the other party responsible.

Home Assistance Validation and Entry (HAVEN) Computer software for the collection and submission of the data elements in the Outcome Assessment Information Set (OASIS). HAVEN is used in the home health prospective payment system (HHPPS).

Home health agency (HHA) Organization that provides services in the home. These services include skilled nursing care, physical therapy, occupational therapy, speech therapy, and personal care by home health aides.

Home health resource group (HHRG) Classifications (groups) for the home health prospective payment system (HHPPS) derived from the data elements in the Outcome Assessment Information Set (OASIS). The HHRG is a six-character alphanumeric code that represents a severity level in three domains.

Hospice Interdisciplinary program of palliative care and supportive services that addresses the physical, spiritual, social, and economic needs of terminally ill patients and their families. *See* Palliative care.

Hospital within hospital (HwH) Long-term care hospital physically located within another hospital.

ICD-10-CM Coordination and Maintenance Committee Committee composed of representatives from the National Center for Health Statistics (NCHS) and the Centers for Medicare and Medicaid Services (CMS) that is responsible for maintaining the US clinical modification version of the *International Classification of Diseases, 10th Revision, Clinical Modification and Procedure Coding System* (ICD-10-CM/PCS) code sets.

Impairment group code (IGC) Multidigit code that represents the primary reason for a patient's admission to an inpatient rehabilitation facility.

Improper payment review Evaluation of claims to determine whether the items and/or services are covered, correctly coded and medically necessary.

Indemnity health insurance Traditional, fee-for-service healthcare plan in which the policyholder pays a monthly premium and a percentage of the usual, customary, and reasonable healthcare costs, and the patient can select the provider.

Independent practice association (IPA) or organization (IPO) Type of health maintenance organization (HMO) in which participating physicians maintain their private practices, and the HMO contracts with the independent practice association. The HMO reimburses the IPA on a capitated basis; the IPA may reimburse the physicians on a fee-for-service or a capitated basis.

Indian Health Service (IHS) An agency within the Department of Health and Human Services (DHHS) responsible for upholding the federal government's obligation to promote healthy American Indian and Alaskan native people, communities, and cultures.

Indirect medical education (IME) adjustment Percentage increase in Medicare reimbursement to offset the costs of medical education that a teaching hospital incurs.

Individual (single) coverage Healthcare insurance benefits that cover only one individual, the member (enrollee, subscriber, certificate holder).

Individual therapy Therapy delivered one-on-one between a physical, occupational, or speech therapist and a resident, patient, or client.

In-network Set of physicians, hospitals, and other providers who have formal agreements with health insurers under which patients and clients receive services at a discounted rate; preferred set of providers. *See* Out-of-network.

Inpatient psychiatric facility (IPF) A hospital or hospital unit that provides psychiatric care for patients.

Inpatient rehabilitation facility (IRF) Inpatient facility that provides intense multidisciplinary rehabilitation services. Facility specializing in the restorative processes and therapies that develop and maintain self-sufficient functioning consistent with individuals' capabilities. Rehabilitative services restore function after an illness or injury. Services are provided by psychiatrists, nurses, and physical, occupational, and speech therapists. The facility may be freestanding or a specialized unit in an acute-care hospital.

Inpatient rehabilitation facility patient assessment instrument (IRF PAI) Data collection tool specific to rehabilitation facilities.

Inpatient Rehabilitation Validation and Entry (IRVEN) Computer software for data entry in inpatient rehabilitation facilities (IRFs). Captures data for the IRF patient assessment instrument (IRF PAI) and supports electronic submission of the IRF PAI. Also allows data import and export in the standard record format of the Centers for Medicare and Medicaid Services (CMS).

Insurance Reduction of a person's (insured's) exposure to risk of loss by having another party (insurer) assume the risk.

Insured Individual or entity that purchases healthcare insurance coverage. *See* Certificate holder, Member, Policyholder, *and* Subscriber.

Integrated delivery system (IDS) Generic term for the separate legal entity that healthcare providers form to offer a comprehensive set of healthcare services to a population. Other terms are health delivery network, horizontally integrated system, integrated services network (ISN), and vertically integrated system.

Integrated provider organization (IPO) Corporate, managerial entity that includes one or more hospitals, a large physician group practice, other healthcare organizations, or various configurations of these businesses.

Integrated revenue cycle (IRC) The coordination of all revenue cycle activities (facility and physician) under a single leadership and team structure.

***International Classification of Diseases, 9th Revision, Clinical Modification* (ICD-9-CM)** Coding and classification system used to report diagnoses in all healthcare settings and inpatient procedures and services.

***International Classification of Diseases, 10th Revision, Clinical Modification* (ICD-10-CM/PCS)** Coding and classification system used to report diagnoses in all healthcare settings and inpatient procedures and services. The procedure code set is separate from the diagnosis code set and is referred to as Procedure Coding System (PCS).

Interrupted stay Discharge in which the patient was discharged from the inpatient rehabilitation facility but returned within three calendar days.

Key performance indicator Area identified for needed improvement through benchmarking and continuous quality improvement.

Labor-related share (portion, ratio) Sum of facilities' relative proportion of wages and salaries, employee benefits, professional fees, postal services, other labor-intensive services, and the labor-related share of capital costs from the appropriate market basket. Labor-related share is typically 70–75 percent of healthcare facilities' costs. Adjusted annually and published in the *Federal Register*.

Late enrollee Individual who does not enroll in a group healthcare plan at the first opportunity but enrolls later if the plan has a general open enrollment period.

Length of stay (LOS) Number of days a patient remains in a healthcare organization. The statistic is the number of calendar days from admission to discharge, including the day of admission but not the day of discharge. This statistic may have an impact on prospective reimbursement.

Limitation Qualification or other specification that reduces or restricts the extent of the healthcare benefit.

Local Coverage Determination (LCD) Reimbursement and medical-necessity policies established by regional fiscal intermediaries. New format for Local Medical Review Policies (LMRPs). LCDs and LMRPs vary from state to state.

Locality Geographic payment area based on differences in the cost of resources; currently about 90 localities exist, formed by state boundaries, political or economic subdivisions within a state, or a group of states (defined at 42 CFR 405.505).

Long-term care hospital (LTCH) Hospitals that provide general acute-care and specialized services to patients who have longer-than-average lengths of stay. These patients may have chronic diseases or acute diseases that require long-term therapies. The Centers for Medicare and Medicaid Services (CMS) has two ways to categorize hospitals as LTCHs. First, an LTCH has an average length of stay for Medicare patients that is 25 days or longer. Second, an LTCH can be a hospital excluded from the inpatient prospective payment system that has an average length of stay for all patients that is 20 days or longer.

Long-term care hospital Continuity Assessment and Record Evaluation (CARE) Data Set Uniform and standardized instrument to assess patients.

Low-utilization payment adjustment (LUPA) Payment adjustment applied when a home health agency provides four or fewer visits in an episode of care.

Major complication/comorbidity (MCC) Diagnosis codes classified as MCCs reflect the highest level of severity. *See* Complications/comorbidities (CC).

Major diagnostic category (MDC) Highest level in hierarchical structure of the federal inpatient prospective payment system (IPPS). The 25 MDCs are primarily based on body system involvement, such as MDC No. 06, Diseases and Disorders of the Digestive System. However, a few categories are based on disease etiology—for example, Human Immunodeficiency Virus Infections.

Malpractice (MP) Element of the relative value unit (RVU); costs of the premiums for professional liability insurance. *See also* professional liability insurance.

Managed care Payment method in which the third-party payer has implemented some provisions to control the costs of healthcare while maintaining quality care. Systematic merger of clinical, financial, and administrative processes to manage access, cost, and quality of healthcare.

Managed care organization (MCO) Entity that integrates the financing and delivery of specified healthcare services. Characterized by (1) arrangements with specific providers to deliver a comprehensive set of healthcare services, (2) criteria for selecting providers, (3) quality assessment and utilization review, and (4) incentives for members to use plan providers. Also known as coordinated care organization.

Management (medical) service organization (MSO) Specialized entity that provides management services and administrative and information systems to one or more physician group practices or small hospitals. An MSO may be owned by a hospital, physician group, physician-hospital organization, integrated delivery system, or investors.

Manager's amendment Legislative mechanism in which a package of numerous individual amendments is added to a bill. The "managers" are the majority and minority members who led their respective legislative factions in the bill's debate.

Market basket Mix of goods and services appropriate to the setting, such as home health services or skilled nursing facilities.

Market basket index Relative measure that averages the costs of a mix of goods and services.

Maximum out-of-pocket cost Specific amount, in a certain timeframe, such as one year, beyond which all covered healthcare services for that policyholder or dependent are paid at 100 percent by the healthcare insurance plan. *See* Catastrophic expense limit *and* Stop–loss benefit.

Meaningful use Providers' use of electronic health records to achieve significant improvement in health services. Included are activities such as entering basic patient data, using software applications to improve safety and quality, exchanging health information, and submitting clinical quality and other measures.

Measure (indicator) 1. The quantifiable data about a function or process. 2. An activity, event, occurrence, or outcome that is to be monitored and evaluated to determine whether it conforms to standards; commonly relates to the structure, process, and/or outcome of an important aspect of care; also called a criterion. (3) A measure used to determine an organization's performance over time. (4) Activity that affects an outcome (types include process measures and quality measures). (5) Compliance with treatment guidelines or standards of care.

Measurement Systematic process of data collection, repeated over time or at a single point in time.

Medicaid Part of the Social Security Act, a joint program between state and federal governments to provide healthcare benefits to low-income persons and families.

Medical emergency Severe injury or illness (including pain); definition depends on the healthcare insurer.

Medical foundation Multipurpose, nonprofit service organization for physicians and other healthcare providers at the local and county levels. As managed care organizations, medical foundations have established preferred provider organizations, exclusive provider organizations, and management service organizations. Emphases are freedom of choice and preservation of the physician–patient relationship.

Medical necessity Healthcare services and supplies that are proved or acknowledged to be effective in the diagnosis, treatment, cure, or relief of a health condition, illness, injury, disease, or its symptoms and to be consistent with the community's accepted standard of care. Under medical necessity, only those services, procedures, and patient care are provided that are warranted by the patient's condition.

Medical tourism Traveling across borders to receive healthcare, other terms include health tourism and medical travel.

Medically uninsurable An individual who has a pre-existing health condition, a chronic disease, or both, who cannot obtain healthcare insurance through the usual mechanisms because of his or her high risk and high cost.

Medicare Federally funded healthcare benefits program for those persons 65 years old and older, as well as for those entitled to Social Security benefits.

Medicare Administrative Contractor (MAC) Newly established contracting authority to administer Medicare Part A and Part B as required by section 911 of the Medicare Modernization Act of 2003. Fifteen Medicare Administrative Contractors will replace Medicare Carriers and Fiscal Intermediaries by 2011. Each MAC will process and manage both Part A and Part B claims.

Medicare Advantage (Part C) Optional managed care plan for Medicare beneficiaries who are entitled to Part A, are enrolled in Part B, and live in an area with a plan. Types of plans available include health maintenance organization, point-of-service plan, preferred provider organization, and provider-sponsored organization (formerly Medicare1Choice).

Medicare carrier Contractor with Medicare to process Medicare Part B claims; determines charges allowed by Medicare and makes payment to physicians and suppliers on behalf of Medicare.

Medicare Integrity Program First comprehensive federal strategy to prevent and reduce provider fraud, waste, and abuse.

Medicare Modernization Act (MMA) of 2003 Most significant legislative change to the Medicare Program since its creation; the law created the outpatient prescription drug benefit and provided expanded coverage choices and improved benefits.

Medicare Part A The portion of Medicare that provides benefits for inpatient hospital services.

Medicare Part B An optional and supplemental portion of Medicare that provides benefits for physician services, medical services, and medical supplies not covered by Medicare Part A.

Medicare Part C Also known as Medicare Advantage, this is a managed care option that includes services under Parts A, B, and D and additional services that are not typically covered by Medicare; Medicare Part C requires an additional premium; plan known formerly as Medicare1Choice.

Medicare Part D Medicare drug benefit created by the Medicare Modernization Act (MMA) of 2003 that offers outpatient drug coverage to beneficiaries for an additional premium.

Medicare physician (provider) fee schedule (MPFS) The maximum amount of reimbursement that Medicare will allow for a service; consists of a list of payments (fees) for services defined by a service coding system, for example, the Healthcare Common Procedure Coding System (HCPCS). *See* Physician (provider) fee schedule (PFS).

Medicare-severity diagnosis-related group (MS-DRG) Medicare refinement to the diagnosis-related group (DRG) classification system, which allows for payment to be more closely aligned with resource intensity.

Medicare-severity long-term care diagnosis-related group (MS-LTC-DRG) Inpatient classification that categories patient discharges with similar clinical characteristics (diagnoses and treatments, age, resources used, and lengths of stay). Used in the federal payment system to reimburse long-term care hospitals (LTCHs) a set fee for patients for treating patients in a single MS-LTC-DRG category, regardless of the actual cost of care for the individual. MS-LTC-DRGs are structurally identical to the acute-care Medicare-severity diagnosis-related groups (MS-DRGs); differences occur in weights and distribution.

Medicare Summary Notice (MSN) Statement that describes services rendered, payment covered, and benefits limits and denials for Medicare beneficiaries.

Medigap Type of private insurance policy available for Medicare beneficiaries to supplement Medicare Part A and/or Part B coverage.

Member Individual or entity that purchases healthcare insurance coverage. *See* Certificate holder, Insured, Policyholder, *and* Subscriber.

Minimum data set (MDS) Standardized, comprehensive assessment instrument that the Centers for Medicare and Medicaid Services (CMS) requires be completed for residents of skilled nursing facilities. The MDS collects administrative and clinical information. States have the option of having supplemental data collected with the approval of CMS.

Modifier Two-digit alpha/alphanumeric/numeric code that provides the means by which a physician or facility can indicate that a service provided to the patient has been altered by some special circumstance(s), but for which the basic code description itself has not changed.

Moral hazard Any change in behavior that occurs as a result of becoming insured.

Mortality The incidence of death.

Motor Related to movement of muscles and coordination and includes both large motor skills, such as walking, and fine motor skills, such as buttoning and zipping clothing.

National Center for Health Statistics (NCHS) Organization that developed the clinical modification to the *International Classification of Diseases, 9th Revision* (ICD-9); responsible for maintaining and updating the diagnosis portion of the *International Classification of Diseases, 9th revision, Clinical Modification* (ICD-9-CM).

National Correct Coding Initiative (NCCI) A set of coding regulations to prevent fraud and abuse in physician and hospital outpatient coding; specifically addresses unbundling and mutually exclusive procedures.

National Coverage Determination (NCD) National medical necessity and reimbursement regulations.

National health service (Beveridge) model Method of health systems financing in which there is a single payer that owns the healthcare facilities, pays the healthcare providers, and is funded by a country's general revenues from taxes.

National standardized episode rate Set dollar amount (conversion factor, constant, across-the-board multiplier), unadjusted for geographic differences, that is multiplied with the weights of the Health Insurance Prospective Payment System (HIPPS) codes in the home health prospective payment system (HHPPS). The amount for each year is published in the *Federal Register*.

National unadjusted copayment Set dollar amount, unadjusted for geographic differences, that beneficiaries pay under the Hospital Outpatient Prospective Payment System (HOPPS).

National unadjusted payment Product of the conversion factor multiplied by the relative weight, unadjusted for geographic differences.

Network Physicians, hospitals, and other providers who provide healthcare services to members of a managed care organization. Providers may be associated through formal or informal contracts and agreements.

Network model Type of health maintenance organization (HMO) in which the HMO contracts with two or more medical groups and reimburses the groups on a fee-for-service or capitation basis. *See* Group practice model.

New technology Advance in medical technology that substantially improves, relative to technologies previously available, the diagnosis or treatment of Medicare beneficiaries. Applicants for the status in new technology must submit a formal request, including a full description of the clinical applications of the technology and the results of any clinical evaluations demonstrating that the new technology represents a substantial clinical improvement, together with data to demonstrate the technology meets the high-cost threshold.

Non-case-mix-adjusted component Amount comprising the non-case-mix component and the non-case-mix therapy component.

Non-case-mix component Standard amount added to the rate for each refined resource utilization group (RUG)-III group to cover administrative and capital-related costs; this standard amount is added to all groups.

Non-case-mix therapy component Standard amount to cover the costs of assessing the needs for therapy of residents who subsequently were determined not to need continued therapy services.

Nonlabor share (portion, ratio) Facilities' operating costs not related to labor (typically 25–30 percent). *See* Labor-related share.

Nonparticipating physicians (NonPARs) Physicians who treat Medicare beneficiaries but do not have a legal agreement with the program to accept assignment on all Medicare services and who, therefore, may bill beneficiaries more than the Medicare reasonable charge on a service-by-service basis. Nonparticipating physicians receive 95 percent of the full Medicare physician fee schedule amount. *See* Medicare physician fee schedule.

Nonroutine medical supplies (NRS) Supplies that are not bundled into typical (routine) medical care for home health, such as catheter bags, urinary and stool collection pouches, irrigation trays, and appliance cleaners.

Nonsingle coverage Healthcare insurance that covers at least one person in addition to the policyholder or employee. *Also known* as dependent coverage.

Normalization Step in assuring budget neutrality in which the Centers for Medicare and Medicaid Services (CMS) isolates the impact of the recalibration of relative weights of prospective payment systems. The average of all proposed relative weights is compared with the average of existing relative weights. The resulting ratio is used to reduce (or increase) all proposed relative weights proportionately to maintain budget neutrality.

Notice of proposed rulemaking (NPRM) Legally required process by which federal departments and agencies make known intended rules, through publication in the *Federal Register*, and allow public review and comment. Government experts then analyze and use the comments to make any necessary changes before the proposed rule is published as a final rule in the *Federal Register*.

Nursing component Amount comprising nursing per diem amount and nursing index.

Nursing index Ratio based on the amount of staff time, weighted by salary levels, associated with each refined resource utilization group (RUG)-III group; applying this ratio to the nursing per diem is case-mix adjustment.

Nursing per diem amount Standard amount that includes direct nursing care and the cost of nontherapy ancillary services.

Observation Service in which providers observe and monitor a patient to decide whether the patient needs to be admitted to inpatient care or can be discharged to home or an outpatient area, usually charged by the hour.

Office of Inspector General (OIG) A division of the Department of Health and Human Services (DHHS) that investigates issues of noncompliance in the Medicare and Medicaid programs, such as fraud and abuse.

Office of Inspector General (OIG) Workplan Yearly plan released by the OIG that outlines the focus for reviews and investigates in various healthcare settings.

Open enrollment (election) period Period during which individuals may elect to enroll in, modify coverage, or transfer between healthcare insurance plans, usually without evidence of insurability or waiting periods (Medicare uses the term *election*).

Open panel Type of health maintenance organization that uses incentives, such as increased cost sharing, to influence members to select providers within the plan.

Operation Restore Trust A 1995 joint effort of the Department of Health and Human Services (DHHS), Office of Inspector General (OIG), the Centers for Medicare and Medicaid Services (CMS), and the Administration of Aging (AOA) to target fraud and abuse among healthcare providers.

Other party liability (OPL) Method of determining responsibility for health expenses when nonhealth insurance sources are involved.

Out-of-network Set of physicians, hospitals, and other providers who lack formal discounted-rate agreements with health insurers. Patients and clients receive no discount and pay increased cost-sharing. *See* In-network.

Out-of-pocket Payment made by the policyholder or member.

Outcome Assessment Information Set (OASIS) Set of data elements that represents core items of a comprehensive assessment for an adult home-care patient. OASIS is used to measure patient outcomes in outcome-based quality improvement (OBQI). This assessment is performed on every patient who receives services from home health agencies that participate in the Medicare or Medicaid programs. The OASIS is the basis of the home health prospective payment system (HHPPS).

Outlier Cases in prospective payment systems with unusually long lengths of stay or exceptionally high costs; day outlier or cost outlier, respectively. *See also* High-cost outlier.

Outpatient Code Editor (OCE) *See* Editor.

Outpatient service-mix index (SMI) The sum of the weights of ambulatory payment classification groups for patients treated during a given period, divided by the total volume of patients treated.

Packaging Combination of an ancillary service with its related procedure or service for one lump-sum payment in the Hospital Outpatient Prospective Payment System.

Palliative care Type of medical care designed to relieve the patient's pain and suffering without attempting to cure the underlying disease.

Partial hospitalization Program of intensive psychotherapy that is provided in a day outpatient setting and is designed to keep patients with severe mental conditions from being hospitalized in an inpatient unit.

Participating physician (PAR) Physician who signs an agreement with Medicare to accept assignment for all services provided to Medicare beneficiaries for the duration of the agreement.

Pass-through Exception to the Medicare prospective payment systems (PPSs) for a high-cost service. The exception minimizes the negative financial impact of the lump-sum payments of the PPSs. Pass-throughs are not included in the PPSs and are passed through to cost-based (retrospective) payment mechanisms. In the Hospital Outpatient Prospective Payment System (HOPPS), the Centers for Medicare and Medicaid Services (CMS) created exceptions for some expensive drugs, pharmaceuticals, biologicals, and devices. Rather than being bundled or packaged, these exceptions to CMS's HOPPS are "passed through" the HOPPS to other payment mechanisms (payment status indicators F, G, H, and J). The inpatient prospective payment system (IPPS) passes through the costs of medical education and organ acquisition and some capital costs.

Patient-centered medical home (PCMH) Model of healthcare delivery in which patients receive structured, proactive, and coordinated care rather than episodic treatments for illnesses. The primary care physician serves as a home for patients, overseeing all aspects of patients' health and coordinating care with specialists (also known as medical home and advanced medical home).

Patient Protection and Affordable Care Act of 2010 (P.L. 111-148) *See* Affordable Care Act (ACA).

Payer A payer is an entity that pays for health services, such as an insurance company, workers' compensation, Medicare, or an individual.

Pay-for-performance (P4P) Type of providers' payment system that is based on performance and incentives. *See* Value-based purchasing.

Pay-for-reporting Federal program in which the action of reporting data in the proper format within the given timeframe is what allows facilities to receive full reimbursement.

Payment status indictor (PSI) Alphabetic code that provides payment information in the Hospital Outpatient Prospective Payment System (HOPPS). There are two types of indicators. The first type designates one of three major categories of reimbursement *outside* the ambulatory patient classification (APC) system (A, C, and E). The second type gives directions related to payment rules for APC payments (D, F, G, H, K, L, N, P, S, T, V, and X).

Per diem (per day) payment Type of prospective payment method in which the third-party payer reimburses the provider a fixed rate for each day a covered member is hospitalized.

Per member per month (PMPM) Amount of money paid monthly for each individual enrolled in a capitation-based health insurance plan.

Pharmacy (prescription) benefit manager (PBM) A specialty benefit management organization that provides comprehensive pharmacy (prescription) services; PBMs administer healthcare insurance companies' prescription drug benefits for healthcare insurance companies or for self-insured employers.

Physician-hospital organization (PHO) Hybrid type of integrated delivery system that is a legal entity formed by a hospital and a group of physicians.

Physician (provider) fee schedule (PFS) Maximum allowed amount of reimbursement based on a list of payments (fees) for services defined by a service coding system. *See* Medicare physician fee schedule.

Physician Quality Reporting System (PQRS) System of reporting quality initiative under the Tax

Relief and Health Care Act (TRHCA) of 2006 (P.L. 109-432). Initiative includes an incentive payment to eligible professionals whose services are paid under the Medicare physician fee schedule.

Physician work (WORK) Component or element of the relative value unit (RVU) that should cover the physician's salary. This work is the time the physician spends providing a service and the intensity with which that time is spent. The four elements of intensity are (1) mental effort and judgment, (2) technical skill, (3) physical effort, and (4) psychological stress.

Point-of-service (POS) healthcare insurance plan Plan in which the determination of the type of care, provider, or healthcare service is made at the time (point) when the service is needed.

Policy Binding contract issued by a healthcare insurance company to an individual or group in which the company promises to pay for healthcare to treat illness or injury (also known as health plan agreement and evidence of coverage).

Policyholder Individual or entity that purchases healthcare insurance coverage. *See* Insured, Certificate holder, Member, *and* Subscriber.

Postacute care (PAC) Settings in which patients receive healthcare services for their recuperation and rehabilitation after an illness or injury.

Postacute care transfer Under IPPS, a transfer to a nonacute-care setting for designated MS-DRGs is treated as an IPPS-to-IPPS transfer when established criteria are met.

Practice expense (PE) Element of the relative value unit (RVU) that covers the physician's overhead costs, such as employee wages, office rent, supplies, and equipment. There are two types: facility and nonfacility.

Practice without walls (PWW) *See* Group practice without walls (PWW).

Preadmission certification *See* Prior approval (authorization).

Preadmission review *See* Prior approval (authorization).

Preauthorization *See* Prior approval (authorization).

Preauthorization (precertification) number Control number issued when a healthcare service is approved.

Preclaims submission activities One of the four components of the revenue cycle; includes tasks and functions from the admitting and case management areas that occur at the onset of admission, before services are provided to the patient.

Precertification *See* Prior approval (authorization).

Pre-existing condition Disease, illness, ailment, or other condition (whether physical or mental) for which, within six months before the insured's enrollment date of coverage, medical advice, diagnosis, care, or treatment was recommended or received. The Health Insurance Portability and Accountability Act (HIPAA) constrains the use of exclusions for pre-existing conditions and establishes requirements that exclusions for pre-existing conditions must satisfy.

Pre-existing condition exclusion Plan provision that limits or excludes benefits or plan coverage based on a condition's presence before the effective date of the coverage.

Preferred drug list Continually updated list of safe, effective, and cost-effective drugs, generic and brand name, which the health plan prefers insureds to use. *See also* formulary.

Preferred provider organization (PPO) Entity that contracts with employers and insurers, through a network of providers, to render healthcare services to a group of members. Members can choose to use the healthcare services of any physician, hospital, or other healthcare provider. Members who choose to use the services of in-network (in-plan) providers have lower out-of-pocket expenses than members who choose to use the services of out-of-network (out-of-plan) providers.

Premium Amount of money that policyholder or certificate holder must periodically pay a healthcare insurance plan in return for healthcare coverage.

Prescription management Cost-control measure that expands the use of a formulary to include patient education; electronic screening, alert, and decision-support tools; expert and referent systems; criteria for drug utilization; point-of-service order entry; electronic prescription transmission; and patient-specific medication profiles.

Pricer Software module in Medicare claims processing systems, specific to certain benefits, used in pricing claims and calculating payment rates and payments, most often under prospective payment systems.

Primary care physician Physician who provides, supervises, and coordinates the healthcare of a member. Family and general practitioners, internists, pediatricians, and obstetricians/gynecologists are primary care physicians. *See* Primary care provider.

Primary care provider (PCP) Healthcare provider who provides, supervises, and coordinates the healthcare of a member. The PCP makes referrals to specialists and for advanced diagnostic testing. Family and general practitioners, internists, pediatricians, and obstetricians/gynecologists are primary care physicians. Other PCPs include nurse practitioners and physician assistants. *See* Primary care physician.

Primary insurer (payer) Entity responsible for the greatest proportion or majority of the healthcare expenses. *See* Secondary insurer.

Principal diagnosis Reason established after study to be chiefly responsible for occasioning the admission of the patient to the hospital for care.

Prior approval (authorization) Process of obtaining approval from a healthcare insurance company before receiving healthcare services (also known as precertification).

Private health insurance model Method of health systems financing in which many competing private health insurance companies exist, collect premiums to create a pool of money, and pay for health claims of their subscribers.

Professional liability insurance (PLI) Element of the relative value unit (RVU); costs of the premiums for malpractice insurance liability insurance. *See* also malpractice.

Programs of All-Inclusive Care for the Elderly (PACE) A joint Medicare–Medicaid venture that allows states to choose a managed care option for providing benefits to the frail elderly population.

Proposed rule Regulation published by a federal department or agency in the *Federal Register* for the public's review and comment prior to its adoption. Does not have the force of law.

Prospective payment method Type of episode-of-care reimbursement in which the third-party payer establishes the payment rates for healthcare services in advance for a specific time period.

Prospective payment system (PPS) Method of reimbursement in which payment rates for healthcare services are established in advance for a specific time period. The predetermined rates are based on average levels of resource use for certain types of healthcare.

Provider Physician, clinic, hospital, nursing home, or other healthcare entity (second party) rendering the care.

Provider-sponsored organization (PSO) Type of point-of-service plan in which the physicians who practice in a regional or community hospital organize the plan.

Prudent layperson standard Standard for determining the need for emergency care based on what a prudent layperson (ordinary person) would believe or decide. A prudent layperson, possessing average knowledge about health and medicine, would expect that a condition could jeopardize the patient's life or seriously impair future functioning.

Purchaser Entity that subsidizes, arranges, and contracts for the cost of healthcare services received by a group.

Qualifying life event (QLE) Changes in an individual's life that make him or her eligible for a special enrollment period. Examples include moving to a new state, certain changes in income, and changes in family size.

Quality Alliance Consumer Assessment of Healthcare Providers and Systems (HCAHPS) First national, standardized, publicly reported survey to collect data regarding patients' perspectives of hospital care.

Quintile Portion of a frequency distribution containing a fifth of the total cases.

Rate year (RY) The 12-month period during which a payment rate is effective. The RY may or may not match the calendar year (CY) or fiscal year (FY). *See* Calendar year *and* fiscal year.

Recovery Audit Contractor (RAC) The result of a successful a demonstration project required by the Medicare Modernization Act of 2003. RACs ensure that correct payments are made to providers and facilities by Medicare for Part A and Part B claims.

Referral Process in which a primary care provider or physician makes a request to a managed care plan on behalf of a patient to send that patient to receive medical care from a specialist or provider outside the managed care plan.

Regression analysis Statistical technique that uses an independent variable to predict the value of a dependent value. In the inpatient psychiatric facility prospective payment system (IPF PPS), patient demographics and length of stay (independent variables) were used to predict cost of care (dependent variable).

Rehabilitation impairment category (RIC) Clusters of impairment group codes (IGCs) that represent similar impairments and diagnoses. RICs are the larger umbrella division within the inpatient rehabilitation facility prospective payment system (IRF PPS). From the RICs, the case-mix groups (CMGs) are determined.

Reimbursement Compensation or repayment for healthcare services already rendered.

Relative value scale (RVS) System designed to permit comparisons of the resources needed or appropriate prices for various units of service. It takes into account labor, skill, supplies, equipment, space, and other costs for each procedure or service.

Relative value unit (RVU) Unit of measure designed to permit comparison of the amount of resources required to perform various provider services by assigning weights to such factors as personnel time, level of skill, and sophistication of equipment required to render service. In the resource-based relative value scale (RBRVS), the RVU reflects national averages and is the sum of the physician work, practice expenses, and malpractice. RVUs are adjusted to local costs through the geographic practice cost indexes (GPCIs). *See* Physician work, Practice expenses, Malpractice, *and* Geographic practice cost index.

Relative weight (RW) Assigned weight that reflects the relative resource consumption associated with a payment classification or group. Higher payments are associated with higher relative weights.

Remittance advice Report sent by third-party payer that outlines claim rejections, denials, and payments to the facility; sent via electronic data interchange.

Request for Anticipated Payment (RAP) First of two transactions submitted to the Medicare Administrative Contractor to obtain partial payment (first split percentage) for an episode of care under the home health prospective payment system.

Resource-based relative value scale (RBRVS) Type of retrospective fee-for-service payment method that classifies health services based on the cost of providing physician services in terms of effort, practice expense (overhead), and malpractice insurance.

Resource utilization group (RUG) Classification for resources used in nursing homes. Patients are classified into one of 44 possible RUGs based on resident information collected in the minimum data set (MDS). The RUG subsequently classifies residents into seven payment categories.

Respite care Short-term care provided during the day or overnight to individuals in the home or institution to temporarily relieve the family home caregiver.

Retrospective payment method Type of fee-for-service reimbursement in which providers receive recompense after health services have been rendered.

Revenue code Three or four digit billing code that categorizes charges based on type of service, supply, procedure, or location of service.

Revenue cycle The regularly repeating set of events that produces revenue.

Revenue cycle management (RCM) The supervision of all administrative and clinical functions that contribute to the capture, management, and collection of patient service revenue.

Rider Document added to a healthcare insurance policy that provides details about coverage or lack of coverage for special situations that are not usually included in standard policies. May function as an exclusion or limitation.

Risk Probability of incurring loss.

Risk pool Group of people who will be covered by a healthcare insurance plan.

Rural area Geographic area outside an urban area and its constituent counties or county equivalents. *See* Core-based statistical area (CBSA) *and* Metropolitan statistical area (MSA).

Rural health clinic (RHC) Healthcare organization located in nonurbanized area with health professional shortage or governor designation with the purpose of increasing access to primary and preventive healthcare in rural areas.

Safety-net provider Healthcare provider who, by mandate or mission, organizes and delivers a significant level of healthcare and other health-related services to uninsured, underinsured, low-income, Medicaid, and other vulnerable populations or patients.

Scrubber Internal claim auditing system used to ensure that claims are complete and accurate before submission to third-party payers.

Second opinion Cost containment measure to prevent unnecessary tests, treatments, medical devices, or surgical procedures.

Secondary insurer (payer) Entity responsible for the remainder of the healthcare expenses after the primary insurer pays. *See* Primary insurer.

Self-insured plan Method of insurance in which the employer or other association itself administers the health insurance benefits for its employees or their dependents, thereby assuming the risks for the costs of healthcare for the group.

Self-pay Type of fee-for-service reimbursement in which the patients or their guarantors pay a specific amount for each service received.

Short-stay outlier Hospitalization that is five-sixths of the geometric length of stay for the Medicare-severity long-term care diagnosis-related group (MS-LTC-DRG).

Single coverage Health insurance covering the policyholder or employee only.

Single-payer health system One method of financing of health services. One entity acts as an administrator of a single insurance pool. The entity collects all health fees (taxes or contributions) and pays all health costs for an entire population. The single entity can be an agency of the government or a government-run organization.

Site neutral payment Harmonization of Medicare reimbursement rates for equivalent services across healthcare settings.

Skilled nursing facility (SNF) Facility that is certified by Medicare to provide 24-hour skilled inpatient nursing care and rehabilitation services in addition to other medical services.

Sliding scale A method of billing in which the cost of healthcare services is based on the patient's income and ability to pay

Social insurance (Bismarck) model Method of health systems financing, based upon universal healthcare coverage, in which all workers and employers contribute, proportionate to their income, to a set of competing funds that collect and redistribute money for healthcare per government regulations.

Social Security Act Federal legislation providing support for state public health activities and healthcare services for mothers and children; amended in 1965 to establish the Medicare and Medicaid programs.

Sole-community hospital Hospital that, by reason of factors such as isolated location, weather conditions, travel conditions, or absence of other hospitals (as determined by the Secretary of the Department of Health and Human Services [DHHS]) is the sole source of patient hospital services reasonably available to individuals in a geographic area who are entitled to benefits.

Special enrollment (election) period Period during which individuals may elect to enroll in, modify coverage, or transfer between healthcare insurance plans, usually without evidence of insurability or waiting periods, because of specific work or life events, without regard to the healthcare insurance company's regular open enrollment period (Medicare uses the term *election*).

Special needs plan (SNP) Form of Medicare Advantage (MA) plan for persons dually eligible for both Medicare and Medicaid, for institutionalized persons, or for persons with severe chronic or disabling conditions. *See* Managed care organization.

Staff model Type of health maintenance organization (HMO) that provides hospitalization and physicians' services through its own staff and facilities (also known as closed panel).

Standard federal rate National base payment amount in the prospective payment system for long-term care hospitals (PPS for LTC). This amount is multiplied with the relative weight of the Medicare-severity long-term care diagnosis-related group (MS-LTC-DRG) to calculate the unadjusted payment. Published annually in the *Federal Register*.

Standard payment conversion factor National base rate that converts the case-mix group weight into an unadjusted payment in the inpatient rehabilitation facility prospective payment system (IRF PPS) and that covers all operating and capital costa that an IRF would be expected to incur to efficiently provide intensive rehabilitation services. Published annually in the *Federal Register*.

State Children's Health Insurance Program (SCHIP) A state–federal partnership created by the Balanced Budget Act of 1997 that provides health insurance to children of families whose income level is too high to qualify for Medicaid but too low to purchase healthcare insurance (also known as CHIP).

State healthcare insurance plan Nonprofit association or governmental agency created by a state to provide healthcare insurance for people without coverage, usually because of pre-existing health conditions or chronic diseases; called health insurance association, comprehensive health insurance association, or simply high-risk pool. *See* Medically uninsurable.

STEEEP (safe, timely, effective, efficient, equitable, and patient-centered) Characteristics described as key to the Institute of Medicine's redesigned healthcare system.

Stop–loss benefit Specific amount, in a certain timeframe, such as one year, beyond which all covered healthcare services for that policyholder or dependent are paid at 100 percent by the healthcare insurance plan. *See* Maximum out-of-pocket cost *and* Catastrophic expense limit.

Subcapitation Portion of capitated rate that is based to specialists for carved-out services.

Subscriber Individual or entity that purchases healthcare insurance coverage. *See* Certificate holder, Insured, Member, *and* Policyholder.

Summary of Benefits and Coverage (SBC) Document that concisely details, in plain language, simple and consistent information about a health plan's benefits and its coverage of health services.

Supplemental insurance Additional healthcare insurance that fills in gaps (supplements) in comprehensive insurance or Medicare benefits; may be a cash benefit, per diem, or other form.

Sustainable growth rate (SGR) system Formula to establish yearly targets for controlled growth in aggregate Medicare expenditures for physicians' services.

Target Specific, measurable objective against which performance can be judged.

Teaching hospital Hospital engaged in an approved graduate medical education residency program in medicine, osteopathy, dentistry, or podiatry.

Temporary Assistance for Needy Families (TANF) Program Replaced the Aid to Families with Dependent Children program; this program provides states with grant money designated to provide low-income families with assistance.

Therapy component Amount comprising the therapy per diem amount and therapy index.

Therapy index Ratio based on the amount of staff time, weighted by salary levels, associated with each refined resource utilization group (RUG)-III group; applying this ratio to the therapy per diem is case-mix adjustment.

Therapy per diem amount Standard amount that includes physical, occupational, and speech-language therapy services provided to beneficiaries in a Part A stay.

Third opinion Cost containment measure to prevent unnecessary tests, treatments, medical devices, or surgical procedures.

Third-party payer Insurance company or health agency that pays the physician, clinic, or other healthcare provider (second party) for the care or services to the patient (first party). An insurance company or healthcare benefits program that reimburses healthcare providers and/or patients for covered medical services.

Third-party payment Payments for healthcare services made by an insurance company or health agency on behalf of the insured.

Tier Level of healthcare benefit.

Title Short name of a diagnosis-related group (DRG), such as DRG 1, Craniotomy Age > 17 Except for Trauma.

Transfer Discharge of a patient from a hospital and readmission to a post-acute-care or another acute-care hospital on the same day.

Transparency Making available to the public, in a reliable and understandable manner, information on a healthcare organization's quality, efficiency, and consumer experience with care, which includes price and quality data, to influence the behavior of patients, providers, payers, and others to achieve better outcomes.

TRICARE The healthcare program for active duty and retired members of one of the seven uniformed services administered by the Department of Defense; formerly known as Civilian Health and Medical Program of the Uniformed Services (CHAMPUS).

Trim point Numeric value that identifies atypically long lengths of stay (LOS) or high costs (long-stay outliers and cost outliers, respectively). Commonly trim points are plus or minus three standard deviations from the mean. *See* Outlier.

Triple aim Goal of better quality of care for individuals, greater health for populations, and lower growth in healthcare costs.

Unbundling The fraudulent process in which individual component codes are submitted for reimbursement rather than one comprehensive code.

Uncompensated care Overall measure of services provided for which no payments were received from the patient, client, or third-party payer.

Underserved area Area or population designated by the federal Health Resources and Services Administration (HRSA) as having the following characteristics: (1) too few primary care providers, (2) high infant mortality, (3) high poverty, (4) high elderly population, or (5) a combination of these characteristics. Also commonly known as medically underserved area (MUA) or medically underserved population (MUP).

Universal healthcare coverage Minimum level of healthcare insurance that includes coverage for preventive and primary care, hospitalization, mental health benefits, and prescription drugs.

Upcoding The fraudulent process of submitting codes for reimbursement that indicates more complex or higher-paying services than those that the patient actually received.

Urban area Core-based statistical area (CBSA).

Usual, customary, and reasonable (UCR) Type of retrospective fee-for-service payment method in which the third-party payer pays for fees that are usual, customary, and reasonable, wherein *usual* means usual for the individual provider's practice, *customary* means customary for the community, and *reasonable* is reasonable for the situation.

Utilization management Program that evaluates the healthcare facility's efficiency in providing necessary care to patients in the most effective manner.

Utilization review Process of determining whether a patient's medical care is necessary according to established guidelines and regulations. Cost containment measure that assesses the appropriateness of the setting for the healthcare service in the continuum of care and the level of service.

Utilization review committee Consists of representatives from health information management (HIM), quality, utilization, and medical staff responsible for determining whether a patient's medical care is necessary according to established guidelines and regulations.

Value Characteristic of healthcare that represents services, service delivery, and outcomes that are of high quality, efficient, appropriate, safe, timely, and cost-effective.

Value-based purchasing (VBP) Strategy that links payment to the quality of care, rewarding providers for delivering high-quality, efficient clinical care.

Veterans Health Administration Integrated healthcare delivery system dedicated to providing healthcare services to American veterans.

Wage index Ratio that represents the relationship between the average wages in a healthcare setting's geographic area and the national average for that healthcare setting. Wage indexes are adjusted annually and published in the *Federal Register*.

Waiting period Period, generally not exceeding 90 days, that must pass before coverage for an employee or dependent who is otherwise eligible to enroll under the terms of a group health plan can become effective.

Wellness program Program to promote health and fitness offered by employers and health insurance plans.

Withhold Portion of providers' capitated payments that managed care organizations deduct and hold to create an incentive for efficient or reduced use of healthcare services (also known as physician contingency reserve [PCR]).

Withhold pool Aggregate amount withheld from all providers' capitation payments as an amount to cover expenditures in excess of targets.

Workers' compensation Medical and income insurance coverage for employees who suffer from a work-related injury or illness.

World Health Organization (WHO) Organization that created and that maintains the International Classification of Diseases (ICD) used throughout the world to collect morbidity and mortality information.

Wraparound Supplemental type of insurance policy that covers the gaps in other types of health insurance. *See* Medigap and Supplemental insurance.

Write-off 1. Amount deducted from a provider's claim; difference between the actual charge and the allowable charge. Some agreements between providers and healthcare insurance companies prohibit providers from charging patients this excess difference. *See also* adjustment. 2. The action taken to eliminate the balance of a bill after the bill has been submitted and partial payment has been made or payment has been denied and all avenues of collecting the payment have been exhausted.

Appendix B
Answer Key for
Check Your Understanding Questions

Check Your Understanding 1.1

1. True

2. Four characteristics of the US healthcare sector are its large size, complexity, intricate payment methods and rules, and programs' broad scopes.

3. False

4. Insurers receive premiums in return for assuming the insureds' exposure to risk or loss.

5. b

Check Your Understanding 1.2

1. In 1929 in Texas, when Blue Cross first created a plan for school teachers

2. Individual or single coverage

3. Reimbursement

4. c

5. d

6. Resource-based relative value scale (RBRVS)

7. Global surgical package, including the procedure, local/topical anesthesia, preoperative visit, and postoperative care/follow-up; special-procedure package, including costs associated with a diagnostic or therapeutic procedure; ambulatory-visit package, including physicians' charges, laboratory tests, and x-rays

Check Your Understanding 2.1

1. Health Insurance Portability and Accountability Act of 1996 (HIPAA)

2. c

3. National Center for Health Statistics (NCHS) and the Centers for Medicare and Medicaid Services (CMS), which together compose the ICD-10-CM/PCS Coordination and Maintenance Committee

4. Official Coding Guidelines can be downloaded from the NCHS and CMS websites. Additional guidance and advice is available in *Coding Clinic for ICD-10-CM and ICD-10-PCS*.

5. Current Procedural Terminology (CPT)

Check Your Understanding 2.2

1. Abuse, the submission of unintentionally inaccurate charges on a claim for reimbursement

2. c

3. IPERA and IPERIA

4. RACs are paid on a contingency fee basis instead of a contract basis.

5. Policies and procedures, education and training, and auditing and monitoring

Check Your Understanding 3.1

1. False

2. True

3. Large-employer pools are the type of risk pool with the greatest diversity and the greatest ability to balance risks.

4. False

5. Blue Cross and Blue Shield. Blue Cross and Blue Shield is one of the most influential organizations in the healthcare sector because the Blue Companies insure nearly one in three Americans.

Check Your Understanding 3.2

1. A healthcare plan offering dependent coverage includes benefits for legally married spouses, children, and young adults until they reach the age of 26, and dependents of the insured individual who have disabilities.

2. Comprehensive policies and essential benefits policies provide coverage for most healthcare services but may have deductibles that must be met before the insurance company pays expenses, and the insured must also pay cost-sharing for all covered expenses until the maximum out-of-pocket cost is reached.

3. c

4. Generic

5. Prior approval is typically required for outpatient surgeries; diagnostic, interventional, and therapeutic outpatient procedures; physical, occupational, and speech therapies; mental health and dependency care; inpatient care, including surgery, home health, private nurses, and nursing homes; and organ transplants.

6. A dependent child's primary insurer is the insurance of the parent whose birthday comes first in the calendar year ("birthday rule").

Check Your Understanding 3.3

1. Guarantor

2. False

3. c

4. False

5. Adjustment or write-off is the term for the difference between the provider's actual charge and the allowable charge.

Check Your Understanding 4.1

1. a. Inpatient hospital services
   b. Supplemental medical insurance
   c. Medicare Advantage
   d. Medicare drug benefit

2. Insurance for excluded Part A/B services is included in Medicare Advantage, so services such as long-term nursing care, dental services, vision services, and hearing aids are covered and provided at a covered rate for Medicare Advantage (Part C) beneficiaries.

3. Medigap policies offer supplemental insurance covering the cost-shared expenses such as the deductibles and 20 percent of durable medical equipment costs that patients otherwise pay.

4. ACA reduces the market basket in two ways. First there is a scheduled reduction and second is the multifactor productivity reduction.

5. Coverage differs among the states because Medicaid allows states to maintain a unique program adapted to state residents' needs and average incomes. Although state programs must meet coverage requirements for groups such as recipients of adoption assistance and foster care, other types of coverage, such as vision and dental services, are determined by the states' Medicaid agencies.

Check Your Understanding 4.2

1. a. TRICARE Standard Network
   b. TRICARE for ADSMs, Extra Nonnetwork
   c. TRICARE Prime
   d. TRICARE for Life (TFL)

2. True. CHAMPVA becomes a secondary payer when another health insurance benefit is available.

3. b

4. To enhance the quality of life for the frail elderly population by allowing them to receive care close to home.

5. d

Check Your Understanding 5.1

1. Preventive, wellness-oriented, acute, and chronic

2. To have visits to an oncologist—or any other specialist—a managed care organization (MCO) member obtains a referral from the primary care provider.

3. Wellness program

4. Primary care physicians are often family practitioners, general practitioners, internists, pediatricians, or obstetricians/gynecologists

5. Sources of evidence-based clinical practice guidelines include the Agency for Healthcare Research and Quality, the Centers for Disease Control and Prevention, the United States Preventive Services Task Force, and specialty organizations such as the American College of Cardiology, the American Academy of Family Physicians, and the American College of Obstetricians and Gynecologists

Check Your Understanding 5.2

1. Cost, quality, and outcomes of care (with others), the health status of the population served

2. True

3. Group practices without walls (GWWs) or clinics without walls (CWWs) share administrative systems and have greater leverage in negotiating reimbursement with managed care organizations (MCOs). Management service organizations (MSOs) provide management services and administrative and information systems to multiple group practices or small hospitals, thereby distributing overhead costs.

4. Group (practice) without walls (also known as clinic without walls)

5. Management service organization

Check Your Understanding 6.1

1. Payment rates are to be established in advance and fixed for the fiscal period to which they apply.

   Payment rates are not automatically determined by the hospital's past or current actual cost.

   Prospective payment rates are considered to be payment in full.

   The hospital retains the profit or suffers a loss resulting from the difference between the payment rate and the hospital's cost, creating an incentive for cost control.

2. Ignored

3. Is a complication/comorbidity (CC) present? Is a major complication or complex diagnosis present? Is the patient older or younger than 17? What is the patient's sex? What is the patient's discharge disposition? For neonates, what is the birth weight?

4. The market basket index is applied, which is based on the mix of goods and services included in the prospective payment system (PPS).

5. The discharge disposition identifies where the patient goes for care after discharge. If the discharge disposition indicates that the patient is to receive post-acute care (i.e., home health) then the encounter is routed through the PACT pathway for possible payment reduction if all criteria are satisfied.

Check Your Understanding 6.2

1. Balanced Budget Refinement Act of 1999. Requirements were to develop a per diem system that reflects the cost differences (resource consumption patterns) among the various inpatient psychiatric facilities (IPFs).

2. Per diem with adjustments

3. ECT formula: (ECT payment × labor % × WI) + (ECT payment × nonlabor %)

   ($315.55 × .69294 × .9812) + ($315.55 × .30706)

   ($215.55) + ($96.90)

   $312.45 *note that this amount is calculated using FY 2015 figures*

4. Patient-level adjustments and facility-level adjustments

5. **Outlier provision:** Outlier add-on payments are provided for high-cost encounters where the cost exceeds the threshold.

   Stop-loss provision: Was used as the phase-in period for this prospective payment system (PPS).

   Initial stay provision: Higher payment is provided for initial days of stay to compensate for the higher costs associated with new admissions.

   Readmission provision: Because facilities have a higher adjustment at the beginning of the admission, the Centers for Medicare and Medicaid Services (CMS) implemented the readmission provision to prevent premature discharge and then readmittance of patients. If a patient is discharged and then readmitted within two days, the two admissions count as one admission.

   Medical necessity provision: Medical necessity must be established for each patient on admission to the inpatient psychiatric facility (IPF).

Check Your Understanding 7.1

1. Dr. William Hsaio of Harvard University

2. Professional liability insurance

3. Conversion factor

4. Geographic Practice Cost Index

5. False

Check Your Understanding 7.2

1. Packaging occurs when reimbursement for minor ancillary services associated with a significant procedure are combined into a single payment for the procedure. Bundling occurs when payment for multiple significant procedures or multiple units of the same procedure related to an outpatient encounter or episode of care is combined into a single unit of payment.

2. APC (prospective payment), fee schedule, reasonable cost, average sale price of drugs

3. True

4. Pass-through for drugs and biological (G); Pass-through for devices (H); Non-pass-through drugs (K); Partial hospitalization (P), Blood and blood products (R); Significant procedures, no reduction (S); Significant procedures, reduction applies (T); Brachytherapy services (U); Medical visits (V).

5. To allow for new technologies and services to be reimbursement in a timely fashion. This allows for Medicare beneficiaries to maintain access to new and innovate services and supplies.

Check Your Understanding 7.3

1. False

2. Revising the ASC List (allowed procedures for the ASC setting)

3. The second procedure is discounted or reduced by 50%.

4. 73, 74, and 52

5. False

Check Your Understanding 7.4

1. True

2. False

3. True

4. False

5. False

6. Routine home care (RHC)

Check Your Understanding 8.1

1. Minimum data set (MDS)

2. The market basket index, which is based on the mix of goods and services included in the SNF prospective payment system (PPS)

3. An inpatient deductible must be paid for the 90-day benefit period; plus, a daily coinsurance payment applies for the 61st through 90th days.

4. True

5. Standard federal rate

Check Your Understanding 8.2

1. Inpatient rehabilitation facility patient assessment instrument (IRF PAI)

2. False. Staff members do not enter rehabilitation impairment categories (RICs); the grouper calculates the appropriate categories from the impairment group codes (IGC) entered on the PAI.

3. Consolidated into a single payment are all therapy (speech, physical, and occupational) sessions, skilled nursing visits, home health aide visits, medical social services, and all medical supplies, including nonroutine medical supplies within a 60-day episode of care.

4. The low-utilization payment adjustment (LUPA) is applied when an agency provides four or fewer visits in an episode; reimbursement in this case is made for each visit rather than for the 60-day episode.

5. Clinical severity, functional status, and service utilization

Check Your Understanding 9.1

1. Preclaims submission activities such as collecting responsible parties' information, educating patients about their ultimate financial responsibility for services rendered, collecting appropriate waivers, and verifying data about procedures before they are performed and their charges submitted.

2. Electronic order entry systems help to capture charges at their point-of-service delivery. If facilities lack electronic systems, staff collect paper-based charges on charge tickets, superbills, or encounter forms to be entered by billing staff into the patient accounting system.

3. Scrubbers edit claims to locate and flag for correction any data that may contain errors, such as dates of service that are incompatible, inaccurate diagnosis and procedure codes, lack of substantiation of medical necessity, and inaccurate assignment of revenue codes.

4. Charge code—facility-specific, Department number—facility-specific, Description—facility-specific, HCPCS code—nationally recognized, Revenue code—nationally recognized, Charge—facility-specific

5. NCDs establish coverage or noncoverage for services. LCDs communicate the circumstances under which covered services are deemed medically necessary.

Check Your Understanding 9.2

1. Can be measured to gauge performance improvement

2. See tables 9.14 and 9.15 in text.

3. Reduced cost to collect, performance consistency, and coordinate strategic goals

4. The Medicare Outpatient Code Editor (OCE)

5. Complication and comorbidity (CC) and major complication and comorbidity (MCC) codes

Check Your Understanding 10.1

1. Quality, performance, and payment

2. *To Err Is Human: Building a Safer Health System*, Kohn, L. T., J.M. Corrigan, and M.S. Donaldson, eds., Committee on the Quality of Health Care in America, Institute of Medicine; *Crossing the Quality Chasm: A New Health System for the 21st Century*, the Committee on Quality of Health Care in America of the Institute of Medicine; and *Rewarding Provider Performance: Aligning Incentives in Medicare*, the Committee on Redesigning Health Insurance Performance Measures, Payment, and Performance Improvement Programs, Board on Health Care Services of the Institute of Medicine

3. False

4. False

5. Reward-based models and penalty-based models

6. Most significant problems in terms of quality or cost, proportion of population covered by the service or provider, and availability of valid and reliable performance measures

Check Your Understanding 10.2

1. Two percent reduction in the annual payment update

2. Moved from a per-encounter reduction to an all-encounter reduction (all encounters in the payment year).

3. 2015—Heart Failure, Acute Myocardial Infarction, Pneumonia. 2016 add—Chronic Obstructive Pulmonary Disease and Total Hip Arthroplasty and Total Knee Arthroplasty. 2017 add—Coronary Artery Bypass Graft surgery.

4. Safety domain, clinical care domain, efficiency and cost reduction domain and patient experience of care domain

5. Physician data is reviewed and shared placing emphasis on quality rather than quantity. The value modifier (VN) adjusts reimbursement based on the physician's quality and efficiency of care.

Appendix C
CMS 1500 Claim Form

1500

HEALTH INSURANCE CLAIM FORM

APPROVED BY NATIONAL UNIFORM CLAIM COMMITTEE 08/05

| | PICA | | | | | | | | | | PICA | | |

1. MEDICARE ☐ (Medicare #)   MEDICAID ☐ (Medicaid #)   TRICARE CHAMPUS ☐ (Sponsor's SSN)   CHAMPVA ☐ (Member ID#)   GROUP HEALTH PLAN ☐ (SSN or ID)   FECA BLK LUNG ☐ (SSN)   OTHER ☐ (ID)   **1a. INSURED'S I.D. NUMBER**   (For Program in Item 1)

2. PATIENT'S NAME (Last Name, First Name, Middle Initial)   **3. PATIENT'S BIRTH DATE** MM ¦ DD ¦ YY   **SEX** M ☐ F ☐   **4. INSURED'S NAME** (Last Name, First Name, Middle Initial)

5. PATIENT'S ADDRESS (No., Street)   **6. PATIENT RELATIONSHIP TO INSURED**   Self ☐ Spouse ☐ Child ☐ Other ☐   **7. INSURED'S ADDRESS** (No., Street)

CITY   STATE   **8. PATIENT STATUS**   Single ☐ Married ☐ Other ☐   CITY   STATE

ZIP CODE   TELEPHONE (Include Area Code) (   )   Employed ☐ Full-Time Student ☐ Part-Time Student ☐   ZIP CODE   TELEPHONE (Include Area Code) (   )

9. OTHER INSURED'S NAME (Last Name, First Name, Middle Initial)   **10. IS PATIENT'S CONDITION RELATED TO:**   **11. INSURED'S POLICY GROUP OR FECA NUMBER**

a. OTHER INSURED'S POLICY OR GROUP NUMBER   **a. EMPLOYMENT?** (Current or Previous) YES ☐ NO ☐   **a. INSURED'S DATE OF BIRTH** MM ¦ DD ¦ YY   **SEX** M ☐ F ☐

b. OTHER INSURED'S DATE OF BIRTH MM ¦ DD ¦ YY   **SEX** M ☐ F ☐   **b. AUTO ACCIDENT?** PLACE (State) YES ☐ NO ☐   **b. EMPLOYER'S NAME OR SCHOOL NAME**

c. EMPLOYER'S NAME OR SCHOOL NAME   **c. OTHER ACCIDENT?** YES ☐ NO ☐   **c. INSURANCE PLAN NAME OR PROGRAM NAME**

d. INSURANCE PLAN NAME OR PROGRAM NAME   **10d. RESERVED FOR LOCAL USE**   **d. IS THERE ANOTHER HEALTH BENEFIT PLAN?** YES ☐ NO ☐ *If yes,* return to and complete item 9 a-d.

READ BACK OF FORM BEFORE COMPLETING & SIGNING THIS FORM.
12. PATIENT'S OR AUTHORIZED PERSON'S SIGNATURE I authorize the release of any medical or other information necessary to process this claim. I also request payment of government benefits either to myself or to the party who accepts assignment below.

SIGNED _____   DATE _____

13. INSURED'S OR AUTHORIZED PERSON'S SIGNATURE I authorize payment of medical benefits to the undersigned physician or supplier for services described below.

SIGNED _____

14. DATE OF CURRENT: MM ¦ DD ¦ YY   ILLNESS (First symptom) OR INJURY (Accident) OR PREGNANCY(LMP)   **15. IF PATIENT HAS HAD SAME OR SIMILAR ILLNESS.** GIVE FIRST DATE MM ¦ DD ¦ YY   **16. DATES PATIENT UNABLE TO WORK IN CURRENT OCCUPATION** FROM MM ¦ DD ¦ YY TO MM ¦ DD ¦ YY

17. NAME OF REFERRING PROVIDER OR OTHER SOURCE   17a. ____ 17b. NPI ____   **18. HOSPITALIZATION DATES RELATED TO CURRENT SERVICES** FROM MM ¦ DD ¦ YY TO MM ¦ DD ¦ YY

19. RESERVED FOR LOCAL USE   **20. OUTSIDE LAB?** YES ☐ NO ☐ $ CHARGES

21. DIAGNOSIS OR NATURE OF ILLNESS OR INJURY (Relate Items 1, 2, 3 or 4 to Item 24E by Line)
1. |___.___| 3. |___.___|
2. |___.___| 4. |___.___|

22. MEDICAID RESUBMISSION CODE   ORIGINAL REF. NO.

23. PRIOR AUTHORIZATION NUMBER

24. A. DATE(S) OF SERVICE						B. PLACE OF SERVICE	C. EMG	D. PROCEDURES, SERVICES, OR SUPPLIES (Explain Unusual Circumstances)		E. DIAGNOSIS POINTER	F. $ CHARGES	G. DAYS OR UNITS	H. EPSDT Family Plan	I. ID. QUAL.	J. RENDERING PROVIDER ID. #
From			To					CPT/HCPCS	MODIFIER						
MM	DD	YY	MM	DD	YY										
1														NPI	
2														NPI	
3														NPI	
4														NPI	
5														NPI	
6														NPI	

25. FEDERAL TAX I.D. NUMBER SSN ☐ EIN ☐   **26. PATIENT'S ACCOUNT NO.**   **27. ACCEPT ASSIGNMENT?** (For govt. claims, see back) YES ☐ NO ☐   **28. TOTAL CHARGE** $ **29. AMOUNT PAID** $ **30. BALANCE DUE** $

31. SIGNATURE OF PHYSICIAN OR SUPPLIER INCLUDING DEGREES OR CREDENTIALS (I certify that the statements on the reverse apply to this bill and are made a part thereof.)

SIGNED _____ DATE _____

32. SERVICE FACILITY LOCATION INFORMATION
a. NPI   b.

33. BILLING PROVIDER INFO & PH # (   )
a. NPI   b.

NUCC Instruction Manual available at: www.nucc.org   *PLEASE PRINT OR TYPE*   APPROVED OMB-0938-0999 FORM CMS-1500 (08/05)

CARRIER — PATIENT AND INSURED INFORMATION — PHYSICIAN OR SUPPLIER INFORMATION

BECAUSE THIS FORM IS USED BY VARIOUS GOVERNMENT AND PRIVATE HEALTH PROGRAMS, SEE SEPARATE INSTRUCTIONS ISSUED BY APPLICABLE PROGRAMS.

NOTICE: Any person who knowingly files a statement of claim containing any misrepresentation or any false, incomplete or misleading information may be guilty of a criminal act punishable under law and may be subject to civil penalties.

REFERS TO GOVERNMENT PROGRAMS ONLY

MEDICARE AND CHAMPUS PAYMENTS: A patient's signature requests that payment be made and authorizes release of any information necessary to process the claim and certifies that the information provided in Blocks 1 through 12 is true, accurate and complete. In the case of a Medicare claim, the patient's signature authorizes any entity to release to Medicare medical and nonmedical information, including employment status, and whether the person has employer group health insurance, liability, no-fault, worker's compensation or other insurance which is responsible to pay for the services for which the Medicare claim is made. See 42 CFR 411.24(a). If item 9 is completed, the patient's signature authorizes release of the information to the health plan or agency shown. In Medicare assigned or CHAMPUS participation cases, the physician agrees to accept the charge determination of the Medicare carrier or CHAMPUS fiscal intermediary as the full charge, and the patient is responsible only for the deductible, coinsurance and noncovered services. Coinsurance and the deductible are based upon the charge determination of the Medicare carrier or CHAMPUS fiscal intermediary if this is less than the charge submitted. CHAMPUS is not a health insurance program but makes payment for health benefits provided through certain affiliations with the Uniformed Services. Information on the patient's sponsor should be provided in those items captioned in "Insured"; i.e., items 1a, 4, 6, 7, 9, and 11.

BLACK LUNG AND FECA CLAIMS

The provider agrees to accept the amount paid by the Government as payment in full. See Black Lung and FECA instructions regarding required procedure and diagnosis coding systems.

SIGNATURE OF PHYSICIAN OR SUPPLIER (MEDICARE, CHAMPUS, FECA AND BLACK LUNG)

I certify that the services shown on this form were medically indicated and necessary for the health of the patient and were personally furnished by me or were furnished incident to my professional service by my employee under my immediate personal supervision, except as otherwise expressly permitted by Medicare or CHAMPUS regulations.

For services to be considered as "incident" to a physician's professional service, 1) they must be rendered under the physician's immediate personal supervision by his/her employee, 2) they must be an integral, although incidental part of a covered physician's service, 3) they must be of kinds commonly furnished in physician's offices, and 4) the services of nonphysicians must be included on the physician's bills.

For CHAMPUS claims, I further certify that I (or any employee) who rendered services am not an active duty member of the Uniformed Services or a civilian employee of the United States Government or a contract employee of the United States Government, either civilian or military (refer to 5 USC 5536). For Black-Lung claims, I further certify that the services performed were for a Black Lung-related disorder.

No Part B Medicare benefits may be paid unless this form is received as required by existing law and regulations (42 CFR 424.32).

NOTICE: Any one who misrepresents or falsifies essential information to receive payment from Federal funds requested by this form may upon conviction be subject to fine and imprisonment under applicable Federal laws.

NOTICE TO PATIENT ABOUT THE COLLECTION AND USE OF MEDICARE, CHAMPUS, FECA, AND BLACK LUNG INFORMATION
(PRIVACY ACT STATEMENT)

We are authorized by CMS, CHAMPUS and OWCP to ask you for information needed in the administration of the Medicare, CHAMPUS, FECA, and Black Lung programs. Authority to collect information is in section 205(a), 1862, 1872 and 1874 of the Social Security Act as amended, 42 CFR 411.24(a) and 424.5(a) (6), and 44 USC 3101;41 CFR 101 et seq and 10 USC 1079 and 1086; 5 USC 8101 et seq; and 30 USC 901 et seq; 38 USC 613; E.O. 9397.

The information we obtain to complete claims under these programs is used to identify you and to determine your eligibility. It is also used to decide if the services and supplies you received are covered by these programs and to insure that proper payment is made.

The information may also be given to other providers of services, carriers, intermediaries, medical review boards, health plans, and other organizations or Federal agencies, for the effective administration of Federal provisions that require other third parties payers to pay primary to Federal program, and as otherwise necessary to administer these programs. For example, it may be necessary to disclose information about the benefits you have used to a hospital or doctor. Additional disclosures are made through routine uses for information contained in systems of records.

FOR MEDICARE CLAIMS: See the notice modifying system No. 09-70-0501, titled, 'Carrier Medicare Claims Record,' published in the <u>Federal Register</u>, Vol. 55 No. 177, page 37549, Wed. Sept. 12, 1990, or as updated and republished.

FOR OWCP CLAIMS: Department of Labor, Privacy Act of 1974, "Republication of Notice of Systems of Records," <u>Federal Register</u> Vol. 55 No. 40, Wed Feb. 28, 1990, See ESA-5, ESA-6, ESA-12, ESA-13, ESA-30, or as updated and republished.

FOR CHAMPUS CLAIMS: <u>PRINCIPLE PURPOSE(S):</u> To evaluate eligibility for medical care provided by civilian sources and to issue payment upon establishment of eligibility and determination that the services/supplies received are authorized by law.

<u>ROUTINE USE(S):</u> Information from claims and related documents may be given to the Dept. of Veterans Affairs, the Dept. of Health and Human Services and/or the Dept. of Transportation consistent with their statutory administrative responsibilities under CHAMPUS/CHAMPVA; to the Dept. of Justice for representation of the Secretary of Defense in civil actions; to the Internal Revenue Service, private collection agencies, and consumer reporting agencies in connection with recoupment claims; and to Congressional Offices in response to inquiries made at the request of the person to whom a record pertains. Appropriate disclosures may be made to other federal, state, local, foreign government agencies, private business entities, and individual providers of care, on matters relating to entitlement, claims adjudication, fraud, program abuse, utilization review, quality assurance, peer review, program integrity, third-party liability, coordination of benefits, and civil and criminal litigation related to the operation of CHAMPUS.

<u>DISCLOSURES:</u> Voluntary; however, failure to provide information will result in delay in payment or may result in denial of claim. With the one exception discussed below, there are no penalties under these programs for refusing to supply information. However, failure to furnish information regarding the medical services rendered or the amount charged would prevent payment of claims under these programs. Failure to furnish any other information, such as name or claim number, would delay payment of the claim. Failure to provide medical information under FECA could be deemed an obstruction.

It is mandatory that you tell us if you know that another party is responsible for paying for your treatment. Section 1128B of the Social Security Act and 31 USC 3801-3812 provide penalties for withholding this information.

You should be aware that P.L. 100-503, the "Computer Matching and Privacy Protection Act of 1988", permits the government to verify information by way of computer matches.

MEDICAID PAYMENTS (PROVIDER CERTIFICATION)

I hereby agree to keep such records as are necessary to disclose fully the extent of services provided to individuals under the State's Title XIX plan and to furnish information regarding any payments claimed for providing such services as the State Agency or Dept. of Health and Human Services may request.

I further agree to accept, as payment in full, the amount paid by the Medicaid program for those claims submitted for payment under that program, with the exception of authorized deductible, coinsurance, co-payment or similar cost-sharing charge.

SIGNATURE OF PHYSICIAN (OR SUPPLIER): I certify that the services listed above were medically indicated and necessary to the health of this patient and were personally furnished by me or my employee under my personal direction.

NOTICE: This is to certify that the foregoing information is true, accurate and complete. I understand that payment and satisfaction of this claim will be from Federal and State funds, and that any false claims, statements, or documents, or concealment of a material fact, may be prosecuted under applicable Federal or State laws.

According to the Paperwork Reduction Act of 1995, no persons are required to respond to a collection of information unless it displays a valid OMB control number. The valid OMB control number for this information collection is 0938-0999. The time required to complete this information collection is estimated to average 10 minutes per response, including the time to review instructions, search existing data resources, gather the data needed, and complete and review the information collection. If you have any comments concerning the accuracy of the time estimate(s) or suggestions for improving this form, please write to: CMS, Attn: PRA Reports Clearance Officer, 7500 Security Boulevard, Baltimore, Maryland 21244-1850. This address is for comments and/or suggestions only. DO NOT MAIL COMPLETED CLAIM FORMS TO THIS ADDRESS.

Appendix D
UB-04 Form

1		2			3a PAT. CNTL #		4 TYPE OF BILL
					b. MED. REC. #		
					5 FED. TAX NO.	6 STATEMENT COVERS PERIOD FROM THROUGH	7

8 PATIENT NAME	a	9 PATIENT ADDRESS	a			
b		b		c	d	e

10 BIRTHDATE	11 SEX	12 DATE	ADMISSION 13 HR 14 TYPE 15 SRC	16 DHR	17 STAT	18 19 20 21 CONDITION CODES 22 23 24 25 26 27 28	29 ACDT STATE	30

31 OCCURRENCE CODE DATE	32 OCCURRENCE CODE DATE	33 OCCURRENCE CODE DATE	34 OCCURRENCE CODE DATE	35 OCCURRENCE SPAN CODE FROM THROUGH	36 OCCURRENCE SPAN CODE FROM THROUGH	37

38			39 VALUE CODES CODE AMOUNT	40 VALUE CODES CODE AMOUNT	41 VALUE CODES CODE AMOUNT

42 REV. CD.	43 DESCRIPTION	44 HCPCS / RATE / HIPPS CODE	45 SERV. DATE	46 SERV. UNITS	47 TOTAL CHARGES	48 NON-COVERED CHARGES	49

PAGE ___ OF ___   CREATION DATE   TOTALS ➡

50 PAYER NAME	51 HEALTH PLAN ID	52 REL INFO	53 ASG. BEN.	54 PRIOR PAYMENTS	55 EST. AMOUNT DUE	56 NPI
						57 OTHER PRV ID

58 INSURED'S NAME	59 P.REL	60 INSURED'S UNIQUE ID	61 GROUP NAME	62 INSURANCE GROUP NO.

63 TREATMENT AUTHORIZATION CODES	64 DOCUMENT CONTROL NUMBER	65 EMPLOYER NAME

66 DX	67 A B C D E F G H I J K L M N O P Q	68

69 ADMIT DX	70 PATIENT REASON DX a b c	71 PPS CODE	72 ECI a b c	73

74 PRINCIPAL PROCEDURE CODE DATE	a. OTHER PROCEDURE CODE DATE	b. OTHER PROCEDURE CODE DATE	75	76 ATTENDING NPI QUAL
				LAST FIRST
c. OTHER PROCEDURE CODE DATE	d. OTHER PROCEDURE CODE DATE	e. OTHER PROCEDURE CODE DATE		77 OPERATING NPI QUAL
				LAST FIRST
80 REMARKS	81CC a b c d			78 OTHER NPI QUAL
				LAST FIRST
				79 OTHER NPI QUAL
				LAST FIRST

UB-04 CMS-1450   APPROVED OMB NO. 0938-0997   NUBC National Uniform Billing Committee   THE CERTIFICATIONS ON THE REVERSE APPLY TO THIS BILL AND ARE MADE A PART HEREOF.

UB-04 NOTICE: THE SUBMITTER OF THIS FORM UNDERSTANDS THAT MISREPRESENTATION OR FALSIFICATION OF ESSENTIAL INFORMATION AS REQUESTED BY THIS FORM, MAY SERVE AS THE BASIS FOR CIVIL MONETARTY PENALTIES AND ASSESSMENTS AND MAY UPON CONVICTION INCLUDE FINES AND/OR IMPRISONMENT UNDER FEDERAL AND/OR STATE LAW(S).

Submission of this claim constitutes certification that the billing information as shown on the face hereof is true, accurate and complete. That the submitter did not knowingly or recklessly disregard or misrepresent or conceal material facts. The following certifications or verifications apply where pertinent to this Bill:

1. If third party benefits are indicated, the appropriate assignments by the insured /beneficiary and signature of the patient or parent or a legal guardian covering authorization to release information are on file. Determinations as to the release of medical and financial information should be guided by the patient or the patient's legal representative.

2. If patient occupied a private room or required private nursing for medical necessity, any required certifications are on file.

3. Physician's certifications and re-certifications, if required by contract or Federal regulations, are on file.

4. For Religious Non-Medical facilities, verifications and if necessary re-certifications of the patient's need for services are on file.

5. Signature of patient or his representative on certifications, authorization to release information, and payment request, as required by Federal Law and Regulations (42 USC 1935f, 42 CFR 424.36, 10 USC 1071 through 1086, 32 CFR 199) and any other applicable contract regulations, is on file.

6. The provider of care submitter acknowledges that the bill is in conformance with the Civil Rights Act of 1964 as amended. Records adequately describing services will be maintained and necessary information will be furnished to such governmental agencies as required by applicable law.

7. For Medicare Purposes: If the patient has indicated that other health insurance or a state medical assistance agency will pay part of his/her medical expenses and he/she wants information about his/her claim released to them upon request, necessary authorization is on file. The patient's signature on the provider's request to bill Medicare medical and non-medical information, including employment status, and whether the person has employer group health insurance which is responsible to pay for the services for which this Medicare claim is made.

8. For Medicaid purposes: The submitter understands that because payment and satisfaction of this claim will be from Federal and State funds, any false statements, documents, or concealment of a material fact are subject to prosecution under applicable Federal or State Laws.

9. For TRICARE Purposes:

   (a) The information on the face of this claim is true, accurate and complete to the best of the submitter's knowledge and belief, and services were medically necessary and appropriate for the health of the patient;

   (b) The patient has represented that by a reported residential address outside a military medical treatment facility catchment area he or she does not live within the catchment area of a U.S. military medical treatment facility, or if the patient resides within a catchment area of such a facility, a copy of Non-Availability Statement (DD Form 1251) is on file, or the physician has certified to a medical emergency in any instance where a copy of a Non-Availability Statement is not on file;

   (c) The patient or the patient's parent or guardian has responded directly to the provider's request to identify all health insurance coverage, and that all such coverage is identified on the face of the claim except that coverage which is exclusively supplemental payments to TRICARE-determined benefits;

   (d) The amount billed to TRICARE has been billed after all such coverage have been billed and paid excluding Medicaid, and the amount billed to TRICARE is that remaining claimed against TRICARE benefits;

   (e) The beneficiary's cost share has not been waived by consent or failure to exercise generally accepted billing and collection efforts; and,

   (f) Any hospital-based physician under contract, the cost of whose services are allocated in the charges included in this bill, is not an employee or member of the Uniformed Services. For purposes of this certification, an employee of the Uniformed Services is an employee, appointed in civil service (refer to 5 USC 2105), including part-time or intermittent employees, but excluding contract surgeons or other personal service contracts. Similarly, member of the Uniformed Services does not apply to reserve members of the Uniformed Services not on active duty.

(g) Based on 42 United States Code 1395cc(a)(1)(j) all providers participating in Medicare must also participate in TRICARE for inpatient hospital services provided pursuant to admissions to hospitals occurring on or after January 1, 1987; and

(h) If TRICARE benefits are to be paid in a participating status, the submitter of this claim agrees to submit this claim to the appropriate TRICARE claims processor. The provider of care submitter also agrees to accept the TRICARE determined reasonable charge as the total charge for the medical services or supplies listed on the claim form. The provider of care will accept the TRICARE-determined reasonable charge even if it is less than the billed amount, and also agrees to accept the amount paid by TRICARE combined with the cost-share amount and deductible amount, if any, paid by or on behalf of the patient as full payment for the listed medical services or supplies. The provider of care submitter will not attempt to collect from the patient (or his or her parent or guardian) amounts over the TRICARE determined reasonable charge. TRICARE will make any benefits payable directly to the provider of care, if the provider of care is a participating provider.

SEE http://www.nubc.org/ FOR MORE INFORMATION ON UB-04 DATA ELEMENT AND PRINTING SPECIFICATIONS

Index